Clinical Reasoning
for Physician Assistants

A Workbook for Certification Review
and Practice Readiness

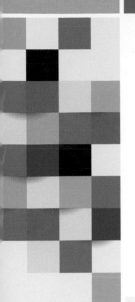

Clinical Reasoning for Physician Assistants

A Workbook for Certification Review and Practice Readiness

Robin D. Risling, EdD, PA-C
Formerly, Program Director
Physician Assistant Studies
University of New England
Portland, Maine
Director of Didactic Education
Physician Assistant Studies
University of South Alabama
Mobile, Alabama

Noelle M. Hammerbacher, MS
Medical Editor and Writer
Philadelphia, Pennsylvania
Formerly, Managing Editor
National Commission on Certification of Physician
Assistants
Johns Creek, Georgia

Daniel L. McNeill, PhD, PA-C
Clinical Professor (ret.)
Physician Assistant Studies Program
Northeastern State University
Muskogee, Oklahoma

ELSEVIER

Elsevier
3251 Riverport Lane
St. Louis, Missouri 63043

CLINICAL REASONING FOR PHYSICIAN ASSISTANTS:
A WORKBOOK FOR CERTIFICATION REVIEW AND PRACTICE READINESS   ISBN: 978-0-323-77568-7

Content Strategist: James T. Merritt/Lauren Willis
Content Development Manager: Luke Held/Danielle Frazier
Senior Content Development Specialist: Sarah Vora
Publishing Services Manager: Julie Eddy
Project Manager: Becky Langdon
Design Direction: Margaret Reid

Printed in India

Last digit is the print number: 9 8 7 6 5 4 3 2 1

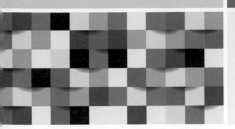

Contributors

Adrian A. Andrews, DHSc, PA-C
Commander
Florida Air National Guard
125th Medical Group
Jacksonville, Florida;

Physician Assistant
Emergency Medicine
University of Florida, Jacksonville
Jacksonville, Florida

Lora-Emily Banks, MHS, PA-C
Assistant Professor
Department of Physician Assistant Studies
Faulkner University
Montgomery, Alabama

Christine Burns, PA-C
Physician Assistant
Internal Medicine
University of Nevada, Reno
Reno, Nevada

Crystal Crowder, MSPAS, PA-C
Physician Assistant
Family Medicine
Alabama

JoAnn Deasy, MPH, PA-C
Former Faculty
Joint MPAS/MPH Program
Touro University, California
Vallejo, California

Yolonda Freeman-Hildreth, PhD, MBA, MS, PA-C
Assistant Professor
College of Health Professions
University of Detroit Mercy
Detroit, Michigan

Larissa L. Garth, DMSc, MPH, PA-C
Family Medicine, Urgent Care
Killeen, Texas

Thomas H. Hansen, MS, PA-C
Clinical Faculty
Physician Assistant Department
Rosalind Franklin University
North Chicago, Illinois

Amy Hendee, MHS, PA-C
Physician Assistant
Hospital Medicine
CarolinaEast Medical Center
New Bern, North Carolina

Jason Bret Largue, MHS, MBA, PA-C
Assistant Professor, Director of Didactic Education
Department of Physician Assistant Studies
University of South Alabama
Mobile, Alabama

Rayne Loder, MHS, PA-C
Assistant Professor, Site Director
Division of Physician Assistant Studies
Department of Family and Preventive Medicine
University of Utah
St. George, Utah

Erin Nicole Lunn, MHS, PA-C
Assistant Professor
Director of Clinical Education
Physician Assistant Studies
University of South Alabama
Mobile, Alabama

Jessica Mattson, CDCES, PAC-C
Endocrinology
Pacific Diabetes and Endocrine Center
Honolulu, Hawaii

Camille Miller, MPAS, PA-C
Physician Assistant
Prime Care Providers/Prodigy Dialysis
Johnstown, Pennsylvania

Bonnie Minton, MHS, PA-C
Director of Clinical Education and Assistant Professor
Physician Assistant Studies
University of South Alabama
Mobile, Alabama

Mark Daniel Minton, DMSc, RN, NRP, PA-C
Assistant Professor
Physician Assistant Studies
University of South Alabama
Mobile, Alabama

Leticea Newton, MD
Guest Lecturer
NSU Physician Assistant Studies
Northeastern State University
Muskogee, Oklahoma;

Medical Director
Green Country Behavioral Health
Muskogee, Oklahoma

Mark W. Perdue, MHS, PA-C
Program Director
Physician Assistant Program
Northeastern State University
Muskogee, Oklahoma

Stephanie Podolski, MPH, MSPA, PA-C
Hospitalist Physician Assistant
Maine General Health
Augusta, Maine

Nikki Quinley, PA-C
Physician Assistant
Compass Urgent Care
Mobile, Alabama

Christopher Roman, DMS, PA-C
Associate Professor
Medical Science and Physician Assistant Studies
Butler University
Indianapolis, Indiana

Janice V. Tramel, MS-HPE, PA-C Emeritus
Instructor of Clinical Family Medicine
Family Medicine
Keck School of Medicine of USC Primary Care
Physician Assistant Program
Los Angeles, California

Narisha Velazquez, MS, MPAS, PA-C
Physician Assistant
Virtual Urgent Care
Baylor Scott & White Health
Temple, Texas

Dana L. Villmore, PhD, PA-C
Assistant Clinical Professor
Physician Assistant Program
University of New England
Portland, Maine;

Physician Assistant
IDEXX Workplace Health Services
Intermed Physician Assistant
Westbrook, Maine

Elsevier and the Authors thank Technical/Layout Reviewer:

Ilaria S. Gadalla, DMSc, MS, PA-C
Physician Assistant, Department Chair of the Physician
Assistant Program
South University
West Palm Beach, Florida

Elsevier and the Authors thank Content Reviewer:

Margaret A. Henderson, RPh, CPh
Mobile, Alabama

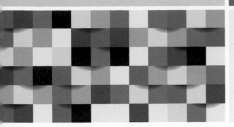

Preface

The purpose of the first edition of *Clinical Reasoning for Physician Assistants: A Workbook for Certification Review and Practice Readiness* is to provide a resource to Physician Assistant (PA) students and practicing PAs when preparing for the Physician Assistant National Certification and Recertification Examinations (PANCE and PANRE). Most important is the robust compilation of quality practice questions that are similar to the PANCE and PANRE items. We believe that every item should be easy to understand and that all the information that is necessary in an item is provided to answer a specific question. As a bonus, we have prepared several case studies with detailed rationales that will benefit all PAs, newly graduated and seasoned PA practitioners. These cases will help sharpen and refine the clinical reasoning skills necessary to deliver impactful and evidence-based, patient-centered care.

TO PHYSICIAN ASSISTANT FACULTY MEMBERS

This clinical practice workbook serves to provide a supplemental resource to your students so they can be as prepared as possible to successfully take the PANCE and begin their journey as competent health care providers. It is a proud moment for faculty and instructors who have watched their students grow from novices in the classroom to students who are knowledgeable and capable of providing appropriate health care to patients after passing the PANCE. However, we know that a cohort of graduating PA students whose next step is taking the PANCE can be stressful for faculty members. They want to know that they guided their students toward a successful path in health care, and they want students to feel confident in their knowledge and skills to succeed in passing the examination.

To ease these concerns, we have provided multiple-choice questions in similar format to PANCE items. If a student has a weakness in one area of the NCCPA PANCE Content Blueprint, faculty members can guide students to the appropriate chapter to review a specific organ system to take some practice items in that specialty. The students can then read the accompanying rationales for each item in which they did not get the answer correct and perhaps have a discussion for clarification with their faculty member, mentor, or fellow students.

If students have a difficult time taking examinations, they can work through each chapter, pretending that each chapter is an actual examination to test their abilities. The more familiar students are with the format of NCCPA items and the more they practice their test-taking skills, the more comfortable they will be in the testing setting.

As you prepare your students to not only pass the PANCE but to be able to function successfully in clinical situations, consider assigning students content from the section of cases that require a higher level of thinking. These case studies will enhance your students' clinical reasoning and critical thinking skills and reinforce best practices for safe and effective medical practice.

TO STUDENTS AND RECERTIFYNG PHYSICIAN ASSISTANTS

A major goal of this review book is to make the examinee feel at ease taking the PANCE or PANRE. The authors and contributors of this book are advocates for the examinee. We are on your side! Experienced item writers who formerly wrote examination questions for the NCCPA certifying examinations and the former Managing Editor of the NCCPA examinations are major contributors.

We have provided some test-taking strategies in Part I of this book. Most important is the robust compilation of multiple-choice practice questions that are similar to the PANCE and PANRE items in Part II of this valuable resource. Finally, Part III allows you to think and process like PAs with the inclusion of clinical case studies where we incorporate patient demographics, cultural aspects of patients, ethics, and professional practice in decision making.

To the newly graduated PA student, use this book as a valuable resource as you prepare yourself for taking the PANCE and to begin working professionally in a health care setting. To the seasoned practicing PA, use this book to brush up on areas in which you have not practiced in preparation for the PANRE.

It is important to note the following about the items in this book:
- Trade names are not used unless the drug in an item is obscure.
- Normal values are provided for all laboratory values; we do NOT provide normal values for vital signs unless they are necessary to the construct of the question.

- Race and ethnicity in Part II of this book are only mentioned if they are pertinent to answering the question.
- More patient information (demographics, ethnicity, religious affiliations, familial situations, etc.) are provided in the case studies in Part III of this book. Our goal with this is to help you take the whole patient into effect and not just the presenting symptoms. It also allows for a higher level of thinking and processing of information to make appropriate decisions regarding the care of patients.
- Note that this workbook was based on the PANCE Content Blueprint that was approved in 2019.
- Some items can be categorized into two Task Codes, especially in the case studies in Part III. Note that we did our best to choose one most relevant Task Code per item within this workbook.
- For more detailed information on the Organ Systems and Task Codes included in this workbook, see the NCCPA website (www.nccpa.net).

We hope this workbook serves as a valuable tool to instructors, students, and certifying PAs as they begin to prepare themselves to take the PANCE and PANRE.

ACKNOWLEDGMENTS

We would like to take this opportunity to thank everyone who was involved in the process of making this first edition possible. Thanks to the folks at Elsevier for encouraging us and believing that this book was a needed resource in the PA profession. Thank you to our mentors and colleagues for listening to our concerns and guiding us through this venture in publishing. Also, thanks to our family and friends for encouraging us to continue working toward the publication of this book. And, most important, thank you to all of the contributors of the items and cases in this book, without whom we could not have succeeded. It was not easy writing medical items for a medical-type book in your spare time while many of you were trying to keep yourselves, your family members, and your patients healthy during the COVID-19 pandemic. Your patience with this process and willingness to write, rewrite, and peer review these items and cases during a difficult time in history are incredible. We are forever indebted to you and your dedication to this task.

Robin D. Risling
Noelle M. Hammerbacher
Daniel L. McNeill

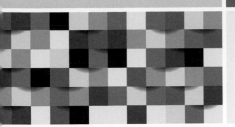

Contents

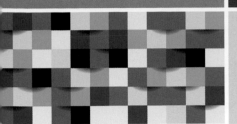

Clinical Reasoning for PANCE/PANRE Success and Safe Clinical Practice

INTRODUCTION

This PANCE/PANRE review book prepares you to successfully pass the National Commission on Certification of Physician Assistants (NCCPA) national certifying board examination. It serves as a valuable companion, accompanying you on your journey to becoming a physician assistant (PA). For those experienced PAs having to recertify, this resource helps in maintaining your licensure so you can continue to serve as a valued member of the health care team. This review book is purposefully designed to reinforce medical knowledge, enhance your clinical reasoning and critical thinking skills, and reinforce best practices for safe and effective medical practice.

Strategic planning and careful consideration are the foundation of this work. Heart and soul have been poured into this body of work by the authors, who consider themselves to be staunch advocates of the examinee. A major goal of this review book is to make the examinee feel at ease taking the PANCE or PANRE. Experienced item writers who formerly wrote examination questions for the NCCPA certifying examinations as well as the former Managing Editor of the NCCPA examinations are major contributors to this book.

The design of this review book has been carefully crafted to meet the needs of the new graduate examinee. The authors recognize and honor the journey you have already undertaken to get to this point. They understand the undergraduate preparation, the arduous admissions process to gain entrance into an accredited program, the dedication and focus it took to graduate from a PA program, and the enormous efforts and sacrifices made along the way. This review book is targeted to the specifics of what it takes for PANCE preparedness. It uses the NCCPA PANCE Content Blueprint organ systems and task categories of known examination areas. This work is also influenced by the Physician Assistant Education Association (PAEA) "Core Competencies for the New Graduate" and the American Academy of Physician Assistants (AAPA) "Competencies for the Physician Assistant Profession."

This review book constitutes three major parts. Part I of this book introduces you to the key clinical reasoning and critical thinking skills for PANCE/PANRE success. It also focuses on safe clinical practice and key test-taking skills and strategies. Part II of this book encompasses chapters for each organ system with items formulated in multiple-choice PANCE/PANRE style, which are organized according to the most current NCCPA PANCE Content Blueprint publication. In each chapter, questions are tracked to a corresponding task category. Part III of the book consists of case-oriented multiple-choice questions broadening the examinee's preparation for entry into practice with careful attention to diversity and professional practice issues. At the end of each chapter in Parts II and III, the answers for all questions are provided, as well as the rationale for why one option is correct and the others are incorrect. Providing a rationale for why options are either correct or incorrect enables the examinee to assess strengths and weaknesses and self-reflect.

HOW BEST TO USE EACH SECTION OF THIS BOOK

In general, Parts II and III of this book prepare the examinee for success by providing the opportunity to answer hundreds of PANCE-style questions. An answer key is given at the end of each chapter of the book, which not only indicates what the correct answer is but also provides a rationale for why the other options are not the best answer. Many of the multiple-choice questions are written by former item writers of the NCCPA PANCE/PANRE examinations. The former Managing Editor of the NCCPA examinations has also provided input for all of the questions in this book that were written by experienced PAs. Furthermore, all questions have been tracked back to the NCCPA PANCE Content Blueprint organ systems and task categories. With regard to pharmaceutical names, generic names for medications are used rather than trade names unless the item refers to a drug that is obscure.

For Students

Students will benefit from this review book in the following manner. Part I deals with preparing for the PANCE. However, you may also find it helpful in preparing for your PA course examinations while in school. You will be able to gain from this book information regarding preparing for taking tests and applying test-taking skills to help you be successful during your time in a PA program. Part I also gives PA students some resources that are useful to enhance and support study. Part II is helpful for PA students to test themselves on selected NCCPA PANCE Content Blueprint areas. Students can gain practice in test-taking skills and be able to self-assess their knowledge base. The answer key and rationales at the end of each chapter in Part II will provide the student with not only the correct answer for the question but also a rationale for why the correct answer is the best answer choice and why the other answer choices, although plausible, are not the correct option. Part III of this review book is helpful to students because not only is the student able to gain more practice in answering multiple-choice questions, they are able to direct their focus on a particular patient presentation. Part III frames multiple-choice questions in a patient-case format to make questions relatable to the real-life clinic environment. Some of the cases provide patient demographics for consideration of care. Furthermore, this chapter purposely involves questions related to professional practice outside of the body systems, science, diagnostic, and pharmaceutical treatment plans.

For PANCE/PANRE Examinees

Part I of this review book has been especially designed for PANCE/PANRE examinees. This section orients the examinee to the critical thinking and clinical reasoning skills necessary for successfully passing PANCE/PANRE-style questions. It also provides some background information regarding the NCCPA's role and policies for administering the examination. Examinees will benefit from the critical thinking and clinical reasoning skills section to enhance their test-taking abilities. They will also benefit from the test-taking preparation, strategies, and skills outlined that specifically prepare the examinee for taking the PANCE/PANRE examinations. Furthermore, resources for enhancing evidence-based knowledge needed for the examination are provided. After acquainting oneself with Part I of this book, examinees can take advantage of Part II of the book which includes a myriad of multiple-choice questions in the PANCE editorial style that are available for practice and review. The more practice gained from answering questions, the better prepared one will be for the actual examination. In Part III of this review book, PANCE-style questions are framed in a patient presentation format of an unfolding case. This part also focuses on patient demographics and professional practice questions as they relate to the NCCPA PANCE Content Blueprint. At the end of each chapter in Parts II and III, you are provided with the correct answer choices as well as a clear rationale for why other plausible options are not correct or not the best option.

For Instructors

Instructors may benefit from this book as well. This review book serves as a great resource for instructors by helping them to provide additional resources available to students, didactic or clinical year, to supplement learning, or as support in remediation plans. Part I is especially helpful, serving students as a guide for test-taking preparation and skills. Part I also highlights other resources students may benefit from using to support and enhance knowledge. Part I

prompts students to continue to apply critical thinking and clinical reasoning skills to their assignments. It also reminds students of the critical role the four institutional pillars play in building, maintaining, and advocating for the PA profession. Furthermore, a section of Part I, called "Pearls for Clinical Practice," helps to prepare clinical year students for starting their first job as a PA, positioning safety and quality care at the forefront, and giving useful tips on documents needed to be gathered and filed as well as how to grow and develop in their profession. Parts II and III are useful for instructors to be able to assign tasks for completion, either to a class or to address a specific student's deficiencies. The answer keys and rationales at the end of each chapter in these two parts of this book are helpful for instructors because they already provide the rationale for why the correct answer is the best choice and why the other options, although plausible, are not correct. Parts II and III are also useful for instructors by providing samples of items that are very similar to the NCCPA PANCE/PANRE examination items. This will help instructors to devise their own multiple-choice questions and answer choices for their examinations. All content in Parts II and III have been mapped back and tracked to the NCCPA PANCE Content Blueprint organ systems and task categories.

INFORMATION ABOUT NCCPA

The NCCPA is considered one of the four pillars upholding the PA profession. It sets the professional standards of knowledge and attitudes PAs should possess as medical providers. The NCCPA is the gate keeper for practice entry and the continuation of practice as a PA. Compliance with NCCPA standards is denoted by the "C" after the PA initials PA-C. NCCPA achieves these standards by administering a certifying board examination which currently all practicing PAs must pass to become certified to practice as a PA-C in all 50 states. To be eligible to take the PANCE, you must be a graduate from an accredited PA program. Program accreditation is granted by the Accreditation Review Commission on Education for the Physician Assistant (ARC-PA). Eligibility limitations in taking the PANCE include the Six-Years-Six Attempts rule. This rule mandates that the PANCE can only be taken a total of six times during the first six-year period after graduation from an accredited PA program. The PANCE examination format is multiple choice. To sit for the examination requires submission of an application, payment to NCCPA, and selecting a site for test taking.

The PANCE multiple-choice examination assesses the applicant's ability for essential clinical reasoning and critical thinking skills especially as they apply to patient evaluation and care. Clinical reasoning and critical thinking skills are applied to specific areas of testing published in the PANCE Content Blueprint on the NCCPA website. The NCCPA PANCE Content Blueprint breaks down assessment into two broad categories. These categories are knowledge of the diseases and disorders PAs will commonly encounter and knowledge and skills related to tasks PAs perform when treating patients.

ESSENTIAL CLINICAL REASONING SKILLS

Essential clinical reasoning skills are considered a competency of practice. Therefore these skills must be successfully demonstrated before entry into practice. They involve the ability of a clinician to integrate and apply appropriate knowledge, use evidence-based medicine, critically weigh evidence, and evaluate the process used to arrive at a diagnosis and treatment plan. At the core of this competency is patient-centered care. Patient-centered care takes into consideration the goals and priorities of the patient and the patient's loved ones and caregivers to arrive at a diagnosis and treatment plan.

A pertinent clinical reasoning skill is the ability to decide if a piece of data is important or irrelevant. This skill is dependent on the types of questions the clinician knows to ask the patient as well the objective data the clinician obtains from patient encounters. Once data are gathered, the clinician must evaluate the data by asking the following types of questions: What aspect of the data is most critical? How does a piece of data interrelate to other data gathered? Does a new piece of data make the working diagnosis more or less likely?

To help PAs practice this skill, this review book helps to fortify their clinical reasoning abilities. It is designed to be able to identify problems with clinical reasoning in the realms of inadequate knowledge, faulty integration of knowledge, and insufficient application of knowledge. This is done by providing PAs with exposure to a wide variety of multiple-choice questions in the NCCPA style, which follow the NCCPA PANCE Content Blueprint. The book further addresses this competency by offering practice in a textual environment to engage your knowledge base and apply it to a wide variety of clinical vignettes in different clinical settings. Part III of this book involves integrating patient demographics, cultural aspects, ethics, and professional practice in decision making. These elements bolster a patient-centered approach to clinical practice.

ESSENTIAL CRITICAL THINKING SKILLS

Essential critical thinking skills involve complex cognitive functioning to arrive at a well-informed conclusion or judgment. The process involves the ability to identify key components, comprehend these components, synthesize data, weigh evidence, analyze findings, and evaluate conclusions used to reach conclusions or judgments. Essential critical thinking skills on the test-taking level require the individual to master the tasks of analysis, evaluation, and creation. In the education world, these three items are what is known as Bloom's Taxonomy. Bloom's Taxonomy is the common standard applied to learning and

acquisition of knowledge in a graduated stepwise process in which attainment of the next level up requires mastery of the levels below. In graduate school training, assessment of knowledge and skills are predominantly at these three top levels. To achieve acquisition of knowledge and skills at the top level requires the individual to first master the ability to remember by recognition and recall, understand by interpreting and explaining, and apply by execution and implementation. Successful performance on the PANCE requires mastery of all Bloom's Taxonomy levels. However, successful critical thinking on the PANCE relies on mastery of Bloom's top tiers: analysis, evaluation, and creation.

Analysis involves the ability to break down a concept to its basic parts and analyze the relationships among these parts. Mastery at this level requires the examinee to understand the rudimentary notions relating to and/or making up the concept.

The next step up from analysis is evaluation. Evaluation involves judgment. To arrive at a judgment there must be defined criteria upon which judgment is based. Usually the criteria involve values and/or knowledge. Once judgment is made, a conclusion is determined. In the test-taking environment, critical thinking comes into play when the individual is asked to come to the best conclusion of a case or scenario. This is achieved by evaluating knowledge of medicine and standards of practice as they apply to the most appropriate answer choice.

Creation occupies the top level in Bloom's Taxonomy, because mastering this area requires competency in all other preceding cognitive areas. Generating something new requires creation, production, and planning. In the test-taking environment, this translates to the ability to integrate learning from different areas of knowledge to come to an interpretation or solution for a medical problem or scientific concept. When examinees are able to master the top three tiers of Bloom's Taxonomy, they successfully overcome plausible yet incorrect distractors. Plausible incorrect distractors within the options of an item are purposefully crafted options that are meant to deflect the examinee from the correct answer. Selecting the right option requires careful and deliberate discernment among possible plausible answers to arrive at the option that is the correct answer.

PATIENT EVALUATION AND CARE

The primary goal of patient evaluation is to arrive at diagnosis and treatment plans derived from clinical practice experience and current research/evidence. Essential components of patient care are ones that include professionalism, include quality and safety considerations, and involve the patient's perspective. At the heart of patient evaluation and care is prioritizing outcomes with patient preferences in mind. In developing this review book with patient evaluation and care in mind, the authors of this book went beyond the scope of solely using the NCCPA PANCE Content Blueprint as a guide to creating this test-taking resource.

They have also included key components of both the AAPA's Competencies for the Physician Assistant profession (https://www.aapa.org/career-central/employer-resources/employing-a-pa/competencies-physician-assistant-profession/) and the PAEA's Core Competencies for New PA Graduates (https://paeaonline.org/our-work/current-issues/core-competencies). Both documents outline the core areas in which PAs should be able to demonstrate clinical competency for the management and care of patients. These include medical knowledge, interpersonal and communication skills, patient care, professionalism, practice-based learning and improvement, and systems-based practice. Both documents, the AAPA's Competencies for the Physician Assistant Profession and the PAEA's Core Competencies for New PA Graduates, indeed have overlapping information that appears redundant. The reason for this has to do with the audience for which each document is intended. The AAPA's publication is geared toward the practicing PA, whereas the PAEA's publication is geared toward the new graduate. Both documents have been created in collaboration with and endorsed by the NCCPA, PAEA, ARC-PA, and AAPA. Because these documents serve as a relevant backdrop for PANCE/PANRE examination questions, the authors included key concepts of these documents in the writing of this book.

KEY TEST-TAKING SKILLS

Preparation, anxiety management, and strategic planning are great ways to sharpen test-taking skills. Preparation is key to successfully passing the PANCE. Exactly what type of preparation is needed and in what form and manner is dependent on the needs of the individual examinee. Therefore the first step in test preparation is to assess your strengths and weaknesses in terms of medical content and task areas. You can do this by analyzing the results of pretests that you have already taken. For instance, the PACKRAT is a good place to start. The PACKRAT is commonly administered in PA schools. It mimics the PANCE and provides individual test results for analytical purposes. PACKRAT feedback provides data about one's areas of strengths and weaknesses. It also allows an individual to assess one's performance against the national average of PACKRAT test scorers. Once feedback performance of the examination is evaluated, preparation for successfully passing the PANCE can begin. Ideally, preparation involves review of content in weaker areas and then retesting knowledge. This review book serves that purpose. This book optimizes PANCE preparation by bolstering content knowledge where performance was weak on the PACKRAT examination. This review book enables you to answer multiple-choice questions that are very similar to the PANCE questions to further assess your performance in organ systems and task areas. A rationale is given for every question to further supplement your understanding and performance. The more practice, the better the results.

Practice also helps to reduce stress and anxiety. Anxiety is one of the most common barriers for successful standardized test taking. This is especially true when you feel the mounting pressure of having to score high enough to pass an examination where just on the other side lies your ability to enter the practice of medicine. The key to managing anxiety performance is first to recognize that anxiety exists, which requires being self-aware and self-reflective. Identify sources of anxiety such as fear, self-doubt, and any other negative emotion or self-talk. Once these factors are identified, seek to manage the anxiety they create. Successfully managing test anxiety varies from person to person. It can manifest in one's physical, behavioral, cognitive, and emotional states. Some physical signs of anxiety are sweating, feeling dizzy, having heart palpitations, rapid breathing, and feeling nauseous. Ways to combat these symptoms are with breathing exercises, meditation, avoiding ingesting stimulants, positive self-talk, and exercise. The way anxiety affects behavior can be seen in emotional outbursts, inability to focus, and avoiding taking the examination. Ways to help deal with behavioral and emotional reactions of anxiety are to recognize the behavior and choose to react in a positive manner, avoid self-medicating with any illegal substances, use positive self-talk, and seek professional help and guidance as needed. Cognitive effects of anxiety can be blanking out, struggling with memory or recall of information, and difficulty concentrating. Help for cognitive symptoms is to use calming techniques such as regulated, conscious breathing, meditating, and self-affirmations. In addition, using your support system such as talking with friends and family can help to bolster confidence and assuage fears.

Overall ways to cope with anxiety are to redirect negative thoughts, images, scenarios, fear of failure, and self-doubt to positive reaffirming self-efficacy focuses. Self-affirming thoughts start with recognizing that anxiety is natural and normal to everyone. A little nervousness can even boost your performance on the examination. If, despite all the self-help measures you used, you are still feeling excessive anxiety, seek help through a licensed professional.

Strategic planning is also essential to desired PANCE/PANRE performance. It relies heavily on an abundance of taking practice examinations and assessing the results. However, there are other considerations in a strategic approach to a successful PANCE score. For instance, schedule the examination when you feel confident about the material. Plan to take the PANCE or PANRE at a time that optimizes your performance. If you are eligible for testing accommodations, plan to use those. Plan to take the examination at a time when there is not significant stress occurring in your life. Take the test at the time of day that best reflects your prime state of attentiveness. Choose a test site location that is easy to access according to your choice of transportation. The night before the examination, rest, get plenty of sleep, eat healthy, exercise, and remain in a positive state of mind.

Lastly, another way to ensure successful test performance involves using a strategy for answering multiple-choice questions. The PANCE/PANRE multiple-choice examinations have two basic components to them: a problem focused stem and possible solutions. Multiple-choice questions are written with a distinct stem in mind (i.e., a clearly defined problem to solve with the options provided). Your job on the PANCE/PANRE is to clearly understand what is being asked of you, what is the problem to solve, and what is the best answer among the options. Many times, once you have determined the objective of the stem of the question, the answer comes to mind before you have ever looked at the options. This is why we recommend that you try to answer the lead-in question of the item before looking at all of the options. Most if not all of the options in NCCPA items are plausible, but only one option is correct—the answer. The other options, called distractors, appear to be correct at first glance but are not, or are partially correct but are not the best answer choice. They are meant to challenge your understanding of the most likely solution. They are not meant to confuse an examinee, although this may happen if an examinee is not familiar with the topic of the item. Therefore do not allow all of the options to distract you from the stem of the question. Identify the problem to solve, see if you can answer the question without looking at the options, choose the best answer from the options provided, and move on to the next item.

Inevitably there will be some questions on the examination that you are uncertain about. Because the PANCE/PANRE are timed examinations, make an educated guess when you are unsure of the answer and move on. In times of uncertainty, usually your first inclination is the best choice. Note that you may mark any questions you would like to revisit, time permitting, within each block of 60 questions. This test-taking strategy helps to ensure you complete the questions within each block on time by not spending more time than you have trying to answer one question.

PATIENT SAFETY AND QUALITY HEALTH CARE

Although the majority of the NCCPA PANCE/PANRE national certifying examinations do not consist of testing specific knowledge and skills in patient safety and quality health care areas, the importance of highlighting aptitude in these areas is important to everybody. In 1999, the Institute of Medicine released its landmark report entitled "To Err Is Human." This report elucidated the vast amount of people who die each year in hospital systems due to preventable medical errors. It further estimated that the national cost of these preventable adverse effects was in the billions of dollars. The report suggested that most medical errors are not done on purpose or by intent and malice but rather from broken processes and systems under which health professionals work and operate. These faulty environments led to these life-costing mistakes. This report led to key policy and system changes. It also led to the Patient Safety and Quality Improvement Act of 2005. This act created a federal system of patient safety organizations and a broad database for reporting medical errors resulting in adverse patient outcomes.

Another policy influencer for the approach and delivery of quality care was an initiative called the Triple Aim from the Institute for Healthcare Improvement (IHI Triple Aim). At the core of this initiative is patient-centered care. The IHI Triple Aim states that improvement in health care systems requires three aims or purposes. These goals are to improve the experience of care (including quality and satisfactions), improve health of populations, and lower per capita costs of health care. Since the release of the IHI Triple Aim, health care organizations have suggested and even implemented fourth and fifth aims which address needs of the provider to prevent burnout and to ensure equity in health care.

How do research and policy translate to the PA profession and the PANCE/PANRE examinations? As mentioned earlier, there are four national PA organizations: AAPA, ARC-PA, NCCPA, and PAEA. All four of these organizations have approved of the position paper called "Competencies for the PA profession." This paper details the core competencies PAs are expected to demonstrate as learned in their training and through their experience as a practicing clinician. These competencies include expectations and accountability for PAs to practice quality care and patient-centered care. Furthermore, the PAEA has published the "Core Competencies for New PA Graduates," which focuses on guiding PA education programs to incorporate uniform practice readiness outcomes of the new graduate. The sixth domain of competencies in this paper deals with Health Care Finance and Systems including the essential skills for patient and personal safety, practice-based improvement, and quality improvement. The NCCPA has proportioned a component of the certifying examinations with special focus questions on professional practice. Some of this involves testing knowledge of risk management in quality improvement and patient safety with the skill in ensuring safety and avoiding medical errors. Another component of this task category is patient care and communication, ensuring patient satisfaction and knowledge of affordable and effective health care that is specific to the patient.

PEARLS FOR CLINICAL PRACTICE

Clinical Pearl #1—New to Practice

It is both exciting and nerve wracking to start a first job. For the new PA graduate, there is often fear as well. The prevailing thought often is: "Am I really prepared for this?" Although you may not have all the experience and knowledge of a well-seasoned clinician, you do have the knowledge, skill, and ability to enter into practice confidently and competently. One of the most important things you can do is to find a mentor. A mentor is someone experienced in the field who can guide and support you. A mentor will help you to further develop knowledge and skills. They can "show you the ropes" by giving you information about your workplace and can show you the best way to navigate the clinic. A mentor can give you more "clinical pearls" of practice specific to your clinic area. They will be able to help guide you through difficult and complex patient care situations. They can also serve as a confidant for expressing your fears or concerns and support you in gaining confidence.

Where can you find a mentor? This can be done by seeking out individuals who can help to further enrich the application of your knowledge and help you to build your acumen in areas of applying more complex diagnostics, imaging, and treatment plans. Health care professionals such as other PAs, nurses, laboratory technicians, specialty trained medical doctors, pharmacists, and social workers are among the key mentors to obtain.

Consistent note taking is another key element that will start you off on good footing when entering practice. Most of the notes you will take will come from the clinical pearls gained by working with your mentors. These notes will serve as fast and easy reference for areas you are sure to encounter in practice. Types of notes to take are how to work the clinical documentation systems, where to find community resources useful for patient care, what medications are used most frequently along with their duration and dosages, and what are some of the most important elements to look for in diagnostic and imaging studies. This type of information will help to ensure fast and efficient patient flow until these things become second nature to you as a seasoned clinician.

Maintaining a good filing system for record keeping is paramount. Maintaining your license and ability to perform certain procedures or prescribe some medications requires documentation. For instance, currently to maintain NCCPA certification, you will need to acquire continuing medical education (CME) credits of category type one and type two (CME 1, CME 2). It is always a good idea to keep records of the CME 1 events you attended and to keep a log of CME 2 activities you have completed. If you are ever audited, you will be able to easily provide evidence of your credentialling and licensing compliance.

Maintaining and developing your knowledge is another key to successful practice. Go beyond the necessity of gaining the CME required to keep your certification and license: be a life-long learner. Take advantage of attending medical lectures and other learning activities offered to expand your knowledge, and keep current on trends and new developments. Volunteer in events that serve the community, which will also help to expand your network. Become a member of the AAPA; this goes farther than supporting the PA profession. The AAPA provides great resources for PAs in practice. It produces a journal full of cases and information to support practice. The AAPA also holds a conference every year where you will be able to meet PAs from all over the nation, gain CME credits, and find out the latest trends in practice. There is a discounted conference rate for those who are AAPA members. The AAPA also offers free CME credit from its JAAPA website: https://journals.lww.com/jaapa/pages/default.aspx. Lastly, AAPA is the advocating body for the PA profession, helping to move the profession forward in the legislative arena of regulations and laws. Becoming a member serves to strengthen the profession and ensure its relevancy and representation in the ever-changing health care delivery system.

Clinical Pearl #2—Resource Gathering

Gather resources that will support your practice and ensure that you are practicing evidence-based medicine. Depending on your practice, there are several downloadable apps for your electronic devices from reliable sources. Some of these apps are free, and others come with a subscription fee. ClincalKey® is an excellent resource to have on hand for consistent, evidence-based information for point-of-care information. It provides materials and information needed for all types of specialty settings. More information about this useful clinical guide can be found at https://www.us.elsevierhealth.com/clinicalkey.

Websites can also serve as a clinical resource. Some of the most useful web-based clinical information sites to know about are the US Preventive Services recommendations for preventative medicine, Centers for Disease Control and Prevention (CDC) guidelines for vaccination status, and Healthy People 2030. As mentioned previously, AAPA members also have access to practical guidance and information for PAs. It also publishes a peer-reviewed journal, JAAPA, which is free to members.

Clinical Pearl #3—Precepting and Growing Your Profession

One of the greatest ways to give back and help to grow the profession is through precepting students. This is due to the fact that one of the biggest obstacles facing the ability to train and grow the PA profession is lack of clinical preceptors for students. Once you become comfortable in clinical practice, one of the biggest contributions you can make is to help train the next generation of PAs.

If you like teaching, then this is also a good way to eventually transition into academia. Becoming a professor in a PA program is, indeed, one of the rewarding professional growth possibilities for practicing PAs. For PAs who like working in the clinic and teaching at a university, this is a possibility as well. Many universities with a PA program allow and even encourage PA professors to continue practicing in their field while teaching. When considering transitioning into the academic setting, the PAEA website is a great place to go for listings of current university job openings from all over the nation. PAEA also publishes numerous resources to help with transitioning from clinical practice into academia. It offers information such as data about salaries and work environment. Its publication on data and statistics is free and is useful for negotiating salary and gaining insight into the world of PA education. These PAEA publications are called By the Numbers and Faculty & Director's Report. For more information visit PAEA online at: https://paeaonline.org/.

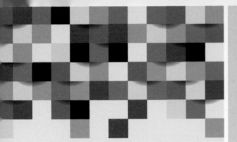

CHAPTER 1
Cardiovascular System

Questions

1. A 62-year-old man comes to the emergency department because he has intermittent pain in his anterior chest that has been increasing in frequency and intensity over the past month. He says the pain often occurs without strenuous activity. The patient rates his current chest pain as 8 on a 10-point scale. Pulse rate is 96/min; all other vital signs are within normal limits. Physical examination shows moderate diaphoresis and no other abnormalities. Electrocardiography shows ST depression in anterior leads and a narrow complex QRS with every QRS preceded by a P wave. Cardiac-specific troponin levels and creatine kinase-MB isoenzyme level are within normal limits. Which of the following is the most likely diagnosis?
   A. Accelerated idioventricular rhythm
   B. Cor pulmonale
   C. Non–ST-segment elevation myocardial infarction
   D. Supraventricular tachycardia
   E. Unstable angina

2. A 74-year-old man comes to the emergency department because he has had worsening pain and cramping in his legs and intermittent blue discoloration of his toes during the past two months. Medical history includes hypertension, hyperlipidemia, and type 2 diabetes mellitus, for which he is taking lisinopril, atorvastatin, and metformin, respectively. He has a history of cigarette smoking 30 years ago. Physical examination shows a dusky, gray-colored left lower extremity and cyanosis to the first and second toe. Dorsalis pedis pulse on the left is absent, and posterior tibialis pulse on the left is faint. Ankle-brachial indexes (ABIs) are 0.4 in the left lower extremity and 0.5 in the right lower extremity (N = 1.0–1.4). CT scan shows a completely occluded common iliac artery. Which of the following is the most appropriate next step?
   A. Discharge to home and schedule follow-up for repeat measurement of ABIs
   B. Initiate therapy with enoxaparin sodium
   C. Perform bedside fasciotomy
   D. Refer for consultation with a cardiologist
   E. Refer for emergency vascular surgery

3. A 25-year-old woman comes to the primary care office for routine physical examination. Medical history includes no chronic disease conditions, and she takes no medications. Vital signs are within normal limits. Physical examination shows a systolic ejection murmur heard best in the second left intercostal space. Based on this finding, which of the following studies is the most appropriate next step in diagnosis?
   A. Chest x-ray study
   B. Creatine kinase-MB test
   C. Echocardiography
   D. Electrocardiography
   E. Troponin test

4.

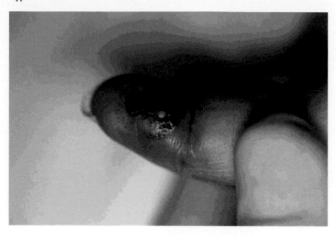

A 52-year-old woman comes to the clinic because she has a two-day history of fever, night sweats, fatigue, anorexia, myalgia, and arthralgia. She says that she noticed a tender lesion on the index finger yesterday. The patient has no history of similar symptoms. Medical history includes end-stage renal disease that is treated with hemodialysis via a right-arm arteriovenous graft. Temperature is 39.4°C (103.0°F), and mild tachycardia is noted; all other vital signs are within normal limits. On physical examination, heart sounds are within normal limits, and no murmur is noted. Auscultation of the lungs shows bibasilar crackles. No tenderness to palpation of the arteriovenous graft is noted. Bruit is normal, and no distal edema is noted. Radial pulse is 1+. Erythrocyte sedimentation rate is 90 mm/hr (N = 0–20 mm/hr). Complete blood cell count shows stable anemia of chronic disease. A photograph of the index finger is shown. Which of the following is the most likely diagnosis?
A. Bacterial endocarditis
B. Cholesterol embolism
C. Nephrotic syndrome
D. Rheumatic fever
E. Septic pneumonia

5. A 54-year-old man is brought to the emergency department by ambulance because he had onset of altered mental status 30 minutes ago. His wife says that he was not acting like himself and had epigastric discomfort four hours before onset. The patient has not eaten or had anything to drink except water during the past 10 hours. He has no history of trauma. Medical history includes poorly controlled type 2 diabetes mellitus. Pulse rate is 108/min, respirations are 20/min, and blood pressure is 80/56 mmHg; he is afebrile. Oxygen saturation is 100% on 2 L of oxygen via nasal cannula. The patient is diaphoretic and only alert and oriented to person.

Laboratory findings include the following:

Fasting serum glucose	154 mg/dL (N = 70–99 mg/dL)
Hematocrit	40.7% (N = 38.3–48.6%)
Hemoglobin	12.3 g/dL (N = 13.5–17.5 g/dL)
White blood cell count	8400/mm³ (N = 4500–11,000/mm³)

Electrocardiography shows sinus tachycardia of 105/min with ST elevations in V_1 through V_4.
Which of the following abnormal findings on physical examination is most likely?
A. Costovertebral angle tenderness
B. Hemiplegia
C. Jugular venous distension
D. Rebound tenderness
E. Turner sign

6. A 56-year-old man comes to the clinic for routine follow-up of stable ischemic heart disease, type 2 diabetes mellitus, and hypertension. During the interview, the practitioner recommends initiating high-intensity statin therapy to decrease the patient's risk for atherosclerotic cardiovascular disease. Which of the following medications is most appropriate to prescribe?
A. Fluvastatin
B. Lovastatin
C. Pravastatin
D. Rosuvastatin
E. Simvastatin

7. A 34-year-old woman comes to the office to establish care with a new primary care provider. She feels well and has no history of fatigue, chest pain, difficulty breathing, or dizziness. Medical history includes seasonal allergic rhinitis. The patient drinks one glass of wine daily and does not use illicit drugs. She says she is currently training for a half marathon. Body mass index is 22 kg/m² (N = 18.5–24.9 kg/m²). Vital signs are within normal limits. On cardiac auscultation, a midsystolic click is heard. Subsequent echocardiography shows that the leaflets of the mitral valve bulge into the left atrium. The leaflets are thin (<5 mm), and no significant mitral regurgitation is noted. Based on these findings, which of the following is the most appropriate advice to give this patient?
A. Avoidance of all alcoholic beverages is required
B. Avoidance of vigorous aerobic exercise such as running is required
C. Endocarditis prophylaxis is required for dental and other procedures
D. Referral to a vascular surgeon is needed for consideration of mitral valve replacement
E. No change in lifestyle is required due to the benign nature of this condition

8. A 16-year-old boy is brought to the office by his mother as a new patient for routine well-child examination. Medical history includes a small ventricular septal defect that was diagnosed when he was a child. Physical examination shows no evidence of jugular venous distention, lower extremity edema, or central or peripheral cyanosis. The lungs are clear to auscultation. Cardiac auscultation shows a holosystolic murmur at the left sternal border. Recent cardiac catheterization shows a normal ejection fraction and no evidence of pulmonary hypertension. Based on this patient's history and physical examination findings, which of the following is the most appropriate next step in management?
   A. Immediate surgical repair of the defect
   B. Percutaneous coronary intervention
   C. Placement of a pericardial patch
   D. Use of antibiotic prophylaxis prior to dental procedures
   E. No intervention is necessary

9. An 88-year-old woman comes to the office for routine physical examination. Medical history includes mitral valve regurgitation; the patient is otherwise healthy and takes no medications. Cardiac auscultation is most likely to show which of the following?
   A. An S_4 gallop
   B. Diastolic rumble to the left lower sternal border that increases with inspiration
   C. Multiple midsystolic clicks
   D. Pansystolic murmur heard best at the apex
   E. Systolic murmur heard best at the second intercostal space and right sternal border that transmits to the neck

10. A 68-year-old man comes to the clinic for a routine physical examination. The patient has no concerns. Medical history includes hypertension, for which he is compliant with taking his medications. He also has a history of myocardial infarction and a popliteal artery aneurysm. He has a 50-pack-year history of smoking cigarettes. Vital signs are within normal limits. On physical examination, a pulsatile abdominal mass is noted on palpation of the abdomen. Ultrasonography shows an abdominal aortic aneurysm that is 4 cm in diameter. Which of the following is the most appropriate management?
   A. Continue the current medical management for hypertension; no further monitoring is required
   B. Immediately refer the patient to the nearest emergency department
   C. Initiate therapy with daily doxycycline
   D. Refer the patient to a cardiothoracic surgeon for urgent repair
   E. Repeat ultrasonography every 12 months to assess for expansion of the aneurysm

11. A 60-year-old man comes to the emergency department because he has had swelling of the lower extremities for the past four weeks. He says that his right leg is more swollen than the left and that he has been more winded lately with any movement. Medical history includes newly diagnosed metastatic lung cancer, hypertension, sleep apnea, and recent embolic stroke. Current medications include metoprolol, lisinopril, aspirin, and atorvastatin. The patient is morbidly obese and says that he is normally not very ambulatory. On physical examination, the right calf is 3 mm larger than the left. Erythema of the right lower extremity is noted, as well as pitting edema and tenderness to palpation of the calves, bilaterally. Pretest probability is performed using the Wells criteria, and it is determined that this patient has an increased risk for thromboembolism. Which of the following studies is the most appropriate next step?
   A. CT angiography with bifemoral runoff
   B. CT pulmonary angiography
   C. MR venography
   D. Venous duplex ultrasonography of the lower extremities
   E. X-ray studies of the right lower extremity

12. A 72-year-old man ccomes to the clinic because he has had episodes of fatigue and light-headedness lasting several minutes and occurring several times a week during the past six months. He says he currently is experiencing both symptoms. The patient also has had episodes of rapid heart palpitations occurring one to two times a week during this time. His wife says that he became so light-headed on two recent occasions that he passed out for several minutes. Medical history includes coronary artery disease for which he had three stents placed approximately one year ago. Daily medications include an 81-mg aspirin, clopidogrel, and simvastatin. Pulse rate is regular at 48/min, and blood pressure is 118/68 mmHg; all other vital signs are within normal limits. Physical examination shows no abnormalities. Electrocardiography shows regular and narrow QRS complexes with each one preceded by a P wave at a rate of 44/min. Which of the following is the most likely diagnosis?
   A. Agonal rhythm
   B. Complete heart block
   C. Junctional bradycardia
   D. Sick sinus syndrome
   E. Wenckebach phenomenon

Answer Key for this chapter begins on p. 23

13. A 15-year-old boy is brought to the clinic by his mother immediately after he fainted at home. The episode occurred after his sister showed him her toe where an ingrown nail had been removed at the same clinic earlier that day. The mother says that the patient looked at the nailbed, became pale and sweaty, and then immediately lost consciousness and fell to the floor. He was unconscious for a minute or two, followed by a few more minutes of grogginess before he eventually regained his normal faculties. The patient has never fainted before and is otherwise healthy. Vital signs are within normal limits. Physical examination shows no abnormalities. Which of the following is the most likely physiologic etiology of the syncopal event in this patient?
   A. Atrioventricular node reentry phenomenon
   B. Hypocapnia
   C. Increased afterload
   D. Increased parasympathetic tone
   E. Uncinate fit

14. A 67-year-old woman comes to the office because she has had worsening fatigue and headaches over the past month. She also has had jaw pain and discomfort with eating. Temperature is 37.4°C (99.4°F), pulse rate is 82/min, respirations are 18/min, and blood pressure is 147/76 mmHg. Physical examination shows tenderness to palpation of the scalp and over the temporal areas. Electrocardiography shows no abnormalities. Temporal arteritis is suspected. Which of the following laboratory results of serum is most likely to confirm this diagnosis?
   A. Elevated creatinine level
   B. Elevated hemoglobin level
   C. Elevated troponin level
   D. Increased erythrocyte sedimentation rate
   E. Increased white blood cell count

15. A 45-year-old man comes to the emergency department because he has had diaphoresis and shortness of breath for the past 12 hours. Medical history includes hypertension and type 2 diabetes mellitus. Current medications include lisinopril and glipizide. Temperature is 36.8°C (98.2°F), pulse rate is 98/min, respirations are 20/min, and blood pressure is 128/72 mmHg. On physical examination, diaphoresis is noted. The lungs are clear to auscultation, and cardiac examination shows no abnormalities. The abdomen is soft, and no tenderness to palpation or distention is noted. Laboratory studies show elevated serum troponin levels. Electrocardiography shows a sinus rhythm with T wave inversion in leads II, III, and aVF. Chest x-ray study shows no abnormalities. Which of the following is the most likely diagnosis?
   A. Inferior wall non–ST-elevation myocardial infarction (non-STEMI)
   B. Inferior wall STEMI
   C. Lateral wall non-STEMI
   D. Lateral wall STEMI
   E. Posterior wall STEMI

16.

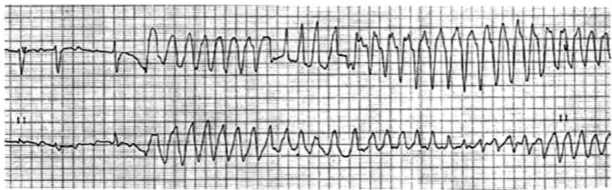

A 55-year-old woman comes to the emergency department because she has had vomiting and diarrhea during the past 48 hours. Medical history includes major depressive disorder, for which she takes citalopram. During the examination, the patient has sudden development of light-headedness and palpitations. Electrocardiography is shown. Which of the following electrolyte abnormalities is most likely in this patient?
   A. Hypercalcemia
   B. Hyperkalemia
   C. Hypernatremia
   D. Hypomagnesemia
   E. Hypophosphatemia

17. A female infant who was delivered prematurely is undergoing an initial examination in the NICU. Birth weight is less than 3.3 lb. Physical examination shows a continuous, rough, machinelike murmur, and echocardiography confirms patent ductus arteriosus (PDA). After one week of mechanical ventilation, repeat echocardiography confirms a persistent PDA. Closure of the PDA is planned. Which of the following is the most appropriate method of closure for this patient?
    A. Course of intramedullary corticosteroids
    B. Infusion of prostaglandin E1
    C. Intravenous nonsteroidal anti-inflammatory drugs
    D. Patch repair
    E. Surgical ligation

18. A 64-year-old woman with a long-standing history of hypertension is admitted to the hospital because she has had worsening shortness of breath and hypoxia over the past two weeks. Oxygen saturation is 83% on room air; all other vital signs are within normal limits. Chest x-ray study shows increased vascular markings and bilateral pleural effusions. Results of complete blood cell count and complete metabolic panel are within normal limits. Initiation of therapy with which of the following medications is most appropriate?
    A. Digoxin
    B. Diphenhydramine
    C. Furosemide
    D. Propranolol
    E. Verapamil

19. An 80-year-old woman has been treated in the hospital for the past three days for pneumococcal pneumonia. Treatment consisted of intravenous fluids and antibiotics. The patient calls the nurse to say that she has pain and swelling at her intravenous site. Pulse rate is 82/min, and blood pressure is 130/72 mmHg. Physical examination shows linear erythema and a tender palpable cord near the intravenous site. Which of the following is the most likely diagnosis?
    A. Cellulitis
    B. Erythema nodosum
    C. Lymphangitis
    D. Panniculitis
    E. Thrombophlebitis

20.

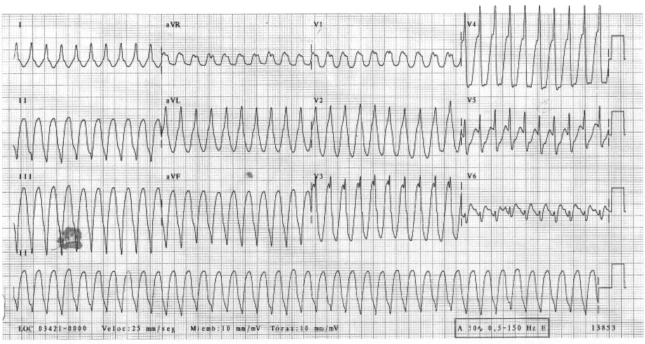

A 48-year-old man is brought to the emergency department because he has had palpitations, light-headedness, and shortness of breath for the past 30 minutes. Pulse rate is approximately 250/min. Twelve-lead electrocardiography is shown. Which of the following is the most likely diagnosis?
A. Atrial flutter
B. Junctional escape rhythm
C. Sick sinus syndrome
D. Torsades de pointes
E. Ventricular tachycardia

    Answer Key for this chapter begins on p. 23

21. A 50-year-old man comes to the emergency department because he has had intermittent chest pain during the past two hours. The pain is located in the retrosternal region of the chest and is sharp and pleuritic in nature. The pain is worse when he lies down and improves when he sits forward. The patient says that he was discharged from the hospital two weeks ago after he had an acute myocardial infarction. On physical examination, cardiac auscultation shows a pericardial friction rub. Electrocardiography is ordered. Which of the following findings on electrocardiography is most likely?
    A. Convex ST elevations with reciprocal ST depressions in opposite leads
    B. Diffuse ST elevations in all leads except aVR and V_1
    C. $S_1Q_3T_3$ pattern with unexplained tachycardia
    D. ST changes and new left bundle branch block
    E. ST depressions and T-wave inversions in the primary leads

22. A 50-year-old man comes to the emergency department because he has had the worst headache of his life for the past 12 hours. He says he needs to refill his prescription for blood pressure medication, and he only remembers that he takes a water pill. Temperature is 37.1°C (98.7°F), pulse rate is 98/min, respirations are 18/min, and blood pressure is 220/140 mmHg. Physical examination shows no abnormalities. CT scan of the head shows encephalopathy. Intravenous antihypertensive therapy is administered, and the patient's blood pressure begins to decrease. At this time, it is most appropriate to admit this patient to which of the following units of the hospital?
    A. Intensive care
    B. Medical/Surgical
    C. Neurology
    D. Neurosurgery
    E. Telemetry

23. A 45-year-old man comes to the emergency department because he had sudden onset of pain in his right foot on awakening this morning. He says the pain is dull and constant, and he rates the pain as a 5 on a 10-point scale, but it improves to a 2 if he sits and keeps the foot in a dependent position. Medical history includes hypertension and type 2 diabetes mellitus, for which he takes metoprolol and metformin, respectively. He has a 25-pack-year history of cigarette smoking. On physical examination, the foot appears pale and is cool to touch below the ankle. Femoral pulse is 3+, and popliteal pulse is 1+. Posterior tibial and popliteal pulses are absent. Ankle and toe strength is 3/5, and loss of sensation to light touch distal to the midcalf is noted. Which of the following findings most likely indicates the need for an emergent consultation with a vascular surgeon?
    A. Absent pulses
    B. Pain
    C. Pallor

D. Paralysis
E. Paresthesia

24. A 67-year-old man is brought to the emergency department by ambulance after he passed out while shoveling the snow. When Emergency Medical Services staff arrived at the scene, an automated external defibrillator showed ventricular fibrillation. A shock was delivered, and the patient's heart rate converted to sinus rhythm. The patient's wife says that he was discharged from the hospital one week ago after undergoing coronary angioplasty. Which of the following is most appropriate to recommend to this patient to decrease the likelihood of ventricular fibrillation occurring again in the future?
    A. Insertion of an implantable cardioverter-defibrillator
    B. Long-term anticoagulation therapy with warfarin
    C. Serial electrocardiography
    D. Therapeutic hypothermia
    E. Transcutaneous pacing

25. A 66-year-old woman comes to the clinic because she has had intermittent substernal chest pain during the past six months. She says the pain is only present with exertion and resolves with rest. The patient is not currently having symptoms. Medical history includes hypertension and hyperlipidemia, for which she takes lisinopril and atorvastatin, respectively. Vital signs are within normal limits. On physical examination, cardiac auscultation shows regular rate and rhythm with no murmurs, gallops, or rubs. The pain is not reproducible with palpation of the chest wall. Electrocardiography shows no ST-segment elevations or depressions. Which of the following is the most likely diagnosis?
    A. Acute coronary syndrome
    B. Costochondritis
    C. Pericarditis
    D. Pulmonary embolism
    E. Stable angina

26. A 65-year-old man comes to the office for follow-up three months after he initiated lifestyle modifications for the treatment of dyslipidemia. He says that he changed his diet, lost weight, started doing aerobic exercise, and decreased his consumption of alcoholic beverages. He is otherwise healthy and has no chronic disease conditions. Laboratory studies show total cholesterol level of 180 mg/dL ($N \leq 200$ mg/dL), high-density lipoprotein cholesterol level of 65 mg/dL ($N \geq 60$ mg/dL), and triglycerides of 935 mg/dL ($N \leq 150$ mg/dL). Which of the following medications is the most appropriate initial management?
    A. Atorvastatin
    B. Cholestyramine
    C. Fenofibrate
    D. Icosapent ethyl
    E. Nicotinic acid

27. A 60-year-old man comes to the clinic because he has had two episodes of constant, tearing pain in the retrosternal aspect of his chest over the past two months. He says the episodes have lasted 15 to 20 minutes, and he rates the pain as a 6 on a 10-point scale. The first episode was two months ago and was associated with a few hours of loss of speech and weakness in the left upper extremity. Currently, the patient is asymptomatic. Medical history includes hypertension and type 2 diabetes mellitus, for which he takes atenolol and metformin, respectively. He also has a history of alcohol and cocaine use disorders. Pulse rate is 88/min, respirations are 16/min, and blood pressure is 150/90 mmHg in the right upper extremity and 130/70 mmHg in the left upper extremity. On physical examination, no carotid bruits are noted. Cardiac auscultation shows a grade 3/6 blowing diastolic murmur heard best during end-expiration at the upper sternal borders with the patient leaning forward in the seated position. Auscultation of the lungs and abdominal examination show no abnormalities. Trace 2+ edema is noted in the tibias, bilaterally. Neurologic examination shows no focal deficits. Which of the following is the most likely diagnosis?
    A. Acute left atrial dissection
    B. Chordae tendineae disruption
    C. Chronic bacterial endocarditis
    D. Impending aortic aneurysm rupture
    E. Ventricular outflow tract obstruction

28. A 44-year-old man comes to the emergency department because he has had several episodes of sudden onset of chest pain with exertion over the past several weeks. Medical history includes migraine. He has a 5-pack-year history of cigarette smoking. Pulse rate is 120/min. Electrocardiography shows acute ST elevation. Coronary angiography shows nonobstructive coronary vessels. Sublingual nitroglycerin is administered, and the patient's symptoms resolve. Which of the following is the most appropriate next step to prevent the recurrence of these episodes in this patient?
    A. Initiate therapy with a beta-blocker
    B. Initiate therapy with a calcium channel blocker
    C. Initiate therapy with a statin drug
    D. Refer for percutaneous coronary intervention
    E. Refer for revascularization

29. A 35-year-old woman is referred to the cardiology clinic because she has had dyspnea on exertion, fatigue, exercise intolerance, light-headedness, and dizziness for the past four weeks. She is a competitive trail runner in New England and has no history of recent international travel. The patient says that she has had three to four tick bites over the past few months, none of which resulted in a rash that she noticed. She says that each tick was on her for less than 12 hours. She is otherwise healthy, does not smoke cigarettes, and does not drink alcoholic beverages. Physical examination shows tachycardia, tachypnea, a laterally displaced apical pulse, a loud S_3 heart sound, and crackles at the bases of both lungs. Which of the following is the most likely diagnosis?
    A. Asthma
    B. Chagas disease
    C. Chronic congestive heart failure
    D. Dilated cardiomyopathy
    E. Sarcoidosis

30. A 50-year-old white man comes to the family medicine clinic for routine physical examination. He feels well and has no history of chronic disease conditions. He says he drinks an occasional alcoholic beverage with dinner, and he does not smoke cigarettes. Family medical history includes the death of his father at 75 years of age from a ruptured abdominal aneurysm. Temperature is 36.8°C (98.2°F), pulse rate is 88/min, respirations are 16/min, and blood pressure is 130/80 mmHg. The patient is concerned about his risk of developing an abdominal aneurysm. It is appropriate to tell the patient that which of the following risk factors has the strongest correlation with the development of this condition?
    A. Age
    B. Alcohol intake
    C. Ethnicity
    D. Family history
    E. Tobacco use

31. A 13-year-old boy comes to the office for his first sports physical examination. During the interview, the patient says that he has occasional chest pain, shortness of breath, and dizziness after running, but says that he has never actually passed out. Family medical history includes sudden unexplained death in an uncle at 42 years of age. On physical examination, a harsh crescendo-decrescendo systolic murmur is heard at the left sternal border and apex. The murmur decreases when the patient is in the squatting position. No other abnormalities are noted. Which of the following findings is most likely on echocardiography?
    A. Coarctation of the aorta
    B. Large patent ductus arteriosus
    C. Mitral valve prolapse
    D. Thickened aortic leaflets
    E. Thickened left ventricular wall

32. A 47-year-old man comes to the emergency department because he has had chest pain for the past two days. He says that he recently had bronchitis but felt like he recovered several days ago. Pulse rate is 122/min, respirations are 20/min and labored, and blood pressure is 89/46 mmHg. Oxygen saturation is 96%. Physical examination shows dyspnea with pale, cool, and moist skin. Heart sounds are muffled, and jugular venous distention is noted. Twelve-lead electrocardiography shows widespread ST-segment elevation with low QRS voltage. Chest x-ray study shows an enlarged cardiac silhouette with clear and fully inflated lung fields. Which of the following is the most likely diagnosis?
    A. Acute myocardial infarction
    B. Cardiac tamponade
    C. Mediastinal tumor
    D. Pulmonary thromboembolism
    E. Tension pneumothorax

33. A 75-year-old man comes to the office because he has had extreme fatigue during the past three days and says that he passed out last night while walking from his kitchen to his bedroom. Medical history includes hypertension and hyperlipidemia, for which he takes lisinopril and atorvastatin. Temperature is 37.1°C (98.7°F), pulse rate is 44/min, respirations are 18/min, and blood pressure is 100/60 mmHg. Twelve-lead electrocardiography shows a complete atrial ventricular disassociation. Which of the following is the most appropriate definitive management for this patient?
    A. 24-Hour ambulatory cardiac monitoring
    B. Placement of a defibrillator
    C. Placement of a pacemaker
    D. Replacement of the aortic valve
    E. Replacement of the mitral valve

34. A 53-year-old man comes to the clinic because he has measured and recorded his blood pressure at retail stores several times during the past six months and found it to be consistently around 150/98 mmHg. Medical history includes recurrent episodes of gout, for which he takes medicine prophylactically, and benign colon polyps discovered and removed during a screening colonoscopy three years ago. The patient has no history of blood pressure abnormalities or cardiovascular disease. He has never smoked cigarettes and consumes alcoholic beverages rarely. Body mass index is 27 kg/m² (N = 18.5–24.9 kg/m²), and the patient exercises regularly and maintains a healthy diet. Current blood pressure is 150/95 mmHg in both arms. Physical examination shows no abnormalities. Which of the following medications is most appropriate to initiate at this time?
    A. Clonidine
    B. Hydralazine
    C. Hydrochlorothiazide
    D. Isosorbide dinitrate
    E. Lisinopril

35.

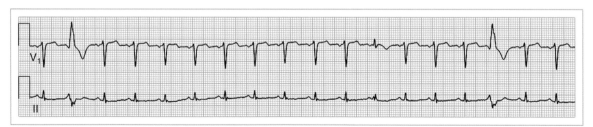

A 22-year-old woman comes to the clinic because her smart watch alerted her that she had an irregular heartbeat eight hours ago. She says she has felt fine but occasionally feels like her heart skips a beat. The patient is a local college student who is taking pre-Physician Assistant classes. She does not smoke cigarettes, use illicit drugs, or take any medications. The patient admits to drinking a lot of coffee and energy drinks to help her get through the long hours of study. Electrocardiography is shown. Which of the following is the most likely diagnosis?
A. Atrial fibrillation
B. Second-degree atrioventricular (Mobitz type I) block
C. Sinus arrhythmia
D. Sinus rhythm with preventricular contractions
E. Ventricular tachycardia

36. A 45-year-old man comes to the clinic because he has had chronic leg fatigue that does not change with standing as well as prominent veins in his legs for the past seven years. Medical history includes hypertension and type 2 diabetes mellitus, for which he takes lisinopril and glipizide, respectively. Which of the following findings, if noted on physical examination, is most likely associated with the venous status of this patient?
    A. Digital paresthesia
    B. Elevated blood pressure
    C. Hyperpigmentation of skin
    D. Irregular distribution of hair on the legs
    E. Subungual dermatophytosis

37. A 32-year-old man comes to the emergency department because he has had a recurrent fever for the past three weeks. He has not had a cough, shortness of breath, sore throat, rhinorrhea, or gastrointestinal symptoms. Temperature is 39.3°C (102.8°F), pulse rate is 98/min, respirations are 18/min, and blood pressure is 108/60 mmHg. Physical examination shows Osler nodes on the palms and soles and splinter hemorrhages of the nails. Cardiac auscultation shows a significant murmur. Several recent and remote venipunctures are noted on the upper and lower extremities. Which of the following is the most appropriate initial step in diagnosis?
    A. Echocardiography
    B. Electroencephalography
    C. Electromyography
    D. Electrophoresis
    E. Endoscopic retrograde cholangiopancreatography

38.

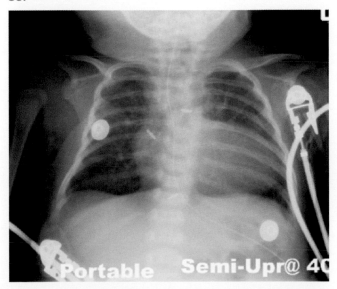

A 7-week-old female infant is brought to the clinic by her parents because she has been irritable, has development of blue-tinted lips after crying, and appears to be short of breath when breastfeeding. Vital signs are within normal limits except for an oxygen saturation of 84%. On physical examination, a loud, harsh systolic murmur is heard at the upper left sternal border. Chest x-ray study is shown. Which of the following is the most likely diagnosis?
    A. Aortic stenosis
    B. Patent ductus arteriosus
    C. Pulmonary atresia
    D. Tetralogy of Fallot
    E. Ventricular septal defect

39. A 57-year-old man comes to the emergency department with his wife because he had onset of chest pain early this morning around five hours ago that recently subsided one hour ago. He is currently asymptomatic, but his wife insisted that he seek medical care. Two weeks ago, he was evaluated at a different emergency department because he had an episode of chest pain that began when he was mowing the lawn and subsided with rest. The patient says that chest x-ray studies and electrocardiography obtained at that time showed no abnormalities, and serum troponin levels were within normal limits; he was advised to follow up with his primary care physician as soon as possible. Medical history includes hypertension and type 2 diabetes mellitus. Medications include hydrochlorothiazide 25 mg once daily, extended-release metformin 500 mg once daily, and sitagliptin 50 mg once daily. Current electrocardiography shows deeply inverted T waves in leads V_2 and V_3. This finding is highly specific for stenosis of which of the following coronary arteries?
    A. Left anterior descending
    B. Left circumflex
    C. Posterior descending
    D. Right coronary
    E. Right marginal

40. A 14-year-old boy is brought to the pediatric office for sports physical examination. He has been healthy and is asymptomatic. Medical history includes surgical repair of coarctation of the aorta at 5 years of age. Pulse rate is 68/min and regular. Blood pressure is 120/60 mmHg in the right upper extremity and 118/64 mmHg in the left. Physical examination shows a normal S_1 and S_2 with no murmurs, and the lungs are clear to auscultation. Radial and pedal pulses are symmetrical at 3+. Which of the following studies is most appropriate to obtain prior to clearing this patient for participation in a sport?
    A. Anterior and lateral chest x-ray studies
    B. Aortic angiography
    C. Arterial Doppler ultrasonography
    D. Exercise stress testing
    E. Transesophageal echocardiography

41. A 56-year-old man with a history of myocardial infarction two years ago comes to the office because he has had shortness of breath with exertion and worsening dependent edema over the past six weeks. Medications include metoprolol, aspirin, lisinopril, and atorvastatin. Temperature is 36.7°C (98.0°F), pulse rate is 82/min, respirations are 16/min, and blood pressure is 138/84 mmHg. Physical examination shows diminished breath sounds bilaterally with an S_3 gallop and regular rate and rhythm. The abdomen is soft and nontender to palpation, and 2+ dependent edema is noted over the anterior shins, bilaterally. Exercise stress testing with myocardial perfusion is planned. Which of the following findings of this study is most likely to support a diagnosis of systolic heart failure in this patient?
    A. Decreased pulmonary artery pressure
    B. Fixed ischemia of the right ventricular wall
    C. Left ventricular ejection fraction of 25%
    D. Reversible ischemic changes in the cardiac apex
    E. Ventricular bigeminy

42. A 74-year-old white man comes to the emergency department because he has had increasing episodes of chest pain on exertion during the past six weeks that are now occurring at rest. Medical history includes hyperlipidemia, for which he takes pravastatin. He has a 35–pack-year history of cigarette smoking. Vital signs are within normal limits, and physical examination shows no acute abnormalities. Cardiac enzymes are within normal limits. Electrocardiography shows no acute ST changes. Which of the following is the most likely diagnosis?
    A. Dyspepsia
    B. Myocardial infarction
    C. Myocarditis
    D. Pulmonary embolism
    E. Unstable angina

43. An 84-year-old woman comes to the emergency department because she has had chest pain for the past two hours that improved after she vomited two times. She currently does not have chest pain but has persistent nausea. Medical history includes hypertension and hypercholesterolemia. Current medications include lisinopril 10 mg once daily and pravastatin 10 mg once daily. Temperature is 36.8°C (98.2°F), pulse rate is 48/min, respirations are 20/min, and blood pressure is 130/70 mmHg. Oxygen saturation is 90% on room air. Physical examination shows an S_3 gallop. Electrocardiography shows ST-segment elevations in leads II, III, and aVF with reciprocal depressions in leads I and aVL. Which of the following is the most appropriate next step?
    A. Cardiac catheterization
    B. Coronary artery bypass grafting
    C. Intravenous beta-blocker
    D. Intravenous glycoprotein IIb/IIIa inhibitor
    E. Sublingual nitroglycerine

44. A 78-year-old man with a long-standing history of bilateral edema of the lower extremities comes to the clinic for routine examination. He says he has had worsening edema and changes to the color of the skin on his lower extremities. On physical examination, hypopigmented white patches with focal red punctate dots are noted on the lower extremities. Based on these findings, which of the following is the most likely diagnosis?
    A. Atrophie blanche
    B. Hyperpigmentation
    C. Lipodermatosclerosis
    D. Varicose eczema
    E. Vascular ulceration

45.

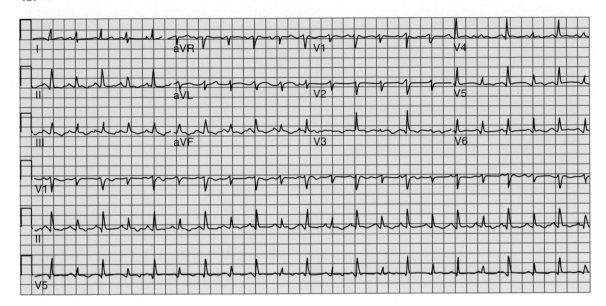

A 26-year-old man comes to the emergency department because he has had chest pain and shortness of breath since he was involved in a motor vehicle collision one hour ago. Pulse rate is 150/min, and blood pressure is 86/60 mmHg. Physical examination shows bruising over the precordium, muffled heart sounds, and jugular venous distention. The airway is patent, and lung sounds are clear, bilaterally. The abdomen is soft and nontender to palpation. Ultrasonography shows a large pericardial effusion. Electrocardiography is shown. Which of the following is the most appropriate initial management?

A. Chest tube insertion
B. Diagnostic peritoneal lavage
C. Endotracheal intubation
D. Needle decompression
E. Pericardiocentesis

46. A 55-year-old man comes to the emergency department because he had sudden onset of pain in the right lower extremity with associated numbness and tingling two hours ago. Medical history includes atrial fibrillation, for which he takes warfarin. On physical examination, the right lower extremity is pale and cool to palpation. Popliteal, dorsal pedis, and posterior tibial pulses are diminished. Laboratory studies show an international normalized ratio of 1.1 (N ≤ 1.1). Based on these findings, which of the following is the most appropriate treatment?

A. Initiate aspirin/dipyridamole therapy twice daily
B. Initiate cilostazol therapy immediately
C. Initiate a daily aspirin regimen
D. Initiate therapy with unfractionated heparin
E. Initiate a trial of clopidogrel therapy

    Answer Key for this chapter begins on p. 23

47. A 68-year-old man returns to the clinic for follow-up eight months after hypertension was diagnosed. He has returned for follow-up four times over the past eight months and has added several medications to his regimen, but his blood pressure has not decreased satisfactorily. Despite his increased blood pressure, the patient says that he feels well and has no physical complaints. Current medications include hydrochlorothiazide 25 mg once daily, amlodipine/benazepril 10 mg/40 mg once daily, and simvastatin 20 mg once daily for treatment of hypercholesterolemia. Pulse rate is 64/min, respirations are 12/min, and blood pressure is 180/102 mmHg in both arms. Ankle-brachial index is 1.1 (N = 1.0–1.4). Physical examination shows persistent bruits in the carotid, abdominal, and iliac vessels. On laboratory studies, thyroid-stimulating hormone level, complete blood cell count, and cholesterol level are within normal limits. Complete metabolic panel shows no abnormalities except for a serum potassium level of 3.0 mEq/L (N = 3.5–5.0 mEq/L). Which of the following is the most likely diagnosis?
    A. Coarctation of the aorta
    B. Hypercortisolism
    C. Pheochromocytoma
    D. Renal artery stenosis
    E. Thyrotoxicosis

48. A 55-year-old woman comes to the emergency department because she had acute onset of palpations, shortness of breath, tremors, anxiety, and insomnia 24 hours ago. Medical history includes Hashimoto thyroiditis. One week ago, the patient was evaluated by her primary care provider because she had fatigue and a thyroid-stimulating hormone level of 0.5 µU/mL (N = 0.5–5.0 µU/mL). Liothyronine 20 µg daily was initiated at that time. Based on these findings, which of the following arrhythmias is most likely to be noted on electrocardiography of this patient?
    A. Atrial fibrillation
    B. Long QT syndrome
    C. Premature ventricular contractions
    D. Ventricular tachycardia
    E. Wolff-Parkinson-White syndrome

49. A 57-year-old man comes to the office because he has had light-headedness, palpitations, and blurred vision for the past two hours since he woke up this morning. He says that the symptoms are worse when he gets out of bed. He also spent the past week resting in bed because he injured his knee while playing tennis. Medical history includes mild hypertension and nephrolithiasis three years ago. His only medication is hydrochlorothiazide 25 mg. Pulse rate is 98/min, and blood pressure is 122/65 mmHg. Which of the following is the most appropriate next step?
    A. Blood pressure measurement with the patient supine and then standing
    B. Echocardiography
    C. Electrocardiography
    D. Exercise stress test
    E. Tilt-table testing

50.

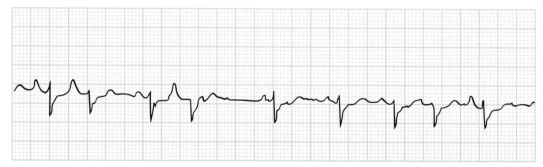

An 89-year-old woman is undergoing intensive rehabilitation in an acute rehabilitation facility 10 days after she sustained a left middle cerebral artery stroke. The source of the stroke remains unknown despite extensive inpatient workup. Medical history includes hypertension, hyperlipidemia, and a recent stroke, for which she takes aspirin, clopidogrel, atorvastatin, lisinopril, and amlodipine. The patient is placed on telemetry monitoring to determine the cause of the stroke, and the rhythm shown is obtained from 24-hour cardiac monitoring. Based on this image, which of the following rhythms is a precursor to the cause of the stroke in this patient?
A. Atrial flutter
B. First-degree atrioventricular block
C. Paroxysmal supraventricular tachycardia
D. Premature atrial contractions
E. Right bundle branch block

51. A 65-year-old woman with a long-standing history of hypertension comes to the office because she has had chronic dependent edema and worsening shortness of breath on exertion over the past six months. Current medications include lisinopril and amlodipine. Temperature is 37.0°C (98.6°F), pulse rate is 80/min, respirations are 14/min, and blood pressure is 130/78 mmHg. Physical examination shows regular rate and rhythm, and breath sounds are diminished bilaterally. Trace pedal edema is noted. Diastolic heart failure is suspected. Which of the following studies is most likely to confirm this diagnosis?
    A. Chest x-ray study
    B. CT coronary angiography
    C. Echocardiography
    D. Electrocardiography
    E. Exercise stress test

52. A 65-year-old man comes to the emergency department because he has had constant pain in the midabdomen and back for the past 20 minutes. He rates the pain as a 6 on a 10-point scale. Medical history includes hypertension, for which he takes lisinopril. Although he is unable to recall the condition, he says he has a family medical history of a condition that includes similar symptoms. The patient has a 45–pack-year history of cigarette smoking. Pulse rate is 90/min, respirations are 16/min, and blood pressure is 100/60 mmHg; he is afebrile. The patient appears to be in mild distress. On physical examination, auscultation of the chest and lungs shows no abnormalities. The abdomen is soft and diffusely tender; no rebound or guarding is noted. Which of the following organs is the most likely source of the symptoms in this patient?
    A. Aorta
    B. Colon
    C. Gallbladder
    D. Pancreas
    E. Stomach

53. A 35-year-old woman is brought to the emergency department by a friend immediately after she had a seizure while at work. Her friend says that the seizure lasted approximately 60 seconds, and the patient seemed confused for several minutes after the seizing stopped. Medical history does not include a seizure disorder, but the patient says that multiple people on her mother's side of the family have a history of seizures and strokes. Vital signs are within normal limits, and neurologic examination shows no focal deficits. MRI of the brain shows an arteriovenous malformation, which is thought to have contributed to the new onset of seizure. Based on these findings, this patient most likely has which of the following genetic conditions?
    A. Alpha$_1$-antitrypsin deficiency
    B. Charcot-Marie-Tooth disease
    C. Fabry disease
    D. Familial adenomatous polyposis
    E. Hereditary hemorrhagic telangiectasia

54. A 60-year-old man comes to the primary care office because he has had swelling of his lower extremities, shortness of breath, and audible wheezing during the past four weeks. Medical history includes recent infectious endocarditis, stage 3 chronic kidney disease, and ischemic heart disease, for which he is taking aspirin, atorvastatin, metoprolol, lisinopril, and isosorbide mononitrate. On physical examination, cardiac auscultation shows a blowing, high-pitched holosystolic murmur that is loudest at the apex and radiates to the axilla. Which of the following diagnoses is most likely to be determined on echocardiography of this patient?
    A. Aortic regurgitation
    B. Aortic stenosis
    C. Mitral regurgitation
    D. Mitral stenosis
    E. Tricuspid regurgitation

55. A 65-year-old man comes to the office for routine physical examination. Medical history includes no chronic disease conditions. Pulse rate is 84/min, respirations are 20/min, and blood pressure is 140/80 mmHg. On physical examination, cardiac auscultation shows a pulsus parvus et tardus. This patient most likely has which of the following valvular abnormalities?

A. Aortic regurgitation
B. Aortic stenosis
C. Mitral regurgitation
D. Pulmonary regurgitation
E. Pulmonary stenosis

56.

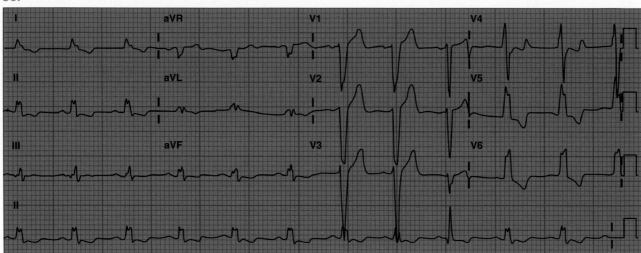

A 65-year-old man comes to the office for preoperative testing prior to undergoing elective cholecystectomy. Medical history includes type 2 diabetes mellitus, which is well-managed with oral metformin 500 mg twice daily. Electrocardiography is shown. Which of the following is the most likely diagnosis?

A. Anterior wall myocardial infarction
B. Inferior wall myocardial infarction
C. Left bundle branch block
D. Left ventricular hypertrophy
E. Right bundle branch block

57.

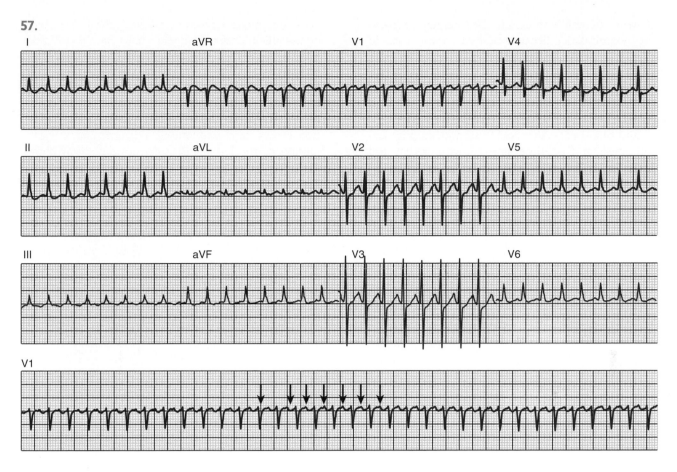

A 72-year-old woman comes to the emergency department because she has had light-headedness, fatigue, and chest discomfort for the past hour. Medical history includes no chronic disease conditions, and she says she has never had an episode of syncope or similar symptoms in the past. Pulse rate is 186/min, respirations are 20/min, and blood pressure is 100/64 mmHg; she is afebrile. Oxygen saturation is 97% on room air. Electrocardiography is shown. Valsalva maneuver, coughing, and breath holding provide no relief of symptoms. Which of the following intravenous medications is most appropriate to administer to this patient?

A. Adenosine
B. Amiodarone
C. Diltiazem
D. Metoprolol
E. Verapamil

58. A 60-year-old man is brought to the emergency department by ambulance because he had abrupt onset of pain in the upper abdomen that radiated to his back after he ate a hamburger at a local restaurant. When he stood up to walk to the ambulance, the patient passed out; he is currently unconscious. Five minutes ago, pulse rate was 130/min, respirations were 24/min, and blood pressure was 80/50 mmHg. Physical examination at that time showed weak radial and femoral pulses. Current pulse rate is 150/min, respirations are 24/min, and blood pressure is 70/50 mmHg. Electrocardiography shows sinus tachycardia. Which of the following is the most likely acute diagnosis?
    A. Aortic aneurysm
    B. Aortic dissection
    C. Appendicitis
    D. Diverticulitis
    E. Myocardial infarction

59. A 72-year-old man comes to the emergency department because he has had heart palpitations for the past three hours. He also has had shortness of breath, light-headedness, and dizziness. Temperature is 36.7°C (98.1°F), pulse rate is 180/min, respirations are 18/min, and blood pressure is 100/60 mmHg. On physical examination, no bruits or jugular venous distention is noted. The lungs are clear to auscultation. Cardiac auscultation shows an irregular heart rhythm without murmurs, rubs, or clicks. Atrial flutter or atrial fibrillation is suspected. To help distinguish between atrial flutter and atrial fibrillation in this patient, it is most appropriate to examine the heart rhythm via which of the following physical examination techniques?
    A. After the patient performs a Valsalva maneuver
    B. After performing a carotid sinus massage
    C. With the patient in the squatting position
    D. With the patient sitting up and leaning forward
    E. With the patient supine in the left lateral position

60. A 42-year-old woman comes to the stroke center by private transportation because she had numbness, tingling, and weakness in the left hand while driving 20 minutes ago. She says she also became slightly disoriented and had difficulty talking. Medical history includes hyperthyroidism and a transient ischemic attack 20 years ago. She has no history of hypertension, diabetes mellitus, or heart or lung disease. The patient does not smoke cigarettes, drink alcoholic beverages, or use illicit drugs. Temperature is 36.6°C (97.8°F), pulse rate is 80/min, respirations are 16/min, and blood pressure is 118/78 mmHg. The patient appears well-developed and well-nourished, and she has an athletic build. Slight aphasia is noted. Cardiopulmonary examination shows no abnormalities. Neurologic examination shows decreased muscle strength and range of motion of the left hand. Electrocardiography shows a regular sinus rate and rhythm. Echocardiography shows a slight bulge of the atrial wall. CT scan of the head shows an old infarct in the left frontal lobe, and an MRI of the brain shows a new infarct in the right cortex. Which of the following congenital heart defects is most likely responsible for the findings in this patient?
    A. Atrial septal defect
    B. Coarctation of the aorta
    C. Patent ductus arteriosus
    D. Pulmonary valve stenosis
    E. Ventricular septal defect

61. A 60-year-old woman comes to the urgent care clinic because she had acute onset of pain in the right lower extremity that woke her from sleep three hours ago. She says she tried to get an appointment with her primary care physician, but the pain was too intense, so she decided to come to urgent care. She has no history of recent injury, stings, or bites and has no history of similar pain. Medical history includes hypertension and type 2 diabetes mellitus, for which she takes lisinopril and metformin, respectively. She does not smoke cigarettes. On physical examination, the right lower extremity is cool to touch. Decreased sensation is noted, and dorsalis pedis and posterior tibial pulses are absent. Which of the following is the most appropriate initial management?
    A. Change lisinopril to a calcium channel blocker
    B. Initiate oral ropinirole 0.25 mg every evening, and then titrate upward to the most effective dose over the coming weeks
    C. Order measurement of serum creatine kinase level, serum lactic acid level, and complete metabolic panel
    D. Order outpatient venous Doppler ultrasonography
    E. Send the patient to the emergency department for arterial Doppler ultrasonography and consultation with vascular surgery

Answers

1. **Answer: E** This patient describes intermittent anterior chest pain occurring in the absence of strenuous activity. The recent onset of his symptom along with an increase in frequency and intensity are characteristic of unstable angina, option E.

   Accelerated idioventricular (or junctional) rhythm, option A, is characterized by an absence of P waves on electrocardiography. Cor pulmonale, option B, is a condition whereby cardiac disease results in clinical symptoms related to respiratory compromise such as dyspnea, fatigue, and crackles. None of these symptoms are observed in the scenario presented. Although similar in presentation to unstable angina, non–ST-segment elevation myocardial infarction, option C, results in damage to cardiac tissue, rather than ischemia alone, thus producing elevations in cardiac biomarkers. Supraventricular tachycardia (SVT), option D, is a re-entry or pre-excitation phenomenon resulting in tachycardia typically with a pulse rate of greater than 150/min. The characteristic feature of SVT is an absence of discernable P waves. **Task:** C—Formulating Most Likely Diagnosis

2. **Answer: E** This patient has atherosclerosis, or peripheral artery disease of the extremities, which is one of the leading causes of cardiovascular disability and death in the United States. Risk factors include cigarette smoking, hypertension, abnormal blood glucose and low-density lipoprotein cholesterol levels, and other chronic inflammatory processes. Claudication is common and includes pain, aching, cramping, numbness, or fatigue of muscles that occurs with exercise and is relieved at rest. On physical examination, an absent or diminished pulse is likely distal to the obstruction. Consultation with a vascular surgeon (option E) is vitally important, as limb ischemia can result from a lack of urgent intervention or revascularization.

   Discharge to home and schedule follow-up for repeat measurement of ABIs, option A, is incorrect because this would indicate that the patient has stable vascular disease. The absence of pulses suggests life-threatening limb ischemia. Initiate therapy with enoxaparin sodium, option B, is a treatment choice best used for acute deep venous thrombosis and is often not a therapy that is used alone in crucial limb ischemia. Perform bedside fasciotomy, option C, is a technique used for compartment syndrome and not critical limb ischemia. Refer for consultation with a cardiologist, option D, is not correct since cardiology is not the specialty of choice to manage this patient's condition. **Task:** D2—Clinical Intervention

3. **Answer: C** This patient most likely has an atrial septal defect, as noted by the findings on physical examination. In most cases, transesophageal echocardiography, option C, is required to more closely examine the interatrial septum to determine both the type and size of the atrial septal defect. These factors become important when considering therapeutic options with respect to closure and repair of the defect.

   Chest x-ray study, option A, is used to identify chest pathology and is not useful in diagnosing a cardiac murmur. Creatine kinase-MB test, option B, measures the level of an isoenzyme of creatine kinase in the blood; it cannot evaluate cardiac blood flow and is not useful in diagnosing a cardiac murmur. Electrocardiography, option D, will evaluate the cardiac electrical flow through the cardiac cycle, but it cannot evaluate blood flow. Troponin test, option E, will evaluate for the death of cardiac cells but will not assess cardiac flow. **Task:** B—Using Diagnostic and Laboratory Studies

4. **Answer: A** Option A, bacterial endocarditis, is correct because the patient has signs and symptoms such as a common predisposing factor (arteriovenous graft), high fever, embolic lesion, and supporting laboratory findings. Up to 6% of patients on hemodialysis will develop infective endocarditis, the most common pathogen (*Staphylococcus aureus*) presents with an acutely elevated fever and is accompanied by the systemic list of symptoms in the vignette. Cardiac murmurs are not necessarily present in the initial acute early presentation of infective endocarditis. Embolic lesions occur in up to half of the affected patients. An increased erythrocyte sedimentation rate is noted in up to 90% of patients.

   Cholesterol embolism, option B, does not present as an acute systemic illness. Nephrotic syndrome, option C, does not present with acute fever or embolic events. Rheumatic fever, option D, is not common in this age group, and patients with this disease do not have the predisposing factor of arterial access. Patients with septic pneumonia, option E, present with prominent respiratory symptoms and would have more significant and oftentimes unilateral findings of consolidation. Also, this disease is not commonly associated with embolic skin lesions of this nature. **Task:** C—Formulating Most Likely Diagnosis

5. **Answer: C** This patient's altered mental status, hypotension, and tachycardia indicate that he is in cardiogenic shock. The ST elevations on electrocardiography, diaphoresis, and epigastric discomfort are consistent with myocardial infarction as the source of cardiogenic

shock. Jugular venous distension, option C, occurs because of elevated venous pressures, which is pathognomonic for cardiogenic shock when compared with neurogenic shock, hypovolemic shock, and septic shock.

Costovertebral angle tenderness, option A, is consistent with pyelonephritis, which is a source of septic shock. Hemiplegia, option B, is found in patients with spinal cord injury, which causes neurogenic shock. This patient, however, has no history of known trauma. Rebound tenderness, option D, is more consistent with peritonitis, which is a cause of septic shock. This patient is afebrile, and his white blood cell count is within normal limits. Turner sign, option E, is a blue discoloration that occurs on the flanks as a result of retroperitoneal bleeding. This is a cause of hypovolemic shock due to blood loss; however, this patient's hemoglobin level and hematocrit are within normal limits. **Task:** A—History Taking and Physical Examination

6. **Answer: D** This question requires the examinee to determine which therapy is a high-intensity statin. Only option D, rosuvastatin, is a high-intensity statin. The other four options (options A, B, C, and E) are moderate-intensity statins. **Task:** D3—Pharmaceutical Therapeutics

7. **Answer: E** No change in lifestyle is required due to the benign nature of this condition, option E, is the correct answer. Patients with only a mid-systolic click usually have no immediate clinical issues, although mitral regurgitation may develop in the future.

Avoidance of all alcoholic beverages, option A, is not necessary. Avoidance of vigorous aerobic exercise such as running, option B, is incorrect because exercise is recommended to keep the heart muscle strong. Endocarditis prophylaxis for dental procedures, option C, was previously recommended, but current American College of Cardiology and American Heart Association guidelines state that prophylaxis is not necessary. Referral to a vascular surgeon for surgery, option D, is incorrect because at this point the patient's condition is benign. If significant valvular disease develops in this patient, mitral valve repair rather than replacement is usually the recommended procedure. **Task:** D1—Health Maintenance, Patient Education, and Disease Prevention

8. **Answer: E** No intervention is necessary, option E, is the correct answer. Small ventricular septal defects in asymptomatic patients do not require surgery or other interventions.

Immediate surgical repair of the defect, option A, is only indicated if there is evidence of the development of cyanosis or elevated pulmonary artery pressure.

Percutaneous coronary intervention and placement of a pericardial patch, options B and C, are incorrect. Small asymptomatic ventricle septal defects do not require surgery or other interventions. Antibiotic prophylaxis for dental procedures, option D, is recommended when the ventricular septal defect is associated with pulmonary hypertension and cyanosis. This is not the case with this patient. **Task:** D2—Clinical Intervention

9. **Answer: D** Mitral regurgitation is clinically noted as a pansystolic murmur heard best at the apex, option D. An S_4 gallop, option A, does not indicate mitral valve regurgitation; this indicates increased resistance within the ventricle such as in ventricular hypertrophy. A diastolic rumble to the left lower sternal border that increases with inspiration, option B, indicates tricuspid stenosis. Multiple mid systolic clicks, option C, indicates mitral valve prolapse. Aortic stenosis is indicated by a systolic murmur heard best at the second intercostal space and right sternal border that transmits to the neck, option E. **Task:** B—Using Diagnostic and Laboratory Studies

10. **Answer: E** This patient has an asymptomatic abdominal aortic aneurysm (AAA) that is less than 5.5 cm. The current recommendation for an AAA of this size is to monitor yearly to assess for any changes, growth, or risk of rupture as well as to concurrently decrease cardiovascular risk (i.e., blood pressure management, smoking cessation, antiplatelet therapy, statin therapy). Therefore, option E is correct.

This patient should continue to take his hypertension medications, option A. However, based on the diagnosis of AAA, he should be monitored for expansion yearly, thus option A is not adequate management. This patient's AAA is small, asymptomatic, and does not show evidence of rupture. Therefore, it does not need a referral for a higher level of care, option B. Taking doxycycline, option C, does not decrease AAA expansion and is not appropriate to recommend. Patients who have an AAA greater than 5.5 cm or rapid expansion (i.e., >5 mm in six months or >10 mm in one year) should be referred to a cardiothoracic surgeon for repair, option D. **Task:** D2—Clinical Intervention

11. **Answer: D** Clinical diagnosis of venous thromboembolism cannot be made using only history and physical examination findings. Pretest probability must be performed using the Wells criteria or an alternative risk stratification method. If pretest probability is low, then a D-dimer assay should be obtained. If pretest probability is intermediate or high as in this patient, then venous duplex ultrasonography of the lower extremities, option D, is the most appropriate next step.

CT angiography with bifemoral runoff, option A, is a test that is best used in critical limb ischemia or with moderate to severe claudication associated with peripheral arterial disease. CT pulmonary angiography, option B, is the test of choice when pulmonary embolism is suspected. MR venography, option C, is used to assess lower extremity veins and is often used to assess varicose veins or other venous insufficiencies. MR venography can be used to evaluate for deep venous thrombosis. However, this test is much more costly than venous duplex ultrasonography and is not as readily available. X-ray studies of the right lower extremity, option E, do not visualize vasculature and as a result, are not the test of choice. **Task:** B—Using Diagnostic and Laboratory Studies

12. **Answer: D** This patient with known cardiovascular disease is experiencing frequent symptoms consistent with bradyarrhythmia with intermittent episodes of tachycardia. Sinus bradycardia intermixed with episodes of tachyarrhythmia in the presence of coronary artery disease are characteristic of sick sinus syndrome, option D. Ambulatory cardiac monitoring will help confirm the diagnosis, and in this patient's case, permanent pacemaker placement is likely the eventual outcome.
An agonal rhythm, option A, is observed when resuscitation following cardiac arrest fails to establish a return of spontaneous circulation. Agonal is not an organized rhythm, thus P waves and narrow QRS complexes are absent. Complete heart block, option B, is also characterized by a pulse rate of around 40/min with narrow QRS complexes. On electrocardiography, P waves are present but are not functionally driving the QRS. Junctional bradycardia, option C, produces a pulse rate of around 40/min. However, since the impulse originates in the atrioventricular node, the characteristic feature of this rhythm disturbance is an absence of P waves. In this patient, every QRS is preceded by a P wave, thus eliminating junctional bradycardia as the correct answer. The Wenckebach phenomenon, option E, is characterized by a progressively elongating PR interval until a P wave fails to produce a QRS. This characteristic feature is not noted in electrocardiography of this patient. **Task:** C—Formulating Most Likely Diagnosis

13. **Answer: D** When presented with the sight of a toe after a nail removal, this patient experienced an episode of vasovagal syncope. Activation of cranial nerve X can occur in response to a stressful trigger, such as the unsightly toe. The resultant increase in parasympathetic tone (option D) to the heart induces a decrease in pulse and blood pressure, which can lead to syncope. Wolff-Parkinson-White syndrome and supraventricular tachycardia (SVT) are examples of atrioventricular node reentry phenomena, option A.

Hypocapnia (option B), or a decrease in the partial pressure of carbon dioxide ($PaCO_2$) dissolved in the blood, is commonly found in patients with anxiety or panic disorder. The tachypnea associated with these disorders blows off carbon dioxide resulting in a decrease in $PaCO_2$. A common presenting symptom is paresthesia in the circumoral area and in a glove-like pattern in the distal upper extremities. Syncope may certainly occur with both disorders but is not typically associated with a visual trigger. Increased afterload, option C, refers to an increase in pressure the ventricles must contract against to eject blood during systole. As aortic and pulmonary pressures increase, the afterload of the left and right ventricles increase, respectively. An uncinate fit, option E, is a type of temporal lobe epilepsy characterized by a prodrome consisting of taste and/or smell hallucinations. Chewing movements are also characteristic of psychomotor seizure activity. **Task:** E—Applying Basic Scientific Concepts

14. **Answer: D** Increased erythrocyte sedimentation rate (ESR), option D, is correct. With temporal arteritis, the ESR is increased due to the presence of cytokines and inflammation in the blood and arteries.
An elevated creatinine level, option A, indicates kidney injury. An elevated hemoglobin level, option B, is incorrect because temporal arteritis is associated with normocytic anemia rather than elevated hemoglobin levels. An elevated troponin level, option C, will indicate myocardial injury. An increased white blood cell count, option E, is incorrect. In contrast to patients with an infection, patients with temporal arteritis have a low-grade fever and a white blood cell count that is within normal limits. **Task:** B—Using Diagnostic and Laboratory Studies

15. **Answer: A** Non-STEMI is characterized by the presence of biomarkers indicative of myocardial injury in the absence of ST elevation on electrocardiography (ECG). The key difference from STEMI is myocardial ischemia in the absence of significant coronary obstruction, such as occurs with acute plaque rupture. The myocardial ischemia in this patient is due to a transient reduction in coronary blood flow that causes an imbalance in myocardial oxygen supply and demand, often with shortness of breath and decompensated heart failure. The ECG demonstrates nonspecific T-wave inversion or ST depression, and the key to diagnosis is the presence of circulating biomarkers (creatine kinase-MB, troponin I, troponin T) indicative of myocardial cellular necrosis. Leads II, III, and aVF correlate with the inferior wall of the heart, thus the answer is inferior wall non-STEMI, option A.
The other options (B through E) are incorrect because of the location of the infarction or the presence of

ST-segment elevation. **Task:** C—Formulating Most Likely Diagnosis

16. **Answer: D** This patient has the classic symptoms of torsades de pointes. Acute gastrointestinal losses of magnesium and potassium, coupled with chronic use of a selective serotonin reuptake inhibitor, lends itself to the development of this condition. Therefore, hypomagnesemia, option D, is the answer.
Electrocardiography of patients with hyperkalemia, option B, shows a classic tall T wave, which is not evident in the image provided. Hypercalcemia, hypernatremia, and hypophosphatemia, options A, C, and E, are not commonly associated with torsades de pointes. **Task:** B—Using Diagnostic and Laboratory Studies

17. **Answer: C** In utero, the ductus arteriosus directs blood from the pulmonary artery to the aorta and typically closes after birth to become the ligamentum arteriosum. Preterm infants and infants with a mother who had rubella while pregnant are at increased risk for the ductus arteriosus not closing. This results in a left-to-right shunt that may lead to congestive heart failure and pulmonary hypertension. Intravenous administration of nonsteroidal anti-inflammatory drugs (option C), such as ibuprofen or indomethacin, can be used to close it pharmacologically.
A course of intramedullary corticosteroids, option A, would have been appropriate to administer to the mother while pregnant. Women between 34 and 37 weeks' gestation who are at increased risk for preterm labor usually receive this therapy to help improve the infant's lung function. It is not appropriate to administer to this patient and will not help to close the PDA. Prostaglandin E1, option B, is inappropriate because it will keep the PDA open. This therapy is an appropriate treatment for coarctation of the aorta. Patch repair, option D, is an appropriate treatment option for a persistent ventricular septal defect. Surgical ligation, option E, is reserved for infants who have failed initial pharmacologic treatment with nonsteroidal anti-inflammatory drugs and have a persistent, hemodynamically significant PDA. **Task:** D2—Clinical Intervention

18. **Answer: C** This patient has acutely decompensated congestive heart failure with volume overload. The hypoxia is due to the volume overload, and treatment with diuretics is likely to be most effective. Therefore, initiation of furosemide therapy, option C, is correct. Digoxin, option A, has been shown to prevent hospitalization in patients with congestive heart failure, but it is not as important as furosemide at this time. Diphenhydramine, option B, is useful in treating allergic reactions but is not needed in this patient scenario. Propranolol and verapamil, options D and E, should not be initiated in this patient prior to

furosemide since the patient requires diuresis first to address volume overload. **Task:** D3—Pharmaceutical Therapeutics

19. **Answer: E** Thrombophlebitis, option E, usually occurs in the upper extremity due to the placement of an intravenous catheter. The inflammation of the vein causes a tender linear palpable cord, as in this patient. Cellulitis, option A, does not typically cause linear erythema. Typical findings of this condition include an enhancing area of erythema, warmth, edema, and tenderness at the site of infection. Erythema nodosum, option B, is characterized by tender red nodules and not linear erythema. In patients with lymphangitis, option C, lymph nodes associated with the infected lymphatic channels are often swollen, which is not true of thrombophlebitis. Panniculitis, option D, is characterized by tender erythematous subcutaneous nodules surrounding the intravenous site. **Task:** A—History Taking and Performing Physical Examination

20. **Answer: E** This question tests the examinee's ability to recognize that the arrhythmia on the electrocardiography shown is ventricular tachycardia, option E. Characteristics of ventricular tachycardia include rapid rhythm with wide-complex QRS complexes.
Option A, atrial flutter, is characterized by rapid P waves, or flutter waves, with a variable ventricular response. Option B, junctional escape rhythm, is a bradycardic rhythm characterized by narrow QRS complexes and the absence of P waves. Sick sinus syndrome, option C, is a bradycardic rhythm caused by dysfunction of the sinus node and is characterized by prolonged intervals or "pauses" between cardiac cycles. Option D, torsades de pointes, is a type of ventricular tachycardia that has a classic "twisted ribbon" appearance due to alternating amplitudes of R waves, which is not seen in the electrocardiogram shown. **Task:** C—Formulating Most Likely Diagnosis

21. **Answer: B** Option B, diffuse ST elevations in all leads except aVR and V_1, is the correct answer. The classic findings on electrocardiography (ECG) associated with pericarditis include diffuse ST elevation and PR depression, with PR elevation in lead aVR.
Convex ST elevations with reciprocal ST depressions in opposite leads, option A, is incorrect because this ECG finding is typical of acute myocardial infarction. $S_1Q_3T_3$ pattern with unexplained tachycardia, option C, is associated with pulmonary embolism. ST changes and new left bundle branch block, option D, is associated with ST-elevation myocardial infarction. ST depressions and T-wave inversions in the primary leads, option E, is incorrect because this ECG finding indicates cardiac ischemia. **Task:** B—Using Diagnostic and Laboratory Studies

22. **Answer: A** Although therapy with parenteral antihypertensive agents may be initiated in the emergency department, patients with a hypertensive emergency should be admitted to an ICU, option A, for continuous blood pressure monitoring, clinical surveillance, and continued parenteral administration of an appropriate agent.
Medical/Surgical units, option B, are not the best equipped to manage the care this patient will require. A standard neurology unit, option C, will not have the capabilities to care for this patient. A neurosurgery unit, option D, is not indicated, as this patient does not have any surgical indications at this time. Telemetry units, option E, typically observe cardiac patients, and this patient does not have a cardiac issue requiring monitoring. **Task:** E—Applying Basic Scientific Concepts

23. **Answer: E** Option E, paresthesia, is correct because limb viability depends on rapid revascularization in this setting. The loss of sensation to light touch is a late finding suggestive of significant ischemia with a poor prognosis.
Pulses that are absent to palpitation, option A, and even to Doppler do not specify the extent of ischemia. Options B and C, pain and pallor, are not specific enough indicators to gauge the extent of injury to determine the immediate necessity for revascularization of arterial ischemia. Paralysis, option D, often occurs prior to paresthesia. **Task:** A—History Taking and Performing Physical Examination

24. **Answer: A** Ventricular fibrillation is an irregular ventricular rhythm that contains no discernible QRS complexes, ST segments, or T waves. Patients who survive sudden cardiac arrest have an increased risk of recurrence. In the absence of reversible causes, such as an opioid overdose, insertion of an implantable cardioverter-defibrillator, option A, is recommended as primary prevention.
Long-term anticoagulation therapy with warfarin, option B, is used for treating atrial tachyarrhythmias such as atrial fibrillation and atrial flutter to prevent thromboembolism. It is not used to prevent the reoccurrence of ventricular fibrillation. Although serial electrocardiography, option C, evaluates conduction abnormalities related to ventricular fibrillation such as prolonged Q-T intervals or ST-T wave changes, this test is not beneficial in preventing the reoccurrence of ventricular fibrillation. Therapeutic hypothermia, option D, is used to help decrease the risk of brain injury following cardiac arrest rather than preventing the reoccurrence of ventricular fibrillation. Transcutaneous pacing, option E, is indicated for monitoring bradycardic arrhythmias such as heart block and is not indicated for the prevention of ventricular fibrillation. **Task:** D1—Health Maintenance, Patient Education, and Disease Prevention

25. **Answer: E** This question is asking the examinee to consider the differential diagnosis of chest pain. The cardiovascular risk factors of hypertension and hyperlipidemia make ischemic heart disease a possible diagnosis. Because the pattern of pain is predictable, is worse with exertion, and resolves with rest, the most likely diagnosis is stable angina, option E.
Acute coronary syndrome, option A, is characterized by acute chest pain and sometimes shows changes on electrocardiography. Because this patient is currently pain-free, this is not the most likely diagnosis. Costochondritis, option B, is caused by inflammation of the costochondral joints and is characterized by pain that is reproducible on palpation during physical examination. Pericarditis, option C, is inflammation of the pericardial sac and is often accompanied by fever, friction rub on examination, and diffuse ST-segment elevation on electrocardiography. Pulmonary embolism, option D, typically causes acute chest pain and dyspnea, which does not match this patient scenario. **Task:** C—Formulating Most Likely Diagnosis

26. **Answer: C** This patient has isolated hypertriglyceridemia and is healthy with no known cardiovascular risk factors. Patients with triglyceride levels greater than 885 mg/dL are at increased risk of pancreatitis. The decision to use drug therapy is based on the potential risk of atherosclerosis or pancreatitis. Fenofibrate, option C, is an appropriate initial treatment for this patient because it may lower triglycerides by up to 70% with continued lifestyle modifications.
Therapy with atorvastatin, option A, typically lowers triglycerides by 5% to 30% based on the dose. This medication would be a good alternative if the patient had cardiovascular risk factors. Cholestyramine, option B, is a bile acid resin that should be used with caution in adults 60 years of age or older. Icosapent ethyl, option D, is increasing in popularity based on the 2019 REDUCE-IT trial. However, this drug is recommended for use as adjunctive therapy to decrease the risk of cardiovascular events in adults with triglyceride levels greater than 150 mg/dL. Nicotinic acid, option E, decreases triglyceride levels by 15% to 25%; however, it is rarely used as monotherapy. **Task:** D3—Pharmaceutical Therapeutics

27. **Answer: D** Impending aortic aneurysm rupture, option D, is correct because of the patient's age, history of hypertension, and cocaine use. While hypertension is the major predisposing factor, the incidence of cocaine use in this patient is another predisposing factor. Furthermore, the differences between upper extremity blood pressure measurements are indicative of possible aortic dissection. Fifteen to 20% of aortic aneurysm dissections may present with transient cerebral ischemia. An aortic regurgitation murmur is common in patients with ascending aortic aneurysms.

Answer Key for this chapter begins on p. 23

Acute left atrial dissection, option A, is a rare complication of surgery. Chordae tendineae disruption, option B, presents with congestive heart failure and a murmur at the apex associated with a thrill. Patients with options C and E, chronic bacterial endocarditis and ventricular outflow tract obstruction, have significantly different clinical presentations and physical examination findings. **Task:** C—Formulating Most Likely Diagnosis

28. **Answer: B** Initiating therapy with a calcium channel blocker, option B, is the most appropriate treatment for this patient who has Prinzmetal angina, which is defined as chest pain with documented ST elevation in the setting of normal or near-normal angiography. Treatment of symptoms resulting from coronary artery vasospasm includes administration of nitroglycerin and therapy with calcium channel blockers. Initiating therapy with a beta-blocker, option A, is incorrect because beta-blockers may exacerbate coronary spasms in this patient. Option C, initiate therapy with a statin drug, is incorrect because this drug is used to treat coronary artery disease (CAD). The same is true of options D and E—percutaneous coronary intervention or revascularization are only warranted in patients with obstructive CAD. **Task:** D2—Clinical Intervention

29. **Answer: D** This patient has dilated cardiomyopathy, option D, which is a heterogeneous group of myocardial disorders characterized by ventricular dilation with reduced myocardial contractility. It is usually identified in the absence of coronary artery disease and is characterized by left ventricular dilatation as well as a left ventricular ejection fraction of 40% or less. Lyme disease is commonly linked to an infectious dilated cardiomyopathy, which is likely the cause in this patient. Common physical examination findings include tachypnea, tachycardia, jugular venous distention, positive hepatojugular reflux, laterally displaced apical impulse, peripheral edema, cool extremities, narrow pulse pressure, and ascites. Findings on auscultation include a loud S_3, presence of an S_3 gallop, and crackles or wheezes. Asthma and sarcoidosis, options A and E, are incorrect because these conditions are primary pulmonary processes, and this patient is experiencing cardiac abnormalities. Chagas disease, option B, is most commonly found in South America, Central America, and Mexico. This is a disease caused by a triatomine bug that transmits a parasite called *Trypanosoma cruzi*. Chronic congestive heart failure, option C, is incorrect because this patient is otherwise healthy, and her symptoms are acute. **Task:** A—History Taking and Performing Physical Examination

30. **Answer: E** Each of the options listed in this item are risk factors for abdominal aortic aneurysms. However, tobacco use, option E, as well as hypertension have the strongest correlation with the development of abdominal aneurysms. **Task:** D1—Health Maintenance, Patient Education, and Disease Prevention

31. **Answer: E** This patient has hypertrophic cardiomyopathy, which causes an enlarged left ventricle muscle, option E. Patients can be asymptomatic or present with several symptoms including chest pain, palpitations, fatigue, presyncope/syncope, and dyspnea. The physical examination can show no abnormalities, but a crescendo-decrescendo murmur that improves with squatting should increase suspicion of this disorder. Patients are at increased risk for sudden cardiac death, and providers should have a high index of suspicion for this condition on sports physical examinations. Symptoms of coarctation of the aorta, option A, include chest pain, cold extremities, claudication with activity, and decreased pulses and blood pressure in the lower extremities on examination. Patients with patent ductus arteriosus, option B, have shortness of breath and tire easily. A short systolic ejection murmur, signs of cyanosis, and clubbing on physical examination are typical findings. Mitral valve prolapse, option C, includes a nonejection click noted on auscultation and shows mitral valve regurgitation on echocardiography. Aortic stenosis is indicated by a systolic ejection murmur heard best at the base of the heart in the right intercostal space. The murmur radiates to the carotid arteries and will show thickened and calcified aortic leaflets, option D, on echocardiography. **Task:** B—Using Diagnostic and Laboratory Studies

32. **Answer: B** This patient is presenting with symptoms of cardiac tamponade, option B, which is noted by the widespread ST-segment elevation with low QRS voltage on electrocardiography. Acute myocardial infarction, option A, is incorrect. Although ST-segment elevation is indicative of cardiac injury, when it is widespread it is more likely to indicate pericarditis. Mediastinal tumor, option C, is not likely to cause acute onset of cardiac tamponade symptoms. Pulmonary thromboembolism, option D, is incorrect as well. Given this patient's symptoms of jugular venous distention and muffled heart sounds, the first concern should be that of cardiac tamponade. Tension pneumothorax, option E, is incorrect because the patient has full, clear breath sounds and has no signs of pneumothorax on chest x-ray study. **Task:** C—Formulating Most Likely Diagnosis

33. **Answer: C** For symptomatic atrioventricular (AV) block or high-grade AV block, such as second-degree type II AV block or third-degree heart block not caused by congenital AV block, permanent pacemaker placement, option C, is the treatment of choice. This patient had a syncopal episode because of AV block; therefore, a permanent pacemaker is indicated.

Option A, 24-hour ambulatory cardiac monitoring, will capture the arrhythmia, but the arrhythmia is already known as a third-degree heart block. Placement of a defibrillator, option B, is helpful when there is the presence of ventricular fibrillation or pulseless ventricular tachycardia. Replacement of the aortic or mitral valve, options D and E, will help to address electrical disassociation between the atria and ventricle. **Task:** D2—Clinical Intervention

34. **Answer: E** This patient has recorded an increased blood pressure on several occasions prior to being seen in the clinic. His age and history are suggestive of essential hypertension. Blood pressure measurements in the clinic confirm the increase, and since the patient already is exercising, eating properly, refrains from smoking, and rarely consumes alcoholic beverages, there is likely no benefit to further lifestyle modifications.

In many cases, hydrochlorothiazide (HCTZ), option C, is an excellent choice for initiating pharmacotherapy for essential hypertension. However, HCTZ has been shown to increase the incidence of exacerbations of gout. As a compelling contraindication, initiating pharmacotherapy with an angiotensin-converting enzyme inhibitor such as lisinopril, choice E, is preferred.

Use of an alpha$_2$-agonist such as clonidine, option A, or nitrates such as hydralazine and isosorbide dinitrate, options B and D, are not considered first- or second-line agents in the treatment of essential hypertension. **Task:** D3—Pharmaceutical Therapeutics

35. **Answer: D** A previously healthy young patient whose only symptom of an irregular heartbeat has been an occasional palpitation (skipping a single beat) and who consumes an above-average amount of caffeine is most likely to have the occurrence of single ectopic beats such as preventricular contractions, option D.

Atrial fibrillation, option A, provides a sustained irregular pattern and, because of the loss of atrial kick, should cause more severe systemic symptoms such as dizziness or weakness. Second-degree atrioventricular (Mobitz type I) block, option B, produces irregularity in the overall rhythm; however, the rhythm is sustained and is not likely in an otherwise healthy young patient. Sinus arrhythmia, option C, is a slight change in rhythm accompanying the change in intrathoracic pressure with breathing and does not usually have any associated symptoms. Ventricular tachycardia, option E, may be pulseless and is therefore associated with a sudden loss of consciousness. Ventricular tachycardia with a pulse still produces severe symptoms of weakness, chest pain, dizziness, or even shortness of breath and would not go unnoticed by the patient. **Task:** C—Formulating Most Likely Diagnosis

36. **Answer: C** Hyperpigmentation of the skin, option C, is correct because this finding is a common result of the venous insufficiency that causes varicose veins. Digital paresthesia, option A, is more often associated with diabetes mellitus. Elevated blood pressure, option B, is not the primary cause of varicose veins. Irregular distribution of hair on the legs, option D, is mostly related to arterial circulation. Option E, subungual dermatophytosis, is more common in patients with diabetes mellitus and is not related to venous insufficiency. **Task:** A—History Taking and Performing Physical Examination

37. **Answer: A** Based on this patient's presentation, infective endocarditis is suspected. Echocardiography, option A, is used to evaluate for abscess formation, leaflet damage, and pseudoaneurysm as well as signs of heart failure.

Electroencephalography, option B, is used to record brain activity and therefore is not useful in this situation. Electromyography, option C, is used to evaluate the firing of nerve and muscle tissue and is not useful in this patient's case. Electrophoresis, option D, employs adding an electric current to separate molecular particles within a gel. Therefore, it is not used in the initial evaluation of infective endocarditis. Endoscopic retrograde cholangiopancreatography, option E, is used to evaluate problems within the liver, pancreas, and bile/pancreatic ducts; therefore, this study is not helpful in the initial evaluation of suspected infective endocarditis. **Task:** B—Using Diagnostic and Laboratory Studies

38. **Answer: D** X-ray study of this patient shows a boot shape of the heart which results from right ventricular hypertrophy and is a common finding in tetralogy of Fallot (TOF), option D.

Aortic stenosis, option A, is rarely symptomatic in children less than 5 years of age, and echocardiography of a patient with aortic stenosis shows no defining characteristics of TOF. Chest x-ray study of a patient with patent ductus arteriosus, option B, shows prominent pulmonary vasculature but does not show the classic boot-shaped heart. Pulmonary atresia, option C, is incorrect because there are no audible murmurs heard in patients with this disorder. Chest x-ray study of a patient with ventricular septal defect, option E, is not likely to show the classic sign of a boot-shaped heart that is evident in this patient. **Task:** C—Formulating Most Likely Diagnosis

39. **Answer: A** Wellens syndrome includes a preinfarction state that occurs as a result of significant stenosis of the left anterior descending coronary artery, option A, due to rupture of an atherosclerotic plaque. Risk factors for Wellens syndrome include hypertension,

Answer Key for this chapter begins on p. 23

atherosclerosis, hyperlipidemia, obesity, and tobacco use. Patients with Wellens syndrome have symptoms consistent with acute coronary syndrome as well as a history of chest pain with activity that is relieved by rest. This patient has a history of chest pain, is currently pain-free, has findings on electrocardiography that show inverted T waves in leads V_2 and V_3, and has serum cardiac enzyme levels that are within normal limits. Based on these findings, he is at increased risk for a large acute anterior wall myocardial infarction. **Task:** E—Applying Basic Scientific Concepts

40. **Answer: D** Exercise stress testing, option D, is the most appropriate next step. This patient has a history of repair of a coarctation of the aorta, and exercise stress testing is necessary in order to clear this patient for participation in competitive sports.

Anterior and lateral chest x-ray studies, aortic angiography, arterial Doppler ultrasonography, and transesophageal echocardiography (options A, B, C, and E) are incorrect because these studies do not appropriately evaluate the cardiovascular response to exercise that is common in competitive sports. **Task:** D1—Health Maintenance, Patient Education, and Disease Prevention

41. **Answer: C** This question tests the examinee's understanding of systolic heart failure and cardiac diagnostic testing. Systolic heart failure, or heart failure with reduced ejection fraction, is characterized by left ventricular ejection fraction of less than 40% (option C).

Decreased pulmonary artery pressure, option A, is not associated with systolic heart failure. Fixed ischemic changes, option B, suggest a prior myocardial infarction but do not suggest systolic heart failure. Reversible ischemic changes in the cardiac apex, option D, are suggestive of cardiac ischemia and likely coronary artery disease that is amenable to potential intervention, such as balloon angioplasty or stenting. Ventricular bigeminy, option E, is an arrhythmia but does not support the diagnosis of systolic heart failure. **Task:** B—Using Diagnostic and Laboratory Studies

42. **Answer: E** This patient has extensive risk factors for cardiac ischemia, and his symptoms of episodic chest pain on exertion and at rest are most consistent with a diagnosis of unstable angina, option E. Dyspepsia, option A, is incorrect because this patient's symptoms and history are more consistent with a cardiac disease origin rather than a gastrointestinal one. Results of electrocardiography and cardiac enzyme tests do not show evidence of myocardial infarction or myocarditis, options B and C. Pulmonary embolism, option D, is unlikely considering this patient's overall presentation. Pulmonary embolism is more commonly associated with acute onset of chest pain and shortness of breath as well as electrocardiography showing right-sided heart strain with a prominent S wave in lead I and Q wave and inverted T wave in lead III. **Task:** C—Formulating Most Likely Diagnosis

43. **Answer: A** In 80% of patients, the inferior myocardium is supplied by the right coronary artery. Approximately 40% to 50% of all myocardial infarctions are inferior wall myocardial infarctions. Symptoms include chest pain, sweating, nausea, fatigue, and light-headedness. Bradycardia on physical examination could be indicative of a heart block. This patient has ST-segment elevation in leads II, III, and aVF, which indicates an inferior wall myocardial infarction. Therefore, cardiac catheterization, option A, is the most appropriate next step.

Option B, coronary artery bypass grafting (CABG), is preferred for high-risk patients with left main stem artery stenosis and severe three-vessel or diffuse disease. Option C, intravenous beta-blockers are indicated early in the course of patients with acute myocardial infarction, but according to the American Heart Association, they are contraindicated in patients with a heart rate of less than 60/min. The American Heart Association currently recommends the use of glycoprotein IIb/IIIa inhibitors, option D, in acute coronary syndrome when a patient arrives at a non-percutaneous coronary intervention (PCI) hospital and requires transport to a PCI-capable hospital for reperfusion. Nitroglycerin, option E, is a vasodilator that the American Heart Association does not recommend in patients with a heart rate of less than 50/min or greater than 100/min or a systolic blood pressure less than 90 mmHg. **Task:** D2—Clinical Intervention

44. **Answer: A** This patient has atrophie blanche, option A, which occurs in the cutaneous stage of chronic venous insufficiency (CVI) and is characterized by hypopigmented white patches with focal red punctate dots or telangiectasia surrounded by hyperpigmentation. At this stage, the skin is avascular and is at increased risk of ulceration.

Hyperpigmentation, option B, is characterized by dark staining of the skin without hypopigmented patches. The stage of CVI that includes lipodermatosclerosis, option C, presents as chronic, brawny induration of the skin and underlying fat, with the appearance of an inverted champagne bottle. Varicose eczema, option D, is an early sign of CVI and is characterized by red, scaling eczematous patches and plaques. Option E, vascular ulceration, occurs in the later stages of CVI and includes ulceration of the skin. **Task:** A—History Taking and Performing Physical Examination

45. **Answer: E** This patient has chest pain and shortness of breath after sustaining trauma. He is hypotensive, has jugular venous distention, and muffled heart

sounds. These three symptoms are referred to as the Beck triad, which is suggestive of cardiac tamponade. This diagnosis is further supported by pericardial effusion on ultrasonography and the presence of electrical alternans on electrocardiography. Because this patient is hemodynamically unstable with hypotension and tachycardia, emergent pericardiocentesis, option E, is the most appropriate initial management.

Chest tube insertion, option A, and needle decompression, option D, are interventions in the treatment of pneumothorax. This patient has clear lung sounds bilaterally, which makes pneumothorax an unlikely diagnosis. Option B, diagnostic peritoneal lavage, is used in patients suspected of having intraabdominal bleeding. This patient has a soft abdomen that is not tender to palpation, which makes intraabdominal bleeding an unlikely diagnosis. Also, the patient has a patent airway, therefore there is no clear indication for endotracheal intubation, option C. **Task:** D2—Clinical Intervention

46. **Answer: D** Initiate therapy with unfractionated heparin, option D, is the correct answer. The initial treatment of acute embolism/thrombosis is aimed at the prevention of extension of the thrombosis and providing hemodynamic stabilization. Initiating unfractionated heparin therapy will help to decrease clot formation and extension of the thrombosis. In this case, the INR is subtherapeutic, which increases this patient's risk for an embolism.

Initiate aspirin/dipyridamole therapy twice daily, option A, is a therapy regimen used primarily for the prevention of strokes. Initiating cilostazol therapy immediately, initiate a daily aspirin regimen, and initiate a trial of clopidogrel therapy (options B, C, and E), are incorrect. Although cilostazol, aspirin, and clopidogrel are used in the treatment of chronic peripheral vascular disease, these drugs are not sufficient to address the urgent need to decrease clot formation and extension of the thrombosis in this patient. **Task:** D3—Pharmaceutical Therapeutics

47. **Answer: D** This patient has persistent hypertension despite taking three agents to decrease his blood pressure. Such a scenario, especially with the patient developing this after 55 years of age, is suggestive of secondary hypertension. Note that all the options presented are indeed causes of secondary hypertension. However, the patient's presentation eliminates all but one choice. Renal artery stenosis, option D, is the correct answer because of the patient's age, history of hypercholesterolemia, presence of an abdominal bruit (present in 50% of cases), and mild hypokalemia due to activation of the renin-angiotensin system.

Coarctation of the aorta, option A, is incorrect because blood pressures in both arms are equal, and the ankle-brachial index is less than 1.0, which indicates that blood flow into the femoral arteries is not compromised. Hypercortisolism (option B), or Cushing syndrome, is not correct because this condition is usually accompanied by a host of general and specific symptoms, which this patient does not have. Pheochromocytoma, option C, is not a likely diagnosis because this patient is asymptomatic, and his age is older than the young- to middle-aged group in whom pheochromocytomas typically occur. Finally, a thyroid-stimulating hormone that is within normal limits eliminates the possibility of thyrotoxicosis (option E) as a diagnosis. **Task:** C—Formulating Most Likely Diagnosis

48. **Answer: A** This patient has thyrotoxicosis, which can be spontaneous or result from exogenous thyroid ingestion. This patient is at increased risk for thyrotoxicosis because she is taking liothyronine. Atrial fibrillation, option A, occurs in 9% to 22% of patients with thyrotoxicosis. Over half of patients with atrial fibrillation associated with thyroid disease will convert to normal sinus rhythm when the thyrotoxicosis is treated.

Long QT syndrome, option B, can be associated with various drug therapies, but it is not associated with thyroid hormone replacement. Symptoms associated may consist of syncope, palpations, and sudden cardiac death. Premature ventricular contractions (PVCs), option C, are a common occurrence. The incidence of PVCs increases with age, dehydration, electrolyte abnormalities, and chronic medical conditions. Ventricular tachycardia, option D, is not associated with thyroid disease. Wolff-Parkinson-White syndrome, option E, is a pre-excitation syndrome associated with an accessory pathway located in the bundle of Kent. **Task:** B—Using Diagnostic and Laboratory Studies

49. **Answer: A** Blood pressure measurement with the patient supine and then standing, option A, is the correct answer. This patient is most likely experiencing orthostatic hypotension related to his decreased activity and use of hydrochlorothiazide, a diuretic. History and physical examination findings are the most important components in evaluating a patient with syncope or near-syncope.

Echocardiography, option B, should be reserved for patients suspected of having structural heart disease. Electrocardiography, option C, should be performed after conducting a thorough physical examination of this patient, which includes testing for orthostatic hypotension. Exercise stress test, option D, is incorrect because this testing is recommended in patients with syncope or presyncope after physical exertion. Also, this patient has a sore knee and cannot participate in this type of test. Tilt-table testing, option E, is not performed unless the initial evaluation and diagnosis are unclear. **Task:** D2—Clinical Intervention

Answer Key for this chapter begins on p. 23

50. **Answer: D** The rhythm identified above in this patient is premature atrial contractions (PACs), option D, which are defined as early depolarizations of atrial tissue distinct from the sinus node. PACs are precursors to atrial fibrillation, which is the cause of stroke in this patient. The electrical impulse for a PAC originates from an area different than the sinus node. As a result, the P wave will often have a different morphology than a P wave originating from the sinus node.

    Atrial flutter, option A, is an irregular tachyarrhythmia that is identified by a sawtooth pattern on the telemetry strip. First-degree atrioventricular (AV) block, option B, is identified on the telemetry strip as a rhythm where every atrial impulse is conducted to the ventricles with the outcome of a regular ventricular rate. However, the PR interval exceeds 0.20 seconds. Paroxysmal supraventricular tachycardia, option C, is a group of rapid regular tachyarrhythmia that is broken down into three major categories of supraventricular tachycardia: atrial tachycardia, AV nodal reentrant tachycardia, and AV reentrant tachycardia. Right bundle branch block, option E, is defined as a conduction delay resulting from the right bundle branch of the electrical conduction system of the heart. It is not usually symptomatic and on rare occasion progresses to advanced AV block. **Task: C—Formulating Most Likely Diagnosis**

51. **Answer: C** The correct answer is echocardiography, option C, as this modality allows evaluation of the structure and function of the heart and determination of left ventricular ejection fraction.

    Chest x-ray study, option A, may suggest volume overload and cardiac enlargement but cannot differentiate systolic versus diastolic dysfunction. CT coronary angiography, option B, evaluates the structure of the coronary arteries to see if there is evidence of blockage, but it does not indicate ejection fraction. Electrocardiography, option D, is useful for evaluated heart rhythm, but it also does not evaluate ejection fraction, which is necessary for confirming diastolic heart failure. Exercise stress test, option E, is best used for the evaluation of potential coronary ischemia. **Task: B—Using Diagnostic and Laboratory Studies**

52. **Answer: A** This patient has a history and clinical presentation of an acutely symptomatic abdominal aortic aneurysm (AAA). Option A, aorta, is correct because the most significant risk factors for an abdominal aortic aneurysm are older age, male sex, history of cigarette smoking, and a family history of AAA. The clinical presentation of this condition also commonly includes constant pain in the midabdomen and back as well as a decrease in blood pressure.

    The acute presentations of conditions related to the colon, gallbladder, pancreas, and stomach (options B through E) do not commonly have this particular combination of risk factors and clinical presentation. **Task: A—History Taking and Performing Physical Examination**

53. **Answer: E** The most common genetic cause of arteriovenous malformation (AVM) is hereditary hemorrhagic telangiectasia, option E. The patient has a new-onset seizure thought to be secondary to a brain AVM diagnosed via MRI. She has a family history of seizures and strokes, both of which can be caused by AVMs.

    Alpha$_1$-antitrypsin deficiency, option A, is an inherited disorder that affects primarily the lungs and liver. Charcot-Marie-Tooth disease, option B, includes a spectrum of disorders that cause neurologic dysfunction. Option C, Fabry disease, is an inherited lysosomal storage disorder. Option D, familial adenomatous polyposis, is a genetic condition linked to the development of colorectal cancer. **Task: E—Applying Basic Scientific Concepts**

54. **Answer: C** Echocardiography of this patient is most likely to indicate that mitral regurgitation, option C, is the diagnosis. Mitral regurgitation is defined as the backflow of blood from the left ventricle to the left atrium during ventricular contraction. This valvular issue is often caused by structural or functional mitral valve abnormalities, of both acute and chronic pathologies. If left untreated, mitral regurgitation can lead to increased left atrial pressure, left ventricle dilation and dysfunction, and eventual left ventricle failure. This condition is diagnosed on physical examination findings on auscultation of the heart as well as echocardiography. The classic murmur heard on auscultation associated with mitral regurgitation is a blowing, high-pitched holosystolic murmur heard loudest at the apex and radiating to the axilla. Echocardiography is vitally important in establishing the diagnosis, cause, and hemodynamic severity of mitral regurgitation, as well as the impact on left ventricle size and function.

    Heart sounds for the other options are not detected on cardiac auscultation of this patient. Aortic regurgitation, option A, includes a soft, high-pitched early diastolic decrescendo murmur heard best with the patient sitting upright and leaning forward. Aortic stenosis, option B, is defined as a crescendo-decrescendo or systolic ejection murmur, heard loudest with a thrill in the aortic area and radiating toward the carotid arteries. Mitral stenosis, option D, includes an opening snap with a low-pitched early diastolic murmur heard best with the patient lying in the left lateral position over the apex. Tricuspid regurgitation, option E, is usually not heard and is best identified on echocardiography. When heard, it is described as a holosystolic murmur heard best at the left middle or lower sternal border with the patient sitting. **Task: C—Formulating Most Likely Diagnosis**

55. **Answer: B** Aortic stenosis, option B, is associated with the finding of pulsus et tardus parvus, or a slow-rising pulse, on cardiac auscultation. Aortic stenosis is the most common valvular heart disease associated with calcification and age. The murmur is a harsh systolic crescendo-decrescendo murmur heard best at the right upper sternal border with radiation to the carotid arteries. Aortic regurgitation, option A, is a blowing diastolic murmur heard best at Erb point. The murmur may be amplified by having the patient lean forward and exhale fully. Physical examination shows pulsus bifurans. Mitral regurgitation, option C, is a holosystolic murmur heard best at the apex with radiation to the back or axilla. Pulmonary regurgitation, option D, is a high-pitched early diastolic murmur heard best at the left upper sternal border that is amplified by deep inspiration. Pulmonary stenosis, option E, includes a harsh systolic murmur heard best at the left upper sternal border with radiation to the carotid arteries. **Task: A—History Taking and Performing Physical Examination**

56. **Answer: C** The findings on electrocardiography (ECG) of this patient are consistent with a left bundle branch block (LBBB), option C. The ECG of an LBBB typically shows a wide QRS complex ≥120 ms and a broad notched R wave in leads V_5 and/or V_6. A new LBBB in patients who are more than 45 years of age should be evaluated for cardiovascular disease. Patients with LBBBs have an increased incidence of coronary artery disease, left ventricular dysfunction, and heart failure.

An anterior wall myocardial infarction, option A, involves the left anterior descending artery. Typical ECG findings include ST elevation in leads V_1 through V_4. Inferior wall myocardial infarction, option B, usually involves the right coronary artery. ECG changes include ST elevations in the inferior leads of II, III, and aVF. For left ventricular hypertrophy, option D, findings on ECG consist of increased QRS voltage. Findings on ECG of a right bundle branch block, option E, include rSR pattern in leads V_1 or V_2 with an M shape in V_1 and V_2. **Task: C—Formulating Most Likely Diagnosis**

57. **Answer: A** This patient has paroxysmal supraventricular tachycardia (PSVT) and has failed mechanical treatment. Intravenous adenosine, option A, is the most appropriate first-line medication to administer to this patient because it has a very rapid onset and brief duration of action, though enough to block the electrical conduction through the AV node which effectively terminates PSVTs. It also has minimal negative ionotropic effects; therefore it will have a minimal effect on decreasing blood pressure.

Intravenous amiodarone, option B, is usually not required and not effective in converting PSVTs into normal sinus rhythm. Diltiazem and verapamil, options C and E, are calcium-channel blockers. Although they are effective in terminating PSVTs, these medications should be used with caution in a 72-year-old patient with a blood pressure of 100/64 mmHg. Intravenous metoprolol, option D, is a beta-blocker that has limited effectiveness in terminating PSVTs. Use of this drug may also lower the patient's blood pressure. **Task: D3—Pharmaceutical Therapeutics**

58. **Answer: B** This patient has symptoms suggestive of aortic dissection, option B. Such symptoms include chest pain that has a sudden onset, migratory pain, neurologic deficits or syncope, and decreased pulses. Aortic aneurysms, option A, usually include hypertension unless they rupture or dissect, as in this patient; they also do not include decreased pulses distally. Acute appendicitis, option C, includes periumbilical pain or pain in the right lower quadrant of the abdomen. Acute diverticulitis, option D, includes pain in the left lower abdomen. Myocardial infarction, option E, does not include decreased distal pulses. **Task: C—Formulating Most Likely Diagnosis**

59. **Answer: B** Examining the rhythm after performing carotid sinus massage, option B, will slow the ventricular rate of this patient. Slowing the ventricular rate will help unmask the characteristic sawtooth pattern associated with atrial flutter. Carotid massage is contraindicated in patients with a history of cerebrovascular disease or carotid bruits.

Examining the rhythm after the patient performs a Valsalva maneuver, option A, will accentuate murmurs associated with mitral valve prolapse and hypertrophic cardiomyopathy, not atrial flutter. Examining the rhythm with the patient in the squatting position, option C, will not accentuate atrial flutter but will accentuate most cardiac murmurs except mitral valve prolapse and hypertrophic cardiomyopathy. Examining the rhythm with the patient sitting up and leaning forward, option D, will accentuate aortic valve murmurs. Examining the rhythm with the patient supine in the left lateral position, option E, is known to accentuate mitral valve disorders. **Task: A—History Taking and Performing Physical Examination**

60. **Answer: A** This patient has an atrial septal defect, option A, which is the most prevalent congenital heart defect in adults. Patients with this defect have symptoms of arrhythmias or thromboembolic events. This patient, who is otherwise healthy, has no significant risk factors for ischemia or strokes such as hypertension, diabetes mellitus, hyperlipidemia, or a smoking history. The patient's medical history and physical

Answer Key for this chapter begins on p. 23

examination findings are consistent with an atrial septal defect.

Mild coarctation of the aorta in adults, option B, is usually associated with upper extremity hypertension, exertional headaches, epistaxis, and cramping of the legs. An adult patient with patent ductus arteriosus, option C, may have a continuous murmur heard at the upper left sternal border or symptoms of left heart overload such as palpitations and dyspnea. Pulmonary valve stenosis, option D, in an adult includes signs and symptoms that vary depending on the degree of obstruction. The patient with pulmonary valve stenosis can have a heart murmur, fatigue, dyspnea, exertional dyspnea, chest pain, or fainting. Ventricular septal defect, option E, diagnosed in late adolescence or adult life usually results in difficulty breathing, fatigue, and cyanosis secondary to the development of high pulmonary vascular resistance. **Task:** C—Formulating Most Likely Diagnosis

61. **Answer: E** This patient has symptoms of a blood clot, and a suspected loss of arterial blood flow to the lower extremity is an emergency. This patient requires urgent evaluation by arterial Doppler ultrasonography and consultation with vascular surgery, option E. If arterial embolism is confirmed, this patient will require emergent revascularization.

While calcium channel blockers, option A, can be used to treat vascular spasm associated with Raynaud disease, they are not indicated in the event of acute arterial occlusion. Ropinirole, option B, can be used to treat restless legs syndrome; however, this drug has no role in acute arterial occlusion. Since muscle tissue dies secondary to acute lack of blood supply, there can be an elevation in the creatine kinase and lactic acid levels with a possible subsequent effect on renal function. Awaiting results of these tests in an outpatient setting, option C, takes too long and is therefore inappropriate. Finally, the use of venous Doppler ultrasonography, option D, is the gold standard for the evaluation of arterial and venous flow within an extremity. However, in an outpatient setting, the results may not be returned to the provider in a timely fashion after being read by a radiologist. Emergent evaluation by Doppler is the appropriate initial step. **Task:** D2—Clinical Intervention

BIBLIOGRAPHY

Akhtar, S. (2018). Ischemic heart disease. In R. Hines & K. Marschall (Eds.), *Stoelting's anesthesia and coexisting disease* (7th ed., pp. 79-84). Philadelphia, PA: Elsevier, Inc.

Akhtar, S. Ischemic heart disease. Stoelting's anesthesia and co-existing disease, Chapter 5, 79-106.

Al-Assaf, O., Abdulghani, M., Musa, A., & AlJallaf, M. (2019). Wellen's syndrome: The life-threatening diagnosis. *Circulation*, *140*, 1851-1852.

Al-Khatib, S. M., Stevenson, W. G., Ackerman, M. J., Bryant, W. J., Callans, D. J., Curtis, A. B., et al. (2018). 2017 AHA/ACC/HRS guideline for management of patients with ventricular arrhythmias and the prevention of sudden cardiac death. *Journal of the American Academy of Cardiology*, *72*(14), e91-e220.

Alpert, J. S., & Klotz, S. A. Infective endocarditis. In: V. Fuster, R. A. Harrington, J. Narula & Z. J. Eapen (Eds.), *Hurst's the heart* (14th ed.). McGraw-Hill.

Ankel, F. K., & Stanfield, S. C. Aortic dissection. Rosen's emergency medicine: Concepts and clinical practice, Chapter 75, pp. 1021-1026.e1.

Baddour, L. M., Wilson, W. R., Bayer, A. S., Fowler, V. G., Jr, Tleyjeh, I. M., Rybak, M. J., et al. (2015). Infective endocarditis in adults: Diagnosis, antimicrobial therapy, and management of complications: A scientific statement for healthcare professionals from the American Heart Association. *Circulation*, *132*, 1435.

Bashore, T. M., Granger, C. B., Jackson, K. P., & Patel, M. R. (2021). Atrial flutter. In M. A. Papadakis, S. J. McPhee, & M. W. Rabow (Eds.), *Current medical diagnosis & treatment 2021*. New York, NY: McGraw-Hill.

Bashore, T. M., Granger, C. B., Jackson, K. P., & Patel, M. R. (2021). Ventricular fibrillation & sudden death. In M. A. Papadakis, S. J. McPhee, & M. W. Rabow (Eds.), *Current medical diagnosis & treatment 2021*. McGraw-Hill.

Bashore, T. M., Granger, C. B., Jackson, K. P. & Patel, M. R. Aortic stenosis. In: M. A. Papadakis, S. J. McPhee, & Rabow, M. W. (eds.) *Current medical diagnosis & treatment 2021*. McGraw-Hill.

Bashore, T. M., Granger, C. B., Jackson, K. P., & Patel, M. R. Paroxysmal supraventricular tachycardia (PSVT). In: M. A. Papadakis, S. J. McPhee, & M. W. Rabow (Eds.), *Current medical diagnosis & treatment 2021*. McGraw-Hill.

Bashore, T. M., Granger, C. B., Jackson, K. P., & Patel, M. R. PSVT due to accessory AV pathways (preexcitation syndromes). In: M. A. Papadakis, S. J. McPhee & M. W. Rabow. (Eds.), *Current medical diagnosis & treatment 2021*. McGraw-Hill.

Bashore, T. M., Granger, C. B., Jackson, K., P. & Patel, M. R. Syncope. In: M. A. Papadakis, S. J. McPhee, M. W. Rabow (Eds.), *Current medical diagnosis & treatment 2021*. McGraw-Hill.

Bern, C., & Montgomery, S. P. (2009). An estimate of the burden of Chagas disease in the United States. *Clinical Infectious Diseases*, *49*(5), e52-e54.

Bradley, E. A., & Zaidi, A. N. (2020). Atrial septal defect. *Cardiology Clinics*, *38*(3), 317-324.

Caforio, A. L., Tona, F., Bottaro, S., Vinci, A., Dequal, G., Daliento, L., et al. (2008). Clinical implications of anti-heart autoantibodies in myocarditis and dilated cardiomyopathy. *Autoimmunity*, *41*(1), 35-45.

Calkins, H., &; Zipes, D. P. (January 1, 2019) Braunwald's heart disease: A textbook of cardiovascular medicine. 11th Edition.

Cheitlin, M. D., Sokolow, M., & McIlroy, M. B. (1993). *Clinical cardiology* (6th ed.). Norwalk, CT: Appleton & Lange publishers.

Clinical overview. Tetralogy of Fallot. Elsevier Point of care. Updated August 9, 2019.

Conte, M., Pomposelli, F., Clair, D. G., Geraghty, P. J., McKinsey, J. F., Mills, J. L., et al. (2015). Society for Vascular Surgery practice guidelines for atherosclerotic occlusive disease of the lower extremities: Management of asymptomatic disease and claudication. *Journal of Vascular Surgery, 61,* 1-41S.

Cox, B. (2020). Congestive heart failure. *Conn's Current Therapy,* 114-117.

Creager, M. A., Kaufman, J. A., & Conte, M. S. (2012). Clinical practice. Acute limb ischemia. *The New England Journal of Medicine, 366,* 2198.

Creager, M. A., & Loscalzo, J. Chronic venous disease and lymphedema. In: J. Jameson, A. S. Fauci, D. L. Kasper, S. L. Hauser, D. L. Longo & J. Loscalzo (Eds.), *Harrison's principles of internal medicine* (20th ed.), McGraw-Hill.

Dalman, R. L., & Mell, M. (2020). Management of asymptomatic abdominal aortic aneurysm. In T. Post (Ed.), *UpToDate.* Waltham, MA: UpToDate.

d'Arcy, J. L., Coffey, S., Loudon, M. A., Kennedy, A., Pearson-Stuttard, J., Birks, J., et al. (2016). Large-scale community echocardiographic screening reveals a major burden of undiagnosed valvular heart disease in older people: The OxVALVE population cohort study. *European Heart Journal, 37*(47), 3515-3522.

Disorders of smell and taste. In: A. H. Ropper, M. A. Samuels, J. P. Klein & S. Prasad (Eds.), *Adams and Victor's principles of neurology* (11th ed.). McGraw-Hill.

Domino, F. J., Baldor, R. A., Golding, J., & Stephens, M. B. (2019). *The 5-minute clinical consult 2020.* Lippincott Williams & Wilkins.

Dubin, D. (2000). *Rapid interpretation of EKG's* (pp. 264-266). Tampa, FL: Cover Publishing Company.

Elefteriades, J., A., Olin, J. W., Halperin, J. L., & Ziganshin, B. A. Diseases of the aorta. In: V. Fuster, R. A. Harrington, J. Narula & Z. J. Eapen (Eds.), *Hurst's the heart* (14th ed.). McGraw-Hill.

Epocrates [online]. (2013). San Francisco, CA: Epocrates, Inc. http://www.epocrates.com. Updated continuously.

Ferri, F. (2021). Hypercholesterolemia. In F. Ferri (Ed.), *Ferri's Clinical Advisor 2021* (pp. 709-713). Philadelphia, PA: Elsevier, Inc.

Fort, F. G. (January 1, 2021). *Ferri's clinical advisor 2021.* 1141-1142.

Gasper, W. J., Iannuzzi, J. C., & Johnson, M. D. Abdominal aortic aneurysm. In: M. A. Papadakis, S. J. McPhee & M. W. Rabow (Eds.), *Current medical diagnosis & treatment 2021.* McGraw-Hill.

Gasper, W. J., Iannuzzi, J. C., & Johnson, M. D. Shock. In: M. A. Papadakis, S. J. McPhee & M. W. Rabow (Eds.), *Current medical diagnosis & treatment 2021.* McGraw-Hill.

Gasper, W. J., Iannuzzi, J. C., & Johnson, M. D. Varicose veins. In: M. A. Papadakis, S. J. McPhee, M. W. Rabow (Eds.), *Current medical diagnosis & treatment 2021.* McGraw-Hill.

Gasper, W. J., Rapp, J. H., & Johnson, M. D. Acute arterial occlusion of a limb. In: M. A. Papadakis, S. J. McPhee, M. W. Rabow (Eds.), *Current medical diagnosis and treatment 2020.* McGraw-Hill.

Gerhard-Herman, M. D., et al. (2017). 2016 AHA/ACC guideline on the management of patients with lower extremity peripheral artery disease: A report of the American College of Cardiology/American Heart Association Task Force on Clinical Practice Guidelines. *Circulation, 135*(12), e726-e779.

Giuliano, R. P., & Braunwald, E. (January 1, 2019). *Braunwald's heart disease: A textbook of cardiovascular medicine.* 60, 1181-1208.

Giuseppe, P. Postoperative management. *Rutherford's vascular surgery and endovascular therapy,* Chapter 34, pp. 424-440.e3.

Goldberger, A. L., Goldberger, Z. D., & Shvilkin, A. (2017). *Clinical electrocardiography: A simplified approach e-book.* Elsevier Health Sciences.

Grupke, S. L., & Fraser, J. F. (2021). AV malformations, cerebral. In F. Ferri (Ed.), *Ferri's clinical advisor 2021* (pp. 222-223). Philadelphia, PA: Elsevier, Inc.

Healthy patient. In: S. C. Stern, A. S. Cifu & D. Altkorn (Eds.), *Symptom to diagnosis: An evidence-based guide* (4th ed.), McGraw-Hill.

Jameson, J., Fauci, A. S., Kasper, D. L., Hauser, S. L., Longo, D. L., & Loscalzo, J. (Eds.). (2018). *Harrison's principles of internal medicine* (20th ed). McGraw-Hill.

John, R. M., & Stevenson, W. G. (2018). Polymorphic ventricular tachycardia and ventricular fibrillation. In J. Jameson, A. S. Fauci, D. L. Kasper, S. L. Hauser, D. L. Longo, & J. Loscalzo (Eds.), *Harrison's principles of internal medicine* (20th ed.). McGraw-Hill.

Jone, P., Kim, J. S., Alvensleben, J., & Burkett, D. Cardiovascular diseases. In: W. W. Jr. Hay, M. J. Levin, M. J. Abzug, & M. Bunik (Eds.), *Current diagnosis & treatment: Pediatrics* (25th ed). McGraw-Hill.

Jones, E. C., Devereux, R. B., Roman, M. J., Liu, J. E., Fishman, D., Lee, E. T., et al. (2001). Prevalence and correlates of mitral regurgitation in a population-based sample (the strong heart study). *The American Journal of Cardiology, 87*(3), 298-304.

Karchmer, A. W. Infective endocarditis. In: J. Jameson, A. S. Fauci, D. L. Kasper, S. L. Hauser, D. L. Longo & J. Loscalzo (Eds.), *Harrison's principles of internal medicine,* (20th ed). McGraw-Hill.

Kasper, D. L., Fauci, A. S., Hauser, S. L., Longo, D. L., Jameson, J., & Loscalzo, J. (2016). *Harrison's manual of medicine* (19th ed.). McGraw-Hill Education.

Khan, M. G. (Eds.). (2008) Bundle branch block. Rapid ECG interpretation. *Contemporary cardiology.* Humana Press.

Khan, R. (2021). Ventricular tachycardia. In F. Ferri (Ed.), *Ferri's clinical advisor 2021* (pp. 1447.e2-1447.e11). Philadelphia, PA: Elsevier, Inc.

Landenhed, M., Engstrom, G., & Smith, G. (2015). Risk profiles for aortic dissection and ruptured or surgically treated aneurysms: A prospective cohort study. *Journal of American Heart Association.*

Leavitt, A. D., & Minichiello, T. (2019). *Current medical diagnosis & treatment.* New York: McGraw-Hill.

Lindman, B. R., et al. (2019). Aortic valve disease. In D. P. Zipes (Ed.), *Braunwald's heart disease: A textbook of cardiovascular medicine* (11th ed., pp. 1389-1414). Philadelphia, PA: Elsevier.

Lopes, A., & Mesquita, S. (2014). Atrial septa defect in adults: Does repair always mean cure? *Arquivos Brasileiros de Cardiologia, 103*(6), 446-448.

Maisch, B., Noutsias, M., Ruppert, V., Richter, A., & Pankuweit, S. (2012). Cardiomyopathies: classification, diagnosis, and treatment. *Heart failure clinics, 8*(1), 53-78.

Maron, M. S. (2020). Hypertrophic cardiomyopathy: Clinical manifestations, diagnosis and evaluation. In T. Post (Ed.), *UpToDate.* Waltham, MA: UpToDate.

McPhee, S. J., & Papadakis, M. A. (2020). *Current medical diagnosis and treatment* (pp. 386-387). New York: McGraw Hill.

McPhee, S. J., & Papadakis, M. A. (2020). *Current Medical Diagnosis and Treatment* (pp. 340-342). New York: McGraw Hill.

National Institute for Health and Care Excellence: Peripheral arterial disease: Diagnosis and management. Clinical guideline (CG147). *Updated February* 2018.

Nayor, M., & Maron, B. A. (2014). Contemporary approach to paradoxical embolism (review). *Circulation, 129*(18), 1892-1897.

Nishimura, R. A., Otto, C. M., Bonow, R. O., Carabello, B. A., Erwin, J. P., 3rd, Guyton, R. A., et al. (2014). 2014 AHA/ACC guideline for the management of patients with valvular

Answer Key for this chapter begins on p. 23

heart disease: A report of the American College of Cardiology/ American Heart Association task force on practice guidelines. *Circulation, 129*(23), e521-e643.

Olgin, J. E., & Zipes, D. P. Bradyarrhythmias and atrioventricular block. Braunwald's heart disease: A textbook of cardiovascular medicine, 40, pp. 772-779.

Olgin, J. E., & Zipes, D. P. *Bradyarrhythmias and atrioventricular block.* Retrieved from: https://www.clinicalkey.com/#!/content/book/3-s2.0-B9780323463423000402?scrollTo=%23top.

Otto, C. M., & Bonow, R. O. (2015). Valvular heart disease. In D. L. Mann & Eugene Braunwald (Eds.), *Braunwald's heart disease: A textbook of cardiovascular medicine* (10th ed., pp. 1446-1523). Philadelphia, PA: Saunders.

Papadakis, M. A., McPhee, S. J., & Rabow, M. W. (2020). *Current medical diagnosis & treatment.* McGraw-Hill.

Papadakis, M. A., & McPhee, S. J. (2020). *Current medical diagnosis & treatment.* 355-357.

Phillips, J. B. (2020). Patent ductus arteriosus in preterm infants: Management. In T. Post (Ed.), *UpToDate.* Waltham, MA: UpToDate.

Pickett, C. (2021). Torsades de Pointes. *Ferri's Clinical Advisor,* 1372-1374.S2.

Rosenson, M. D., Robert S., Eckel, M. D., & Robert, H. Hypertriglyceridemia. *UpToDate.* October 2020.

Sarafidis P. A. & Bakris, G. L. Evaluation and treatment of hypertensive emergencies and urgencies. *Comprehensive Clinical Nephrology,* 37, pp. 444-452.e1.

Shah, S. N., Gangwani, M. K., & Oliver, T. I. (2021). Mitral valve prolapse. [Updated 2020 Nov 20]: *StatPearls [Internet].* Treasure Island (FL): StatPearls Publishing.

Society for Vascular Surgery Lower Extremity Guidelines Writing Group, Conte, M. A., Pomposelli, F. B., Clair, D. G., Geraghty, P. J., McKinsey, J. F., et al. (2015). Society for Vascular Surgery practice guidelines for atherosclerotic occlusive disease of the lower extremities: Management of asymptomatic disease and claudication. *Journal of Vascular Surgery, 61*(3 Suppl), 2S-41S.

Spodick, D. H. (2003). Acute cardiac tamponade. *The New England Journal of Medicine, 349,* 684.

Tritschler, T., Kraaijpoel, N., Le Gal, G., & Wells, P. S. (2018). Venous thromboembolism: Advances in diagnosis and treatment. *The Journal of the American Medical Association, 320*(15), 1583-1594.

Trivedi, V., & Kokkirala, A. (2021). Cardiac tamponade. In F. Ferri (Ed.), *Ferri's clinical advisor 2021* (pp. 298-299). Philadelphia, PA: Elsevier, Inc.

Vahdatpour, C., Collins, D., & Goldberg, S. (2019). Cardiogenic shock. *Journal of the American Heart Association, 8*(8). e011991.

Warner, M. J., & Tivakaran, V. S. (2020). *Inferior myocardial infarction (Updated 2020 Aug 8).* Treasure Island (FL): Stat Pearls Publishing.

Wells, P., & Anderson, D. (2013). The diagnosis and treatment of venous thromboembolism. *Hematology: the Education Program of the American Society of Hematology, 2013,* 457-463.

Yancy, C., Januzzi, J. L., Jr, Allen, L. A., Butler, J., Davis, L. L., Fonarow, G. C., et al. (2017). ACC expert consensus decision pathway for optimization of heart failure treatment: Answers to 10 pivotal issues about heart failure with reduced ejection fraction. *JACC, 71,* 201-230.

Yarnell, S., & Conroy, M. (2015). Cocaine abuse in the elderly. *The American Journal of Geriatric Psychiatry, 23*(3).

Yealy, D. M., & Kosowsky, J. M. (2018). Rosen's Emergency medicine: *Concepts and clinical practice.* Published January 1, 2018. pp. 929-958.e2.

Zile, M. (Ed.). Heart Failure with a preserved ejection fraction. *Braunwald's heart disease: A textbook of cardiovascular medicine, 26,* 523-542.e2.

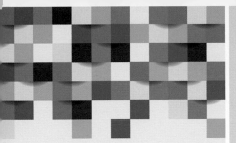

CHAPTER 2
Dermatologic System

Questions

1. A 32-year-old woman comes to the emergency department because she has had a rash on her face and trunk for the past two days. She says the rash started as red spots but now has developed into skin blisters; she feels feverish. The patient has never had a similar rash and has no history of using new bathing or cleaning products. Medical history includes no chronic disease conditions. Her only current medication is trimethoprim-sulfamethoxazole for treatment of a urinary tract infection. Temperature is 38.3°C (101.0°F), pulse rate is 110/min, respirations are 20/min, and blood pressure is 120/70 mmHg. Physical examination shows erythematous macules of various sizes, some of which are quite large, on the face and trunk. Ulcers are noted on the buccal mucosa. Flaccid blisters are noted on the trunk associated with large macules. Slight rubbing causes exfoliation of the outer layer of skin. Which of the following is the most likely diagnosis?
   A. Herpes simplex virus type 1 infection
   B. Rhus dermatitis
   C. Stevens-Johnson syndrome
   D. Urticaria
   E. Varicella-zoster virus

2. A 24-year-old man comes to the urgent care clinic because he has had intense pruritus and dry, cracking skin lesions on his elbows, knees, forehead, hands, neck, and feet for the past three weeks. He says he had a similar rash as a child, that was treated for years with a topical cream. Physical examination shows no signs of infection, and the lesions do not seem severe in nature. Which of the following is the most appropriate treatment?
   A. Acyclovir cream
   B. Calamine lotion
   C. Clobetasol cream
   D. Ketoconazole cream
   E. Oral cefalexin

3. A 69-year-old woman with a history of chronic obstructive pulmonary disease is transferred to an extended care facility after recovering from COVID-19. Transfer records show that she was on a ventilator for two weeks before she recovered. During the initial history and physical examination at the extended care facility, a shallow, open 2-mm ulcer is noted on the right heel. There are no signs of exposed subcutaneous fat, bone, tendon, or muscle. Based on this description, which of the following is the most likely stage of this ulcer?
   A. Stage 1
   B. Stage 2
   C. Stage 3
   D. Stage 4
   E. Unstageable

4. A 7-year-old girl is brought to the emergency department by her parents because she has had worsening pain in the left lower extremity that has recently become generalized, as well as muscle spasms during the past 12 hours. The patient has not had any recent changes in activities of daily living, and the parents say she played at an outdoor park yesterday, which is part of her routine. Vital signs are within normal limits. Physical examination shows a focal area of erythema and edema on the distal, left lateral leg. The site is markedly tender to palpation, and no necrosis is noted. Muscle rigidity is in the left lower extremity. Which of the following is the most likely cause?
   A. Black widow spider bite
   B. Brown recluse spider bite
   C. Scabies
   D. Scorpion sting
   E. Tick-borne illness

5. A 50-year-old woman comes to the dermatology clinic because she has had a lesion on her nose for the past four weeks. She says the lesion bleeds often and has not healed. The patient has worked as a landscaper for the past 30 years and uses topical sun-blocking agents intermittently. She has had a history of smoking one pack of cigarettes daily for the past 30 years. Physical examination shows a well-differentiated, pearly white dome-shaped papule located on the left side of the nose. Slight dimpling in the middle is noted, and the lesion is less than 5 mm in diameter. Which of the following is the most appropriate next step?
   A. Perform excisional biopsy with histopathology
   B. Recommend oral doxycycline therapy
   C. Recommend topical hydrocortisone cream
   D. Refer for radiation therapy
   E. Schedule follow-up in six months to monitor for growth of the lesion

6. A 36-year-old man comes to the clinic for routine physical examination. He says he has been healthy and has no concerns. He has no history of chronic disease conditions and takes no medications or over-the-counter supplements. Vital signs are within normal limits; physical examination shows a bright red, well-demarcated plaque with silvery scales. Psoriasis is suspected. In which of the following areas was this plaque most likely found?
   A. Posterior shoulder
   B. Lower abdomen
   C. Anterior knee
   D. Posterior calf
   E. Dorsal foot

7.

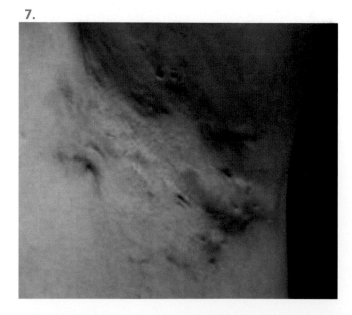

A 31-year-old woman comes to the office because she has had recurrent, painful nodular lesions in the axilla and groin regions for the past six months. She says she is self-conscious about her skin and wears long sleeves to cover her axillae. Body mass index is 33 kg/m² (N = 18.5–24.9 kg/m²). The patient has smoked one pack of cigarettes daily for the past five years. Findings on physical examination are shown. No other abnormalities are noted. Which of the following is the most likely diagnosis?
   A. Behçet disease
   B. Erythema nodosum
   C. Granuloma inguinale
   D. Hidradenitis suppurativa
   E. Prurigo nodularis

8. A 16-year-old girl comes to the clinic for routine well-child examination and says that she has had a rash on her forehead, cheeks, and chin for the past eight weeks. The rash does not itch and is not painful. She wears cosmetic products daily. The patient has no history of dietary changes, new medications, or hygiene products. Physical examination shows a few scattered comedones, pustules, and areas of hyperpigmentation on the face; no cystic lesions are noted. The remainder of the examination shows no abnormalities. Which of the following is the most appropriate initial treatment?
   A. Combined oral contraception
   B. Oral antibiotics
   C. Oral isotretinoin
   D. Topical retinoids
   E. Topical spironolactone

9. A 32-year-old man comes to the local urgent care because he has had worsening pain near his buttocks for the past week. He says his symptoms started with a boil in that area that began to bleed two days ago. The pain is most prominent with ambulation and sitting, which has hindered his ability to work. Two years ago, he had to miss work for a few days due to similar symptoms. He has not used any new cosmetic or hygiene products, but he says he sweats a lot due to having a lot of hair on his back. Medical history includes no chronic disease conditions, and he takes no medications. Temperature is 37.0°C (98.6°F), pulse rate is 86/min, respirations are 16/min, and blood pressure is 126/74 mmHg. Body mass index is 26 kg/m² (N = 18.5-24.9 kg/m²). Physical examination shows tenderness to palpation and foul-smelling purulent drainage immediately superior to the natal cleft. No edema or active bleeding is noted. Which of the following is the most appropriate next step?
   A. Bone scan of the sacrococcygeal area
   B. Incision and drainage
   C. Opioid prescription for pain management
   D. Routine consultation with a dermatologist
   E. Surgical excision

10.

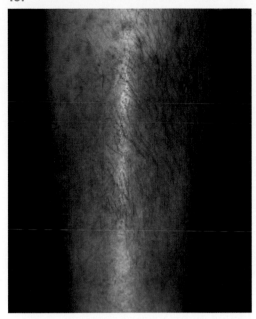

A 38-year-old man who works as a gardener comes to the office because he has had a rash on his right leg for the past three days. He says the rash began as a small patch and has been enlarging. It is now painful but not itchy. The patient has never had a similar rash and has no history of trauma to the leg. Medical history includes no chronic disease conditions. Temperature is 37.2°C (99.0°F), pulse rate is 90/min, and respirations are 16/min. On physical examination, the area is tender to palpation and warm to touch. The remainder of the skin is clear. A photograph of the rash is shown. Which of the following is the most likely diagnosis?

A. Cellulitis
B. Contact dermatitis
C. Erythema nodosum
D. Kaposi sarcoma
E. Sporotrichosis

11. A 31-year-old man comes to the office because he has had a worsening rash on his face over the past week. On physical examination, severe, greasy scales overlying erythematous patches are noted in the nasolabial folds. Similar greasy scales are noted on the eyebrows, eyelids, and scalp as well as the beard region. These findings most likely increase this patient's risk of having which of the following conditions?

A. Addison disease
B. Autoimmune thyroiditis
C. Dermatomyositis
D. HIV infection
E. Hypoparathyroidism

12. A 45-year-old man is brought to the emergency department by ambulance immediately after he sustained thermal burns to his upper torso, neck, and arms when his wife doused him with hot cooking oil after learning of his recent infidelity. His pulse rate is 100/min, respirations are 32/min, and blood pressure is 160/100 mmHg. Oxygen saturation is 96% on room air. On physical examination, the involved area is shiny, moist, erythematous, edematous, and extremely painful to touch. Scattered blisters are also present. Which of the following descriptions of this patient's burn is most consistent with these findings?

A. The burn extends deep to the subcutaneous layer
B. The burn is characterized as second degree
C. The burn is characterized as superficial
D. The burn is limited to the epidermal layer
E. The depth of the burn is characterized as full thickness

13.

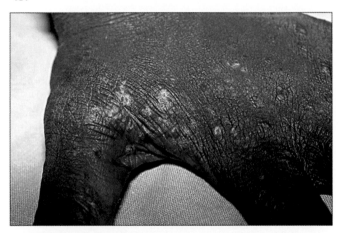

A 13-year-old boy is brought to the clinic because he has had an intensely pruritic rash on his left hand and fingers for the past three days. He attended a basketball camp in Maine last week and noticed the rash appearing the day after he arrived home. The lesions initially appeared on his wrist but quickly spread to other areas of his forearm and hand. He did not participate in any outdoor activities while at the camp. Vital signs are within normal limits. On physical examination, the rash is confined to the left hand and fingers, is raised, and is erythematous. Excoriation due to scratching is evident. No induration or heat is noted. A photograph of the rash is shown. Bites or infection from which of the following is most likely?

A. Chiggers
B. Cutaneous larva migrans
C. Fleas
D. *Pediculus humanus*
E. *Sarcoptes scabiei*

     Answer Key for this chapter begins on p. 43

14. A 21-year-old man who is otherwise healthy comes to the clinic because he has had fatigue, low-grade temperature, and myalgia for the past five days. He says that he woke up this morning with pain, burning, and itching around his penile shaft and anus and noticed a rash in this area. During the interview, the patient says that he has a new sexual partner, and he does not know the partner's status concerning sexually transmitted infections. Physical examination shows vesicles with surrounding erythema and central ulceration of the lesions on the penile shaft and external anus. Which of the following tests is the most appropriate initial step in diagnosis?
   A. Mineral oil preparation of a skin scraping
   B. Potassium hydroxide preparation of a skin scraping
   C. Rapid plasma reagin titer
   D. Tzanck test of an ulcer
   E. Urethral culture

15. A 45-year-old man comes to the office because he has had persistent facial redness with flushing for the past six months. He says he also has had an occasional burning sensation in his eyes. The patient has not had joint pain. Vital signs, including temperature, are within normal limits. Physical examination shows redness on the central portion of the face, forehead, and chin. In addition to pharmacologic treatment and avoidance of triggers that he knows to cause exacerbation of this condition, which of the following nondrug measures is most appropriate to include in the management plan?
   A. Applying sunscreen daily
   B. Eating a diet rich in green vegetables
   C. Initiating an aerobic exercise program
   D. Sleeping with the head elevated
   E. Using an alcohol-based facial cleanser

16. A 28-year-old man comes to the clinic because he has had a red, painful finger for the past two days. He has no history of trauma to the area but says he has a habit of biting his nails and pulling out his hangnails. On physical examination of the affected finger, the lateral nail fold is erythematous, edematous, tender to palpation, and fluctuant over a pus pocket. Which of the following is the most likely diagnosis?
   A. Cellulitis
   B. Felon
   C. Herpetic whitlow
   D. Paronychia
   E. Pyogenic granuloma

17. A 42-year-old man comes to the office because his right great toenail has been discolored and disfigured for the past six months. He is a runner and, for the past month, has had discomfort in the toe, which interferes with his ability to exercise. Medical history includes no chronic disease conditions, and he takes no medications. On physical examination, the nail is 75% yellowish in color and brittle. Subungual hyperkeratosis is noted. No erythema or edema of the surrounding skin is noted. If studies confirm the presence of a dermatophyte, which of the following is the most appropriate therapy?
   A. Oral griseofulvin
   B. Oral terbinafine
   C. Topical clotrimazole
   D. Topical miconazole

18. An 18-year-old woman comes to the office because she has had a mildly pruritic rash for the past two weeks. She says the rash started with an oval-shaped, salmon-colored lesion on her midback that then started to scale and clear in the center. One week later, similar appearing but smaller lesions appeared on her back. Physical examination shows oval-shaped lesions on the back in a triangle pattern. No other lesions are noted. Which of the following is the most likely diagnosis?
   A. Guttate psoriasis
   B. Nummular eczema
   C. Pityriasis rosea
   D. Secondary syphilis
   E. Tinea corporis

19. A 10-year-old girl is brought to the office by her mother because she has had a generalized rash for the past 24 hours. The mother says that the patient was recently diagnosed with streptococcal pharyngitis and had been taking penicillin for treatment. Physical examination shows generalized papules that are pruritic, raised, and erythematous. Based on these findings, it is most appropriate to tell the mother which of the following regarding the use of drug therapy in this patient in the future?
   A. Once the rash is treated, the patient may resume taking the course of penicillin
   B. The patient is likely allergic to all antibiotics, and use should be limited
   C. The patient may have an allergy to cephalosporins
   D. The patient should take diphenhydramine with the penicillin
   E. The patient's reaction to penicillin will decrease with future exposure

20.

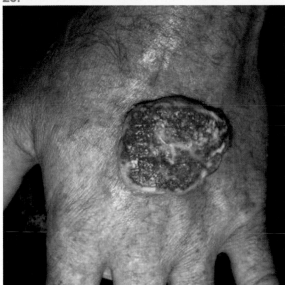

A 68-year-old man comes to the office because he has had a skin lesion on the back of his hand for the past month that does not seem to be healing. He says that he has had several lesions frozen off this area in the past, but this lesion seems different. Medical history includes nonmelanoma skin cancer. The patient golfs and fishes often and does not routinely use sunscreen. A photograph of the lesion is shown. Which of the following is the most appropriate immediate next step?

A. Perform a complete skin examination
B. Perform a shave biopsy of the lesion
C. Prescribe a high-potency corticosteroid cream
D. Refer to a dermatologist for Mohs micrographic surgery
E. Use liquid nitrogen for cryotherapy

21. A 20-year-old woman comes to the office because she has had lesions on her lower abdomen, thighs, and genitals for the past two weeks. The lesions are painless and have not changed in appearance during this time. She says she had sexual intercourse about one month ago with a new partner who had similar-appearing lesions. The patient has not been with this partner since then, and she has no history of using new hygiene products. Physical examination shows several 5-mm flesh-colored, dome-shaped papules with a central indentation. Which of the following is the most appropriate initial treatment?

A. Intramuscular penicillin G benzathine
B. Oral cephalexin
C. Topical liquid nitrogen
D. Topical miconazole
E. Topical triamcinolone cream

22. A 42-year-old man comes to the clinic because he has had a painless mass on his posterior left shoulder for the past two years. The patient says that his spouse told him that the mass has increased in size since onset. Physical examination shows a soft, superficial cutaneous mass that is 4.5 cm in diameter. There is no central punctum, and the skin is not warm to the touch. Which of the following is the most likely diagnosis?

A. Abscess
B. Basal cell carcinoma
C. Benign nevus
D. Epidermal inclusion cyst
E. Lipoma

23. A 16-year-old girl is brought to the office by her father because she has had a rash in her periumbilical region for the past four days. The patient says she recently pierced her navel at the local mall, and the itchy rash has since developed. Physical examination shows the presence of erythematous papules and plaques with sharp demarcation in the periumbilical area. Which of the following is the most likely diagnosis?

A. Contact dermatitis
B. Eczema
C. Psoriasis
D. Tinea corporis
E. Xerosis

24.

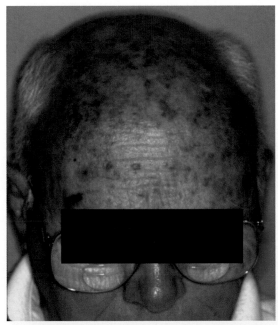

A 72-year-old man comes to the office because he has had spots on his scalp and forehead that have been increasing in number over the past year. He says the spots occasionally feel itchy, but he has no other symptoms. Physical examination of the lesions shows that some are flat and some are raised. A photograph is shown. Which of the following is the most appropriate initial topical treatment?

A. Fluorouracil
B. Metronidazole
C. Mupirocin
D. Terbinafine
E. Triamcinolone

 Answer Key for this chapter begins on p. 43

25. A 30-year-old woman comes to the office because she has had a mole on her right arm that has been increasing in size over the past month. She says that she has had this mole for many years, but over the past few weeks, it has increased in size and become more pigmented with color. On physical examination, a 4-mm nevus is noted with irregular borders and a brownish-pink color. Right axillary lymph nodes are palpable. Which of the following is the most appropriate next step in management?
    A. Cryosurgery of the lesion
    B. Excisional biopsy of the lesion
    C. Sentinel lymph node biopsy
    D. Shave biopsy of the lesion
    E. Wood light examination of a skin scraping

26. A 4-year-old boy is brought to the pediatrician's office by his mother because he has had patchy hair loss for the past two weeks. The mother says that she has tried using antidandruff shampoo, but it did not improve the symptoms. Physical examination shows well-demarcated scaly patches with the appearance of broken hairs above the skin. Potassium hydroxide preparation of a lesion scraping shows the presence of hyphae. Which of the following is the most likely diagnosis?
    A. Acne rosacea
    B. Atopic dermatitis
    C. Contact dermatitis
    D. Psoriasis
    E. Tinea capitis

27.

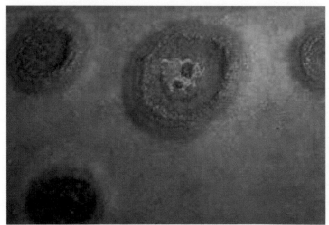

A 33-year-old man comes to the urgent care because he has had a rash on his hands, feet, palms, and soles for the past three days. He has been otherwise healthy and says his only recent medical issue included cold sores around his lips two weeks ago. The sores were fluid-filled and appeared in a cluster. Findings on physical examination of the patient's current rash are shown in the photograph. Which of the following is the most likely diagnosis?
    A. Erythema multiforme
    B. Pityriasis rosea
    C. Rhus dermatitis
    D. Scarlet fever
    E. Urticaria

28. A 3-year-old girl is brought to the office by her parents because she has had a rash on her face for the past three days. The parents say that the patient attends daycare, and multiple children have displayed similar symptoms. The patient appears well nourished, healthy, and playful. Physical examination shows clear conjunctiva with white sclera. Both tympanic membranes are pearly grey, and no erythema is noted. The uvula is midline, and no erythema, exudate, or tonsillar enlargement is noted. Examination of the face shows multiple honey-crusted lesions around both nares and the mouth. Which of the following is the most appropriate treatment?
    A. Hydrocortisone cream
    B. Ketoconazole cream
    C. Mupirocin ointment
    D. Oatmeal baths
    E. Oral amoxicillin

Answers

1. **Answer: C** The correct answer is Stevens-Johnson syndrome, option C, because this patient has an extensive rash that began as erythematous macules and then developed into blisters. She also has mucosal lesions, which is symptomatic of this syndrome. Exfoliating of the skin with rubbing (Nikolsky sign) supports this diagnosis, as does the recent use of a sulfa drug such as trimethoprim-sulfamethoxazole.

   Herpes simplex virus type 1 infection, option A, causes cold sores and blisters around the face and mouth. Rhus dermatitis, option B, is an allergic contact dermatitis that includes red, itchy bumps in a linear distribution with possible blistering. Urticaria, option D, causes pale red bumps and wheals on the skin. Varicella-zoster virus, option E, causes small, itchy blisters that scab over. **Task:** A—History Taking and Performing Physical Examination

2. **Answer: C** This patient has signs and symptoms of eczema, which is also known as atopic dermatitis. It is a chronic, relapsing inflammatory disease resulting in dysfunction of the skin barrier. It is characterized by xerosis, pruritus, erythema, erosions, oozing, and crusting. It can also be seen with other medical conditions such as food allergies, asthma, and allergic rhinitis. This diagnosis is made specifically based on patient history and physical examination. Treatment includes proper hygiene, hydration of the skin with moisturizers, and topical corticosteroids such as clobetasol, option C, in varying strengths depending on the location of eczema on the body and the degree of severity.

   Antiviral drugs such as acyclovir cream (option A), antifungal creams such as ketoconazole (option D), and antibiotics such as oral cephalexin (option E) are inappropriate for treating eczema, as this condition is not viral, fungal, or bacterial. Antipruritic drugs such as calamine lotion, option B, are not appropriate for treating the pruritis that is accompanied by eczema. Corticosteroids are the mainstay of treatment of atopic dermatitis. **Task:** D3—Pharmaceutical Therapeutics

3. **Answer: B** Stage 2 pressure ulcers, option B, include partial-thickness skin loss involving the epidermis and/or dermis. This type of pressure ulcer often occurs over bony prominences or parts of the body subjected to sustained localized pressure. On physical examination, findings include the presence of a shallow open ulcer or blister without the presence of exposed subcutaneous fat, bone, tendon, or muscle.

   Stage 1 ulcers, option A, are associated with non-blanchable erythema and intact skin. Stage 3 ulcers, option C, involve the presence of full-thickness skin loss but not through the fascia. Findings at this stage may show the presence of exposed subcutaneous fat, but bone, tendon, or muscle will remain nonexposed. Stage 4 pressure ulcers, option D, also involve the presence of full-thickness tissue loss, but there is associated exposed bone, tendon, or muscle. A pressure ulcer that is characterized as unstageable, option E, is usually covered by eschar, resulting in difficulty with staging. **Task:** A—History Taking and Performing Physical Examination

4. **Answer: A** The physical examination findings of generalized muscle pain, muscle spasms, and rigidity are characteristic symptoms of a black widow spider bite, option A.

   A brown recluse spider bite, option B, will progress rapidly to necrosis without rigidity. Scabies, option C, present severe itching with a rash commonly found on finger webs and wrist creases. Scorpion stings, option D, generally just cause localized pain. Tick-borne diseases, option E, such as Lyme disease, present with erythema migrans. **Task:** A—History Taking and Performing Physical Examination

5. **Answer: A** This patient has a lesion that is indicative of basal cell carcinoma, which is one of the most common skin malignancies. It is most commonly seen on sun-exposed skin, such as the head or neck, and rarely metastasizes. The usual reported history includes a skin lesion that does not heal within four weeks, has a dimpled midpoint, and grows slowly. Additional common characteristics of this lesion are that it bleeds occasionally or only when localized trauma occurs. The most common basal cell carcinoma is nodular basal cell carcinoma, a classification that includes a lesion described as a pearly white, dome-shaped papule with notable telangiectatic surface vessels. The gold standard for confirming this diagnosis is excisional biopsy with histopathology, option A.

   Recommend oral doxycycline therapy, option B, is incorrect because doxycycline is often used for severe cases of acne vulgaris and acne rosacea. Recommend topical hydrocortisone cream, option C, is used in low doses on the face for treatment of seborrheic dermatitis as well as contact dermatitis. Refer for radiation therapy, option D, is not correct as the current lesion has yet to be clearly identified. Radiation therapy is used in adjunct for known skin cancers that meet certain criteria. Schedule follow-up in six months to monitor for growth of the lesion, option E, is not correct since this patient has warning signs of basal cell carcinoma, including a long history of sun exposure, smoking history, and bleeding of the lesion. **Task:** D2—Clinical Intervention

6. **Answer: C** The most common locations for psoriasis are the knees, elbows, and scalp. Based on the options, the most appropriate location for this patient is on the anterior knee, option C. Options A, B, D, and E are not common locations for psoriasis. **Task:** A—History Taking and Performing Physical Examination

7. **Answer: D** This patient has hidradenitis suppurativa, option D. Patients with this disorder typically have painful nodules in the axilla or groin regions. It commonly affects people in the second or third decade of life who are overweight or who have obesity; cigarette smoking is a risk factor.
Behçet disease, option A, typically causes ulcerations of the mouth and genital areas. Patients with option B, erythema nodosum, have a rash typically seen on the shins and is self-limiting, usually resolving within three to six weeks. Granuloma inguinale, option C, is typically characterized by genital ulcers. Prurigo nodularis, option E, is characterized by pruritic nodules that typically appear on the extremities. **Task:** A—History Taking and Performing Physical Examination

8. **Answer: D** Topical retinoids, option D, are the treatment of choice for mild, primarily comedonal acne. This drug is also known to help prevent hyperpigmentation, which this patient also has.
Oral contraception pills, option A, and topical spironolactone, option E, are reasonable options to treat hormone-related acne in nonpregnant females; however, there is no evidence that the patient's acne flares around menses. Oral antibiotics, option B, are prescribed for moderate comedonal acne. Monotherapy with systemic antibiotics is not recommended due to the potential for developing resistance. Oral isotretinoin, option C, is used to treat severe cystic acne, which this patient does not have. **Task:** D3—Pharmaceutical Therapeutics

9. **Answer: E** This patient has pilonidal disease based on his history and physical examination. This condition occurs when a pilonidal sinus is formed by the forceful entry of hair into the natal cleft. The patient presents with pain and purulent drainage with a foul odor. It is recurrent and often found in males from 16 to 40 years of age. The treatment of choice is surgical excision, option E.
A bone scan of the sacrococcygeal area, option A, is not an appropriate next step in management because the diagnosis can be obtained via physical examination. Incision and drainage, option B, is only appropriate if a superficial abscess is present, but that is not the case with this patient. Opioid prescription for pain management, option C, will only treat this patient's pain and not the condition. Routine consultation with a dermatologist, option D, is not an appropriate treatment due to the active bleeding, drainage, and level of patient discomfort. Treatment should occur prior to a routine consultation. **Task:** D2—Clinical Intervention

10. **Answer: A** This patient has cellulitis, option A, because of the classic symptoms of erythema, spread, warmth, and tenderness to palpation.
Option B, contact dermatitis, also appears as an erythematous rash but is usually pruritic and often has associated vesicles. Erythema nodosum, option C, is a skin condition that appears on the anterior of the legs and is painful but consists of subcutaneous nodules 1 to 10 cm in diameter. Kaposi sarcoma, option D, appears as red or purple plaques or nodules and is associated with HIV infection. Sporotrichosis, option E, is a fungal skin infection that begins as a nodule and then ulcerates and reddens. **Task:** A—History Taking and Performing Physical Examination

11. **Answer: D** HIV infection, option D, is the correct answer. The new onset of severe generalized seborrheic dermatitis in this patient may be a marker for HIV infection regardless of age.
Addison disease, autoimmune thyroiditis, and hypoparathyroidism (options A, B, and E) are associated with vitiligo. Vitiligo is characterized by the presence of depigmented patches of the skin. Dermatomyositis, option C, is associated with the presence of a heliotrope rash. This rash typically consists of violaceous discoloration around the eyes and periorbital edema. **Task:** D1—Health Maintenance, Patient Education, and Disease Prevention

12. **Answer: B** The depth of a burn is categorized from first to the sixth degree. This patient's burn is characterized as a second-degree burn, option B. This type of burn involves the epidermis and dermis layers of the skin, and findings are similar to what is noted in this patient—shiny, moist, erythematous, edematous, and extremely painful to touch with scattered blisters. Second-degree burns are intensely painful and may take weeks to heal. While scarring may occur, the need for skin grafting is not necessary.
A first-degree burn results in erythema and edema of the epithelial layer only, is considered superficial in nature, and lacks blistering. First-degree burns, although painful to touch, are self-limited and typically resolve in a few days. Thus, options C and D are incorrect. A third-degree burn is considered a full-thickness burn, as it extends past the epidermis and dermis into the subcutaneous tissues. The affected area may appear black, brown, white, or yellow and is not painful to touch due to the destruction of sensory nerve endings. The description of this patient's burn is not consistent with a third-degree burn, which makes options A and E incorrect. Third-degree burns typically require skin grafting for proper closer and

healing. **Task:** A—History Taking and Performing Physical Examination

13. **Answer: E** The correct answer is *Sarcoptes scabiei* (scabies), option E. Scabies insects burrow into the superficial skin producing pimplelike lesions that are intensely pruritic. The pathognomonic characteristics of scabies include the appearance of more lesions over time and lesions located in the intertriginous areas between the fingers. Both of these characteristics are present in this patient.

    Chiggers, option A, are larval forms of the mite *Trombiculidae.* The larvae exist in outdoor vegetation and are able to attach to human skin, particularly around pant cuffs, shirt sleeves, and collars. Most bites occur in the axilla, groin, waistline, ankles, and behind the knees. This option is incorrect because there is no indication that this patient was outdoors, and the location of the bites is inconsistent with the patient's presentation. Cutaneous larva migrans, option B, is a skin infection caused by the larvae of various nematode parasites. Although most commonly encountered in tropical climates, infestation does occur in the southwestern United States. The larvae typically burrow into the skin via contact with bare feet and produce an erythematous and serpiginous eruption. This option is incorrect because the location of the camp was in Maine, the patient did not go outdoors, and the lesions are papular rather than serpiginous. Bites from fleas, option C, is a possibility. However, flea bites more commonly occur on the legs and around the ankles. *Pediculus humanus* (option D), or body lice (louse), is a parasitic insect infesting humans worldwide. Bites from lice may appear erythematous and papular but are not typically associated with the hand and intertriginous areas of the fingers. **Task:** A—History Taking and Performing Physical Examination

14. **Answer: D** This patient most likely has the herpes simplex virus based on his clinical history and the findings on physical examination. There are some tests that remain quite useful in the clinical diagnosis and treatment of this virus. Tzanck test of an ulcer, option D, is performed by scraping a fresh vesicular lesion or ulcer base, spreading and drying the collected material on a glass slide, staining the result with Giemsa formula, and examining the material with a microscope for the characteristic presence of multinucleated giant cells. It is an easy-to-perform, low-cost, and rapid office-based test that can allow for more immediate treatment.

    Mineral oil preparation of a skin scraping, option A, is incorrect since this test is specific for microscopic examination of scabies. Potassium hydroxide preparation of a skin scraping, option B, is incorrect since this test is primarily used to evaluate for candidiasis. Rapid plasma reagin titer, option C, is a test used for syphilis and is incorrect since findings on physical examination of this patient do not show a chancre consistent with syphilis infection. Urethral culture, option E, is incorrect since this test is used to screen for gonorrhea and chlamydia in male patients. **Task:** B—Using Diagnostic and Laboratory Studies

15. **Answer: A** This patient has rosacea. The correct answer is applying sunscreen daily, option A, because this will minimize rosacea flare-ups due to sun exposure.

    Eating a diet rich in green vegetables, option B, is incorrect because the only dietary intervention that has been shown to be helpful for some forms of rosacea is avoidance of alcoholic beverages. Initiating an aerobic exercise program, option C, is incorrect because this will cause flare-ups of rosacea due to vasodilatation. Sleeping with the head elevated, option D, is not known to have any effect on rosacea. Using an alcohol-based facial cleanser, option E, is incorrect because this will only irritate rosacea. **Task:** D1—Health Maintenance, Patient Education, and Disease Prevention

16. **Answer: D** Paronychia, option D, is an acute, painful inflammatory process occurring at the lateral fold of the nail that develops from an injury such as biting one's nails. In more severe cases, a pus pocket may develop at the site.

    Cellulitis, option A, is a superficial skin infection that is not painful to palpation. A felon, option B, is a subcutaneous infection occurring at the palm side of the fingertips in the digital pulp space. A herpetic whitlow, option C, is a vesicular lesion on a finger caused by the herpes virus. Ruptured blisters scab over. A pyogenic granuloma, option E, is a benign skin lesion commonly having a raw, minced, or ground beef appearance. Due to the proliferate vascular nature, these lesions tend to bleed easily. **Task:** A—History Taking and Performing Physical Examination

17. **Answer: B** Based on this patient's history and physical examination, he has a fungal infection of the toenail. The correct answer is oral terbinafine, option B, which can penetrate the nail and has shown success in treating fungal infections of the toenail.

    Oral griseofulvin, option A, is incorrect because onychomycosis does not respond to this drug, even though it is antifungal. Topical drugs such as clotrimazole and miconazole, options C and D, have limited value in treating toenail infections and would not be effective for treatment of a toe in which 75% of the nail is involved. **Task:** D3—Pharmaceutical Therapeutics

18. **Answer: C** This patient has the classic presentation of pityriasis rosea, option C, with an oval-shaped, salmon-colored herald patch followed by similar lesions spreading along the lines of cleavage on the back in a triangle or "Christmas tree" pattern. The rash will typically resolve on its own in four to six weeks.

    Answer Key for this chapter begins on p. 43

Guttate psoriasis, option A, will typically have small, erythematous papules and plaques with a drop-like appearance that affects the trunk and proximal extremities. Nummular eczema, option B, typically affects the legs and upper extremities and presents with extremely pruritic coin-shaped patches that start as dull red, exudative, and crusted but then become dry and scaly. Secondary syphilis, option D, typically includes a rash that involves the entire trunk and extremities, including the palms and soles. Tinea corporis, option E, will typically appear as an erythematous, pruritic, ring-shaped patch or plaque that spreads and then develops central clearing with an active advancing border. **Task:** A—History Taking and Performing Physical Examination

19. **Answer: C** It is most appropriate to tell the mother that the patient may have an allergy to cephalosporins, option C. Penicillin belongs to a class of antibacterial drugs called beta-lactam antibiotics that include cephalosporins. Patients who have an allergy to one type of penicillin may have an allergy to other types of penicillin and cephalosporins.
Once the rash is treated, the patient may resume taking the course of penicillin, option A, is incorrect. If there is a confirmed penicillin allergy, then the patient should be educated to avoid future exposure to beta-lactam antibiotics. Option B, the patient is likely allergic to all antibiotics, and use should be limited, is incorrect. If the patient has an allergic reaction to beta-lactam antibiotics such as penicillin and cephalosporins, then the patient should be educated to limit future use of only this class of antibiotics. Option D, the patient should take diphenhydramine with penicillin, is also incorrect. If there is a confirmed penicillin allergy, then the patient should avoid future exposure to beta-lactam antibiotics. The patient's reaction to penicillin will decrease with future exposure, option E, is incorrect. Future exposure to beta-lactam antibiotics will result in antibodies triggering a quicker response. Therefore, future exposure to beta-lactam antibiotics should be avoided. **Task:** D1—Health Maintenance, Patient Education, and Disease Prevention

20. **Answer: A** The lesion in this patient is suspicious of squamous cell carcinoma (SCC). The next step is to perform a complete skin examination to identify any additional lesions that may need evaluation and treatment. Therefore, the correct answer is option A.
A shave biopsy of the lesion, option B, can be used to diagnose SCC; if there is concern for invasive disease, it is recommended that the biopsy extend into the mid reticular dermis. However, the clinician should first perform a skin evaluation to determine if there are any other lesions that need to be biopsied as well. A high-potency corticosteroid cream, option C, does not have any role in the diagnosis or treatment of SCC.

Mohs micrographic surgery, option D, is a tissue-sparing procedure that is used in locations where excision with wide margins may cause cosmetic distress or loss of function, such as the face, hands, feet, and genitalia. This may be appropriate in the management of this patient due to the location of the lesion, but a complete skin examination must be performed first. Liquid nitrogen, option E, is most appropriate to treat skin conditions such as actinic keratosis; it is not an appropriate treatment for SCC. **Task:** D2—Clinical Intervention

21. **Answer: C** This patient has signs and symptoms of molluscum contagiosum. Lesions typically resolve without treatment within two months; however, in a sexually active patient with genital lesions, it is recommended that the lesions be treated to prevent spread. No large placebo-controlled trials have been done; however, cryotherapy, option C, is an accepted first-line treatment due to clinically evident response.
Intramuscular penicillin G benzathine, option A, is an appropriate treatment for primary syphilis. The lesions in this patient are not consistent with the classic chancre with a painless, 1- to 2-cm ulcer with a raised margin and nonexudative base, and she does not have regional lymphadenopathy. Oral antibiotics such as cephalexin, option B, are an appropriate treatment for secondary bacterial infection, but this patient does not have any pustules, purulent discharge, or crusting suggesting this diagnosis. Topical antifungals such as miconazole, option D, are appropriate for a fungal infection, but this patient does not have the itching and burning of a moist, red, beefy patch with satellite lesions consistent with this type of infection. Topical corticosteroids such as triamcinolone, option E, are an appropriate treatment for contact dermatitis, which this patient does not have. **Task:** D3—Pharmaceutical Therapeutics

22. **Answer: E** This patient has a lipoma, option E. Lipomas are benign, soft superficial or cutaneous masses that are typically less than 5 cm in size and grow slowly over time.
Development of an abscess, option A, is usually rapid, and the abscess is often tender to palpation with surrounding erythema, none of which are present in this patient. A basal cell carcinoma, option B, is described as a pearly white nodule. A benign nevus, option C, is a pigmented finding that is typically present since birth. Epidermal inclusion cysts, option D, are usually rounded, firm, and have a central punctum. **Task:** A—History Taking and Performing Physical Examination

23. **Answer: A** This patient's history and physical examination findings indicate that she has contact dermatitis, option A, which is associated with prior exposure to an irritating substance. In this case, the patient's reaction is likely due to nickel in the navel piercing.

With contact dermatitis, the shape, location, and pattern of the rash provide clues to the possible cause of the allergen.

Rashes associated with atopic dermatitis, or eczema (option B), are typically distributed over the flexural areas and less likely to be sharply delineated. Psoriasis, option C, is typically located on extensor skin surfaces and consists of demarcated salmon-colored plaques with a silvery scale. Lesions associated with tinea corporis, option D, are scaly, round, or oval plaques with a central clearing. Xerosis, option E, is a condition that occurs due to dry, rough, cracking skin, usually resulting from a lack of skin moisture or the aging process. **Task:** A—History Taking and Performing Physical Examination

24. **Answer: A** This patient has actinic keratosis, and the correct answer is option A, fluorouracil because this drug is the most appropriate first-line topical treatment for extensive actinic keratosis (AK). Fluorouracil is an antineoplastic drug and is effective in clearing AK lesions that can be precancerous. More isolated lesions would likely be treated with a nonpharmacologic therapy such as cryotherapy.

    Metronidazole, option B, is used to treat rosacea on the face. Option C, mupirocin, is used to treat lesions caused by bacteria such as impetigo. Terbinafine, option D, is used to treat fungal skin lesions such as tinea corporis. Finally, triamcinolone, option E, is a moderate-potency corticosteroid that is used to treat many skin rashes. It is ineffective for clearing actinic keratosis; however, it would likely decrease the itching. Triamcinolone is too potent a corticosteroid to apply initially to the scalp and forehead. A low-potency corticosteroid could be applied in combination with fluorouracil to relieve itching. **Task:** D3—Pharmaceutical Therapeutics

25. **Answer: B** This patient is suspected of having melanoma, and option B, excisional biopsy of the lesion, is correct. A full-thickness excisional biopsy is the gold standard for diagnosing melanoma. Any suspicious moles should be excised. Lesions associated with melanoma tend to have asymmetry, border irregularity, color variation, and diameter enlargement.

    Cryosurgery of the lesion, option A, is used to treat low-risk skin cancers such as basal cell carcinoma and squamous cell carcinoma after a biopsy has confirmed the diagnosis. Sentinel lymph node biopsy, option C, is done to evaluate for micrometastatic melanoma in regional lymph nodes. This procedure is used for staging once the diagnosis is confirmed via excisional biopsy. Shave biopsy of the lesion, option D, should be avoided when confirming the diagnosis of melanoma. Instead, a full-thickness excisional biopsy with 1- to 3-mm margins should be obtained. Wood light examination of a skin scraping, option E, is commonly used to diagnose fungal infections rather than melanoma. **Task:** D2—Clinical Intervention

26. **Answer: E** This patient has tinea capitis, option E, which is a dermatophyte infection commonly noted in children with the presence of well-demarcated scaly lesions and patchy alopecia. Diagnosis is confirmed by potassium hydroxide preparation showing the presence of hyphae.

    Acne rosacea and contact dermatitis, options A and C, are incorrect because neither of these conditions is associated with hair loss or the presence of hyphae. Atopic dermatitis, option B, frequently presents with elevated IgE levels and the presence of erythematous, scaling vesicles involving the flexure area of the body. This condition is not associated with the presence of hyphae. Psoriasis, option D, typically presents with silvery-white, scaly, circumscribed plaques affecting the extensor surfaces of the body. Similar to atopic dermatitis, this condition is not associated with the presence of hyphae. **Task:** C—Formulating Most Likely Diagnosis

27. **Answer: A** This patient has erythema multiforme (EM), option A, based on his history and physical examination. Herpes simplex is the most common cause of EM, and this patient had cold sores prior to development of the current skin lesions. The usual distribution of EM lesions is palms, soles, and extensor surfaces. The typical appearance consists of target lesions with three concentric rings of color change, which is evident in the photograph.

    Pityriasis rosea, option B, appears as an oval, fawn-colored, scaly eruption following the cleavage lines of the trunk. A herald patch precedes the eruption by one to two weeks. Rhus dermatitis, option C, is a contact dermatitis caused by the oil of plants such as poison oak or poison ivy and causes blisters often in a linear pattern. Scarlet fever, option D, is associated with streptococcal pharyngitis, and this patient has no history of this disorder. The rash of scarlet fever is generalized with punctate red lesions. Urticaria, option E, appears as wheals or hives, and pruritis is usually present. The appearance of these lesions may vary in duration from a period of minutes to hours. **Task:** A—History Taking and Performing Physical Examination

28. **Answer: C** This patient has signs and symptoms of impetigo, which is defined as a highly contagious infectious disease that affects the superficial epidermis. The diagnosis is determined by history and physical examination primarily, although localized wound cultures may assist with tailoring treatment if the condition does not improve with standard care. It is most common in children from two to five years of age, although it can occur in any age group. The most common organisms associated with this disease include *Staphylococcus aureus* and/or *Streptococcus pyogenes*. Topical mupirocin, option C, is the treatment of choice in patients with localized disease.

Hydrocortisone cream, option A, is used for seborrheic dermatitis, contact dermatitis, and other localized allergic responses. Ketoconazole cream, option B, is used to treat localized fungal infections, including tinea capitis, corporis, barbae, pedis, cruris, and versicolor. Oatmeal baths, option D, are used as an adjunct therapy for eczema and other irritant dermatitis.

Oral antibiotics such as amoxicillin (option E) can be considered, although oral antibiotics are typically only used for patients with extensive skin lesions or outbreaks associated with poststreptococcal glomerulonephritis, which is not the case with this patient. **Task:** D3—Pharmaceutical Therapeutics

BIBLIOGRAPHY

Bieber, T. (2010). Atopic dermatitis. *Annals of Dermatology, 22*(2), 125-137.

Brodell, R. T., & Helms, S. E. (1991). Office dermatologic testing: The scabies preparation. *American Family Physician, 44*, 505-558.

Cole, C., & Gazewood, J. (2007). Diagnosis and treatment of impetigo. *American Family Physician, 75*(6), 859-864.

Domino, F. J., Baldor, R. A., Golding, J., & Stephens, M. B. (2019). *The 5-minute Clinical Consult 2020*. Philadelphia: Lippincott Williams & Wilkins.

Eichenfield, L. F., Tom, W. L., Chamlin, S. L., Feldman, S. R., Hanifin, J. M., Simpson, E. L., et al. (2014). Diagnosis and assessment of atopic dermatitis. *Journal of the American Academy of Dermatology, 70*(2), 338-351.

Epocrates [online]. (2013). San Francisco, CA: Epocrates, Inc. http://www.epocrates.com. Updated continuously.

Fatahzadeh, M., & Schwartz, R. A. (2007). Human herpes simplex virus infections: epidemiology, pathogenesis, symptomatology, diagnosis, and management. *Journal of the American Academy of Dermatology, 57*, 737-763.

Ferri, F. F., DaSilva, M. F, Fort, G. G., Fricchione, G. L., Goldsmith, C. E., Kass, J. S., et al. (2021). *Ferri's Clinical Advisor 2021*. Philadelphia: Elsevier.

Ferri, F. F., Fort, G. G., Goldberg, R. J., Kass, J. S., Rafeq, S., Rathore, B., et al. (2020). *Ferri's Clinical Advisor*. 27-28.

Goldserin, A. O., & Goldstein, B. G. (2020). Pityriasis Rosea. In T. Post (Ed.), *UpToDate*. Waltham, MA: UpToDate.

Habif, T. B. (2020). Clinical dermatology: A color guide to diagnosis and therapy, 331-375.

Habif, T. P. (2015). *Clinical dermatology e-book*. Elsevier Health Sciences.

Hon, A., & Oakley, A. (1997) What is paronychia? (Gomez, J. updated 2017). *DermNet NZ*.

Hotzenecker, W., Prins, C., & French, L. E. (2018). *Dermatology*, 20; 332-347.

Isaacs, S. N. (2020). Molluscum contagiosum. In T. Post (Ed.), *UpToDate*. Waltham, MA: UpToDate.

Lawley, L. P., McCall, C. O., & Lawley, T. J. (2018). Eczema, psoriasis, cutaneous infections, acne, and other common skin disorders. In J. Jameson, A. S. Fauci, D. L. Kasper, S. L. Hauser, D. L. Longo, & J. Loscalzo (Eds.), *Harrison's principles of internal medicine* (20th ed.). New York: McGraw-Hill.

Leiter, U., Eigentler, T., & Garbe, C. (2014). Epidemiology of skin cancer. *Advances in Experimental Medicine and Biology, 810*, 120-140.

Lim, J. L., & Asgari, M. (2020). Cutaneous squamous cell carcinoma(cSCC): Clinical features and diagnosis: *UpToDate*. Waltham, MA: UpToDate.

Nazzal, M., Osman, M. F., Albeshri, H., Abbas, D. B., & Angel, C. A. (2019). Wound healing. In F. Brunicardi, D. K. Andersen, T. R. Billiar, D. L. Dunn, L. S. Kao, J. G. Hunter, J. B. Matthews, & R. E. Pollock (Eds.), *Schwartz's principles of surgery* (11th ed.). New York: McGraw-Hill.

NCCN: Basal Cell Skin Cancer. NCCN website. Version I.2017. Published October 3, 2016.

Niszczak, J., Forbes, L., & Serghiou, M. Burn rehabilitation, I. B. Maitin, & E. Cruz (Eds),. Current *diagnosis & treatment: Physical medicine & rehabilitation*. New York: McGraw-Hill.

Papadakis, M., McPhee, S., & Rabow, M. (2019). *Current Medical Diagnosis & Treatment 2020* (59th Ed.). Cenveo Publisher Services.

Papadakis, M. A., & McPhee, S. F. (2020). Current Medical Diagnosis & Treatment. 144-145.

Pilonidal Disease.

Smith, C. Infestations and bites. In: C. Soutor, & Hordinsky, M. K. (Eds.), *Clinical dermatology*. McGraw-Hill.

Stevens, D. L., Bisno, A. L., Chambers, H. F., Dellinger, E. P., Goldstein, E. J. C., Gorbach, S. L., et al. (2014). Infectious Diseases Society of America Practice guidelines for the diagnosis and management of skin and soft tissue infections: 2014 update by the Infectious Diseases Society of America [published correction appears in Clin Infect Dis. 60(9): 1448, 2015]. *Clinical Infectious Diseases, 59*(2), e10-e52.

Two, A. M., Wu, W., Gallo, R. L., & Hata, T. R. (2015). Rosacea: part II. Topical and systemic therapies in the treatment of rosacea. *Journal of the American Academy of Dermatology, 72*(5), 761-770.

Wilkison, B. D., Sperling, L. C., Spillane, A. P., & Meyerle, J. H. (2015). How to teach the potassium hydroxide preparation: a disappearing clinical art form. *Cutis, 96*, 109-112.

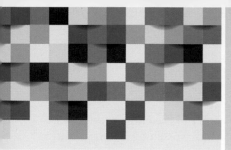

Questions

1. A 48-year-old man comes to the clinic for an annual health insurance physical examination. Medical history includes no chronic disease conditions. He says he has not been evaluated by a primary care physician for the past 20 years. Height is 5 ft 9 in, and weight is 289 lb. Pulse rate is 72/min, respirations are 16/min, and blood pressure is 172/98 mmHg. Oxygen saturation is 98%. Fasting laboratory findings of serum include the following:

Glucose	218 mg/dL (N = 80–110 mg/dL)
Total cholesterol	290 mg/dL (N = 100–199 mg/dL)
Low-density lipoprotein cholesterol	201 mg/dL (N = 0–99 mg/dL)
High-density lipoprotein cholesterol	36 mg/dL (N = >39 mg/dL)
Triglycerides	194 mg/dL (N = 0–149 mg/dL)

Which of the following findings is most likely to be included in the pathophysiology of this patient?
A. Decreased thyroid-stimulating hormone level
B. Hyperprolactinemia
C. Hypoinsulinemia
D. Insulin resistance
E. Pheochromocytoma

2. A 37-year-old woman comes to the office because she has had fullness at the base of her neck for the past six months. She has not had dysphagia, odynophagia, hoarseness, or dyspnea. Physical examination shows enlargement of the thyroid gland with a palpable nodule on the left. Serum thyroid-stimulating hormone and thyroxine levels are within normal limits. Ultrasonography of the thyroid gland shows a 2-cm hypoechoic, solid nodule in the left inferior lobe. Which of the following is the most appropriate next step?
A. Initiate levothyroxine therapy
B. Measure serum thyroglobulin level
C. Perform fine-needle aspiration biopsy of the nodule
D. Perform a thyroid uptake and scan
E. Refer for partial thyroidectomy

3. Type 1 diabetes mellitus commonly results from autoantibodies destroying which of the following types of islet pancreatic cells?
A. Acinar cells
B. Alpha cells
C. Beta cells
D. Delta cells
E. PP cells

4. A 30-year-old man comes to the clinic because he has had a headache for the past two months. He has not had nausea and vomiting or changes in vision. The patient says that he has had a recent change in his glove and shoe size. Physical examination shows enlargement of the jaw, a hollow-sounding voice, and a widened space between the front teeth. Initial measurement of which of the following laboratory values is most likely to determine the diagnosis?
A. Insulin-like growth factor
B. Growth hormone
C. Serum prolactin
D. Serum testosterone
E. Thyroid-stimulating hormone

5. A 72-year-old woman comes to the office for follow-up to discuss the results of a recent central DEXA scan. Her T-score is −2.8 (N = −1.0 and above). Current medications include oral calcium citrate, 1.2 g per day, and vitamin D, 800 IU per day. Adding a drug from which of the following classes of medications is most appropriate?
A. Bisphosphonates
B. Glucocorticoids
C. HMG-CoA reductase inhibitors
D. Proton pump inhibitors
E. Thiazolidinediones

6. A 45-year-old woman with Hashimoto thyroiditis comes to the family medicine clinic because she has had persistent chronic fatigue, hair loss, and decreased appetite for the past three months. Pulse rate is 80/min, and blood pressure is 120/78 mmHg; she is afebrile. On physical examination, there is no tenderness to palpation of the thyroid gland. The gland is diffusely enlarged with a rubbery texture; no palpable nodules are noted. Results of thyroid function tests of serum show decreased thyroxine level, decreased triiodothyronine level, and elevated thyroid-stimulating hormone level. Test for antithyroid peroxidase antibodies is positive. Based on these findings, this patient has an increased risk of developing which of the following malignancies?
   A. Anaplastic carcinoma
   B. Follicular carcinoma
   C. Medullary carcinoma
   D. Papillary carcinoma
   E. Sarcoma

7. A 38-year-old man comes to the outpatient clinic because he has had increased thirst and has been voiding large volumes of urine during the past four months. Medical history includes bipolar disorder. Temperature is 36.6°C (97.8°F), pulse rate is 80/min, respirations are 16/min, and blood pressure is 118/78 mmHg. Physical examination shows no abnormalities. Blood glucose level measured by finger stick is 100 mg/dL. Laboratory studies show serum sodium level of 150 mEq/L (N = 135–145 mEq/L), potassium level of 4.1 mEq/L (N = 3.5–4.5 mEq/L), and glucose level of 89 mg/dL (N = 82–105 mg/dL). Which of the following medications is most likely causing the symptoms in this patient?
   A. Bupropion
   B. Divalproex sodium
   C. Lithium carbonate
   D. Olanzapine
   E. Quetiapine

8. A 33-year-old woman comes to the office because she has had excessive tiredness, muscle weakness, dry skin, and weight gain over the past six months. She also says that her menstrual cycles have become irregular. Laboratory findings of serum include the following:

Thyroxine	2.0 μg/dL (N = 5.4–11.5 μg/dL)
Triiodothyronine, resin uptake	20% (N = 25–35%)
Free thyroxine index	1.0 (N = 1.5–3.8)
Thyroid-stimulating hormone	0.5 μU/mL (N = 0.45–4.5 μU/mL)

Which of the following is the most likely diagnosis?
   A. Hashimoto thyroiditis
   B. Infectious thyroiditis
   C. Pituitary hypothyroidism
   D. Primary hypothyroidism
   E. Riedel thyroiditis

9. A 35-year-old woman comes to the clinic because she has had fever, malaise, and worsening soreness and pain in the anterior neck over the past two days. She says that other than recovering from a summertime cold two weeks ago, she has been otherwise healthy all her life. Current medications include acetaminophen for treatment of fever. Temperature is 38.6°C (101.4°F), pulse rate is 104/min, respirations are 12/min, and blood pressure is 135/90 mmHg. Physical examination shows exquisite tenderness with palpation of both lobes of the thyroid gland up to the angle of the jaw. Which of the following findings is most likely on laboratory studies of serum?
   A. Decreased free thyroxine level
   B. Decreased total triiodothyronine level
   C. Elevated thyroid-stimulating hormone level
   D. Increased erythrocyte sedimentation rate
   E. Presence of thyroid antibodies

10. A 78-year-old woman is brought to the clinic by her daughter because she has struggled with memory loss and poor mentation for the past six months. The patient also has had fatigue, nausea, constipation, and polydipsia during this time. Medical history includes osteoporosis and kidney stones. Physical examination shows no abnormalities. Based on these findings, which of the following is the most likely diagnosis?
    A. Adrenocortical insufficiency
    B. Cushing syndrome
    C. Hyperparathyroidism
    D. Hypothyroidism
    E. Primary aldosteronism

11. Elevation of which of the following serum levels suggests the possibility of malignancy and occurs most often in patients with breast, lung, and renal cancer as well as multiple myeloma?
    A. Aldolase
    B. Bicarbonate
    C. Calcium
    D. Ferritin
    E. Lipase

Answer Key for this chapter begins on p. 55

12. A 74-year-old woman is being treated in the hospital because she had difficulty breathing as a result of small-cell lung cancer. Currently, the patient has increased oral intake, confusion, and decline in neurologic function. Pulse rate is 76/min, and blood pressure is 150/90 mmHg. During physical examination, the patient has a seizure and progresses into a coma. Laboratory findings include the following:

Serum

Calcium	9.2 mg/dL (N = 8.5–10.5 mg/dL)
Sodium	117 mEq/L (N = 135–145 mEq/L)
Potassium	4.2 mEq/L (N = 3.5–5.0 mEq/L)
Fasting glucose	98 mg/dL (N = 65–110 mg/dL)
Urea nitrogen	14 mg/dL (N = 10–20 mg/dL)

Urine

Urine	Hypertonic
Glucose	Negative
Ketones	Negative
24-Hour protein	136 mg/24 hr (N = <150 mg/24 hr)
Specific gravity	1.035 (N = 1.001–1.035)
pH	5.3 (N = 4.5–8.5)

Electrocardiography and echocardiography show no abnormalities. Which of the following is the most likely diagnosis?
A. Central diabetes insipidus
B. Diabetes mellitus
C. Nephrogenic diabetes insipidus
D. Psychogenic polydipsia
E. Syndrome of inappropriate antidiuretic hormone secretion (SIADH)

13. A 56-year-old man is being treated in the hospital after a recent myocardial infarction. Medical history includes type 2 diabetes mellitus, and current medications include metformin, atorvastatin, lisinopril, aspirin, and metoprolol. On laboratory studies, serum creatinine level and glomerular filtration rate are within normal limits, but hemoglobin A_{1c} is 8.5 mg/dL (N = 4–6 mg/dL). In addition to educating the patient about diet and lifestyle changes, the most appropriate next step to decrease the risk of mortality is initiation of therapy with which of the following?
A. Acarbose
B. Empagliflozin
C. Glyburide
D. NPH insulin
E. Pioglitazone

14. A 28-year-old woman with polycystic ovarian syndrome comes to the family medicine clinic to request a pregnancy test. She says she stopped breastfeeding her infant approximately six months ago but still has not had a menses. The patient says that she has gained weight, especially in her abdomen, has had swelling of the feet and legs, and has had fatigue during the past three months. The patient has mild obesity and a flat affect. Physical examination shows increased facial hair and comedones. Abdominal examination shows round protuberance with striae. Result of a pregnancy test is negative. Cushing syndrome is suspected. Which of the following studies is most likely to confirm this diagnosis?
A. Corticotropin-releasing hormone stimulation test
B. Late-night salivary cortisol test
C. Measurement of plasma adrenocorticotropic hormone
D. Measurement of plasma dehydroepiandrosterone-sulfate
E. Urinary 17-ketosteroids test

15. A 24-year-old woman comes to the family medicine clinic as a new patient for routine annual physical examination. Medical history includes hypoparathyroidism diagnosed at 18 years of age and primary adrenal insufficiency diagnosed at 20 years of age. Current physical examination shows no abnormalities. Based on current medical data, which of the following is the most likely etiology of the adrenal insufficiency in this patient?
A. HIV infection
B. Humoral and cell-mediated autoimmune involvement
C. Metastatic cancer
D. Tuberculosis
E. Typhoid fever

16. A 30-year-old woman who is at eight weeks' gestation comes to the clinic because she has had palpitations, easy fatigability, and excessive sweating for the past two months. Medical history includes no chronic disease conditions. Pulse rate is 110/min. Physical examination shows fine tremor in the hands. Laboratory studies of serum show decreased thyroid-stimulating hormone level and elevated free thyroxine level; result of thyroid-stimulating immunoglobulin test is positive. Results of complete metabolic panel and complete blood cell count are within normal limits. The most appropriate treatment for this patient includes therapy with which of the following?
A. Levothyroxine
B. Liothyronine
C. Methimazole
D. Propylthiouracil
E. Radioactive iodine

 Answer Key for this chapter begins on p. 55

17. A 45-year-old man comes to the office because he has had depression, decreased libido, and erectile dysfunction during the past year. He says he also has been exercising at the gym but has had minimal weight loss and/or increase in muscle mass during this time. Body mass index is greater than 30 kg/m^2 (N = 18.5–24.9 kg/m^2). Laboratory studies obtained on two separate mornings show total serum testosterone level of 243 ng/dL and 250 ng/dL (N = 280–1000 ng/dL). Results of all other laboratory studies are within normal limits. Which of the following findings, if present on further physical examination, is most likely to contraindicate the use of testosterone replacement therapy in this patient?
    A. Major depressive disorder
    B. Osteoporosis
    C. Prostate cancer
    D. Thyroid cancer
    E. Type 2 diabetes mellitus

18. A 16-year-old girl is brought to the pediatric office for follow-up of hyperparathyroidism. She also recently received a diagnosis of gastrinoma confirmed via esophagogastroduodenoscopy. Family medical history includes pituitary adenoma in a younger brother and adrenal adenomas in her mother. Vital signs are within normal limits. Physical examination shows no new abnormalities. Genetic testing for a mutation in which of the following proteins is most appropriate to recommend to this patient and her family members?
    A. Aspartoacylase
    B. Hexosaminidase A
    C. Menin
    D. Podocin
    E. Tumor protein p53

19. A 38-year-old woman has muscle spasms and tingling of her lips, hands, and feet 48 hours after undergoing complete thyroidectomy for treatment of papillary thyroid cancer. Which of the following laboratory abnormalities is most likely?
    A. Elevated serum parathyroid hormone level
    B. Hyperkalemia
    C. Hypermagnesemia
    D. Hypocalcemia
    E. Hypophosphatemia

20. A 42-year-old man with type 1 diabetes mellitus for the past 23 years comes to the outpatient clinic for routine examination and follow-up laboratory studies. He says he has no symptoms and feels well. Pulse rate is 64/min, respirations are 18/min, and blood pressure is 126/82 mmHg. The patient is alert and oriented. On physical examination, cardiac auscultation shows a regular rhythm. The lungs are clear to auscultation. The abdomen is soft and nontender to palpation. Diminished sensation is noted over the great toes, bilaterally. Result of microalbumin-to-creatinine ratio test is 45 mg/dL (N = <30 mg/dL). Which of the following medications is most appropriate to initiate at this time?
    A. Amlodipine
    B. Colchicine
    C. Lisinopril
    D. Metformin
    E. Metoprolol

21. A 34-year-old woman comes to the office because she has had weight gain, fatigue, and constipation over the past three months. Medical history includes an uncomplicated pregnancy and delivery six years ago; she takes no medications. Temperature is 36.6°C (97.9°F), pulse rate is 72/min, respirations are 16/min, and blood pressure is 116/78 mmHg. Physical examination shows loss of the lateral third of the eyebrows. Pupils are equal, round, and reactive to light and accommodation; no nystagmus is noted. Cardiac examination shows regular rhythm. The lungs are clear to auscultation. Moderate truncal obesity is noted. The abdomen is soft and nontender to palpation. Mild pretibial edema is noted. Based on these findings, which of the following laboratory results for serum thyroid-stimulating hormone (TSH), free thyroxine (T$_4$), and presence of antibodies are most likely if the etiology of this patient's symptoms is the thyroid gland itself?
    A. Decreased TSH; decreased T$_4$; elevated thyrotropin receptor antibody
    B. Decreased TSH; elevated T$_4$; elevated *Saccharomyces cerevisiae*, IgA
    C. Elevated TSH; decreased T$_4$; elevated antithyroid peroxidase antibody
    D. Elevated TSH; elevated T$_4$; elevated antithyroglobulin antibody
    E. Normal TSH; elevated T$_4$; elevated antibodies to deamidated gliadin peptide

22. A 63-year-old man is brought to the emergency department by his wife and daughter who say that he has had worsening confusion and lethargy and has been acting differently for the past 12 hours. Medical history includes hypertension, hypercholesterolemia, and type 2 diabetes mellitus. All conditions are well managed with lisinopril, simvastatin, and metformin. The patient also has advanced bronchogenic carcinoma for which he has been taking an oral chemotherapy agent for the past month. Vital signs are within normal limits. On physical examination, the patient appears to be in a stupor, and symptoms of neuromuscular hyperexcitability are noted. Results of laboratory studies include a serum sodium level of 112 mEq/L (N = 136–142 mEq/L) and decreased serum osmolality. Urinary sodium and osmolality are elevated. Which of the following is the most likely underlying etiology of this patient's condition?
    A. Diabetic ketoacidosis
    B. Hypercortisolism
    C. Multiple endocrine neoplasia type 1
    D. Primary hyperaldosteronism
    E. Syndrome of inappropriate antidiuretic hormone secretion (SIADH)

23. During routine physical examination of a 56-year-old woman, a solitary 1.5-cm nodule is noted in the left lobe of the thyroid gland. On follow-up laboratory studies, serum thyroid-stimulating hormone level, complete blood cell count, and complete metabolic panel are within normal limits. On ultrasonography, the lesion is round, thin-walled, and cystic with no mural component. Which of the following is the most appropriate next step?
    A. Monitor by routine physical examinations
    B. Obtain laboratory values for free thyroxine, free triiodothyronine, and triiodothyronine uptake
    C. Obtain a radionuclide thyroid scan
    D. Perform fine-needle aspiration biopsy
    E. Refer for lobectomy

24. A 21-year-old man has been in the ICU for the past three weeks being treated for a traumatic brain injury that he sustained when he fell out of the bed of a moving pickup truck. He has not regained consciousness since the incident and is on mechanical ventilation. Vital signs are within normal limits. During the past few days, the patient's urinary output has increased significantly. Laboratory studies show a serum sodium level of 148 mEq/L (N = 136–142 mEq/L), potassium level of 4.8 mEq/L (N = 3.5–5.0 mEq/L), and calcium level of 9.8 mEq/L (N = 8.2–10.2 mEq/L). Serum creatinine, urea nitrogen, and blood glucose levels are within normal limits. Serum osmolality is 310 mOsm/kg H_2O (N = 275–295 mOsm/kg H_2O), and urine osmolality is decreased. Which of the following is the most likely diagnosis?
    A. Diabetes insipidus
    B. Hyperosmolar nonketotic coma
    C. Myxedema coma
    D. Nephritic syndrome
    E. Syndrome of inappropriate antidiuretic hormone secretion (SIADH)

25. A 14-year-old girl is brought to the office because she has had hoarseness and the sensation of a lump in her throat when swallowing for the past three months. Medical history includes radiation of the head at 6 years of age. Family medical history does not include thyroid cancer. Physical examination shows a solitary, 3-cm, firm palpable thyroid nodule and enlarged cervical lymph nodes. Malignancy is suspected. Based on these findings, this patient most likely has which of the following types of carcinoma?
    A. Anaplastic
    B. Follicular
    C. Hürthle cell
    D. Medullary
    E. Papillary

26. A 72-year-old woman who is postmenopausal comes to the office to discuss the results of recent laboratory studies. The patient's serum calcium level is 12.5 mg/dL (N = 8.8–10.4 mg/dL), and serum phosphate level is 2 mg/dL (N = 3.0–4.5 mg/dL). A DEXA scan obtained one year ago showed a T-score of −2.5 (N = −1.0 or above, between −1.0 and −2.5 osteopenia, −2.5 osteoporosis). Which of the following is the most likely cause of the increase in this patient's calcium level?
    A. Breast cancer
    B. Familial hypocalciuric hypercalcemia
    C. Multiple myeloma
    D. Parathyroid adenoma
    E. Sarcoidosis

27. A 42-year-old man comes to the clinic for routine annual physical examination. Height is 6 ft, and weight is 250 lb. Pulse rate is 82/min, respirations are 16/min, and blood pressure is 124/82 mmHg. Other than mild obesity, physical examination shows no abnormalities. Laboratory studies show a fasting blood glucose level of 140 mg/dL (N = 80–110 mg/dL), and hemoglobin A_{1c} of 8.1 (N = <5.6%). Estimated glomerular filtration rate is within normal limits, and urinary albumin level is not detected. In addition to lifestyle modifications, which of the following is the most appropriate initial treatment?
    A. Desmopressin
    B. Insulin detemir
    C. Insulin regular human
    D. Metformin
    E. Metoprolol

28. A 43-year-old woman comes to the office because she has had irritability, unintentional weight loss, and episodes of light-headedness during the past month. Pulse rate is 110/min. On physical examination, heart rate and rhythm are regular. A smooth, tender enlargement of the anterior neck is noted. Laboratory studies show serum thyroid-stimulating hormone level of 0.01 µU/mL (N = 0.4–4.0 µU/mL), thyroxine level of 2.8 µg/dL (N = 0.9–2.3 µg/dL), and triiodothyronine level of 4.9 pg/mL (N = 2.3–4.2 pg/mL). Which of the following is the most likely cause?
    A. Euthyroid state
    B. Hyperparathyroidism
    C. Primary hypothyroidism
    D. Secondary hypothyroidism
    E. Thyrotoxicosis

29. A 52-year-old woman comes to the clinic because she has had numbness and tingling around her mouth and tingling in her hands and feet with severe cramping for the past six hours. Pulse rate is 68/min, respirations are 18/min, and blood pressure is 128/72 mmHg. Oxygen saturation is 99%. Medical history includes thyroidectomy two days ago. Physical examination shows a linear incision with sutures present on the anterior neck. Trousseau and Chvostek signs are positive. Which of the following findings on electrocardiography is most likely?
    A. Bundle branch block
    B. Complete heart block
    C. Peaked T waves
    D. QT prolongation
    E. ST-segment depression

Answers

1. **Answer: D** This patient is most likely to have insulin resistance, option D, on further testing. Considering the obesity, elevated blood glucose level, and hyperlipidemia, this patient is most likely resistant to organic insulin levels.

   A decreased thyroid-stimulating hormone level, option A, would indicate hyperthyroidism, and weight loss would be a symptom, which is unlikely in this patient given his current obesity. Hyperprolactinemia, option B, is incorrect because this condition normally will present in adult males with symptoms of decreased libido, impotence, gynecomastia, and/or galactorrhea. Hypoinsulinemia, option C, is incorrect. Based on this patient's age and body habitus, it is unlikely that he would have this condition. Pheochromocytoma, option E, is unlikely causing the obesity and hyperglycemia secondary to insulin resistance in this patient. **Task:** B—Using Diagnostic and Laboratory Studies

2. **Answer: C** The correct answer is C, perform fine-needle aspiration biopsy of the nodule. This is based on the American Thyroid Association's recommendations for diagnostic fine-needle aspiration of a thyroid nodule based on sonographic pattern. The 2-cm nodule on the left meets criteria by size and sonographic evidence.

   Initiate levothyroxine therapy, option A, is incorrect because this patient has normal laboratory findings, and suppression of the thyroid-stimulating hormone (TSH) with levothyroxine is not indicated unless there is a diagnosis of thyroid cancer. Option B, measure serum thyroglobulin level, is incorrect because measurement of serum thyroglobulin for initial evaluation of thyroid nodules is not recommended. Perform a thyroid uptake and scan, option D, is used when the TSH level is abnormally low. Benign and malignant nodules tend to be hypofunctional on thyroid scan; therefore, it does not differentiate the two. Refer for partial thyroidectomy, option E, is incorrect because there is no diagnosis of cancer or symptoms of compression indicating the need for surgical removal. **Task:** D2—Clinical Intervention

3. **Answer: C** Beta islet cells, option C, secrete insulin. Therefore, this type of cell is destroyed by autoantibodies in patients with type 1 diabetes mellitus.

   The remainder of the options are incorrect. Option A, acinar cells, is incorrect because this type of cell secretes digestive enzymes. Alpha cells, option B, secrete glucagon. Delta cells, option D, secrete somatostatin. PP cells, option E, secrete pancreatic polypeptide. **Task:** E—Applying Basic Scientific Concepts

4. **Answer: A** This patient most likely has acromegaly. Measurement of insulin-like growth factor level, option A, is the best screening test for acromegaly, since the level is elevated in patients with acromegaly. Due to the pulsatile nature of growth hormone, option B, a single random measurement of growth hormone is not useful for diagnosing acromegaly. Nonsuppressible growth hormone levels after a 100 g oral glucose load can assist in the diagnosis of acromegaly, but this would not be the best initial test. Serum prolactin, option C, is primarily used in the workup of patients suspected of having a pituitary tumor, specifically prolactinoma. Patients with prolactinoma are often asymptomatic but do not present with the symptoms described in this patient. Measurement of serum testosterone, option D, is useful in the diagnosis of hypogonadism. Testosterone is the principal male sex hormone produced by the Leydig cells of the testes. Measurement of thyroid-stimulating hormone level, option E, is used when diagnosing patients suspected of having hyperthyroidism or hypothyroidism. **Task:** B—Using Diagnostic and Laboratory Studies

5. **Answer: A** A T-score on a central DEXA scan of ≤ -2.5 is considered diagnostic for osteoporosis. The patient is already taking calcium and vitamin D supplementation at the correct doses. Adding a bisphosphonate, option A, to this regimen will inhibit bone resorption, augment bone density, and decrease fracture rate.

   Glucocorticoids, proton pump inhibitors, and thiazolidinediones (options B, D, and E) are drug classes that contribute to osteoporosis and the risk of fractures. While not contraindicated, none of these drug classes is indicated for the treatment of osteoporosis and would most likely contribute to worsening this patient's condition. HMG-CoA reductase inhibitors (i.e., statins), option C, are used in the treatment of hypercholesterolemia and would serve no purpose in addressing the osteoporosis in this patient. **Task:** D3—Pharmaceutical Therapeutics

6. **Answer: D** This patient has Hashimoto thyroiditis and is at risk for developing papillary thyroid carcinoma, option D, or thyroid lymphoma. Hashimoto thyroiditis is an autoimmune lymphocytic thyroiditis. It is the most common cause of hypothyroidism in women. The risk factors associated with an increased incidence of papillary thyroid carcinoma are Hashimoto thyroiditis and increased iodine intake.

   Anaplastic carcinoma, option A, is a rare form of thyroid cancer that occurs in 2% of patients with thyroid cancer and occurs in people over 60 years of age. The cause is unknown. Follicular carcinoma, option B, is the second most common type of thyroid carcinoma and is a well-differentiated thyroid cancer that occurs in patients between 40 and 60 years of age. Follicular carcinoma occurs more often in areas of the world where diets are low in iodine. Option C, medullary carcinoma, arises from the C cells in the thyroid gland that produce calcitonin and may be associated with a genetic predisposition to medullary carcinoma, familial medullary thyroid cancer, or as a part of the multiple endocrine neoplasia syndrome (MEN type 2A or 2B). Sarcomas, option E, represent less than 1% of all malignant tumors found in the thyroid gland. **Task**: C—Formulating Most Likely Diagnosis

7. **Answer: C** This patient has diabetes insipidus, and lithium carbonate, option C, is the medication most commonly known to cause this disorder.
Bupropion, divalproex sodium, and quetiapine (options A, B, and E) do not commonly cause diabetes insipidus. Olanzapine, option D, may lead to weight gain and hyperglycemia, which are not noted in this patient. **Task**: D3—Pharmaceutical Therapeutics

8. **Answer: C** The laboratory values of this patient indicate that she has a decreased thyroxine (T_4) level and a decreased free thyroxine index, which is most consistent with a diagnosis of hypothyroidism. Her thyroid-stimulating hormone (TSH) level is not elevated, which suggests a secondary cause of hypothyroidism or pituitary hypothyroidism, option C. Therefore, a thorough assessment and evaluation of the pituitary gland is indicated.
In Hashimoto thyroiditis, option A, the TSH level is elevated, and there would be increased circulating levels of antithyroperoxidase (90%) or antithyroglobulin (at least 40%) antibodies. In infectious thyroiditis, option B, the TSH level would be decreased and triiodothyronine (T_3) and T_4 would be increased. If this patient's TSH level were elevated and her T_4 level decreased, the most likely diagnosis would be primary hypothyroidism, option D. In Riedel thyroiditis (option E), also called invasive fibrous thyroiditis, the TSH level is decreased in 90% of cases, and antithyroperoxidase antibodies are present. **Task**: C—Formulating Most Likely Diagnosis

9. **Answer: D** Exquisite tenderness of the thyroid gland after a viral infection during the summertime in a female patient are all characteristics of subacute thyroiditis (de Quervain thyroiditis). Disruption of thyroid parenchymal cells resulting from this inflammatory disorder releases excess thyroid hormone into the circulation. The inflammatory nature of this self-limiting disorder results in a markedly increased erythrocyte sedimentation rate (ESR), option D, often above 100 mm/hr by the Westergren scale.

With the release of excess thyroid hormone into the circulation, free thyroxine (T_4) and total triiodothyronine (T_3) levels would be elevated and not decreased (options A and B). Through negative feedback inhibition, an elevation of T_3 and T_4 results in a suppression of thyroid-stimulating hormone (TSH) level rather than an elevation (option C). Thyroid antibodies are typically present in patients with Graves disease. However, the pathophysiology of subacute thyroiditis involves an inflammatory rather than an autoantibody process. Hence, thyroid-related antibodies are usually not present in subacute thyroiditis (option E). Although de Quervain thyroiditis mimics Graves disease, the thyroid tenderness on palpation, a decreased TSH, increased ESR, and an absence of thyroid-specific antibodies focus the diagnosis on subacute thyroiditis. **Task**: B—Using Diagnostic and Laboratory Studies

10. **Answer: C** The symptoms of hyperparathyroidism, option C, are classically summarized as "stones, bones, abdominal groans, thrones, and psychiatric overtones." This patient has kidney stones, osteoporosis, nausea, constipation, and poor mentation with memory loss, all of which fit into the criteria for this disorder.
Adrenocortical insufficiency, option A, is incorrect because patients with this disorder generally present with extreme fatigue, weight loss, and decreased blood pressure. Patients with Cushing syndrome, option B, typically have weight gain and new onset or worsening diabetes mellitus. Patients with hypothyroidism, option D, generally have weight gain, constipation, and cold intolerance. Primary aldosteronism, option E, includes symptoms such as high blood pressure, muscle cramps, headache, and excessive thirst. **Task**: A—History Taking and Performing Physical Examination

11. **Answer: C** The correct answer is calcium, option C. The differential for hypercalcemia includes malignancy, as the hypercalcemia of malignancy is one of the most common endocrine paraneoplastic syndromes, occurring in up to 10% of all patients with advanced tumors.
Aldolase, option A, is elevated in muscle disease. Bicarbonate, option B, is elevated in electrolyte disorders and acid–base imbalance. Ferritin, option D, is a marker of the body's iron stores. Lipase, option E, is elevated in pancreatic disease; although it can be elevated in pancreatic cancer, it is more commonly elevated in nonmalignant pancreatic disease. Lipase is not elevated in other cancers. **Task**: B—Using Diagnostic and Laboratory Studies

12. **Answer: E** This patient has symptoms and laboratory findings that are consistent with increased amounts of antidiuretic hormone; therefore, syndrome of inappropriate antidiuretic hormone secretion (SIADH),

option E, is correct. ADH is secreted by the pituitary gland and works on the collecting tubules of the kidney to conserve water. In this patient's case, the increased production is caused by small-cell carcinoma of the lung. This syndrome is characterized by hyponatremia, hypoosmolality, and urine osmolality greater than 100 mOsm/kg H_2O. Urine sodium concentration is usually greater than 40 mEq/L. Hyponatremia can cause central nervous system symptoms such as obtundation, seizure, and coma.

Central diabetes insipidus, option A, is characterized by a deficiency in ADH from the pituitary gland. Because of the lack of adrenal function, there is an inability of the kidney to concentrate the urine, which results in a large output of dilute urine and tends to cause hypernatremia, not hyponatremia. Diabetes mellitus, option B, is caused by an absolute or relative insulin deficiency. Symptoms include polyuria, polydipsia, elevated blood glucose level, glucosuria, and the presence of ketones in the urine. Nephrogenic diabetes insipidus, option C, is characterized by an impaired response of the kidney to ADH. This results in a large output of dilute urine. Symptoms include polyuria, polydipsia, and hypernatremia. Nocturia can be a symptom. Psychogenic polydipsia, option D, is a psychological condition in which a patient drinks excessive amounts of water. There is polyuria due to this large water intake, but nocturia is usually absent with psychogenic polydipsia. **Task**: C—Formulating Most Likely Diagnosis

13. **Answer: B** This patient has established cardiovascular disease; therefore, a sodium–glucose cotransporter-2 inhibitor such as empagliflozin, option B, is most appropriate to decrease his risk for mortality. Empagliflozin has been studied and proven to lower cardiovascular risk in patients with type 2 diabetes mellitus and carries an FDA indication for this.

Acarbose, glyburide, NPH insulin, and pioglitazone (options A, C, D, and E) may be used for diabetic management, but they have not been shown to decrease mortality rates in patients with established cardiovascular disease. **Task**: D3—Pharmaceutical Therapeutics

14. **Answer: B** This patient has central obesity, moon face, protuberant abdomen, and amenorrhea, which are all manifestations of Cushing syndrome. The most appropriate study to confirm this diagnosis is late-night salivary cortisol test, option B. Other possible tests include overnight dexamethasone suppression test, low-dose dexamethasone depression test, sleeping midnight serum cortisol, and urinary free cortisol. However, late-night salivary cortisol tests are particularly useful for adrenocorticotropic hormone (ACTH)-dependent hypercortisolism and have a relatively high sensitivity and specificity for Cushing syndrome. Once Cushing syndrome is confirmed, then plasma ACTH and dehydroepiandrosterone-sulfate, options C and D, are used to determine the cause of the excess cortisol.

Option A, corticotropin-releasing hormone stimulation test, is a second-line test used to determine the anatomical cause of hypercortisolism and is not used as a first-line test to diagnose hypercortisolism. Urinary 17-ketosteroids, option E, are byproducts of ketosteroid metabolism of the male and female sex hormones and other hormones released by the adrenal glands. An elevation of urinary 17-ketosteroids is not specific for Cushing syndrome and can be increased in adrenal gland problems, testicular cancer, ovarian cancer, and polycystic ovarian syndrome. **Task**: B—Using Diagnostic and Laboratory Studies

15. **Answer: B** The correct answer is humoral and cell-mediated autoimmune involvement, option B. Based on recent data, the most likely cause of the primary adrenal insufficiency in this patient is autoimmune destruction. When first described by Dr. Thomas Addison in the mid-19th century, tuberculosis was the primary cause. Today, almost all causes are associated with autoantibodies.

Metastatic cancer, option C, is not a common cause of primary adrenal insufficiency. HIV infection, tuberculosis, and typhoid fever (options A, D, and E) are incorrect. As stated above, when first identified, tuberculosis was the primary known cause of adrenal insufficiency. However, since that time, autoimmune destruction has surpassed this condition and is currently the leading cause of primary adrenal insufficiency. **Task**: E—Applying Basic Scientific Concepts

16. **Answer: D** This patient has Graves disease, and propylthiouracil, option D, is correct because this drug is the preferred treatment of choice in the first trimester of pregnancy in a patient with Graves disease. Levothyroxine and liothyronine, options A and B, are prescribed to patients who have hypothyroidism and not hyperthyroidism. For other patients with Graves disease and women beyond the first trimester of pregnancy, methimazole, option C, is the preferred antithyroid drug therapy. If methimazole is prescribed during the first trimester of pregnancy, rare teratogenic effects can occur. Radioactive iodine therapy, option E, is contraindicated in pregnant patients due to adverse effects. **Task**: D3—Pharmaceutical Therapeutics

17. **Answer: C** During workup for hypogonadism in a male patient who is greater than 40 years of age, both measurement of prostate-specific antigen level and digital rectal examination are recommended. If this patient is found to have prostate cancer (option C) via these tests, then testosterone replacement therapy is not recommended because of androgen sensitivity of prostate cancer cells and potential disease progression.

    Answer Key for this chapter begins on p. 55

Testosterone replacement therapy is known to improve symptoms of major depressive disorder, option A. Bone mineral density is increased especially during the first year of treatment in patients with osteoporosis (option B) who undergo testosterone replacement therapy. Testosterone replacement therapy has no effect on patients with thyroid cancer, option D, and therefore is not contraindicated. This type of therapy improves insulin sensitivity and causes improvement in glycemic control in patients with type 2 diabetes mellitus, option E. **Task**: D3—Pharmaceutical Therapeutics

18. **Answer: C** A mutation in menin, option C, causes multiple endocrine neoplasia tumors such as those noted in this patient and her family members. Presentations can vary within a family and present in adulthood or childhood.

    The other options are incorrect because mutations in these proteins cause other diseases. Aspartoacylase, option A, is associated with the neurologic degenerative disease called Canavan disease, which is common in those of Ashkenazi descent. Hexosaminidase A, option B, causes a progressive neurodegenerative disease called Tay-Sachs disease. Podocin, option D, is related to glomerulosclerosis. A mutation in tumor protein p53, option E, causes Li-Fraumeni syndrome and induces uninhibited cell growth that may lead to cancer. **Task**: D1—Health Maintenance, Patient Education, and Disease Prevention

19. **Answer: D** This patient has hypoparathyroidism. The correct answer is D, hypocalcemia. Hypoparathyroidism is a common complication following total thyroidectomy and can present with muscle spasms and tingling of the extremities and lips.

    Elevated serum parathyroid hormone level, option A, is incorrect because hypoparathyroidism is characterized by a decreased or inappropriately decreased parathyroid hormone level. Option B, hyperkalemia, is incorrect because potassium is not typically affected following thyroidectomy. Option C, hypermagnesemia, is incorrect because laboratory testing would most likely show a decreased magnesium level in the setting of hypocalcemia. Hypophosphatemia, option E, is incorrect because the phosphate level typically increases in the setting of hypocalcemia. **Task**: B—Using Diagnostic and Laboratory Studies

20. **Answer: C** Initiation of angiotensin-converting enzyme (ACE) inhibitors or angiotensin II receptor blockers have been shown to prevent and treat patients with diabetic nephropathy. The elevated microalbumin-to-creatinine ratio in this patient is often one of the first signs of nephropathy. Only lisinopril, option C, is an ACE inhibitor and appropriate for treating this patient.

Non-dihydropyridine calcium channel blockers may be used to treat refractory proteinuria, but amlodipine, option A, is a dihydropyridine calcium channel blocker and is not preferable to an ACE inhibitor. Colchicine, option B, is used to treat patients with gout and not nephropathy. Metformin, option D, is not appropriate for use in patients with type 1 diabetes mellitus because it does not address insulin deficiency. Also, metformin would not help improve or correct the microalbuminuria in this patient. Metoprolol, option E, is a beta-blocker and is indicated in the treatment of diabetic nephropathy. **Task**: D3—Pharmaceutical Therapeutics

21. **Answer: C** This patient has many of the classic signs of hypothyroidism. The unusual finding of the lateral one-third of her eyebrow being missing is known as the Hertoghe sign and is commonly associated with hypothyroidism. The most prevalent form of hypothyroidism is primary hypothyroidism of the Hashimoto type, which like most dysfunctions of the thyroid gland has an autoimmune etiology. In primary hypothyroidism, the free thyroxin (T_4) is decreased resulting in a compensatory increase in thyroid-stimulating hormone (TSH) release, option C. Furthermore, regarding autoantibody studies in Hashimoto thyroiditis, elevated antithyroid peroxidase and antithyroglobulin antibody levels are present in 95% and at least 40% of people presenting with primary hypothyroidism, respectively.

    Option A is incorrect not only because the TSH would not be decreased in this patient but because elevated thyrotropin receptor antibodies are present in approximately 90% of patients with primary hyperthyroidism, or Graves disease. Option B is incorrect since T_4 would be decreased in hypothyroidism and once again, TSH would be elevated. The IgA antibodies to *Saccharomyces cerevisiae* in option B make this answer even more incorrect in that these antibodies have nothing to do with thyroid disease but are present in 80% of people with Crohn disease. Options D and E are both incorrect because, once again, T_4 would be decreased in primary hypothyroidism. While antithyroglobulin antibodies is correct in option D, the two other components make this option incorrect. Regarding the antibody listed in option E, elevated antibodies to deamidated gliadin peptide are not associated with thyroid dysfunction but are often present in people with celiac disease or gluten-sensitivity enteropathies. **Task**: B—Using Diagnostic and Laboratory Studies

22. **Answer: E** This patient presents with symptoms related to neuromuscular dysfunction such as changes in mentation and neuromuscular hyperexcitability. As a general rule, nerve and muscle cells that rely on electrical potentials for proper functioning are readily

impacted by disturbances in serum sodium, potassium, and/or calcium (in the case of muscle contraction). Thus, questions related to neuromuscular dysfunction typically have an electrolyte-related answer.

The profound hyponatremia observed in this patient fits the picture of neuromuscular dysfunction, but the question asks for the underlying etiology. Important information comes from this patient's history of having bronchogenic carcinoma. Endocrinopathies occur in 12% of lung cancers, with syndrome of inappropriate antidiuretic hormone secretion (SIADH) arising from ectopic secretion of vasopressin from small cell-type tumors. Laboratory findings of hyponatremia with decreased serum osmolality but elevated urinary sodium and osmolality are hallmarks of SIADH (option E), or excess vasopressin secretion.

Option A, diabetic ketoacidosis (DKA), is not a likely choice as the patient, having been well-managed on metformin alone, apparently has type 2 diabetes mellitus. Furthermore, the volume contraction seen in DKA would result in an increase in serum osmolality. Hypercortisolism (option B), or Cushing syndrome, if primary in nature, is in the differential diagnosis of hypernatremia. If hypercortisolism is due to excess adrenocorticotropic hormone (ACTH) secretion, which may also be ectopically produced by small-cell lung cancers, stimulation of the renin-angiotensin system may occur. In this instance, the resultant excess aldosterone produced would result in hypernatremia and a decreased urinary sodium level. Urinary sodium and osmolality would both be decreased.

The inherited autosomal dominant disorder, multiple endocrine neoplasia type 1 (option C), is characterized by ectopic hormone-secreting tumors, typically associated with parathyroid, pancreas, and pituitary glandular-type secretions. One such hormone, ACTH, would result in the same findings as previously described for hypercortisolism and hyperaldosteronism. The laboratory findings would thus contrast with those observed for the patient in this question.

Primary hyperaldosteronism (option D), or Conn syndrome, results from excess aldosterone secretion directly from the adrenal cortex. Neuromuscular dysfunction in this disorder is typically due to hypokalemia rather than sodium imbalance. Sodium and osmolality levels would mirror the levels described for hypercortisolism. **Task:** C—Formulating Most Likely Diagnosis

23. **Answer: A** This patient's symptoms are characteristic of a benign thyroid nodule because she is a middle-aged female, the nodule is 1.0 to 1.5 cm in size, and the nodule is cystic in nature. Furthermore, ultrasonography shows no mural component, which means there is no cell mass, or potential cancer, hiding in the cyst wall.

The correct approach to the management of this lesion is to continue to monitor it over time by routine physical examinations (option A). If this patient presented with a decreased serum thyroid-stimulating hormone level (TSH), and/or if ultrasonography showed that the nodule was a malignant lesion (i.e., microcalcifications, irregular borders, hypoechoic appearance, increased vascularity, or being taller than wide), a more aggressive approach to management would have been indicated.

Additional laboratory studies of thyroid function, option B, do not alter the decision tree and are thus unwarranted. A radionuclide thyroid scan, option C, would be appropriate management if this lesion were solid and the TSH level were decreased. If the nodule possessed these characteristics, a scan would have identified the nodule as "hot" or "cold." Only "cold" lesions should be further worked up by fine-needle aspiration (FNA) biopsy. The decision tree for workup of a solitary thyroid nodule incorporates only measurement of the serum TSH level. The purpose of an FNA biopsy, option D, is to gather cells for cytologic examination. Since the nodule in this patient is not solid but cystic, there is no reason for an FNA. It is for this reason that ultrasonography precedes an FNA in the workup of a thyroid nodule. Lobectomy, choice E, would be an appropriate choice had thyroid cancer been confirmed by biopsy. However, as this lesion possesses several characteristics of a benign nodule, surgical consultation is unwarranted at this time. **Task:** D1—Health Maintenance, Patient Education, and Disease Prevention

24. **Answer: A** Significant head trauma may lead to damage of the hypothalamus and/or pituitary gland. Diabetes insipidus, option A, is frequently encountered following such an insult to the diencephalon. The presentation of polyuria with an elevated serum sodium level and elevated serum osmolality with a decreased urine osmolality are characteristic of a decrease in antidiuretic hormone.

While serum osmolality would be increased in hyperosmolar nonketotic coma, option B, the condition is precipitated by a significantly elevated serum glucose level and is not associated with traumatic brain injury. Myxedema coma, option C, is the end result of untreated or inadequately treated hypothyroidism. The condition may occur following injury to the hypothalamus-pituitary-thyroid axis but is accompanied by significant hypothermia and hyponatremia. Nephritic syndrome, option D, is characterized by urinary loss of albumin and is associated with poststreptococcal glomerulonephritis. This patient scenario is unrelated to nephritic syndrome. Syndrome of inappropriate antidiuretic hormone secretion (SIADH), option E, is indicated by an excess of antidiuretic hormone. Since SIADH is essentially the opposite of diabetes insipidus, values for serum electrolytes and the osmolality of serum and urine would be opposite of what is noted in this scenario. **Task:** C—Formulating Most Likely Diagnosis

Answer Key for this chapter begins on p. 55

25. Answer: E Papillary thyroid cancer, option E, is the most common form of thyroid cancer in both children and adults, accounting for approximately 80% of malignant thyroid gland tumors. These tumors generally present as firm, solid nodules, and patients, especially children, have enlarged cervical lymph nodes. Anaplastic carcinoma, option A, is incorrect because undifferentiated carcinoma typically occurs in older patients and accounts for approximately 3% of malignant thyroid tumors. Options B and C, follicular carcinoma and Hürthle cell carcinoma, are incorrect because Hürthle cell carcinoma is a variant of follicular carcinoma and only accounts for approximately 10% of malignant thyroid tumors. Option D, medullary carcinoma, is incorrect because this type of cancer accounts for only 5% of malignant thyroid tumors. It is typically more aggressive, invading into surrounding tissues, and is most often familial. **Task:** A—History Taking and Performing Physical Examination

26. Answer: D Primary hyperparathyroidism is the most common cause of hypercalcemia with a prevalence of 1000 to 4000 cases per one million people. It occurs in all ages but is most common in women in the seventh decade. In 80% of cases, hypersecretion of parathyroid hormone is caused by a solitary parathyroid adenoma, option D. In less than 20% of cases, it is caused by hyperplasia of two or more of the parathyroid glands. Breast cancer, multiple myeloma, and sarcoidosis, (option A, C, and E) are secondary causes of hypercalcemia. Familial hypocalciuric hypercalcemia (FHH), option B, is an uncommon autosomal dominant inherited disorder that sometimes can present in the neonatal period with severe primary hyperthyroidism. Adults with hypercalcemia due to FHH are either asymptomatic or have nonspecific symptoms such as fatigue, weakness, or cognitive issues. FHH can also be associated with recurrent pancreatitis. **Task:** C—Formulating Most Likely Diagnosis

27. Answer: D This patient has type 2 diabetes mellitus based on the findings on laboratory studies. Lifestyle modifications in addition to therapy with metformin,

option D, is the most appropriate management. Because of the mild to moderate level of hyperglycemia in this patient, the risk of hypoglycemia associated with insulin use outweighs its benefits. Desmopressin, option A, is used to treat patients with diabetes insipidus and not diabetes mellitus. Insulin detemir and insulin regular human, options B and C, are inappropriate to initiate in this patient because they could cause hypoglycemia. Metoprolol, option E, is not an appropriate treatment for diabetes mellitus and could lead to hypotension in a nonhypertensive patient. **Task:** D3—Pharmaceutical Therapeutics

28. Answer: E Patients with tachycardia, enlargement of the thyroid gland, and unintentional weight loss have the classic symptoms of thyrotoxicosis, option E. Euthyroid state, option A, includes normal function of the thyroid gland, which is not demonstrated in this patient. Patients with hyperparathyroidism, option B, have abnormal serum calcium levels and elevated levels of parathyroid hormone, which are not noted in this patient. Primary hypothyroidism, option C, occurs when the thyroid gland fails and is characterized by elevated levels of thyroid-stimulating hormone (TSH) and decreased levels of thyroxine (T_4) and triiodothyronine (T_3). Secondary hypothyroidism, option D, results from a failure of the pituitary gland to secrete sufficient levels of TSH and is marked by decreased levels of TSH, T_3, and T_4. **Task:** C—Formulating Most Likely Diagnosis

29. Answer: D This patient has symptoms of hypocalcemia after undergoing thyroidectomy, and the most likely finding on electrocardiography is QT prolongation (option D), which is a dangerous anomaly associated with acute hypocalcemia as seen in patients with hypoparathyroidism.
A left or right bundle branch block or complete heart block, options A and B, are not associated with hypocalcemia. Peaked T waves, option C, are associated with hyperkalemia. ST-segment depression, option E, is indicative of cardiac ischemia. **Task:** B—Using Diagnostic and Laboratory Studies

BIBLIOGRAPHY

ADVANCE Collaborative Group. (2008). Intensive blood glucose control and vascular outcomes in patients with type 2 diabetes. *New England Journal of Medicine, 358*(24), 2560-2572.

Behre, H. M., Kliesch, S., Leifke, E., Link, T. M., & Nieschlag, E. (1997). Long-term effect of testosterone therapy on bone mineral density in hypogonadal men. *The Journal of Clinical Endocrinology & Metabolism, 82*(8), 2386-2390.

Bornstein, S. R., Allolio, B., Arlt, W., Barthel, A., Don-Wauchope, A., Hammer, G. D., et al. (2016). Diagnosis and treatment of primary adrenal insufficiency: An endocrine society clinical practice

guideline. *The Journal of Clinical Endocrinology & Metabolism, 101*(2), 364-389.

Braunwald, E., Fauci, A. S., Hauser, S. L., Longo, D. L., & Jameson, J. L. (2005). *Harrison's principles of internal medicine.* McGraw-Hill Companies, Inc.

Brent, G. A., & Weetman, A. P. (2016). Hypothyroidism and thyroiditis: *Williams textbook of endocrinology* (pp. 416-448). Elsevier.

Cascone, T., Gold, K. A., & Glisson, B. S. (2016). Small cell carcinoma of the lung. In H. M. Kantarjian & R. A. Wolff (Eds.),

The MD anderson manual of medical oncology (3rd ed.). New York, NY: McGraw-Hill. Lung cancer, paraneoplastic syndromes, syndrome of inappropriate ADH Cognitive Level: Analyze/Analysis.

Crandall, J. (2020). Diabetes mellitus. *Goldman-Cecil Medicine, 216*, 1490-1510. E3.

Dimitriadis, G. K., Angelousi, A., Weickert, M. O., Randeva, H. S., Kaltsas, G., & Grossman, A. (2017). Paraneoplastic endocrine syndromes. *Endocr Relat Cancer, 24*(6), R173-R190.

Dowell, J. E., Gerber, D. E., & Johnson, D. H. (2015). Small cell lung cancer: Diagnosis, treatment, and natural history. In M. A. Grippi, J. A. Elias, & J. A. Fishman (Eds.), *Fishman's pulmonary diseases and disorders* (5th ed.). McGraw-Hill.

Findling, J. (2014). Diagnostic testing for cushing's disease.

Gardner, D. G., & Shoback, D. (2018). *Greenspan's basic & clinical endocrinology* (10th ed.). McGraw-Hill Education.

Gluvic, Z., Zaric, B., Resanovic, I., Obradovic, M., Mitrovic, A., Radak, D., et al. (2017). Link between metabolic syndrome and insulin resistance. *Current Vascular Pharmacology, 15*(1), 30-39.

Haugen, B. R., Alexander, E. K., Bible, K. C., Doherty, G. M., Mandel, S. J., Nikiforov, Y. E., et al. (2016). 2015 American Thyroid Association management guidelines for adult patients with thyroid nodules and differentiated thyroid cancer: The American Thyroid Association guidelines task force on thyroid nodules and differentiated thyroid cancer. *Thyroid, 26*(1), 1-133.

Kasper, D. L., & Fauci, A. S., Hauser, S. L., Longo, D. L., Jameson, J. L., Loscal, J. (2016). *Harrison's Manual of Medicine* (19th ed.).

Hollenberg, A. (2020). Hyperthyroid disorders. *Williams Textbook of Endocrinology*, 12, 364-403. E9.

Jameson, J. L. (2017). *Harrison's endocrinology* (4th ed.). McGraw-Hill Education Medical.

Khan, A. A., Koch, C. A., Van Uum, S., Baillargeon, J. P., Bollerslev, J., Brandi, M. L., et al. (2019). Standards of care for hypoparathyroidism in adults: A Canadian and International Consensus. *European Journal of Endocrinology, 180*(3), P1-P22.

Kirk, L. F., Jr., Hash, R. B., Katner, H. P., & Jones, T. (2000). Cushing's disease: clinical manifestations and diagnostic evaluation. *American Family Physician, 62*(5), 1119-1127.

Lai, X., Xia, Y., Zhang, B., Li, J., & Jiang, Y. (2017). A meta-analysis of Hashimoto's thyroiditis and papillary thyroid carcinoma risk. *Oncotarget, 8*(37), 62414.

Lopes, M. P., Kliemann, B. S., Bini, I. B., Kulchetscki, R., Borsani, V., Savi, L., et al. (2016). Hypoparathyroidism and pseudohypoparathyroidism: Etiology, laboratory features and complications. *Archives of Endocrinology and Metabolism, 60*, 532-536.

Mayer-Davis, E. J., Lawrence, J. M., Dabelea, D., Divers, J., Isom, S., Dolan, L., et al. (2017). Incidence trends of type 1 and type 2 diabetes among youths, 2002–2012. *New England Journal of Medicine, 376*, 1419-1429.

McDermott, M. T. (2020). *Endocrine ecrets* (7th ed.). Elsevier Inc.

McPhee, S. J., & Papadakis, M. A. (2020). *Current medical diagnosis and treatment*. McGraw Hill.

Multiple Endocrine Neoplasia (MEN). (2021). In M. A. Papadakis, S. J. McPhee, & J. Bernstein (Eds.), *Quick medical diagnosis & treatment* 2021. McGraw-Hill.

Peri, A., Grohé, C., Berardi, R., & Runkle, I. (2017). SIADH: differential diagnosis and clinical management. *Endocrine, 55*(1), 311-319.

Persani, L., Cangiano, B., & Bonomi, M. (2019). The diagnosis and management of central hypothyroidism in 2018. *Endocrine Connections, 8*(2), R44-R54.

Robertson, G. L. (2015). Disorders of the neurohypophysis. In D. Kasper, A. Fauci, & S. Hauser (Eds.), *Harrison's principles of internal medicine* (19th ed.). McGraw-Hill.

Sterns, R., Emmett, M., & Forman, J. (2020). *Pathophysiology and etiology of the syndrome of inappropriate antidiuretic hormone secretion (SIADH)*. UpToDate, Inc.

Verbalis, J. G., & Berl, T. (2008). Disorders of water balance. *Brenner and Rector's the kidney, 1*, 540-594.

    Answer Key for this chapter begins on p. 55

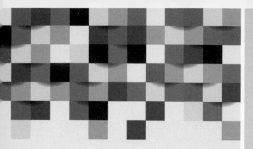

Questions

1. A 28-year-old man comes to the office because he has had increased dizziness, tinnitus, and hearing loss in his right ear for the past week. He says that he also has been falling over to his right side during the past two days. The patient has not had headache, visual disturbances, or dysarthria. On physical examination, the eyes rapidly flicker horizontally toward the left side and slowly move toward the right back to center. Which of the following best describes this type of eye movement?
   A. Exotropia
   B. Myopia
   C. Nystagmus
   D. Ptosis
   E. Strabismus

2.

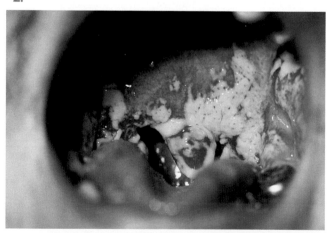

   A 70-year-old man comes to the office because he has had pain in his mouth for the past four days. Medical history includes B-cell lymphoma, for which he has been undergoing chemotherapy. He is afebrile. Findings on oral examination are shown in the photograph. Which of the following is the most appropriate next step?
   A. CEA blood test
   B. Complete blood cell count
   C. HIV antibody test
   D. Microscopic examination of lesion scrapings
   E. Punch biopsy of multiple discolored areas

3. A 7-year-old girl is brought to the clinic because she has had continuous purulent drainage from her right ear for the past two days. Medical history includes at least three visits to the clinic per year since 1 year of age because of otalgia, aural pressure, and fever. Treatment consists of amoxicillin for the first three years and amoxicillin-clavulanic acid thereafter, with complete resolution of symptoms after each course of antibiotics. Current physical examination shows a perforated tympanic membrane on the right. Weber test localizes to the affected ear, and Rinne test shows bone conduction greater than air conduction. Which of the following is the most likely causative organism?
   A. *Bacillus cereus*
   B. *Haemophilus influenzae*
   C. *Klebsiella pneumoniae*
   D. *Pseudomonas aeruginosa*
   E. *Streptococcus pyogenes*

4. A 17-year-old girl comes to the urgent care clinic because she has had mild eye discomfort and light sensitivity for the past 36 hours. She usually wears contact lenses but is currently wearing glasses. Vital signs are within normal limits. Physical examination shows erythema of the left eye with purulent drainage. Minimal yellow crusting is noted on the left superior eyelid. No edema is noted. Eyelid inversion shows that no foreign body is present, and there is no concern for corneal abrasion. Visual acuity is 20/20 bilaterally, and extraocular movements are intact. The pupils are equal, round, and reactive to light. Which of the following is most appropriate to tell this patient about this condition?
   A. Contact lenses can be worn immediately
   B. It is highly contagious, so prevention measures are necessary
   C. It will most likely take six weeks to resolve
   D. Oral antibiotics are the gold standard of treatment
   E. Use of an eye patch is required for appropriate healing

5. A 46-year-old man comes to the office because he has had episodes of ear ringing twice daily for the past five days. Each episode lasts for about four hours. He has no history of similar symptoms. The patient says he was evaluated in the urgent care clinic one week ago because he had sinusitis and nasal congestion; he was prescribed ciprofloxacin 500 mg twice daily for treatment. Medical history includes type 2 diabetes mellitus, elevated triglyceride levels, and allergic rhinitis. Medications include metformin 500 mg twice daily for treatment of type 2 diabetes mellitus, omega-3-acid ethyl esters 2 g twice daily for elevated triglyceride levels, and fluticasone propionate one to two sprays in each nostril daily, as well as levocetirizine 5 mg daily for treatment of allergic rhinitis. Which of the following medications is the most likely cause of the ear ringing episodes in this patient?
   A. Ciprofloxacin
   B. Fluticasone propionate
   C. Levocetirizine
   D. Metformin
   E. Omega-3-acid ethyl esters

6. A 50-year-old man comes to the emergency department because he has had an active nosebleed for the past 40 minutes, and he could not stop the bleeding at home. Physical examination shows blood in the left nostril and the throat. After applying direct pressure, suction, and topical decongestants, the source of the bleed is unable to be identified. Which of the following next steps is most likely to help identify the source of the bleed?
   A. CT scan of the nasal cavity
   B. MR angiography of the brain
   C. MRI of the nasal cavity
   D. Nasal endoscopy
   E. X-ray study of the nasal cavity

7. A 7-year-old girl is brought to the office by her mother because she has had a fever for the past 24 hours. The mother says that the patient's most recent temperature was 38.8°C (101.8°F). The patient says that her throat hurts. She has no history of runny nose, cough, vomiting, or diarrhea. Her appetite is diminished. The patient appears ill but is not in any respiratory distress. Physical examination shows erythema of the posterior pharynx. Petechiae are noted on the soft palate, and exudate is covering the tonsillar pillars. Palpation of the neck shows enlarged anterior cervical lymph nodes. The remainder of the examination shows no abnormalities. Which of the following is the most likely causative agent?
   A. Adenovirus
   B. *Corynebacterium diphtheriae*
   C. *Fusobacterium necrophorum*
   D. Parainfluenzae virus
   E. *Streptococcus pyogenes*

8. A 72-year-old woman comes to the emergency department because she had sudden onset of vision changes one hour ago. She says she sees flashes of light and squiggly lines. The patient has no history of trauma to the eyes, and she does not have pain, discharge, or itchy, watery eyes. Medical history includes type 2 diabetes mellitus, for which she takes metformin 500 mg twice daily. Vital signs are within normal limits. On physical examination, extraocular movements are intact and do not produce pain, and the pupils are equally round and reactive to light and accommodation. No hyperemia or discharge is noted. Visual acuity is 20/20 in the unaffected eye and 20/80 in the affected eye. Intraocular pressure is 15 mmHg (N = 10–21 mmHg). Which of the following is the most likely diagnosis?
   A. Acute angle-closure glaucoma
   B. Cataracts
   C. Keratoconjunctivitis sicca
   D. Macular degeneration
   E. Retinal detachment

9. A 44-year-old man comes to the office because he has had sneezing, runny nose, nasal congestion, and itchy eyes with a watery discharge for the past week. He says that he always has these symptoms at this time of year when the pollen count is high, and they typically improve with use of an antihistamine and nasal spray. Based on this history, which of the following findings is most likely on physical examination of this patient?
   A. Atrophy and thinning of the nasal mucosa with crusting
   B. Erythematous and bulging tympanic membrane with decreased mobility
   C. Pale bluish nasal mucosa and cobblestoning of the posterior pharynx
   D. Perforation of the nasal septum and oropharyngeal ulcers
   E. Swollen and erythematous tonsils with exudate and cervical lymphadenopathy

10. A 14-year-old girl is brought to the office by her father because she has had pain in her right ear for the past 12 hours. On physical examination, an insect is identified in the external auditory canal. The tympanic membrane is visualized and intact. Which of the following liquids is most appropriate to instill into the ear canal to aid in the removal of the insect?
   A. Acetone
   B. Lidocaine
   C. Peroxide
   D. Povidone-iodine
   E. Water

Answer Key for this chapter begins on p. 69

11. A 22-year-old man comes to the emergency department because he has had facial swelling and pain in the right eye since he was hit in the face during a fight 12 hours ago. Physical examination shows significant edema around the eye and some tenderness and crepitus on palpation of the orbit. An orbital blowout fracture is suspected. Which of the following additional findings on physical examination is most likely to confirm this diagnosis?
    A. Enophthalmos and limited upward gaze
    B. Malocclusion of the teeth and tenderness of the cheekbone
    C. Numbness of the forehead
    D. Tear-shaped pupil and severe conjunctival hemorrhage
    E. Widened intercanthal distance

13. A 5-year-old boy is brought to the emergency department by his mother because he has had worsening fever and dysphagia over the past 24 hours. The mother says that they immigrated to the United States from Mexico four months ago. The patient has not received any vaccinations since birth. He appears to be in moderate distress, is drooling, and has a muffled voice. Physical examination shows inspiratory stridor and chest wall retractions. Which of the following is the most appropriate next step in management?
    A. Evaluate the throat with direct visualization
    B. Obtain a throat culture
    C. Obtain white blood cell count
    D. Obtain x-ray studies of the lateral neck
    E. Secure the patient's airway

12.

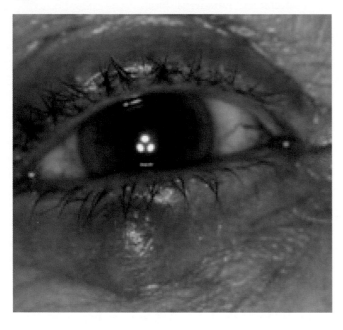

A 50-year-old man comes to the office because he has had a swelling in his lower eyelid that has been increasing in size over the past week. He has not had associated fever or impairment of vision. On physical examination, the edema is firm and nontender. A photograph of the eye is shown. Which of the following is the most likely diagnosis?
A. Blepharitis
B. Chalazion
C. Dacryocystitis
D. Hordeolum
E. Pinguecula

14.

A 32-year-old woman comes to the emergency department because she has had worsening photophobia, foreign body sensation, and blurred vision in her right eye over the past four days. She wears soft, extended-wear contact lenses and recently spent the weekend at the beach. Medical history includes Crohn disease for which she takes cyclosporine. Vital signs are within normal limits. On physical examination, visual acuity is 20/20 bilaterally prior to removing the contact lenses. Slit-lamp examination shows an ulcer that involves the stroma; no hypopyon is noted. A photograph of the eye is shown. Which of the following is the most appropriate next step in diagnosis?
A. Confrontation visual field testing
B. Fluorescein staining
C. Measurement of intraocular pressure
D. Orbital CT scan
E. Scraping of the ulcer for culture

15. A 43-year-old woman comes to the urgent care center because she has had continuous severe dizziness with associated nausea and vomiting for the past two days. One week ago, she had symptoms of an upper respiratory tract infection that has since resolved. On physical examination, horizontal nystagmus is noted with beats toward the right ear, and disequilibrium is noted. Otoscopic examination shows no abnormalities. Weber test shows lateralization toward the left ear. Rinne test shows air conduction is greater than bone conduction, bilaterally. Which of the following is the most likely diagnosis?
    A. Acoustic neuroma
    B. Benign positional vertigo
    C. Labyrinthitis
    D. Meniere disease
    E. Vestibular neuritis

16. A 25-year-old woman who is a graduate student comes to the campus health center because she has had a painful mouth sore for the past three days. She says that the sore is interfering with her ability to eat citrus foods and drink liquids comfortably. Medical history includes no chronic disease conditions. She occasionally smokes cigarettes and does not use illicit drugs. Physical examination shows a 2.5-mm round, yellowish, shallow ulceration with an erythematous halo in the buccal mucosa. When educating the patient regarding this condition, it is most appropriate to recommend which of the following preventative measures to decrease the recurrence of this type of oral ulcer?
    A. Begin oral vitamin B_1 supplementation
    B. Begin using toothpaste that contains sodium lauryl sulfate
    C. Decrease physiological stress
    D. Perform daily oral rinses with warm salt water
    E. Stop smoking cigarettes

17. A 28-year-old woman comes to the office because she has had a hoarse voice for the past three days. She says symptoms started one week ago with runny nose, nasal congestion, sore throat, and cough. The patient is a first-year elementary school teacher, and several of her students have been out sick. Vital signs are within normal limits. During the interview, the patient is whispering. Physical examination shows clear rhinorrhea with postnasal drainage and some mild erythema of the posterior pharynx. Which of the following is the most appropriate treatment?
    A. Prescribe therapy with oral amoxicillin
    B. Recommend conservative therapy such as voice rest, increase in fluids, and use of a humidifier
    C. Recommend she immediately go to the emergency department

    D. Refer the patient for voice therapy
    E. Refer the patient to an otolaryngologist for laryngoscopy

18.

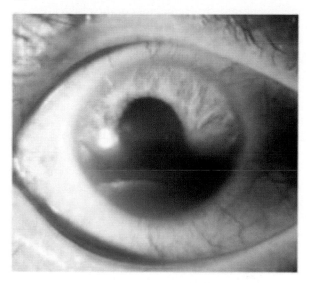

A 16-year-old boy comes to the clinic because he has had pain in his eye since he was directly hit in the eye with a tennis ball one hour ago. He says he has blurry vision in the affected eye and mild tenderness around the ocular orbit. He does not have double vision. On physical examination, extraocular movements are intact and do not produce pain. Pupils are equally round and reactive to light and accommodation. No enophthalmos or exophthalmos is noted. Funduscopic examination shows no abnormalities. A photograph of the eye is shown. Which of the following is the most likely diagnosis?
    A. Blowout fracture
    B. Hyphema
    C. Hypopyon
    D. Retinal detachment
    E. Subconjunctival hemorrhage

19. A 3-year-old girl is brought to the office because her mother suspects that she may have put something in her nose three days ago. The mother thinks this occurred outside while the patient was playing in the yard with an older cousin. Based on this history, which of the following physical examination findings is most likely?
    A. Deviated nasal septum
    B. Erythema overlying the nares
    C. Postnasal drip
    D. Tenderness to palpation of the upper teeth
    E. Unilateral purulent rhinorrhea

Answer Key for this chapter begins on p. 69

20. A 24-year-old man comes to the urgent care clinic because he has had stuffiness in his left ear for the past week. Medical history includes severe allergies managed with cetirizine daily. Otoscopic examination shows a small amount of fluid behind the left tympanic membrane. The remainder of the physical examination shows no abnormalities. A complete hearing test is planned. Which of the following findings on this testing is most likely?
    A. Diminished hearing in the right ear on whisper test
    B. Lateralization to the left ear on Weber test
    C. No lateralization to the left ear on Weber test
    D. Ratio of air conduction to bone conduction in the left ear is equal on Rinne test
    E. Ratio of air conduction to bone conduction in the left ear is greater than 2:1 on Rinne test

21. An 18-year-old man comes to the emergency department because he has had fever up to 38.3°C (100.9°F), severe sore throat, and painful swallowing for the past three days. Temperature is 38.4°C (101.1°F), pulse rate is 112/min, respirations are 18/min, and blood pressure is 108/72 mmHg. Oxygen saturation is 100% on room air. Physical examination shows medial deviation of the soft palate and peritonsillar fold. Which of the following additional findings is most likely on further workup of this patient?
    A. Muffled voice
    B. Red, smooth tongue
    C. Scarlatiniform rash
    D. Steeple sign on x-ray study
    E. Thumb sign on x-ray study

22. A 55-year-old woman comes to the office because she has had worsening blurry vision over the past four months. She says she has had increased difficulty driving at night and reading small print during this time. Medical history includes sarcoidosis that is controlled with prednisone. On physical examination, visual acuity is 20/60 in the right eye and 20/40 in the left eye. Funduscopic examination shows no abnormalities. Cataracts are suspected. Which of the following best describes the physiology associated with the formation of cataracts in this patient?
    A. Formation of drusen bodies
    B. Increased intraocular pressure
    C. Opacity of the lens
    D. Retinal tear
    E. Swelling of the macula

23. A 2-year-old boy is brought to the emergency department by his mother because he has had fever, lethargy, and irritability for the past two days. His mother says that he has a history of ear infections, with the most recent occurring in his left ear. Temperature is 39.4°C (103.0°F). Physical examination shows a protrusion of the left auricle with postauricular erythema and tenderness. A bulging tympanic membrane with pus behind the membrane is noted on the left. Based on these findings, it is most appropriate to further evaluate this patient for which of the following conditions?
    A. Acoustic neuroma
    B. Erysipelas
    C. Eustachian tube dysfunction
    D. Mastoiditis
    E. Necrotizing fasciitis

24. A 22-year-old woman comes to the office because she has had sore and crusty eyelids for the past week. Medical history includes rosacea, and she takes no medications. Physical examination shows crusting and flaking at the base of the outside front edge of both eyelids. Both eyelids are erythematous and edematous. Which of the following is the most appropriate initial treatment?
    A. Antibiotic ointment
    B. Corticosteroid eyedrops
    C. Oral doxycycline
    D. Topical cyclosporine
    E. Warm compresses and gentle scrubbing with baby shampoo

25. A 20-year-old female college student comes to the office because she has had consistent, dull pain on the left side of her face for the past three days. She also has had difficulty chewing and says that the pain radiates up to her left ear and down the left side of her neck. The patient had a sore throat that resolved four days ago, and she also has had fatigue for the past two weeks but attributes this to stress from her current studies. She has not had fever or chills, has no history of trauma to the affected area, and has no sick contacts. Current medications include drospirenone and ethinyl estradiol for birth control and ibuprofen as needed for pain. She is up-to-date on all immunizations. Vital signs are within normal limits. Physical examination of the face shows left-sided edema inferior and anterior to the left auditory canal. Palpation of this area shows warmth and tenderness between the zygomatic arch and the angle of the mandible. There is no tenderness or limitation with opening the mouth or moving the jaw. Anterior cervical lymphadenopathy is noted on the left. The lymph node measures 3 cm, has a rubbery consistency, is nontender to palpation, and is not fixed. Which of the following is the most likely diagnosis?
    A. Parotitis
    B. Peritonsillar abscess
    C. Stomatitis
    D. Temporal mandibular joint dysfunction
    E. Trigeminal neuralgia

26. A 7-year-old boy is brought to the office by his mother because he has had nasal congestion, headache, and sore throat for the past five days. Acute sinusitis is suspected. If found on further examination of this patient, which of the following symptoms is most concerning for a potential complication?
    A. Cough
    B. Dental pain
    C. Fever
    D. Nasal discharge
    E. Periorbital edema

27.

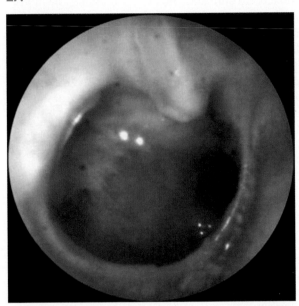

A 36-year-old woman comes to the clinic because she has had pain in her left ear for the past 14 days. She says she woke up this morning with a "whooshing, buzzing noise" inside her left ear. Vital signs are within normal limits. Physical examination of the throat shows no abnormalities. A superficial cervical lymph node is palpable on the left side of the neck. The lymph node measures less than 2 cm and is rubbery, nontender, and not fixed. Findings on otoscopic examination are shown. Ear drops containing which of the following substances is the most appropriate first-line treatment?
A. Benzocaine
B. Carbamide peroxide
C. Chloroxylenol
D. Hydrocortisone
E. Ofloxacin

28. A 52-year-old man comes to the office as a new patient for routine physical examination. He says he feels well and has no history of recent weight loss, dysphagia, numbness, or tingling. The patient has a 35-year history of tobacco chewing. On physical examination, a flat, white lesion about 1 mm in size is noted on the floor of the mouth; the lesion cannot be scraped off with a tongue depressor. No evidence of lymphadenopathy is noted, and cranial nerves II through XII are grossly intact. Which of the following is the most likely diagnosis?
A. Hairy cell leukemia
B. Invasive squamous cell carcinoma
C. Leukoplakia
D. Oral candidiasis
E. Oral lichen planus

29. A 15-year-old boy is brought to the office because he has had pain in his left ear for the past 24 hours. He says he just returned from a surfing vacation. He has no history of recent upper respiratory tract infection, nor does he have a history of ear problems. Physical examination shows erythema and mild edema of the left ear canal. A small amount of discharge is noted in the canal. Which of the following objective findings is most likely to support the suspected diagnosis?
A. Enlargement of the posterior cervical lymph nodes
B. Immobility of the tympanic membrane
C. Pain on palpation of the tragus
D. Presence of vesicles in the external acoustic meatus
E. Temperature >38.3°C (101.0°F)

30. A 54-year-old man comes to the emergency department because he has had fever, restriction of extraocular movements, and proptosis of his left eye for the past four hours. Physical examination shows edema and erythema of the eyelid. Based on these findings, which of the following is the most appropriate immediate treatment?
A. Amoxicillin
B. Isoniazid
C. Metronidazole
D. Solumedrol
E. Vancomycin

31. A 55-year-old woman comes to the office because she has had persistent headache and fever for the past two days. She also has had nausea and vomiting as well as vision changes during this time. She rates her pain as a 9 on a 10-point scale. Medical history does not include any chronic disease conditions, and she does not take any medications. Temperature is 38.9°C (102.0°F), pulse rate is 107/min, respirations are 18/min, and blood pressure is 130/80 mmHg. Physical examination shows nuchal rigidity. Which of the following findings is most likely on funduscopic examination of this patient?
A. Cotton wool spots
B. Papilledema
C. Retinal detachment
D. Retinoblastoma
E. Roth spot

   Answer Key for this chapter begins on p. 69

32.

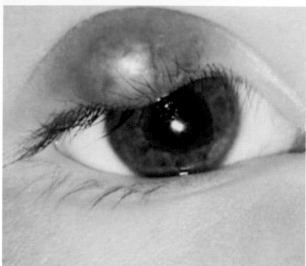

An 8-year-old boy is brought to the clinic by his mother because he has had a lesion on his right upper eyelid for the past two days. The patient says that the lesion is slightly tender to touch. Vital signs are within normal limits. Other than erythema of the lid and the nodular lesion, physical examination of the eyes shows no abnormalities. A photograph is shown. Which of the following is the most appropriate initial course of action to hasten improvement and resolution of the lesion?

A. Apply over-the-counter 1% hydrocortisone ointment

B. Apply a warm compress to the lid several times daily

C. Begin a seven-day course of oral doxycycline

D. Perform incision and drainage of the lesion

E. Perform marsupialization of the lesion

33. A 46-year-old woman comes to the urgent care clinic because she has had recurrent episodes of vertigo lasting from 20 minutes to two hours during the past two weeks. She says she feels as if the room is spinning, and she has associated nausea and vomiting. The patient says she also has had intermittent hearing loss and low-pitched ringing in her ears during this time. She has not had fevers but says that her ear still feels full despite recently recovering from an upper respiratory tract infection. Appropriate initial therapy for this condition includes a low-salt diet and treatment with which of the following types of drugs?

A. Antibiotics

B. Antiemetics

C. Antihistamines

D. Corticosteroids

E. Diuretics

34. A 3-year-old girl is brought to the urgent care clinic by her mother because she has had pain in her right ear for the past day. The mother says that her daughter has been more irritable, has had a decreased appetite, and woke up several times during the night. This morning, the mother said the patient had a low-grade fever and was pulling on her right ear. On physical examination, there are no signs of external edema to the ear or tenderness with palpation. Pneumatic otoscope shows the tympanic membrane to be erythematous with limited mobility. Which of the following is the most likely diagnosis?

A. Acute otitis externa

B. Acute otitis media

C. Cerumen impaction

D. Upper respiratory tract infection

E. Viral otitis externa

35. A 32-year-old man comes to the emergency department because he has had pain in his right eye since he felt something hit the eye while he was in his garage grinding metal parts eight hours ago. Physical examination of the right eye shows hyperemia and excessive blinking. Extraocular movements are intact. No periorbital edema, redness, or tenderness to palpation is noted. No collection of fluid is noted in the anterior chamber of the eye. Visual acuity of the right eye is unable to be assessed due to pain and excessive tearing. Slit-lamp examination with fluorescein staining of the affected eye shows a lighter color stain band projecting down from the suspected site of injury. Which of the following is the most likely diagnosis?

A. Corneal abrasion

B. Globe perforation

C. Herpes simplex keratitis

D. Hyphema

E. Rust stain

Answers

1. **Answer: C** This patient has vertigo. Nystagmus, option C, is described as involuntary, spontaneous rhythmic movement of the eyes that is seen in individuals with peripheral vertigo. Unilateral hearing loss, tinnitus, dizziness, and falling over to the affected side all lead toward this diagnosis. Patients with this disorder have unidirectional horizontal nystagmus.
Exotropia, option A, is a type of strabismus in which one or both eyes turn outward. Myopia, option B, is defined as nearsightedness. Ptosis, option D, is drooping of the upper eyelid. Strabismus, option E, occurs when the eyes do not properly align. **Task:** A—History Taking and Performing Physical Examination

2. **Answer: D** This patient has candidiasis, and the most appropriate next step is to confirm this diagnosis via microscopic examination of lesion scrapings, option D. When a diagnosis of candidiasis is suspected, the lesions can be scraped and examined microscopically under high power. Findings of budding yeast and pseudohyphae support the diagnosis of candidiasis.
CEA blood test, option A, is a marker for various cancers such as colon cancer. Complete blood cell count, option B, will not give any diagnostic information. It might be ordered if an infectious cause of the skin lesions is suspected, which is not the case with this patient since he does not have a fever. HIV antibody test, option C, is not useful for diagnosing candidiasis. It is useful for identifying immunosuppression as a cause of candidiasis; however, this patient has a known risk factor for candidiasis, which is chemotherapy. Punch biopsy, option E, will provide diagnostic information but will not give immediate results. **Task:** B—Using Diagnostic and Laboratory Studies

3. **Answer: D** *Pseudomonas aeruginosa*, option D, is the pathogen that most likely causes chronic otitis media. *Bacillus cereus*, option A, is an enterotoxin that is found in contaminated food and causes food poisoning. *Haemophilus influenzae* and *Streptococcus pyogenes*, options B and E, are most likely to cause acute otitis media. *Klebsiella pneumoniae*, option C, is found in the gastrointestinal tract and causes nosocomial urinary tract infections and aspiration pneumonia with signature currant-jelly sputum. **Task:** E—Applying Basic Scientific Concepts

4. **Answer: B** This patient has signs and symptoms of bacterial conjunctivitis, which is highly contagious. Preventive measures should be discussed with the patient to decrease the risk of spreading the condition. Therefore, the correct answer is option B.

Contact lenses should not be worn until symptoms resolve, which makes option A incorrect. Bacterial conjunctivitis should resolve in seven to 10 days; therefore, waiting six weeks for this condition to resolve (option C) is inappropriate. The treatment of choice is topical antibiotics and not oral antibiotics, option D. An eye patch, option E, is not indicated for this condition to heal. **Task:** D1—Health Maintenance, Patient Education, and Disease Prevention

5. **Answer: A** Although many medications can cause tinnitus, the most likely etiology of the tinnitus in this patient is ciprofloxacin, option A. This patient has been taking ciprofloxacin twice daily, which could account for the new onset of twice daily episodes of tinnitus.
Fluticasone propionate, option B, is a nasal spray dosed once daily and is not likely to cause tinnitus. The patient has been taking levocetirizine, option C, chronically without episodes of tinnitus and it is a once daily medication; therefore, this drug is less likely to be responsible for the new onset of tinnitus in this patient. Although metformin and omega-3-acid ethyl esters, options D and E, are dosed twice daily, the patient has been taking these medications at the same dose chronically; therefore, they are less likely to cause auditory disturbances such as tinnitus. **Task:** D3—Pharmaceutical Therapeutics

6. **Answer: D** Nasal endoscopy, option D, is the most appropriate next step since this will allow direct visualization of the nasal passages and help identify the bleeding site.
CT scan of the nasal cavity, option A, is the most appropriate next step only if a nasal fracture or intranasal soft-tissue injury is suspected. MR angiography of the brain, option B, is appropriate for evaluating arterial blood vessel abnormalities in the brain such as arterial stenosis, thrombosis, or an aneurysm. MRI, option C, is used in cases of recurrent epistaxis when there is suspicion of a nasal neoplasm. X-ray study of the nasal cavity, option E, is an appropriate next step only if a nasal fracture is suspected. It will not help determine the source of the bleed in this patient. **Task:** B—Using Diagnostic and Laboratory Studies

7. **Answer: E** The correct answer is *Streptococcus pyogenes*, option E, the causative agent of streptococcal pharyngitis, which most commonly occurs in patients between 4 and 7 years of age. The onset is acute and is most often accompanied by fever and throat pain. Coryza and cough are absent.

Options A and D, adenovirus and parainfluenzae virus, are viral causes of pharyngitis in which there is a gradual onset and associated coryza and cough. *Corynebacterium diphtheriae*, option B, can cause pharyngitis but includes the hallmark sign of a tenacious gray membrane covering the pharynx and tonsils. Fever is usually absent. *Fusobacterium necrophorum*, option C, is a recently recognized cause of pharyngitis in young adults and is often associated with peritonsillar abscess. **Task:** E—Applying Basic Scientific Concepts

8. **Answer: E** Retinal detachment, option E, can happen to anyone, however, advanced age and diabetic retinopathy are common risk factors. Retinal detachment does not cause eye pain but can cause loss of vision if not treated promptly. Common symptoms include blurry vision, flashes of light, and squiggly lines or floaters. When obstructed vision occurs, the patient will often describe the experience that a curtain suddenly came down over their field of vision.

   Acute angle-closure glaucoma, option A, is a painful eye condition caused by sudden increasing pressure in the eye. It is also an emergency ocular event. Cataracts, option B, are a nonpainful clouding of the normally clear lens of the eye occurring over time as one ages. This condition affects vision in older age. Keratoconjunctivitis sicca, option C, which is also called dry eye, commonly affects older adults or those affected by autoimmune diseases. This condition is caused by the diminished lubricating and nourishing elements of tears, which in effect can cause increased tearing to occur. Macular degeneration, option D, is a painless and insidious eye disease causing gradual central vision loss. It is a leading cause of blindness in older populations. **Task:** C—Formulating Most Likely Diagnosis

9. **Answer: C** This patient's history is consistent with allergic rhinitis, which will typically include pale bluish nasal mucosa and cobblestoning of the posterior pharynx, option C, as well as clear rhinorrhea, visible drainage down the posterior pharynx, edema and discoloration under the eyes, conjunctival injection with clear discharge, and a transverse crease across the nose from pushing up due to itching and drainage.

   Atrophic rhinitis is typically seen in older adults or patients who have had multiple sinus surgeries. These patients have atrophy and thin nasal mucosa as well as crusting, option A. Patients with this disorder may say they smell a persistent bad odor. Otitis media includes an erythematous and bulging tympanic membrane with decreased mobility, option B. Cocaine use causes vasoconstriction and ischemic

necrosis that can present as a perforated nasal septum, option D. Acute streptococcal pharyngitis includes edematous and erythematous tonsils with exudate and cervical lymphadenopathy, option E. **Task:** A—History Taking and Performing Physical Examination

10. **Answer: B** Lidocaine, option B, or mineral oil, are used to kill insects in the ear prior to removing them. Lidocaine is the ideal choice because it provides local anesthesia for the removal process.

    Acetone, option A, is used to dissolve foreign bodies made of extruded polystyrene foam. Peroxide, option C, is most appropriate to use for removal of cerumen from the ear. Use of povidone-iodine, option D, can cause ototoxicity and should be avoided for use in the ear canal. Irrigation of the ear with water, option E, is not advised for use with organic foreign bodies because it can cause edema of the foreign body, making it difficult to remove. **Task:** D2—Clinical Intervention

11. **Answer: A** A fracture of the orbital floor, or blowout fracture, can occur from assault, being struck in the face by a ball, a motor vehicle collision, or a fall. Clinicians must have a high index of suspicion for complications such as entrapment of the inferior rectus muscle, which may cause loss of muscle function. Enophthalmos, or posterior displacement of the eye in the orbit, and an inability to look upwards, option A, as well as numbness below the eye are signs of entrapment.

    A zygomatic fracture is more likely to include malocclusion of the teeth as well as point tenderness over the zygoma, option B. Numbness of the forehead, option C, is more consistent with an orbital rim fracture and damage to the supraorbital nerve. A ruptured globe includes a tear-shaped pupil and hemorrhage, option D. A widened intercanthal distance, option E, is seen with disruption of the medial canthal ligament and a naso-orbito-ethmoid fracture. **Task:** A—History Taking and Performing Physical Examination

12. **Answer: B** The correct answer is chalazion, option B, which is an inflammation of the meibomian gland resulting in a nontender edema of the upper or lower eyelid.

    Blepharitis, option A, is a chronic bilateral inflammation of the lid margins. Dacryocystitis, option C, is an infection of the lacrimal sac. Hordeolum, option D, is an abscess on the upper or lower lid that appears as a localized red, edematous, and acutely tender area. Pinguecula, option E, appears as a yellow, conjunctival nodule. **Task:** A—History Taking and Performing Physical Examination

Answer Key for this chapter begins on p. 69

13. **Answer: E** This patient has signs and symptoms of epiglottitis, a life-threatening bacterial infection caused by narrowing of the glottic opening and airway obstruction. The first step in managing this condition is to ensure that the patient's airway is intact, option E. Evaluate the throat with direct visualization and obtain a throat culture, options A and B, are incorrect. With epiglottitis, it is important to ensure that the airway is secure prior to any interventions, including an intrusive physical examination and throat culture. Obtain white blood cell count and x-ray studies of the lateral neck, options C and D, are incorrect as well. Although these options help determine the diagnosis, these steps should not be completed until it is confirmed that the patient's airway is secure. **Task: D2—Clinical Intervention**

14. **Answer: E** Scraping the ulcer for culture, option E, is the most appropriate next step in diagnosis, because a corneal ulcer represents a serious multiple-layer infection that needs the offending organism identified to assure effective treatment. An ophthalmologist should be consulted to perform the scraping. The use of cyclosporine, an immunosuppressant, also puts this patient at risk for a broader spectrum of pathogens.
Confrontation visual field testing, fluorescein staining, and measurement of intraocular pressure (options A, B, and C) will not add diagnostic support for the corneal ulcer as pictured. Option D, orbital CT scan, is not indicated and is more helpful in the setting of trauma or significant periorbital cellulitis. **Task: B—Using Diagnostic and Laboratory Studies**

15. **Answer: C** Labyrinthitis, option C, is an inflammatory condition caused by bacterial or viral infections affecting the inner ear. Symptoms include sensorineural hearing loss, vertigo, and disequilibrium lasting hours to days.
An acoustic neuroma, option A, is a benign, slow-growing tumor. Pressure from the growing tumor results in unilateral sensorineural hearing loss, disequilibrium, intermittent dizziness, and facial numbness. Benign positional vertigo, option B, is associated with attacks of vertigo that are triggered by a change in head position with respect to gravity. This condition is not associated with hearing loss. Meniere disease, option D, is characterized by episodic vertigo, lasting minutes to hours, with fluctuating hearing loss and tinnitus. Patients often have the sensation of fullness in the affected ear. Vestibular neuritis, option E, is differentiated from labyrinthitis by lack of hearing loss. Labyrinthitis is associated with hearing changes in addition to dizziness and vertigo. Vestibular neuritis is caused by inflammation of the vestibular nerve and associated with vertigo and dizziness. **Task: C—Formulating Most Likely Diagnosis**

16. **Answer: C** This patient has an aphthous ulcer which is a painful, self-limited ulceration that occurs on non-keratinized oral mucosa. Decreasing physiological stress, option C, is correct because stress is a predisposing factor that triggers reoccurrences of aphthous ulcers.
Begin oral vitamin B_1 supplementation, option A, is incorrect because supplementation with vitamin B_{12} rather than vitamin B_1 is known to help decrease the recurrence of aphthous ulcers. Using toothpaste that contains sodium lauryl sulfate, option B, is a risk factor for developing aphthous ulcers. Patients should be encouraged instead to use toothpaste and mouthwash that are free of sodium lauryl sulfate. Performing daily rinses with warm salt water, option D, may provide symptomatic relief by decreasing inflammation. However, this measure is not known to prevent recurrences. Stop smoking cigarettes, option E, is incorrect because nonsmokers have a higher prevalence of recurrent aphthous ulcers than smokers. Smoking cessation, in this case, will not assist with decreasing the recurrence of these ulcers. **Task: D1—Health Maintenance, Patient Education, and Disease Prevention**

17. **Answer: B** This patient has acute laryngitis, a condition typically associated with a viral upper respiratory tract infection lasting less than three weeks. This is best treated with conservative care such as voice rest, increasing fluids, and humidified air, option B.
This patient does not have any evidence of a bacterial infection, and symptoms typically resolve without antibiotic therapy, option A. This patient does not have any concerning symptoms and is stable, so she does not need a higher level of care at an emergency department, option C. Voice therapy, option D, helps patients retrain the vocal muscles and can be helpful in certain conditions such as muscle tension dysphonia, functional dysphonia, and neurologic causes such as Parkinson disease. However, this type of therapy is not helpful in treating acute laryngitis. Referral to an otolaryngologist, option E, is recommended when symptoms last longer than two weeks or if the patient does not have associated symptoms of an upper respiratory tract infection. Concern for malignancy should also prompt a referral, including patients with a history of alcohol or tobacco use, pain, hemoptysis, dysphagia, stridor, mass, or unexplained weight loss. **Task: D2—Clinical Intervention**

18. **Answer: B** This patient has a hyphema, option B, which typically occurs after direct trauma to the eye. A tear occurs in the iris or the pupil creating a collection

of blood anterior to the iris and posterior to the cornea. Hyphemas are painful and can even block vision with significant blood pooling.

A blowout fracture and retinal detachment, options A and D, may accompany a hyphema depending on the nature of the injury. However, there is not enough evidence to make these diagnoses based on this patient's case and the image shown. A blowout fracture is diagnosed with imaging studies. Retinal detachment is diagnosed with a dilated funduscopic examination. Hypopyon, option C, is an accumulation of white, milky sediment in the anterior chamber of the eye visible on physical examination. This finding indicates an underlying inflammatory process taking place such as from uveitis, corneal ulcer, or Behçet disease. The visible layer of exudate occurs from an accumulation of white blood cells. Subconjunctival hemorrhage, option E, occurs when vessels of the conjunctiva break, causing a red spot to accumulate on the affected area of the sclera. Pain and obscured vision are not associated with this type of injury. **Task:** A—History Taking and Performing Physical Examination

19. **Answer: E** The correct answer is unilateral purulent rhinorrhea, option E, caused by the foreign body. Deviated nasal septum, option A, is most often congenital or due to trauma such as a broken nose. Erythema overlying the nares, option B, is a finding suggestive of cellulitis. Postnasal drip, option C, is a drip going down the back of the throat. It is most often associated with sinusitis and allergies and not a nasal foreign body. Tenderness to palpation of the upper teeth, option D, is a symptom of sinusitis. Sinusitis can be a complication of a nasal foreign body, but it is not an expected finding on day three to four. **Task:** A—History Taking and Performing Physical Examination

20. **Answer: B** This patient has suspected conductive hearing loss due to eustachian tube dysfunction. In this case, the Weber test will show lateralization to the affected (left) ear, option B. If this patient is suspected of having sensorineural hearing loss, then the sound would lateralize to the opposite (right) ear.

Diminished hearing in the right ear on whisper test, option A, is incorrect. In this patient's case, the expected finding on whisper test would be diminished hearing on the left side rather than the right side. No lateralization to the left ear on Weber test, option C, is incorrect. In the case of conductive hearing loss, the Weber test will show lateralization to the affected (left) ear. Ratio of air conduction to bone conduction in the left ear is equal to or greater than 2:1 on Rinne test (options D and E) are incorrect. In patients with conductive hearing loss, bone conduction is greater

than air conduction on Rinne test. **Task:** B—Using Diagnostic and Laboratory Studies

21. **Answer: A** This patient has a peritonsillar abscess. A muffled voice (option A), or hot potato voice as it is sometimes called, is one of the pathognomonic findings of this disorder. Other findings include medial deviation of the soft palate and peritonsillar fold on physical examination. A red, smooth tongue, option B, is indicative of glossitis and is not a finding in patients with peritonsillar abscess. Scarlatiniform rash, option C, is noted in patients with streptococcal pharyngitis. Steeple sign and thumb sign, options D and E, are x-ray findings for croup and epiglottitis, respectively. **Task:** A—History Taking and Performing Physical Examination

22. **Answer: C** Cataracts occur due to the opacification or clouding of the eye lens, option C. This can be caused by medications such as prednisone, the normal aging process, trauma, metabolic disorders (hereditary or acquired), or congenital problems.

The formation of drusen bodies, option A, occurs in patients with macular degeneration. Increased intraocular pressure, option B, is associated with acute angle and open-angle glaucoma. Retinal tears, option D, are associated with retinal detachment. Swelling of the macula, option E, is not related to cataract formation. **Task:** E—Applying Basic Scientific Concepts

23. **Answer: D** The correct answer is mastoiditis, option D, based on the patient's history of otitis media, displacement of the auricle, and erythema and tenderness over the mastoid area.

Acoustic neuroma, option A, is a benign tumor that develops in nerves from the inner ear to the brain; the tympanic membrane is not involved in this disorder. Erysipelas, option B, is a superficial form of cellulitis. Patients with this condition do not present with a bulging tympanic membrane. Eustachian tube dysfunction, option C, leads to otitis media but does not involve the mastoid area. Necrotizing fasciitis, option E, is a severe, rapidly spreading infection resulting in death of soft tissue usually marked by red or purple skin and bullae. It is not related to otitis media. **Task:** A—History Taking and Performing Physical Examination

24. **Answer: E** This patient has symptoms of blepharitis. Appropriate initial treatment includes lid hygiene with warm compresses to the affected area and gentle scrubbing with baby shampoo, option E.

Depending on other underlying conditions, pharmaceutical agents such as A through D may be prescribed. If a subsequent bacterial infection is suspected, antibiotic ointment, option A, may be prescribed. If an autoimmune condition is suspected, corticosteroid eyedrops, option B, may be added to the regimen. Oral doxycycline, option C, may be prescribed for meibomian gland dysfunction and infection. Topical cyclosporine, option D, can be used to treat dry eye. **Task: D2—Clinical Intervention**

25. **Answer: A** The parotid gland is the largest salivary gland. It is an exocrine gland situated at either side of the dental occlusal plains and is the most common of the salivary glands to be affected by an inflammatory process. This patient has parotitis, option A, which is inflammation of the parotid gland that occurs from infection, autoimmune disorders, and obstruction. Regardless of the cause, symptoms include pain, tenderness, warmth, and edema over the affected gland. Radiation of pain usually occurs at the ear and down the neck, as in this patient. Associated findings may also include anterior cervical lymphadenopathy. Treatment is aimed at the underlying cause of the inflammation.
Peritonsillar abscess, option B, usually follows a streptococcal pharyngitis infection and is associated with sore throat, fever, deviated uvula, and trismus. These findings are not present in this patient. Stomatitis, option C, is an inflammation of the oral mucosa of the mouth and lips. Typical manifestation includes vesicular, painful lesions. The underlying cause can be from a viral infection, trauma (such as biting the mucosa of the cheek when eating or dental work), and idiopathic causes. Although pain is associated with eating and palpation of the affected area, it is not associated with lymphadenopathy, radiating pain, and warmth and edema of the face. Temporal mandibular joint dysfunction, option D, is primarily caused by musculoskeletal issues of the temporal mandibular joint and/or muscles of mastication. Symptoms include jaw pain, pain with chewing and opening the mouth, and headache. It is not associated with cervical lymphadenopathy. Trigeminal neuralgia, option E, causes excruciating, sharp pain occurring at any of the three branches of the trigeminal nerve. Nerve aggravation triggers the pain event. Pain is intense and sporadic and can be triggered by the most minute event. The cyclic nature of this disorder, and unassociated findings of lymphadenopathy and facial edema, make this diagnosis less likely in this patient. **Task: A—History Taking and Performing Physical Examination**

26. **Answer: E** Periorbital edema, option E, is an indication of worsening acute sinusitis secondary to venous obstruction related to a specific bacterial etiology. Other symptoms of acute sinusitis that could lead to potential complications include erythema of the eyelid, pain with extraocular movements, and proptosis. Cough, dental pain, fever, and nasal discharge (options A through D) are all typical symptoms of acute sinusitis and are not a cause for concern. **Task: A—History Taking and Performing Physical Examination**

27. **Answer: E** This patient has suppurative otitis media with tympanic membrane perforation. Ofloxacin ear drops (option E), which is an antibiotic, is the most appropriate first-line treatment for this condition. Ear drops containing benzocaine, carbamide peroxide, chloroxylenol, or hydrocortisone (options A through D) may all be used to treat other types of ear problems, such as pain and inflammation, but should not be used when the tympanic membrane is compromised as with a rupture or perforation. **Task: D3—Pharmaceutical Therapeutics**

28. **Answer: C** Leukoplakia, option C, is a white plaque or lesion in the oropharynx that cannot be wiped off or diagnosed as any other distinct lesion. Leukoplakia has potential to undergo malignant transformation over time. Risk factors include smoking tobacco, smokeless tobacco use, and excessive alcohol use.
Hairy cell leukemia, option A, is a slow-growing blood cancer characterized by the excessive production of B-cell lymphocytes by the bone marrow. Oral findings include mucosa bruising and bleeding gums resulting from a decreased platelet count. Lesions associated with invasive squamous cell carcinoma, option B, are associated with lymphadenopathy, pain, numbness, dysphagia, or dysarthria. Over time, leukoplakia can transform into squamous cell carcinoma. As opposed to leukoplakia, oral candidiasis, option D, is characterized by white lesions that can be scraped off. Oral lichen planus, option E, results from an immune-mediated reaction characterized by erosive, atrophic, reticular plaquelike white lesions in a symmetrical distribution. These lesions are typically not associated with tobacco or alcohol use but rather an immune response triggered by certain medications or diseases. **Task: A—History Taking and Performing Physical Examination**

29. **Answer: C** The correct answer is option C, pain on palpation of the tragus, which is an objective finding most likely to support a diagnosis of otitis externa. Enlargement of the posterior cervical lymph nodes, option A, is incorrect. An enlarged lymph node in front of the tragus, or occasionally an enlarged anterior cervical node, is consistent with a diagnosis of otitis externa. Immobility of the tympanic membrane, option B, is consistent with otitis media but not otitis externa. Presence of vesicles in the external acoustic meatus, option D, is a finding suggestive of herpes zoster infection (Ramsay Hunt syndrome). Temperature more than 38.3°C (101.0°F), option E, most likely

indicates a complication. If fever is present in patients with otitis externa, it is most often less than 38.3°C (101.0°F). **Task:** A—History Taking and Performing Physical Examination

30. **Answer: E** This patient has orbital cellulitis possibly caused by methicillin-resistant *Staphylococcus aureus* (MRSA), which is an emergent condition. The most appropriate immediate treatment is intravenous administration of vancomycin, option E.

Penicillinase-resistant antibiotics are often used as a treatment option for MRSA; therefore, amoxicillin (option A), a penicillin antibiotic, is inappropriate. Isoniazid, option B, is used for treatment of tuberculosis and not cellulitis. Metronidazole, option C, is used in conjunction with penicillinase-resistant antibiotics or when there is a penicillin hypersensitivity, neither of which are described in this patient scenario. Solumedrol, option D, is a glucocorticoid corticosteroid and is not indicated as first-line treatment of cellulitis caused by MRSA. **Task:** D3—Pharmaceutical Therapeutics

31. **Answer: B** The most likely finding on funduscopic examination of this patient is papilledema, option B. Papilledema occurs with increased intracranial pressure typically caused by direct trauma, encephalitis, or a mass in the brain. Intracranial pressure causes edema of the optic nerve and blurring of the optic disc margins. When papilledema is present, it is most important to find the cause. This patient's presentation suggests encephalitis as the cause.

Cotton wool spots, option A, are caused by damaged nerve fibers on the retina of the eye, not the optic nerve. Cotton wool spots appear as white, fluffy patches on the retina. There are many possible etiologies for cotton wool spots, and their appearance may even be an idiopathic finding. While retinal detachment, option C, causes vision changes, typical presentation does not include edematous changes to the optic nerve. Retinoblastoma, option D, is a type of cancer occurring in the retina most commonly occurring in young children. Roth spots, option E, are red spots on the retina with a characteristic pale center commonly associated with bacterial endocarditis. **Task:** C—Formulating Most Likely Diagnosis

32. **Answer: B** The photograph shows an external hordeolum (stye), which is defined as an infection within a blocked gland of Zeis or Moll. As these glands are associated with a hair shaft (eyelash), an external hordeolum always occurs on the edge of the lid. The correct initial approach to treating a hordeolum is to apply a warm compress to the lid several times daily, option B. The warmth allows the lesion to come to a head, rupture, and spontaneously drain.

Although inflammation often accompanies a hordeolum, topical corticosteroids, option A, do not hasten recovery and are not indicated. Although *Staphylococcus aureus* is the typical infectious organism in a stye, resolution of symptoms appears to occur irrespective of topical or oral antibiotic use, option C. Incision and drainage, option D, is appropriate management for an internal hordeolum but is incorrect in this patient's case, because an external hordeolum is quite superficial and readily responds to much more conservative treatment. If conservative measures are not efficacious, incision and drainage may be a subsequent therapy. Marsupialization of the lesion, option E, includes incising a slit in an abscess and suturing the edges to prevent closure. This technique is most commonly applied to larger lesions such as pilonidal and Bartholin cysts and is certainly not indicated in this case. **Task:** D1—Health Maintenance, Patient Education, and Disease Prevention

33. **Answer: E** This patient has Meniere disease. The most common symptoms of this condition include aural fullness, hearing loss, tinnitus, and vertigo. The most appropriate initial treatment for Meniere disease is a low-salt diet and therapy with a diuretic, option E.

Antibiotics, antiemetics, antihistamines, and corticosteroids (options A through D) are not indicated in the initial treatment of patients with Meniere disease. Options B and C, antiemetics and antihistamines, may be used later in the disease course to treat associated symptoms of nausea and vomiting, if present. **Task:** D3—Pharmaceutical Therapeutics

34. **Answer: B** This patient has acute otitis media, option B, because of the abrupt onset of inflammation of the middle ear. The three most common pathogens of this condition are *Streptococcal pneumoniae*, *Haemophilus influenzae*, and *Moraxella catarrhalis*.

Acute otitis externa, option A, which is also called swimmer's ear, is an inflammation of the external auditory canal. This patient has no tenderness to palpation of the tragus or pinna, which are hallmark signs of acute otitis externa. Cerumen impaction, option C, is usually asymptomatic in adults or is caused by the use of a cotton swab to clean the ears. Upper respiratory tract infection, option D, can often be associated with acute otitis media but usually presents with symptoms of rhinorrhea, cough, and pharyngitis. Viral otitis externa, option E, has a clinical presentation that typically includes facial paralysis along with otalgia. On physical examination, vesicles may be noted in the auditory canal. **Task:** A—History Taking and Performing Physical Examination

35. **Answer: B** The finding on slit-lamp examination of this patient represents a positive Seidel test. A positive Seidel test occurs when fluorescein stain shows a flow of aqueous humor in a waterfall appearance as a lighter stain diluted by aqueous humor at the site of injury. The cause of this finding is a globe perforation, option B.

A corneal abrasion, option A, would show fluorescein stain catching at the site of the denuded cornea, and the stain would not appear lighter in color. Findings on slit-lamp examination of herpes simplex keratitis, option C, includes dendritic lesions, which are not present in this patient. Hyphema as a result of ocular trauma, option D, is indicated by a pooling of blood inside the anterior chamber of the eye. A corneal rust stain, option E, occurs when a metal foreign body is embedded in the cornea; it undergoes oxidation and forms a rust circle around the metal object. Although conditions are favorable for rust ring formation, the characteristic findings described are not consistent with this diagnosis. **Task:** C—Formulating Most Likely Diagnosis

BIBLIOGRAPHY

Anand, J., & Emerson, L. P. (2015). *Current concepts of Otitis Media and recent management strategies.* Jaypee Brothers Medical Publishers.

Bauman, N. (2009). Drugs and tinnitus: Put yourself in the driver's seat. *Tinnitus Today, 34*(1), 21-23.

Deafness, dizziness, and disorders of equilibrium. (2019). In A. H. Ropper, M. A. Samuels, J. P. Klein, & S. Prasad (Eds.), *Adams and victor's principles of neurology* (11th ed.). McGraw Hill.

Del Mar, C. (2016). Acute sinusitis and sore throat in primary care. *Australian Prescriber, 39*(4), 116-118.

deShazo, R. D., & Kemp, S. F. (2020). *Allergic rhinitis: Clinical manifestations, epidemiology and diagnosis.* UpToDate.

Domino, F. J., Baldor, R. A., Golding, J., & Stephens, M. B. (2019). *The 5-minute Clinical Consult 2020.* Lippincott Williams & Wilkins.

Durso, S. C. (2018). Oral manifestations of disease. In J. Jameson, A. S. Fauci, D. L. Kasper, S. L. Hauser, D. L. Longo, & J. Loscalzo (Eds.), *Harrison's principles of internal medicine* (20th ed.). McGraw Hill.

(2013). *Epocrates.* San Francisco, CA: Epocrates, Inc.; http://www.epocrates.com. Updated continuously.

Flores, A. R., & Cossera, M. T. (2020). *Mandell, Douglas and Bennett's principles and practice of infectious diseases* (chap 59, pp. 824-831). Elsevier.

Gariano, R. F., & Kim, C. -H. (2004). Evaluation and management of suspected retinal detachment. *American Family Physician, 69*(7), 1691-1698.

Horton, J. C. (2018). Disorders of the eye. In J. Jameson, A. S. Fauci, D. L. Kasper, S. L. Hauser, D. L. Longo, & J. Loscalzo (Eds.), *Harrison's principles of internal medicine* (20th ed.). McGraw Hill.

Jackson, J. L. (2020). *Pfenninger and Fowler's procedures for primary care* (chap 57, pp. 365-370). Elsevier.

Jung, J. Eye. In W. W. Jr. Hay, M. J. Levin, M. J. Abzug & M. Bunik (Eds.), *Current diagnosis & treatment: Pediatrics* (25th ed.). McGraw Hill.

Lustig, L. R., & Schindler, J. S. (2021). Diseases of the ear canal. In M. A. Papadakis, S. J. McPhee, & M. W. Rabow (Eds.), *Current medical diagnosis & treatment 2021.* McGraw Hill.

Lustig, L. R., & Schindler, J. S. (2021). Diseases of the inner ear. In M. A. Papadakis, S. J. McPhee, & M. W. Rabow (Eds.), *Current medical diagnosis & treatment 2021.* McGraw Hill.

Lustig, L. R., & Schindler, J. S. (2021). Diseases of the Middle Ear. In M. A. Papadakis, S. J. McPhee, & M. W. Rabow (Eds.), *Current medical diagnosis & treatment 2021.* McGraw Hill.

Lustig, L. R., & Schindler, J. S. (2021). Epistaxis. In M. A. Papadakis, S. J. McPhee, & M. W. Rabow (Eds.), *Current medical diagnosis & treatment 2021.* McGraw Hill.

Neuman, M. I., & Bachur, R. G. (2020). Orbital fractures. In T. Post (Ed.), *UpToDate.* Waltham, MA: UpToDate.

Onoh, A., Linnebur, S. A., & Fixen, D. R. (2018). Moxifloxacin-induced tinnitus in an older adult. *Therapeutic Advances in Drug Safety, 9*(4), 219-221.

Papadakis, M. A., & McPhee, S. F. (2020). *Current medical diagnosis & treatment 2020.* McGraw Hill.

Patel, P., Scott, S., & Cunningham, S. (2017). Challenging case of parotitis: A comprehensive approach. *The Journal of the American Osteopathic Association, 117*(12), 137-140.

Pelton, S. I. *Mandell, Douglas, and Bennett's principles and practice of infectious diseases* (9th ed., chap 61, pp. 835-843).

Pflipsen, M., Massaquoi, M., & Wolf, S. (2016). Evaluation of the painful eye. *American Family Physician, 93*(12), 991-998.

Putnam, C. M. (2016). Diagnosis and management of blepharitis: An optometrist's perspective. *Clinical Optometry, 8,* 71.

Rubin, M. A., Ford, L. C., & Gonzales, R. (2018). Sore throat, earache, and upper respiratory symptoms. In J. Jameson, A. S. Fauci, D. L. Kasper, S. L. Hauser, D. L. Longo, & J. Loscalzo (Eds.), *Harrison's principles of internal medicine* (20th ed.). McGraw Hill.

Stevenw, H., & Karenl, M. (2007). Foreign bodies in the ear, nose, and throat. *American Family Physician, 76*(8), 1185-1189.

Templer, J. W. (2020). Parotitis. In A. D. Meyers (Ed.) *Medscape.*

Turbert, D. (2020). *What is hyphema.* American Academy of Ophthalmology.

Usatine, R. P., Gonsalves, W. C., & Díaz, D. (2019). Aphthous ulcer. In R. P. Usatine, M. A. Smith, E. J. MayeauxJr., & H. S. Chumley (Eds.), *The color atlas and synopsis of family Medicine* (3rd ed.). McGraw Hill.

Vagefi, M. Lids & lacrimal apparatus. In P. Riordan-Eva, & J. J. Augsburger (Eds.), *Vaughan & Asbury's general ophthalmology* (19th ed.). McGraw Hill.

Walker, M. F., & Daroff, R. B. Dizziness and vertigo. In J. Jameson, A. S. Fauci, D. L. Kasper, S. L. Hauser, D. L. Longo, & J. Loscalzo

(Eds.), *Harrison's principles of internal medicine* (20th ed.). McGraw Hill.

Walker, R. A., & Adhikari, S. Eye emergencies. In J. E. Tintinalli, O. Ma, D. M. Yealy, G. D. Meckler, J. Stapczynski, D. M. Cline, & S. H. Thomas (Eds.), *Tintinalli's emergency medicine: A comprehensive study guide* (9th ed.). McGraw Hill.

Wolff, K., Johnson, R. A., Saavedra, A. P., & Roh, E. K. (2017). *Fitzpatrick's color atlas and synopsis of clinical dermatology.* McGraw Hill.

Yellon, R. F., & Chi, D. H. (2017). *Zitelli and Davis atlas of pediatric physical diagnosis* (7th ed., chap 24, pp. 868-915). Elsevier.

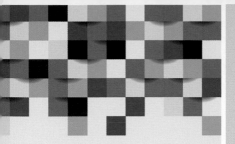

CHAPTER 5
Gastrointestinal System and Nutrition

Questions

1. A 22-year-old woman comes to the emergency department because she has had abdominal pain for the past five hours. She says the pain began in the periumbilical region and has since moved to the right lower quadrant. The pain is sharp and exacerbated by movement. She rates the pain as a 9 on a 10-point scale. Temperature is 38.1°C (100.5°F). On physical examination, the abdomen is firm, bowel sounds are diminished, and there is tenderness and guarding with light and deep palpation in the right lower quadrant. Obturator and psoas signs are positive. Which of the following is the most appropriate management?
A. Antibiotic therapy with follow-up in one week
B. Antibiotic therapy with laparoscopic appendectomy in six weeks
C. CT-guided drainage of an abdominal abscess
D. Laparoscopic appendectomy
E. Serial ultrasonography and then plan for laparoscopic appendectomy if the condition worsens

2. A 9-year-old girl is brought to the office by her mother for routine well-child examination. The mother is concerned because the patient has been gaining weight ever since she and her husband went through a terrible divorce six months ago. The patient is in the 90th percentile for weight. It is most appropriate to recommend which of the following to the mother regarding weight loss in this patient?
A. Consumption of fast food needs to be limited to once a week
B. Consumption of sugary drinks needs to be limited to once daily
C. The entire family needs to adopt a healthy lifestyle along with the patient
D. The patient should strive to achieve rapid weight loss of at least 2 lb per week
E. Unhealthy foods need to be kept out of reach of the patient

3. A 55-year-old man is admitted to the hospital because he has had significant weight loss of 16 lb, polydipsia, polyuria, and blurry vision during the past two months.

Pulse rate is 114/min and blood pressure is 102/60 mmHg. Medical history includes alcohol use disorder and chronic pancreatitis. Physical examination shows dry mucous membranes and poor skin turgor. Findings on laboratory studies of serum include the following:

Calcium	9.4 mg/dL (N = 8.6–10.3 mg/dL)
Sodium	138 mEq/L (N = 135–145 mEq/L)
Potassium	4.2 mEq/L (N = 3.6–5.2 mEq/L)
Glucose	284 mg/dL (N = 80–140 mg/dL)
Hemoglobin A_{1c}	10% (N = < 5.7%)

C-peptide level is within normal limits. Which of the following is the most appropriate treatment regimen?
A. Extended-release metformin therapy once daily
B. Glipizide therapy twice daily with meals
C. Orlistat therapy once daily
D. Semaglutide therapy once per week
E. Sitagliptin therapy once daily

4. A 28-year-old woman comes to the clinic because she has had cramping abdominal pain one to two days per week for the past several years. She says the pain is often associated with diarrhea. At times, defecation makes the pain worse, while at other times it relieves the pain. The patient has been evaluated in multiple emergency departments over the past several years for these symptoms, but results of laboratory studies have always been within normal limits, and CT scans have shown no abnormalities. According to the Rome IV Diagnostic Criteria for Irritable Bowel Syndrome (IBS), this patient has two of the criteria for diagnosing IBS—recurrent abdominal pain related to defecation and associated with a change in stool form. Which of the following is the third criteria that is most likely to confirm a diagnosis of IBS in this patient?
A. Change in color of the stool
B. Change in stool frequency
C. Nocturnal diarrhea
D. Presence of blood in the stool
E. Vomiting

5. A 47-year-old woman who is a health care worker comes to the clinic because she has malaise, nausea and vomiting, fatigue, and an achiness in the right upper quadrant of her abdomen approximately two months after she was exposed to blood while at work. Vital signs are within normal limits. Physical examination shows jaundice to the sclera of the eyes. Tenderness to palpation is noted in the right upper quadrant of the abdomen. Acute hepatitis B infection is suspected. Which of the following laboratory studies is most likely to confirm the diagnosis?
   A. Alanine aminotransferase and aspartate aminotransferase levels
   B. Hepatitis B surface antibody and hepatitis B core antibody
   C. Hepatitis B surface antibody and hepatitis B e antigen
   D. Hepatitis B surface antigen and hepatitis B virus DNA
   E. Hepatitis B surface antigen and IgM antibody to hepatitis B core antigen

6. Emergency medical technicians are called to the home of a 14-year-old boy after he was found unconscious on the floor. Temperature is 36.4°C (97.6°F), pulse rate is 106/min, respirations are 11/min and shallow, and blood pressure is 80/62 mmHg. Blood glucose level is 72 mg/dL (N = 80–100 mg/dL). On physical examination, the pupils are constricted and nonreactive to light and accommodation. The skin is cool, and bowel sounds are decreased. Which of the following is the most likely diagnosis?
   A. Acute subdural hematoma
   B. Alcohol intoxication
   C. Bacterial meningitis
   D. Hypoglycemia
   E. Opioid toxicity

7. A 35-year-old woman is brought to the emergency department because she has had nausea and bilious vomiting for the past day. She also has had diffuse abdominal pain and swelling. The patient has no history of recent travel, change in diet, or sick contacts. Her most recent bowel movement was three days ago, and no blood or melena was noted. Medical history includes endometriosis. Physical examination shows a distended tympanic abdomen with diffuse tenderness and guarding. Bowel sounds are high-pitched. Abdominal x-ray studies show distended loops of small bowel with multiple air-fluid levels. Small-bowel obstruction is confirmed. Which of the following is the most likely cause?
   A. Adhesions
   B. Foreign body
   C. Intussusception
   D. Neoplasm
   E. Volvulus

8. A 34-year-old man with Crohn disease comes to the clinic because he has had rectal pain when sitting and passing stool during the past two weeks. Rectal examination shows a fistula tract. Which of the following conditions is most likely to have preceded these findings in this patient?
   A. Anal condyloma
   B. Anal fissure
   C. Anorectal abscess
   D. Hemorrhoids
   E. Pilonidal cyst

9. An 86-year-old man comes to the emergency department because he has had abdominal pain and constipation for the past five days. His most recent bowel movement was six days ago. Medical history includes a recent diagnosis of lung cancer, for which a "pain medication" was initiated. The patient says that since he has started taking this medication, he has been unable to have a bowel movement. X-ray studies of the abdomen show a nonspecific bowel gas pattern without signs of perforation; a large stool burden is noted. Which of the following pain medications is most likely causing the constipation in this patient?
   A. Acetaminophen
   B. Diclofenac sodium
   C. Ibuprofen
   D. Lidocaine
   E. Oxycodone

10. A 2-year-old girl is brought to the local urgent care by her parents because she developed a rash after snack time at daycare two hours ago. The father says that the patient ate three peanut butter cookies at snack time; he does not know if she has had this type of cookie in the past. The patient has not had vomiting, but she had one incident of loose stool while in the clinic's waiting room. The parents say that she has been playing outside more often with several healthy children in the local neighborhood. Temperature is 37.0°C (98.6°F), pulse rate is 90/min, and respirations are 22/min. Oxygen saturation is 100%. The patient does not appear to be in respiratory distress, but she occasionally scratches her upper extremities and neck. Physical examination shows perioral erythema with no edema or pallor. The airway is patent, and no adenopathy is noted. Which of the following findings on history and physical examination is most suggestive of a food allergy in this patient?
    A. Perioral erythema with no edema or pallor
    B. Potential sick contacts in the neighborhood
    C. Symptoms beginning two hours after snack time
    D. Uncertainty of previous peanut butter ingestion
    E. Vital signs that are within normal limits

11. A 57-year-old woman comes to the office because she continues to have daily symptoms of gastroesophageal reflux disease (GERD) despite initiating twice daily therapy with a proton pump inhibitor (PPI) seven months ago. GERD was initially diagnosed three years ago, and her symptoms of heartburn and regurgitation were responsive to avoidance of aggravating foods and antacids as needed for the first year. Approximately two years ago, once daily PPI therapy was initiated because her symptoms became worse. Current esophagogastroduodenoscopy confirms a hiatal hernia. Which of the following surgical procedures is the most appropriate next step in management?
    A. Indiana pouch procedure
    B. Laparoscopic esophagectomy
    C. Nissen fundoplication
    D. Roux-en-Y procedure
    E. Whipple procedure

12. A 46-year-old woman comes to the emergency department because she has had abdominal pain, fever up to 39.2°C (102.6°F), and yellowing of her eyes during the past two days. The patient's roommate says that she has "not been all there" today and seems confused. Current temperature is 38.8°C (101.9°F), pulse rate is 106/min, and blood pressure is 102/64 mmHg. Oxygen saturation is 99%. Physical examination shows marked tenderness to palpation of the right upper quadrant. Laboratory studies show an increased white blood cell count as well as elevated serum C-reactive protein, bilirubin, and alkaline phosphatase levels. Ultrasonography of the abdomen shows dilation of the bile duct and evidence of stones. Which of the following is the most likely diagnosis?
    A. Acute cholangitis
    B. Acute cholecystitis
    C. Acute pancreatitis
    D. Liver abscess

13. A 16-year-old boy is brought to the emergency department by his mother because he has had fever and several episodes of bloody diarrhea during the past two hours. He also has had pain in the lower abdomen, tenesmus, and worsening diarrhea over the past 24 hours. The patient says he has mild nausea, but he has not vomited. The mother says that he has no history of changes in diet, sick contacts, or illnesses. He recently returned from a mission trip where he spent two weeks in an underdeveloped country where he ate and drank the native food and water. Temperature is

39.2°C (102.6°F), pulse rate is 96/min, respirations are 17/min, and blood pressure is 117/76 mmHg. Oxygen saturation is 100%. The patient appears uncomfortable. Physical examination shows mild generalized abdominal pain. Murphy sign is absent, and there is no tenderness to palpation of McBurney point. Which of the following agents is most likely to be present in the stool culture?
    A. *Bacillus cereus*
    B. *Clostridium difficile*
    C. *Helicobacter pylori*
    D. Rotavirus
    E. *Shigella dysenteriae*

14. A 46-year-old man comes to the clinic because he has had painless, bright red bleeding from his rectum after bowel movements during the past three months. He also has had occasional itching around his perirectal area during this time. Digital rectal examination as well as anoscopy confirm grade 1 internal hemorrhoids. Which of the following findings, if present on history taking, most likely contributed to the development of hemorrhoids in this patient?
    A. Family history of prostate cancer
    B. History of appendicitis at 16 years of age
    C. History of constipation during the past six months
    D. Initiation of a vegetarian diet three months ago
    E. Recent completion of antibiotic therapy for a tooth infection

15. A 42-year-old woman is brought to the emergency department by her family members because she has had frequent falls secondary to an ataxic gait during the past week. It is difficult to obtain a history because the patient is confused and has slurred speech. According to her family members, she has not been acting like herself and has been more irritable lately. Physical examination shows involuntary twisting of the upper arms in a repetitive fashion. Slit-lamp examination shows brown pigmented rings around the periphery. On laboratory studies, the result of indirect Coombs test for hemolytic anemia is negative, serum aspartate aminotransferase and alanine aminotransferase levels are elevated, and serum ceruloplasmin level is decreased. CT scan of the head shows no abnormalities. Which of the following is the most appropriate treatment?
    A. D-penicillamine
    B. Levodopa
    C. Pyrimethamine
    D. Tetrabenazine
    E. Therapeutic phlebotomy

16. A 7-year-old boy is brought to the clinic by his parents because he has had intermittent vomiting, dysphagia, heartburn, and poor weight gain during the past 12 months. Medical history includes eczema, seasonal allergic rhinitis, and peanut allergy. Recent upper endoscopy showed esophageal furrows without erosions. Peripheral blood smear is most likely to show a predominance of which of the following blood cell types?
    A. Basophils
    B. Eosinophils
    C. Lymphocytes
    D. Monocytes
    E. Neutrophils

17. A 40-year-old man comes to the emergency department because he has had generalized abdominal pain, fever to 38.9°C (102.0°F), diarrhea, and nausea for the past 24 hours. He rates the abdominal pain as a 10 on a 10-point scale. Medical history includes ulcerative colitis and hypertension. Current medications include lisinopril. Current temperature is 39.4°C (103.0°F), pulse rate is 122/min, respirations are 22/min, and blood pressure is 96/62 mmHg. Oxygen saturation is 95% on room air. Physical examination of the abdomen shows distention, generalized tenderness to palpation, decreased bowel sounds, and rebound and guarding. CT scan of the abdomen is planned. In the meantime, x-ray studies of the abdomen show significant dilation measuring 8 cm of the ascending and transverse colon. Which of the following is the most likely diagnosis?
    A. Colorectal cancer
    B. Ischemic colitis
    C. Toxic megacolon
    D. Ulcerative colitis

18. A 17-year-old boy comes to the emergency department because he has felt drunk and not well for the past two hours despite not drinking any alcohol. He says he recently ate a meal that his girlfriend prepared consisting of pasta and punch. Results of laboratory studies are pending. While waiting, the patient's mother and several law enforcement officers come to the emergency department to say that the patient's girlfriend admitted to putting some antifreeze in the punch in an attempt to kill him. After hemodialysis, treatment with which of the following drugs is the most appropriate next step?

A. Deferoxamine
B. Fomepizole
C. Hydroxocobalamin
D. Pralidoxime
E. Pyridostigmine

19. A 38-year-old woman comes to the family medicine clinic because she has had gnawing, dull discomfort in the epigastric region for the past four months. She rates the pain as a 4 on a 10-point scale and says that it goes away after taking an antacid but returns after four to five hours. Vital signs are within normal limits, and physical examination shows no abnormalities. Results of laboratory studies are within normal limits. Electrocardiography shows a normal sinus rhythm with no abnormalities. Esophagogastroduodenoscopy shows nonbleeding gastric and duodenal ulcers. Which of the following is the most likely cause of the findings in this patient?
    A. Alcohol use disorder
    B. Caffeine use
    C. Cytomegalovirus
    D. *Helicobacter pylori* infection
    E. Spicy food

20. A 31-year-old woman, gravida 1, para 1, comes to the OB/GYN office because she has had worsening rectal pain during and immediately after defecation for the past three weeks. The patient is one month post partum from a vaginal birth. She rates the pain between 7 and 9 on a 10-point scale and describes it as a tearing sensation, as if she is passing shards of glass. The pain resolves approximately 30 minutes after defecation, but it returns with the next bowel movement. She says she also has had minor rectal bleeding, stool that is streaked with bright red blood, and perianal pruritus. Physical examination with the patient in the Sims position shows a posterior midline elliptical separation in the epithelial lining with fresh mucosal edges and some mild granulation tissue. In addition to a high-fiber diet, which of the following is the most appropriate recommendation?
    A. Acetaminophen suppository
    B. Colonoscopy
    C. Sitz baths
    D. Surgical correction
    E. Topical nitroglycerine

21.

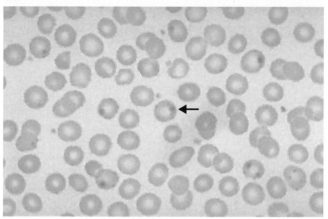

A 47-year-old man comes to the office because he had sudden onset of jaundice, fatigue, increased heart rate, diarrhea, abdominal pain, and dark urine one week after receiving vaccinations and initiating malaria prophylaxis for an upcoming trip to Africa. Current laboratory studies show hemoglobin level of 8.2 g/dL (N = 13.5–17.5 g/dL) and reticulocyte count of 8% of red cells (N = 0.5–1.5% of red cells). A photomicrograph of a peripheral blood smear is shown. Which of the following is the most likely diagnosis?

A. Chronic lymphocytic leukemia
B. Chronic myelogenous leukemia
C. G6PD deficiency
D. Lead poisoning
E. Multiple myeloma

22. A 4-week-old male infant is brought to the emergency department by his mother because he has had recurrent projectile vomiting during the past week. The mother says that the vomiting typically occurs shortly after feeding, and it has progressively become projectile and forceful during the past few days. No bile has been noted in the vomitus. Between feedings, the patient is playful and appears well. On physical examination, a 2-cm firm, movable olive-shaped mass is palpated in the right upper epigastric region of the abdomen. Which of the following is the most likely diagnosis?

A. Duodenum atresia
B. Gastric volvulus
C. Gastroesophageal reflux disease
D. Intussusception
E. Pyloric stenosis

23. A 48-year-old woman comes to the urgent care clinic because she has had intermittent pain in the right upper abdomen during the past six months. She says the pain occurs after she eats fatty foods, and it is often associated with nausea, bloating, and flatulence. Temperature is 37.1°C (98.8°F), pulse rate is 92/min, respirations are 18/min, and blood pressure is 138/70 mmHg. Physical examination shows no abnormalities. Results of laboratory studies and ultrasonography are pending. Cholecystitis is suspected. Which of the following additional findings is most likely to distinguish chronic cholecystitis from acute cholecystitis in this patient?

A. Elevated liver function tests
B. Gallbladder contraction
C. Increased white blood cell count
D. Pericholecystic inflammation
E. Thickened gallbladder wall

24. A 20-year-old woman comes to the primary care office because she has had episodes of diarrhea, bloating, fatigue, and dyspepsia after eating during the past three years. She says she recently noticed bright-red blood in her stool and is concerned. The patient is a college athlete and says that her symptoms are worse after she attends pasta parties prior to game days. Laboratory studies show an abnormal result on tissue transglutaminase 2-IgA antibody titer, and the patient is referred to a gastroenterologist. In the meantime, it is most appropriate to recommend that this patient eat which of the following types of diet?

A. Carbohydrate-controlled
B. Gluten-free
C. High-fiber
D. Ketogenic
E. Low-salt

25. A 55-year-old man with portal hypertension comes to the office for follow-up to discuss the results of an esophagogastroduodenoscopy (EGD) one week ago to evaluate for the presence of esophageal varices. He is told that the EGD shows nonbleeding varices in the esophagus. The patient then asks what can be done to prevent the varices from bleeding in the future. Initiation of therapy with which of the following types of drugs is most appropriate to recommend to this patient?

A. Antibiotics
B. Anxiolytics
C. Nonselective beta-blockers
D. Nonsteroidal anti-inflammatory drugs
E. Vasoconstrictors

Answer Key for this chapter begins on p. 85

26. An 18-month-old girl is brought to the emergency department by her parents because she has had nausea and vomiting as well as grossly bloody stools for the past three hours. The patient is crying and in distress, and she insists on drawing her knees to her chest. Physical examination shows a palpable mass in the abdomen. Ultrasonography of the abdomen shows an area of multiple concentric rings found within the distal ileum/proximal cecum. Intestinal obstruction is suspected. Which of the following is the most likely cause?

A. Adhesions
B. Bezoar
C. Intussusception
D. Pyloric stenosis
E. Volvulus

27. A 78-year-old woman comes to the emergency department because she had acute onset of excruciating abdominal pain one hour ago. She says she also vomited twice during this time. The pain is centered primarily around the umbilicus. Pulse rate is 92/min, respirations are 20/min, and blood pressure is 148/92 mmHg. Oxygen saturation is 98%. On physical examination, bowel sounds are absent. Abdominal distention is noted, and the abdomen is tender to palpation in all quadrants. Contrast-enhanced CT scan of the abdomen and pelvis shows focal wall thickening, intestinal pneumatosis, and mesenteric stranding in the region of the splenic flexure. There is a lack of contrast enhancement noted within the same region. Which of the following is the most appropriate initial management?

A. Admit the patient to the hospital for administration of intravenous antibiotics
B. Admit the patient to the hospital for monitoring once the nausea and pain are controlled
C. Arrange for urgent gastroenterology consultation
D. Arrange for urgent surgical consultation
E. Discharge the patient to home once the pain and nausea are controlled

28. A 42-year-old woman comes to the emergency department because she has had worsening abdominal bloating and swelling of both lower extremities over the past two weeks. She says she drinks about five to six glasses of wine daily and admits that she has been counseled to stop drinking multiple times because of "liver problems." Physical examination shows spider nevi, a firm palpable liver, and positive shifting dullness to percussion. An elevation in which of the following laboratory studies is most likely to indicate that the liver disease in this patient has progressed to cirrhosis?

A. Albumin level
B. Hemoglobin level
C. International normalized ratio
D. Platelet count
E. Sodium level

29. A 34-year-old man comes to the clinic as a new patient to establish care. During the interview, he says that his father died of colon cancer at 55 years of age; he is concerned about the possibility of developing this type of cancer as well. Based on this finding, it is most appropriate to recommend that this patient be screened for colon cancer at which of the following ages?

A. 35
B. 40
C. 45
D. 50
E. 55

30. A 65-year-old man with moderate to severe gastroesophageal reflux disease comes to the primary care office because he has had dysphagia for the past two weeks. He also has had regurgitation of gastric contents as well as worsening heartburn, despite increasing his dose of omeprazole to twice daily. He says he feels as if food is either getting stuck in his esophagus or he cannot swallow. The patient's most recent endoscopy was approximately five years ago. Based on these findings, which of the following is the most likely diagnosis?

A. Barrett esophagus
B. Esophageal stricture
C. Esophageal varices
D. Esophagitis
E. Gastritis

31. A 45-year-old woman comes to the emergency department because she has had pain in the left lower quadrant of her abdomen for the past two days that started after she ate fried chicken. Medical history includes no chronic disease conditions. Body mass index is 40 kg/m² (N = 18.5–24.9 kg/m²), and vital signs are within normal limits. Physical examination shows tenderness to palpation of the left lower quadrant of the abdomen. Contrast-enhanced CT scan of the abdomen and pelvis shows multiple stones located in the gallbladder with no inflammation of the gallbladder wall. Which of the following is the most appropriate immediate next step?

A. Extracorporeal shock wave lithotripsy
B. HIDA radionuclide scan
C. Laparoscopic cholecystectomy
D. Ultrasonography of the gallbladder
E. Weight loss and lifestyle changes

32. A two-year-old boy is brought to the emergency department by his mother because he told her that he swallowed some coins. Vital signs are within normal limits. The patient does not appear to be in distress and is playing with a cellular phone. Physical examination shows no abnormalities. X-ray studies of the abdomen show one radiopaque coin that appears to be a dime in the stomach. Which of the following is the most appropriate management?
    A. Emetic therapy
    B. Endoscopy
    C. Glucagon therapy
    D. Laxative therapy
    E. Observation

33. A 52-year-old man comes to the office because he has had a painful lump in his left groin for the past three days. He says the pain started after he lifted a heavy couch while helping a friend move. The pain started as more of a dull discomfort, then it became a little worse by the end of his shift as a cashier yesterday, and today the pain has become more intense. He currently has a fever, has had three episodes of vomiting, and says that his stomach feels like a balloon. Which of the following findings on physical examination is most likely to indicate that this patient needs immediate surgical exploration and repair?
    A. Bulge that disappears when the patient is supine
    B. Erythema of the skin with inability to reduce the mass
    C. Fluctuance over the area with purulent discharge
    D. Hard, fixed nodules along the inguinal ligament
    E. Soft scrotal mass that feels like a bag of worms

34. An 18-year-old woman comes to the emergency department because she has had nausea and vomiting for the past 12 hours. Pulse rate is 88/min, respirations are 20/min, and blood pressure is 108/72 mmHg. Oxygen saturation is 99% on room air. The patient appears thin. Physical examination shows widespread tooth decay. Cardiac auscultation shows a regular rate and rhythm with no gallops, clicks, rubs, or murmurs. The lungs are clear to auscultation bilaterally. Mild tenderness to palpation of the epigastrium is noted. Bowel sounds are present in all quadrants. Near the end of the physical examination, the patient begins to vomit copious amounts of bright red blood. After establishing intravenous access, baseline laboratory values including hematocrit, hemoglobin, prothrombin time, activated partial thromboplastin time, and type and screen are ordered. In addition to intravenous administration of a proton pump inhibitor and antiemetics, which of the following is the most important next step?

A. Admit the patient to the hospital for general surgery consultation
B. Discharge to home and recommend outpatient follow-up with a gastroenterologist
C. Obtain a CT scan of the chest and abdomen
D. Refer for emergent upper endoscopy
E. Repeat laboratory studies in 24 hours

35. A 22-year-old woman comes to the family medicine clinic for examination prior to going on her first vacation outside of the United States. The patient is healthy, immunizations are up-to-date, and the only medication she takes is a daily oral contraceptive pill. She says she is traveling to a developing country and would like to know what preventative measures she should implement while away. After learning about the common occurrence of traveler's diarrhea and what to expect with this condition, the patient asks for the best preventive measure while traveling. Which of the following is most appropriate to tell this patient?
    A. Avoid engaging with local residents while in country
    B. Avoid ingesting fresh foods and local water sources
    C. Do not travel more than 10 miles from the hotel
    D. Take prophylactic antibiotics prior to departure
    E. Take prophylactic antidiarrheal pills prior to departure

36. A 49-year-old man comes to the emergency department because he had sudden onset of pain in the left lower quadrant of the abdomen three days ago. He also has had nausea and vomiting as well as anorexia. Medical history includes obesity, hypertension, and chronic intermittent constipation. Medications include hydrochlorothiazide and docusate sodium. The patient has smoked one half pack of cigarettes per day for the past 20 years. Temperature is 37.7°C (99.9°F), pulse rate is 102/min, respirations are 14/min, and blood pressure is 145/90 mmHg. Oxygen saturation is 98% on room air. Physical examination shows sweaty, pale skin. Tachycardia is noted on cardiac auscultation. Pain is noted on palpation of the left lower quadrant. No guarding is noted, and bowel sounds are present in all four quadrants. Which of the following imaging studies is the most appropriate next step in diagnosis?
    A. Colonoscopy
    B. Contrast-enhanced CT scan of the abdomen and pelvis
    C. HIDA radionuclide scan
    D. Ultrasonography of the abdomen
    E. X-ray studies of the kidneys, ureter, and bladder

  Answer Key for this chapter begins on p. 85

37. A 60-year-old man comes to the clinic because he has had worsening constipation over the past four weeks. Currently, he says that he feels like he needs to have a bowel movement, but the stool will not come out. The patient also says that he has had a 40-lb unintentional weight loss during the past six months. On physical examination, the abdomen is distended, and there is tenderness to palpation beneath the umbilicus. CT scan of the abdomen and pelvis shows a transition point in the sigmoid colon with significant narrowing of the lumen of the bowel. Which of the following is the most likely diagnosis?
    A. Appendicitis
    B. Cancerous obstruction of the colon
    C. Diverticulitis
    D. Intussusception
    E. Volvulus

38. A 54-year-old woman comes to the emergency department because she has had persistent pain in the epigastric region for the past two days. She has not had nausea and vomiting or hematemesis. She rates the pain as an 8 on a 10-point scale and says that the pain increases to 10 after she eats or is supine. The pain is not relieved with acetaminophen or ibuprofen. Medical history includes alcohol use disorder, but the patient has been sober for the past 10 months. Pulse rate is 118/min, and blood pressure is 92/50 mmHg. All other vital signs are within normal limits. She says that her blood pressure is usually around 110/70 mmHg, and her pulse rate is always less than 70/min. Physical examination shows tenderness to palpation in the epigastric region and abdominal distention. Laboratory studies show an elevated white blood cell count and increased serum aspartate aminotransferase, amylase, and lipase levels. Hemoglobin level, hematocrit, serum alanine aminotransferase, and serum alkaline phosphatase levels are within normal limits. Electrocardiography shows a normal sinus tachycardia. Which of the following is the most likely diagnosis?

    A. Acute pancreatitis
    B. Boerhaave syndrome
    C. Cirrhosis
    D. Duodenal ulcer
    E. Mallory-Weiss tears

39. A 26-year-old woman comes to the family practice office because she has had fatigue for the past month. She says she also has had seven to nine mostly bloody bowel movements on a daily basis during the past two months. The patient has had unintentional weight loss of 19 lb (>10% of her body weight) during this time. She says she waited this long to seek care because she did not have insurance, but she now has full coverage. Colonoscopy shows no evidence of colon cancer. Which of the following findings is most likely on further workup of this patient?
    A. Erythrocyte sedimentation rate within normal limits
    B. Hematocrit >40%
    C. Hypoalbuminemia
    D. Skip lesion on colonoscopy
    E. Terminal ileitis

40. A 4-year-old boy is brought to the emergency department by his mother because she found him with his mouth on the opening of a drain cleaner bottle one hour ago. The mother is not sure how much of the drain cleaner the patient ingested. He has mild pain in the epigastric region and mid chest. The patient is drooling and has had one episode of vomiting. Otherwise, the patient is asymptomatic and hemodynamically stable. The local poison control center is contacted for recommendations. Which of the following is the most appropriate study to assess for damage in this patient?
    A. Abdominal ultrasonography
    B. Chest x-ray study
    C. Contrast-enhanced CT scan of the abdomen
    D. MRI of the abdomen
    E. Upper endoscopy

Answers

1. **Answer: D** This patient has appendicitis. Laparoscopic appendectomy, option D, is the treatment of choice for appendicitis. A laparoscopic appendectomy is associated with improved cosmetic results, decreased length of stay, decreased postoperative pain, and decreased risk of wound infection.

   Antibiotic therapy and then follow-up in one week or laparoscopic appendectomy in six weeks (options A and B) are both incorrect. Broad-spectrum antibiotics are recommended for the treatment of appendicitis, but a prompt appendectomy is the most appropriate management. Scheduling a follow-up evaluation in one week or laparoscopic surgery in six weeks is inappropriate. CT-guided drainage of an abdominal abscess, option C, is incorrect. This intervention is used when there is a suspected abscess; this patient does not have any signs or symptoms of an abdominal abscess. Serial ultrasonography and then plan for laparoscopic appendectomy if the condition worsens, option E, is incorrect. This patient is displaying signs and symptoms related to acute appendicitis. Prompt surgical intervention is the standard treatment for appendicitis. Prolonging the duration of symptoms before surgical intervention increases the patient's risk of perforation and sepsis. **Task:** D2—Clinical Intervention

2. **Answer: C** The entire family needs to adopt a healthy lifestyle along with the patient, option C, is the correct answer. Lifestyle modification is the initial and primary treatment for children with a body mass index greater than or equal to the 85th percentile. For this child to be successful, both parents and the rest of the family will have to adopt healthy lifestyle habits.

   Limiting consumption of fast food to once a week and sugary drinks to once daily (options A and B) are inappropriate. The patient's parents should be counseled to eliminate all fast food and sugary drinks from her diet. Gradual weight loss is encouraged rather than rapid weight loss. Therefore, recommending the patient strive to achieve rapid weight loss of at least 2 lb per week, option D, is incorrect. At 9 years of age, this patient should strive for weight maintenance because she is still growing. Keeping unhealthy foods out of reach of the patient, option E, is not an appropriate recommendation. If possible, all unhealthy foods should be removed from the home. This will allow the family and child to develop healthy eating habits. **Task:** D1—Health Maintenance, Patient Education, and Disease Prevention

3. **Answer: A** This patient has secondary diabetes mellitus due to chronic pancreatitis. Extended-release metformin therapy once daily, option A, is the most appropriate treatment for this patient. In patients with a C-peptide level that is within normal limits, oral hypoglycemic agents may be used instead of insulin. Metformin is preferred, as it may lower the risk of secondary pancreatic carcinoma.

   Glipizide therapy twice daily with meals, option B, is incorrect because glipizide may cause hypoglycemia in patients with brittle diabetes mellitus with pancreatitis and is not preferred over metformin. Orlistat therapy once daily, option C, may cause steatorrhea, which is already a common symptom in patients with chronic pancreatitis. Options D and E are incorrect because semaglutide (a GLP-1 agonist) and sitagliptin (a DPP-4 inhibitor) should be avoided in patients with pancreatitis. **Task:** D3—Pharmaceutical Therapeutics

4. **Answer: B** According to the Rome IV Criteria, IBS is characterized by recurrent abdominal pain with defecation and is associated with a change in stool form and a change in stool frequency, option B.

   Change in color of the stool, nocturnal diarrhea, presence of blood in the stool, and vomiting (options A, C, D, and E) should alert the provider to the possibility of another pathology. Presence of these signs and symptoms could indicate infection, changes in liver function, or even the possibility of gastrointestinal cancer. **Task:** B—Using Diagnostic and Laboratory Studies.

5. **Answer: E** This patient has signs and symptoms of hepatitis B infection after being exposed to blood while at work. A diagnosis of acute hepatitis B is based on the detection of hepatitis B surface antigen and IgM antibody to hepatitis B core antigen, option E.

   Alanine aminotransferase and aspartate aminotransferase levels, option A, may indicate liver disease, but they are not diagnostic of acute hepatitis B. An elevated or positive hepatitis B surface antibody test (options B and C) indicates either the patient has had the disease in the past or has received the vaccine. Hepatitis B virus DNA, option D, is used to assess recovery from infection and candidacy for antiviral therapy. **Task:** B—Using Diagnostic and Laboratory Studies

6. **Answer: E** Opioid toxicity, option E, should be highly suspected in patients with respirations less than 12/min and central nervous system depression secondary to the rise in carbon dioxide, which can lead to

respiratory depression and eventually respiratory arrest. Other physical examination findings associated with opioid toxicity include miosis, hypotension, hypothermia, and bradycardia. Overdose is more common among young males and associated with increased risk of repeat self-harm. Associated risk factors for opioid toxicity consist of mental illness, chronic opioid use, and hepatic and renal impairment. Intravenous naloxone is the standard treatment for opioid overdose.

An acute subdural hematoma, option A, is more likely to occur in an older patient who has had symptoms of dizziness, confusion, or headache prior to losing consciousness. A CT scan of the head will help diagnose this disorder. Alcohol intoxication, option B, is often associated with the use of opiates. Diagnosis is with toxicology or measurement of the patient's blood alcohol level. Alcohol intoxication/poisoning may result in respiratory depression, aspiration, and vomiting. Bacterial meningitis, option C, is typically associated with additional symptoms of headache, vomiting, and fever. A lumbar puncture and CT scan of the head will most likely confirm this diagnosis. Hypoglycemia, option D, can be ruled out in this patient because his blood glucose level is within normal limits. **Task:** A—History Taking and Performing Physical Examination

7. **Answer: A** Adhesions, option A, are the most common cause of a mechanical small-bowel obstruction in 60 to 70% of cases. This implies a physical barrier either partial or complete that impedes normal progress of intestinal contents. Patients with small-bowel obstruction have abdominal pain and profuse vomiting. Vomiting may be feculent if small-bowel obstruction is in the more distant colon. Peristaltic rushes, gurgles, and high-pitched tinkles are audible in coordination with attacks of cramping pain in distal obstructions. Supine and upright abdominal x-ray studies show a ladder like pattern of dilated small bowel loops with air-fluid levels.

Foreign bodies, option B, such as bezoars and ingested foreign bodies may cause obstruction, but this is not the most likely cause of small-bowel obstruction in this patient. Intussusception, option C, is a small-bowel obstruction, but it usually occurs in children less than 2 years of age. Intussusception is the most common cause between the ages of 6 to 36 months of age. Children present with colicky abdominal pain, passage of blood per rectum, and a palpable mass on palpation. Neoplasm, option D, is the second leading cause of small-bowel obstruction. It can progressively occlude the lumen with primary, metastatic, or bulky lymph metastasis as a point for intussusception. A volvulus, option E, results from rotation of bowel loops about a fixed point. Onset is rapid and strangulation develops abruptly. **Task:** C—Formulating Most Likely Diagnosis

8. **Answer: C** This patient with Crohn disease has findings consistent with an anal fistula. The question requires the examinee to recall the natural history of anal fistulae, which are most commonly caused by an antecedent anorectal abscess, option C. This type of abscess drains through a tract that later epithelializes, leading to development of a fistula. The other options (A, B, D, and E) are anorectal disorders that are not associated with the development of an anal fistula. **Task:** E—Applying Basic Scientific Concepts

9. **Answer: C** This patient has severe constipation as a result of taking oxycodone, option E, for treatment of pain associated with lung cancer. Symptoms of constipation often include hard stools, abdominal pain, abdominal bloating/cramping, a feeling of incomplete voiding, straining with defecation, and the need for digital stimulation. A full review of systems should be performed to determine duration of symptoms, change in bowel habits, change in diet, and whether the onset is acute or chronic in nature. The treatment of constipation is focused on symptom relief followed by prevention of future episodes. Opioid medications, option E, are common offending agents for worsening or contributing to constipation. Stool softeners, laxatives, increased mobility, and increased fluid and fiber intake, depending on the patient's condition, remain the mainstay of treatment.

The other medications listed have a much lower risk of causing constipation when compared with oxycodone. Acetaminophen, option A, is generally tolerated well. One of the greatest risk factors of regular acetaminophen use is elevation of liver function tests as well as potential liver damage with high dose use of greater than 3000 to 4000 mg/day depending on age and medical comorbidities. Nonsteroidal anti-inflammatory drugs such as diclofenac sodium and ibuprofen (options B and C) have adverse reactions that are most concerning for inhibition of platelet function, renal impairment, and gastrointestinal bleeding or ulceration. Lidocaine, option D, has not been found to be associated with constipation. Adverse reactions associated with lidocaine include anaphylaxis, cardiac arrest, and bronchospasm. **Task:** D3—Pharmaceutical Therapeutics

10. **Answer: C** This patient most likely has a food allergy to peanut butter. Food allergies are more common in children, and proteins in peanuts are one of the most common causes of acute systemic reactions. The most supportive finding for food allergy on history and physical examination of this patient is that the symptoms occurred within two hours of ingestion of peanut butter cookies, option C.

Perioral erythema with no edema or pallor, option A, may help formulate the diagnosis, but these findings are not diagnostic for this condition. Potential sick contacts in the neighborhood, option B, is an appropriate answer only if there were known sick contacts who had similar symptoms. The uncertain history of previous ingestion of peanut butter, option D, can also help formulate the diagnosis of a food allergy, but it is not most suggestive of this diagnosis. Vital signs that are within normal limits, option E, do not support a diagnosis of food allergy; vital signs would be abnormal (i.e., hypotension and rapid pulse rate) in a patient with a food allergy. **Task:** A—History Taking and Performing Physical Examination

11. **Answer: C** This patient has chronic refractory gastroesophageal reflux disease symptoms that were treated conservatively at first, with once daily proton pump inhibitor (PPI) therapy, and then with twice daily PPI therapy without improvement of symptoms. Therefore, surgery is the most appropriate next step. Laparoscopic Nissen fundoplication, option C, involves wrapping the proximal portion of the stomach around the distal portion of the esophagus to create a valvelike setting between the two structures to prevent reflux of contents from the stomach into the esophagus.
An Indiana pouch, option A, is a urinary diversion that is created using a portion of the bowel. Laparoscopic esophagectomy, option B, includes removal of a portion of or the entire esophagus, usually in the setting of trauma or a tumor. Roux-en-Y procedure, option D, is a type of weight-loss surgery. A Whipple procedure, option E, is a surgical procedure that removes the head of the pancreas, duodenum, gallbladder, and bile duct and is used to treat patients with tumors and other disorders of the pancreas, intestine, and bile duct. **Task:** D2—Clinical Intervention

12. **Answer: A** Acute cholangitis, option A, is a bacterial infection of the biliary tract. Symptoms include fever, abdominal pain, and jaundice, also known as the Charcot triad. In severe cases, this may also include hypotension and mental status changes. Acute cholangitis most commonly occurs due to a stone in the bile duct causing obstruction but can also be secondary to tumors, benign strictures, pancreatitis, inflammatory conditions, or damage to the bile duct during a surgical procedure. Patients have increased white blood cell count and elevated C-reactive protein and bilirubin levels, and elevated results of liver function studies. Ultrasonography or CT scan of the abdomen shows evidence of biliary dilation. It typically is treated with antibiotics but may require surgical intervention if it is a severe case or is not responding to medical therapy. Acute cholecystitis, option B, will not typically include elevated serum bilirubin or alkaline phosphatase levels, and imaging shows a normal bile duct with thickening

of the gallbladder wall. Acute pancreatitis, option C, typically includes acute epigastric pain that radiates to the back and is improved by leaning forward. Serum lipase level will be elevated, and enlargement of the pancreas is noted on imaging studies. Liver abscess, option D, would be obvious on imaging studies; no lesion in the liver was noted on ultrasonography of this patient. **Task:** C—Formulating Most Likely Diagnosis

13. **Answer: E** Bloody diarrhea, pain in the lower abdomen, and tenesmus are findings common in patients with *Shigella dysenteriae* infection, option E.
Bacillus cereus, option A, is a common cause of food poisoning; this patient has no history of recent changes in diet. *Clostridium difficile*, option B, is a common cause of diarrhea associated with taking antibiotic therapy, which this patient has no history of doing. *Helicobacter pylori*, option C, is a common cause of peptic ulcer disease; this patient has no symptoms of this disease. Rotavirus, option D, is a common cause of noninflammatory, watery diarrhea. **Task:** E—Applying Basic Scientific Concepts

14. **Answer: C** Factors that contribute to the development of hemorrhoids include diarrhea, aging, chronic straining, pregnancy, heavy lifting, and constipation, which is option C.
Family history of prostate cancer, history of intra-abdominal surgery, initiation of a vegetarian diet, and recent antibiotic use (options A, B, D, and E) are not contributing factors to the development of hemorrhoids. **Task:** A—History Taking and Performing Physical Examination

15. **Answer: A** This patient has Wilson disease, which is an autosomal recessive metabolic disorder in which impaired copper excretion causes copper accumulation in the liver, cornea, and central nervous system. Patients are usually asymptomatic until hepatitis/cirrhosis, psychosis, and dystonia raise suspicion. Elevated aminotransferase levels, hemolytic anemia, decreased serum ceruloplasmin level, increased free serum copper level, and decreased total serum copper level confirm the diagnosis. Management consists of maintaining a low-copper diet and D-penicillamine therapy, option A, which acts as a chelating agent.
Levodopa, option B, is commonly used to treat patients with Parkinson disease. Pyrimethamine, option C, is used for toxoplasmosis encephalitis and does not have a role in the treatment of Wilson disease. Tetrabenazine, option D, is the first-line treatment for Huntington disease. Therapeutic phlebotomy, option E, has no role in the treatment of Wilson disease; however, it is used to treat disorders such as hemochromatosis. **Task:** D3—Pharmaceutical Therapeutics

 Answer Key for this chapter begins on p. 85

16. Answer: B This patient has signs and symptoms of eosinophilic esophagitis (EoE). EoE is an esophageal disorder characterized by esophageal dysfunction and mucosal infiltration by eosinophils. In children, it is more common in males with an average age of 7 years at diagnosis. EoE is characterized by symptoms of esophageal dysfunction, concurrent atopic conditions, and endoscopic abnormalities including edema, rings, exudates, furrows, and strictures. Laboratory abnormalities include peripheral eosinophilia, option B.

A predominance of basophils (option A) is rare and not associated with EoE. A predominance of lymphocytes, monocytes, and neutrophils (options C, D, and E) are seen in certain types of infectious or inflammatory conditions but are not associated with EoE. **Task:** B—Using Diagnostic and Laboratory Studies

17. Answer: C This patient has toxic megacolon, option C, which is diagnosed based on the combination of symptoms and signs of systemic toxicity in combination with radiologic evidence of colonic distension. It should be suspected in any patient who has diarrhea, abdominal distension, and toxicity, as in this patient. Toxic megacolon guidelines for clinical diagnostic criteria are as follows: (1) radiographic evidence of colonic dilation, transverse colon diameter greater than 6 cm; (2) three of the following clinical signs: temperature greater than 38.0°C (100.4°F), pulse rate greater than 120/min, white blood cell count greater than 10,500/mm³, and/or anemia requiring transfusion; and (3) one of the following: altered mental status, dehydration, electrolyte disturbances, and/or hypotension.

Colorectal cancer, option A, is an unlikely choice specifically because of the clinical findings in this patient. In addition, symptoms of colorectal cancer do not include colonic dilation. Ischemic colitis, option B, includes dilation that does not meet the criteria for toxic megacolon. Finally, there are no specific findings of ulcerative colitis, option D, on the x-ray study. **Task:** C—Formulating Most Likely Diagnosis

18. Answer: B The classic antidote for methanol and ethylene glycol poisoning was ethanol, a preferential substrate for alcohol dehydrogenase. It prevents the metabolism of parent compounds to toxic metabolites. Fomepizole, option B, a potent competitive inhibitor of alcohol dehydrogenase, has almost entirely replaced ethanol because of its ease of administration, lack of central nervous system and metabolic effects, and overall excellent patient tolerability profile.

Deferoxamine, option A, is used for iron intoxication. Hydroxocobalamin, option C, is used for treatment of cyanide poisoning. Pralidoxime, option D, is used for the treatment of organophosphate/insecticide poisoning. Pyridostigmine, option E, is indicated for the treatment of neuromuscular disorders. **Task:** D3—Pharmaceutical Therapeutics

19. Answer: D This patient has peptic ulcer disease (PUD). *Helicobacter pylori* infection is one of the most common causes of PUD; therefore, option D is the correct answer.

Alcohol use disorder, option A, is not a cause of PUD but can worsen ulcers once they have already developed. Caffeine use, option B, increases stomach acid but does not cause PUD. Cytomegalovirus, option C, is found in less than 5 to 10% of patients with PUD and is most often associated with transplant recipients. Spicy food, option E, does not cause PUD but can worsen PUD symptoms including heartburn. **Task:** C—Formulating Most Likely Diagnosis

20. Answer: C This patient has an anal fissure, which is a longitudinal tear in the epithelium of the anal canal. The diagnosis of anal fissure is based on patient history and physical examination. Symptoms associated with an anal fissure are most commonly described as severe pain and bleeding during or after bowel movements. On physical examination, anal fissures are often found extending from the dentate line toward the anal verge. The treatment for an anal fissure is individualized based on the patient presentation and duration of illness. This patient has an acute anal fissure, which will heal with conservative management and symptomatic relief including sitz baths (option C), stool softeners, and a high-fiber diet.

Local pain medications such as acetaminophen suppositories, option A, are not usually recommended due to the inflammatory nature of the anal fissure. If analgesics are needed, oral acetaminophen or nonsteroidal anti-inflammatory drugs are more beneficial. Option B, colonoscopy, is reserved for symptoms associated with rectal bleeding, if there is a significant family history of colon cancer, for general health maintenance after the age of 50, or for acute lower gastrointestinal bleeds. For chronic fissures or acute on chronic anal fissures, conservative therapy plus a topical medication, either nitroglycerin (option E) or a calcium channel blocker, is most appropriate. If conservative treatment fails, then a referral can be made to a general surgery provider (option D). **Task:** D2—Clinical Intervention

21. Answer: C G6PD deficiency, option C, is an X-linked recessive inherited disorder caused by a genetic defect in the red blood cell enzyme G6PD. Three main types of triggers for hemolysis include infection, medication such as antimalarial drugs, and foods such as fava beans. Heinz bodies, which indicate G6PD deficiency, are collections of denatured globin chains attached to the red blood cell membrane.

Chronic lymphocytic leukemia (CLL), option A, is the most common type of leukemia, and patients are usually asymptomatic at the time of presentation. CLL is a chronic lymphoproliferative disorder that causes progressive accumulation of functionally incompetent lymphocytes. Hallmark findings on laboratory studies include isolated lymphocytosis and mature small lymphocytes called smudge cells. Chronic myelogenous leukemia, option B, is a myeloproliferative neoplasm characterized by uncontrolled mature granulocytes. Symptoms consist of a gradual onset of fatigue, night sweats, fevers, and anorexia. Laboratory studies show markedly increased white blood cell counts predominately with neutrophils but also eosinophils and basophils. Lead poisoning, option D, is associated with symptoms of abdominal pain, difficulty with concentration, low intelligent quotient, and ataxic gait. Peripheral blood smear shows basophilic stippling. Multiple myeloma, option E, is caused by plasma cell proliferation. Symptoms consist of bone pain, renal failure, and hypercalcemia. Urine electrophoresis showing Bence-Jones protein is a hallmark sign of multiple myeloma. **Task:** C—Formulating Most Likely Diagnosis

22. **Answer: E** Pyloric stenosis, option E, presents in infants at 3 to 6 weeks of age. Symptoms include recurrent forceful projectile and nonbilious vomiting. Physical examination findings show a palpable olive-shaped mass in the right upper epigastric region, which is noted in this patient.
Duodenum atresia, option A, is also associated with bilious emesis. On abdominal x-ray studies, a double bubble is classically seen with this condition. Gastric volvulus, option B, is more common in adults and is associated with bilious emesis rather than the nonbilious emesis that is seen in patients with pyloric stenosis. In patients with gastroesophageal reflux disease, option C, emesis may occur similarly to pyloric stenosis after feeding, but the emesis is not forceful and is typically less in volume. Intussusception, option D, often includes a sausage-shaped mass in the abdomen with associated colicky abdominal pain, fever, nausea and vomiting, and red currant jellylike stools. **Task:** A—History Taking and Performing Physical Examination

23. **Answer: B** Gallbladder contraction, option B, is correct. When a patient has chronic cholecystitis, ultrasonography will show that the gallbladder is contracted around the stones rather than distended, which is typical of acute cholecystitis.
Elevated liver function tests and increased white blood cell count (options A and C) are incorrect, because results of these two laboratory studies are typically within normal limits in patients with chronic cholecystitis. Option D, pericholecystic inflammation, is

incorrect. Chronic cholecystitis is associated with the absence of pericholecystic inflammation. Thickened gallbladder wall, option E, is associated with acute cholecystitis rather than chronic cholecystitis. Chronic cholecystitis is associated with a shrunken and contracted gallbladder rather than one that is inflamed and distended. **Task:** B—Using Diagnostic and Laboratory Studies

24. **Answer: B** This patient has celiac disease, which is defined as a chronic gastrointestinal disorder caused by an immune-mediated reaction to gluten-containing food products. There is a wide range of clinical signs and symptoms that are associated with celiac disease, including unexplained weight loss, diarrhea, bloating, bloody stool, dyspepsia, and fatigue, among many others. Diagnosis is often made based on history and physical examination, with an emphasis placed on family history. Additional diagnostic tools include serum testing for autoantibodies, specifically tissue transglutaminase 2-IgA and IgA endomysial antibody, followed by an upper endoscopy with duodenal biopsy. Once diagnosed, the mainstay of treatment of celiac disease is a strict gluten-free diet, option B.
A carbohydrate-controlled diet, option A, is most often used for diabetes mellitus or prediabetes to assist with overall glycemic control. A high-fiber diet, option C, is recommended for individuals who have diverticulitis, anal fissures, or constipation. Option D, a ketogenic diet, has been successfully scientifically implemented in patients with epilepsy, cancer, obesity, diabetes mellitus, glucose transfer type 1 deficiency syndrome, traumatic brain injuries, and neurodegeneration. A low-salt diet, option E, is not correct since this diet is used to assist in the overall management of individuals with congestive heart failure, coronary artery disease, cirrhosis, hypertension, and chronic lower extremity edema. **Task:** D2—Clinical Intervention

25. **Answer: C** Nonselective beta-blocker therapy, option C, should be used as primary prophylaxis to prevent variceal bleeding in this patient. This medication has been shown to decrease the rates of a first variceal bleed.
Prophylactic antibiotics, option A, are used once there is a variceal bleed. Prophylactic antibiotics have been shown to reduce the rate of bacterial infection, treatment failure, rebleeding, and mortality in patients with variceal bleeding. Anxiolytic therapy, option B, is plausible but incorrect because medications that alter mental status should be limited in patients with portal hypertension. Nonsteroidal anti-inflammatory drug therapy, option D, is incorrect. Patients with esophageal varices are at increased risk of bleeding and should refrain from medications that pose a bleeding risk, such as nonsteroidal anti-inflammatory

drugs. Vasoconstrictor therapy, option E, is used to reduce the incidence of bleeding reoccurrence. In this patient's case, bleeding from the varices has not yet occurred, therefore this drug is inappropriate. **Task:** D3—Pharmaceutical Therapeutics

26. **Answer: C** Intussusception, option C, is the most common cause of intestinal obstruction in patients from 6 to 36 years of age. Multiple concentric rings, also referred to as a "coiled spring" lesion, is often noted on ultrasonography of the abdomen or during an enema. This is the classic sign of telescoping of multiple layers of intestine.

    Adhesions, option A, typically form secondary to past procedures and are not a typical finding in patients of this age. A bezoar, option B, is made up of foreign material such as hair and is not the most common cause of obstruction in patients this age. Pyloric stenosis, option D, occurs typically in the first six months of life and involves the proximal small intestine. Volvulus, option E, causes intestinal obstruction; however, it is not the most common cause in patients of this age. **Task:** C—Formulating Most Likely Diagnosis

27. **Answer: D** This patient has symptoms of intestinal ischemia, which is an emergency and must be treated promptly, typically with embolectomy or thrombolytics. Therefore, arranging for urgent surgical consultation, option D, is correct.

    Options A, B, C, and E do not properly consider the urgency of the situation or recognize the nature of the emergency. Simply admitting the patient to a Medical/Surgical unit, awaiting gastroenterology consultation, and most certainly discharging the patient to home will greatly delay care and can result in death. **Task:** D2—Clinical Intervention

28. **Answer: C** An elevation in international normalized ratio (INR), option C, is correct. As liver disease progresses to cirrhosis, the INR will increase due to a reduction in the levels of most clotting factors, except for factor VIII.

    An elevated albumin level and an elevated sodium level, options A and E, are incorrect. As liver disease progresses to cirrhosis, the albumin and sodium levels decrease. An elevated hemoglobin level, option B, is incorrect. Cirrhosis is associated with the presence of anemia that results from hemolysis, folate deficiency, and/or splenomegaly. An increased platelet count, option D, is incorrect. Advanced liver disease can cause marrow suppression, folate deficiency, and/or splenic sequestration, resulting in a decreased platelet count. **Task:** B—Using Diagnostic and Laboratory Studies

29. **Answer: B** Patients with a family history of colon cancer in a first-degree relative should undergo screening by colonoscopy at age 40 or 10 years before the age at diagnosis of the affected relative, whichever is earlier. This patient's father was 55 years of age at the time of diagnosis; therefore, screening colonoscopy is most appropriate for this patient at 40 years of age (option B). **Task:** D1—Health Maintenance, Patient Education, and Disease Prevention

30. **Answer: B** Gastroesophageal reflux disease (GERD) includes a broad spectrum of diseases that contribute to a constellation of symptoms. Some of the most common clinical signs and symptoms of GERD include heartburn, acid reflux, substernal chest discomfort after eating, throat clearing, sore throat, as well as other ear, nose, and throat symptoms. Complications from uncontrolled or poorly controlled GERD include visible mucosal damage at the time of endoscopy, esophagitis, esophageal strictures, or Barrett esophagus.

    This patient most likely has esophageal strictures, option B, which are more commonly seen in men, are often related to use of nonsteroidal anti-inflammatory drugs, and can occur in up to 23% of patients with untreated GERD. Esophageal strictures begin to form when the mucosal layer is damaged at the cellular level, leading to edema and inflammation in the esophageal wall, followed by cellular infiltration, vascular congestion, and ending with collagen deposits and fibrosis. The fibrosis of the esophageal tissues is an irreversible process and leads to dysphagia.

    Barrett esophagus, option A, does not usually cause symptoms. However, it is often associated with GERD. Barret esophagus is diagnosed based on endoscopic evaluation and biopsy of the esophageal mucosa. Esophageal varices, option C, are dilated submucosal veins in the lining of the esophagus. Esophageal varices occur in patients with underlying portal hypertension and cirrhosis. If they are exacerbated by trauma or an irritant, they can result in severe upper gastrointestinal bleeding. Esophagitis, option D, is an acute or chronic inflammation of the esophagus and is defined as mucosal inflammation from food, liquid, or chemical irritants. Gastritis, option E, is defined as acute or chronic inflammation of the gastric mucosa associated with food, liquid, or chemical irritants. **Task:** A—History Taking and Performing Physical Examination

31. **Answer: E** This patient has nonspecific left lower quadrant abdominal pain and is found to have gallstones that are noted incidentally on CT scan of the abdomen and pelvis. Patients with symptomatic cholelithiasis would have right upper quadrant pain and tenderness to palpation on examination, which this patient does not have. Patients with asymptomatic gallstones do not require immediate therapeutic intervention. Therefore, no immediate intervention is

necessary, but recommendation for weight loss and lifestyle changes, option E, is most appropriate with regard to management of the gallstones.

Extracorporeal shock wave lithotripsy, option A, is used to break up kidney stones and not gallstones. HIDA radionuclide scan, option B, is used to view the liver, gallbladder, bile ducts, and small intestines; visualization of the stones has already occurred with the CT scan. Laparoscopic cholecystectomy, option C, is a surgical procedure to remove the gallbladder, and this is not indicated for this patient at this time. Ultrasonography of the gallbladder, option D, aids in the diagnosis of gallbladder pathology, but this was already accomplished incidentally in this patient via CT scan of the abdomen. **Task:** D1—Health Maintenance, Patient Education, and Disease Prevention

32. **Answer: E** Once in the stomach, most ingested objects will pass spontaneously, and the risk of complications is much lower, making observation, option E, the most appropriate management for this patient. If a more complex or sharp object progressed beyond the stomach and could not be retrieved, periodic x-ray studies should be obtained to document progression through the gastrointestinal tract.

Emetic therapy, option A, may actually cause more harm to the gastrointestinal tract than allowing the coin to pass on its own. Endoscopy, option B, is a procedure, and as with any procedure, it can present risks. The coin will most likely pass on its own, and the risk does not outweigh the benefit; therefore, this patient does not require endoscopy. Glucagon therapy, option C, is not indicated for an ingested coin. This therapy is more suited for treatment of an impacted food bolus. Laxative therapy, option D, is indicated for constipation and is not indicated for this child, as the coin will pass with normal bowel motility. **Task:** D2—Clinical Intervention

33. **Answer: B** This patient has signs of an acute strangulated hernia. Hernias occur when intra-abdominal tissue protrudes through a defect in the abdominal wall. They can be located in the groin, the umbilicus, or along a previous incision. Since this patient has developed symptoms of a bowel obstruction with overlying skin changes, and the mass is not able to be reduced (option B), this warrants immediate surgical intervention within four to six hours to attempt to prevent bowel loss.

A bulge that disappears when the patient is supine, option A, is consistent with a hernia that has not become incarcerated or strangulated. This may be referred to a surgeon to discuss elective hernia repair, and the patient may receive education about the signs of strangulation and when to go to the emergency department. Fluctuance over the area with purulent

discharge, option C, is consistent with an abscess that can be treated with local incision and drainage. Hard, fixed nodules along the inguinal ligament, option D, are more consistent with a malignancy that warrants further workup and imaging, but immediate surgical intervention is not required. A soft scrotal mass that feels like a bag of worms, option E, is consistent with a varicocele which typically does not require surgical intervention but can be treated with surgical ligation or venous embolization electively. **Task:** A—History Taking and Performing Physical Examination

34. **Answer: D** This patient has symptoms suggestive of a Mallory-Weiss tear. Proper immediate treatment includes intravenous proton pump inhibitors and antiemetics as well as referral for emergent upper endoscopy, option D.

Admitting the patient to the hospital for general surgery consultation and discharging the patient to home with a recommendation to follow-up with a gastroenterologist, options A and B, do not consider the urgency of this patient's condition. A CT scan of the chest and abdomen, option C, is not a recommended modality to diagnose a Mallory-Weiss tear. Repeating laboratory studies in 24 hours, option E, is incorrect because the delay could end in death of the patient. **Task:** D2—Clinical Intervention

35. **Answer: B** In order to decrease her risk of contracting noninfectious traveler's diarrhea, educating this patient about the best preventive measures includes advising her to avoid fresh foods and local water sources, option B. Fresh foods and local water sources in developing countries are likely to be contaminated. Prophylactic medications such as antibiotics and antidiarrheal drugs, options D and E, are not indicated in healthy individuals without comorbid disease. Recommending the patient avoid engaging with local residents, option A, and avoid traveling more than 10 miles from the hotel, option C, are inappropriate and will have no effect on whether or not this patient gets noninfectious traveler's diarrhea. **Task:** D1—Health Maintenance, Patient Education, and Disease Prevention

36. **Answer: B** This patient has symptoms of diverticulitis, which is an inflammatory condition that involves microperforation followed by localized inflammation of a diverticulum or group of diverticula of the colon. Contributing factors of diverticulitis include constipation, diets high in red meat and low in fiber, obesity, sedentary lifestyle, and tobacco and alcohol use. Diagnosis of acute diverticulitis can be made on the basis of history and physical examination, which usually includes tenderness to palpation of the left lower quadrant of the abdomen. The test of choice for confirming this diagnosis is a contrast-enhanced CT scan

of the abdomen and pelvis, option C, as long as allergies and kidney function allows.

Colonoscopy, option A, is sometimes considered in cases of acute diverticulitis because oftentimes gastrointestinal bleeding can be associated. Colonoscopy is not the test of choice for diverticulitis as this procedure can increase the risk of perforation of the bowel during the acute inflammatory state. It is recommended to be deferred four to six weeks until resolution of the diverticulitis. HIDA radionuclide scan, option C, is used to evaluate gallbladder function when other studies, such as right upper quadrant ultrasonography, are not definitive for acute or chronic cholecystitis. Ultrasonography of the abdomen, option D, is often used for evaluation of ascites, gallbladder disease, and diseases of the pancreas and liver. It is not the test of choice for diverticulitis, as it cannot fully evaluate the colon and small bowel. X-ray studies of the kidneys, ureter, and bladder (option E) is a test used to assess for kidney stones and bladder obstruction, but it can also be used to assess for constipation or small-bowel obstruction. **Task:** B—Using Diagnostic and Laboratory Studies

37. **Answer: B** Considering this patient's history of unintended weight loss coupled with worsening symptoms, the most likely diagnosis is cancerous obstruction of the colon, option B. The CT scan shows a significant narrowing of the lumen with a transition point indicating an obstruction. These areas of narrowing are also known as an "apple core sign" or "napkin ring sign."

Appendicitis, option A, is incorrect because this patient does not have the classic signs of nausea, fever, localizing abdominal pain, or tenderness over the right lower quadrant. Option C, diverticulitis, is incorrect because no diverticula with signs of inflammation are noted on CT scan of the abdomen. Options D and E, intussusception and volvulus, would be clearly indicated on the CT scan. Intussusception is identified as areas of bowel within bowel. A volvulus can present in many ways on CT; however, the classic sigmoid volvulus is evident by a largely dilated region of the sigmoid colon twisting upon itself in the shape of a coffee bean. **Task:** C—Formulating Most Likely Diagnosis

38. **Answer A:** This patient has acute pancreatitis, option A. This is the most likely diagnosis based on the history of alcohol use disorder, current epigastric pain, and increased serum amylase and lipase levels.

Boerhaave syndrome, option B, is a transmural esophageal tear causing esophageal perforation that is sometimes found in patients who participate in binge drinking. This patient has been sober for the past 10 months. Cirrhosis, option C, is most commonly caused by alcoholic liver disease. Laboratory findings would indicate elevated liver enzyme levels. Duodenal ulcers, option D, cause pain that is usually relieved with eating. Mallory-Weiss tears, option E, are mucosal tears at the gastroesophageal junction that can also be seen in patients who participate in binge drinking, but hematemesis is usually an indication of this disorder. **Task:** C—Formulating Most Likely Diagnosis

39. **Answer: C** This patient has severe ulcerative colitis (UC) due to the fact that she is having greater than six mostly bloody bowel movements on a daily basis and because she has lost over 10% of her body weight. Also, colonoscopy has ruled out a diagnosis of colon cancer. Hypoalbuminemia, option C, is often seen in patients with severe UC because of impaired nutrition. Erythrocyte sedimentation rate, option A, would be increased, and not within normal limits, in a patient with severe UC. Hematocrit greater than 40%, option B, is a normal laboratory value. In a patient who has had an increased amount of blood loss over two months, expected laboratory findings would include decreased hemoglobin level and a hematocrit usually less than 30%. Skip lesions, option D, noted on colonoscopy are indicative of Crohn disease but not UC. In UC, there is usually continuous involvement of the colonic mucosa. Terminal ileitis, option E, is found in patients with Crohn disease. UC is usually confined to the colon and rectum. **Task:** B—Using Diagnostic and Laboratory Studies

40. **Answer: E** Accidental ingestion of caustic substances is common in children. Typical symptoms include dysphagia, drooling, vomiting, chest pain, hematemesis, and upper airway injury or severe symptoms that indicate a perforation such as severe pain, abdominal rigidity, or fever. Initial management includes getting detailed information on the type and amount of substance ingested and finding out if the ingestion was suspected or witnessed. Then, the local poison control center should be contacted for recommendations. In patients who are symptomatic but hemodynamically stable, an upper endoscopy, option E, is performed to grade the injury and make further recommendations for treatment and follow-up. It is important to note that inducing vomiting and administering neutralizing agents, diluting agents, or activated charcoal are not recommended as initial management.

Abdominal ultrasonography, option A, has no role in evaluation or diagnosis after caustic ingestion. A chest x-ray study, option B, can be done in patients with respiratory symptoms and can be used to evaluate for signs of a perforation, but this imaging study is not used to stage the damage. Contrast-enhanced CT scan or MRI of the abdomen, options C and D, are occasionally used to evaluate patients when there is concern for erosion into vascular structures. **Task:** B—Using Diagnostic and Laboratory Studies.

BIBLIOGRAPHY

Afdhal, N. H. (2020). Acute cholangitis: Clinical manifestation, diagnosis and acute management. In T. Post (Ed.), *UpToDate*. Waltham, MA: UpToDate.

Anderson, M., & Grucela, A. (September 1, 2019). Toxic megacolon. *Seminars in Colon and Rectal Surgery*, *30*(3). Article 100691.

Bachoud-Lévi, A. C., Ferreira, J., Massart, R., Youssov, K., Rosser, A., Busse, M., et al. (2019). International guidelines for the treatment of Huntington's disease. *Frontiers in Neurology*, *10*, 710.

Barkun, A. N., Bardou, M., Kuipers, E. J., Sung, J., Hunt, R. H., Martel, M., et al. (2010). International consensus recommendations on the management of patients with nonvariceal upper gastrointestinal bleeding. *Annals of Internal Medicine*, *152*, 101.

Bharucha, A. E., Pemberton, J. H., & Locke, G. R. (2013). American Gastroenterological Association technical review on constipation. *Gastroenterology*, *144*(1), 218-238.

Brooks, D. C. (2020). Overview of treatment for inguinal and femoral hernia in adults. In T. Post (Ed.), *UpToDate*. Waltham, MA: UpToDate.

Brumbaugh, D., Furuta, G. T., Hoffenberg, E. J., Kobak, G. E., Kramer, R. E., Septer, S., et al. (2020). Gastrointestinal tract. In W. W., Jr., Hay, M. J. Levin, M. J. Abzug, & M. Bunik (Eds.), *Current Diagnosis & Treatment: Pediatrics*, 25e. McGraw Hill.

Carroll, A. G., Kavanagh, R. G., Ni Leidhin, C., Cullinan, N. M., Lavelle, L. P., & Malone, D. E. (2017). Comparative effectiveness of imaging modalities for the diagnosis and treatment of intussusception: A critically appraised topic. *Academic Radiology*, *24*, 521.

Clair, D. G., & Beach, J. M. (2016). Mesenteric ischemia. *New England Journal of Medicine*, *374*, s959.

Clinical Overview: Cholangitis. In *Elsevier Point of Care*. Updated May 2, 2022. Elsevier.

Clinical Overview: Small-bowel obstruction. In *Elsevier Point of Care*. Updated June 25, 2022. Elsevier.

Clinical Overview: Opioid Toxicity. *Elsevier Point of Care*. Updated Nov 8, 2020. Elsevier.

Dalsey, W. C., & Sullivan, W. P. *Narcotic overdose case review*. American College of Emergency Physicians. Acep.org.

Domino, F. J., Baldor, R. A., Golding, J., & Stephens, M. B. (2019). *The 5-minute Clinical Consult 2020*. Lippincott Williams & Wilkins.

Elbright, C. *Opiate overdose: Fact vs. fiction: A case study in opioid overdose complication, management strategies and provider safety*. Limmer Education (July 10, 2019).

(2013). Epocrates [online]. San Francisco, CA: Epocrates, Inc.; http://www.epocrates.com. Updated continuously.

Feingold, D., Steele, S. R., Lee, S., Kaiser, A., Boushey, R., Buie, W. D., et al. Practice parameters for the treatment of sigmoid diverticulitis. *Diseases of the Colon & Rectum*, *57*(3), 284-294.

Ferguson, D. D. (2005). Evaluation and management of benign esophageal strictures. *Diseases of the Esophagus*, *18*, 359-364.

Ferri, F. F. Cholelithiasis. *Ferri's Clinical Advisor 2020*, pp. 335-336.

Feuerstein, J. D., & Falchuk, K. R. (2016). Diverticulosis and diverticulitis. *Mayo Clinic Proceedings*, *91*(8), 1094-1104.

Fishman, D. S. (2020). Caustic esophageal injury in children. In T. Post (Ed.), *UpToDate*. Waltham, MA: UpToDate.

Ford, A. C., Brenner, D. M., & Schoenfeld, P. S. (2013). Efficacy of pharmacological therapies for the treatment of opioid-induced constipation: systematic review and meta-analysis. *American College of Gastroenterology*, *108*(10), 1566-1574.

Forsmark, C. E. (2021). Chronic Pancreatitis. In M. Feldman, L. S. Freidman, & L. J. Brandt (Eds.) *Sleisenger and Fortran's Gastrointestinal and Liver Disease*. (11th ed.). Elsevier.

Francis, N. K., Sylla, P., Abou-Khalil, M., Arolfo, S., Berler, D., Curtis, N. J., et al. (2019). EAES and SAGES 2018 consensus conference on acute diverticulitis management: evidence-based recommendations for clinical practice. *Surgical Endoscopy*, *33*(9), 2726-2741.

Friedman, L. S. (2021). Cirrhosis. In M. A. Papadakis, S. J. McPhee, & M. W. Rabow (Eds.), *Current medical diagnosis & treatment 2021*. New York, NY: McGraw-Hill.

Gallagher, P. F., O'Mahony, D., & Quigley, E. M. (2008). Management of chronic constipation in the elderly. *Drugs Aging*, *25*(10), 807-821.

Gouveia, M., Torres, M., Lins, C., Alves, G., & Silva, P. (2020). Acute diarrhea with blood: Diagnosis and drug treatment. *Jornal de Pediatria*, *96*(1), 20-28.

Grace, N. D., & Minor, M. A. (2016). Portal hypertension & esophageal variceal hemorrhage. In N. J. Greenberger, R. S. Blumberg, & R. Burakoff (Eds.), *Current diagnosis & treatment: Gastroenterology, hepatology, & endoscopy* (3rd ed.). McGraw-Hill.

Green, P. H., & Jabri, B. (2003). Coeliac disease. *Lancet*, *362*(9381), 383-391.

Harcke, S., Rizzolo, D., & Harcke, H. T. (2019). G6PD deficiency: An update. *Journal of the American Academy of Physician Assistants* *32.11*, 21-26.

Jones, M. W., Gnanapandithan, K., Panneerselvam, D., & Ferguson, T. (2020 Oct 1). Chronic cholecystitis: *StatPearls [Internet]*. Treasure Island (FL): StatPearls Publishing.

Kahrilas, P. J., & Hirano, I. Diseases of the esophagus. In: J. Jameson, A. S. Fauci, D. L. Kasper, S. L. Hauser, D. L. Longo & J. Loscalzo (Eds.), *Harrison's principles of internal medicine* (20th ed.). McGraw-Hill.

Katz, P. O., Gerson, L. B., & Vela, M. F. (2013). Guidelines for the diagnosis and management of gastroesophageal reflux disease. *American College of Gastroenterology*, *108*(3), 308-328. quiz 329.

Khan, S. (2020). Eosinophilic esophagitis, pill esophagitis, and infective esophagitis. In R. Kliegman, B. Stanton, N. Schor, J. St Geme, & R. Behrman (Eds.), *Nelson textbook of pediatrics* (21st ed., pp. 1939-1940). Philadelphia, PA: Elsevier, Inc.

Kwaan, M. (2020). Hemorrhoids, anal fissure, and anorectal abscess and fistula. In R. Kellerman & D. Rakel (Eds.), *Conn's current therapy 2020* (pp. 222-226). Elsevier, Inc.

Markogiannakis, H., Messaris, E., Dardamanis, D., Pararas, N., Tzertzemelis, D., Giannopoulos, P., et al. (2007). Acute mechanical bowel obstruction: clinical presentation, etiology, management and outcome. *World Journal of Gastroenterology*, *13*(3), 432.

McQuaid, K. R. Gastroesophageal reflux disease. In M. A. Papadakis, S. J. McPhee & M. W. Rabow (Eds.), *Current medical diagnosis & treatment 2021*. McGraw-Hill.

National Institute for Health and Care Excellence: Coeliac Disease: Recognition, Assessment and Management. NICE Guideline NG20. NICE website. Published September 2015. Reviewed December 2019.

Papadakis, M., McPhee, S., & Rabow, M. *Current medical diagnosis & treatment 2020* (59th ed.). McGraw-Hill.

Answer Key for this chapter begins on p. 85

Pfau, P. R., & Benson, M. *Foreign bodies, bezoars, and caustic ingestions.* Sleisenger and Fordtran's gastrointestinal and liver disease, 28, pp. 399-410.

Pignone, M., & Salazar, R. (2021). Prevention of overweight & obesity. In M. A. Papadakis, S. J. McPhee, & M. W. Rabow (Eds.), *Current Medical Diagnosis & Treatment 2021.* McGraw-Hill.

Radlović, N., Leković, Z., Radlović, V., Simić, D., Ristić, D., & Vuletić, B. (2016). Food allergy in children. *Acad Med Sci Servian Med Soc, 144*(1-2), 99-103.

Rex, D., Boland, R., Dominitz, J., Giardiello, F. M., Johnson, D. A., Kaltenbach, T. et al. (2017). Colorectal Cancer Screening: Recommendations for Physicians and Patients from the U.S. Multi-Society Task Force on Colorectal Cancer. *Gastroenterology., 153*(1), 307-323.

Rubio-Tapia, A., Hill, I. D., Kelly, C. P., Calderwood, A. H., & Murray, J. A. (2013). American College of Gastroenterology. ACG clinical guidelines: diagnosis and management of celiac disease. *The American Journal of Gastroenterology, 108*(5), 656-676. quiz 677.

Schick, P. *Glucose-6-phosphate dehydrogenase deficiency.* Medscape. Updated: Apr 07, 2016.

Schmulson, M. J., & Drossman, D. A. (2017). What is new in Rome IV. *Journal of Neurogastroenterology and Motility, 23*(2), 151.

Stewart, D. B., Sr, Gaertner, W., Glasgow, S., Migaly, J., Feingold, D., & Steele, S. R. (2017). Clinical practice guideline for the management of anal fissures. *Diseases of the Colon & Rectum, 60*(1), 7-14.

The ABCs of Hepatitis-for health Professionals, The Centers for Disease Control. Retrieved from: www.cdc.gov/hepatitis

Theobald, J. L., & Kostic, M. A. *Poisoning.* Nelson textbook of pediatrics, Chapter 77, pp. 490-510.e1.

Thio, C. L., & Hawkins, C. (2015). Hepatitis B virus and hepatitis delta virus. Mandell, Douglas, and Bennett's principles and practice of infectious diseases.

Vakili, B., & Werth, A. (2021). Anorectal fistula. In F. Ferri (Ed.), *Ferri's clinical advisor 2021.* Elsevier, Inc.

Wald, A., Bharucha, A. E., Cosman, B. C., & Whitehead, W. E. (2014). ACG clinical guideline: management of benign anorectal disorders. *American College of Gastroenterology, 109*(8), 1141-1157. (Quiz) 1058.

Yeo, D. M., & Jung, S. E. (August 2018). Differentiation of acute cholecystitis from chronic cholecystitis: Determination of useful multidetector computed tomography findings. *Medicine, 97*(33), e11851.

Youngster, I. *Glucose-6-phosphate dehydrogenase deficiency.* National organization for rare disease.

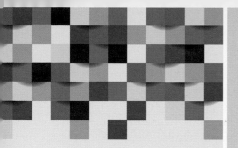

CHAPTER 6
Genitourinary System

Questions

1. A 67-year-old man with prostate cancer comes to the clinic for preoperative evaluation prior to undergoing radical prostatectomy. The patient is concerned about possible complications of radical prostatectomy and is wondering what to expect. It is most appropriate to tell this patient that which of the following is the most common postoperative complication of this procedure?
   A. Anal fissuring
   B. Erectile dysfunction
   C. Fecal incontinence
   D. Testicular injury
   E. Ventral hernia

2. A 12-year-old boy is brought to the clinic by his father because he has had a painless scrotal mass for the past three months. The patient has no history of trauma to the scrotum. Physical examination shows a large, soft scrotal mass. The testicle is firm, and no tenderness to palpation or masses are noted. Which of the following is the most likely diagnosis?
   A. Epididymitis
   B. Orchitis
   C. Testicular torsion
   D. Testicular tumor
   E. Varicocele

3. A 34-year-old woman comes to the clinic because she has had urinary frequency, urinary urgency, and dysuria for the past two days. This is the seventh time this year that this patient has had these symptoms. Physical examination shows tenderness to palpation in the suprapubic region and no costovertebral angle tenderness. Results of urinalysis are positive for leukocyte esterase and nitrites, and numerous red blood cells are noted. Which of the following recommendations is most appropriate to provide to this patient in

order to prevent the recurrence of this condition in the future?
   A. Do not urinate before sexual intercourse and hold urine for at least two hours after sexual intercourse
   B. Drink plenty of fluids and void immediately before and after sexual intercourse
   C. Hold urine for at least two hours after sexual intercourse and drink plenty of fluids
   D. Limit fluid intake and do not urinate before intercourse
   E. Limit fluid intake and empty the bladder frequently and completely

4. A 74-year-old man comes to the office because he has had worsening nocturia and increasing daytime urinary frequency over the past year. He says he has had to strain to initiate his urinary stream during this time, and there is dribbling at the end of the stream. The patient had similar symptoms at his annual physical examination nine months ago, but now his symptoms are worse and interfering with daily activities. Medical history includes hypertension, for which he takes hydrochlorothiazide 25 mg/day. Temperature is 37.0°C (98.6°F), pulse rate is 83/min, and blood pressure is 160/94 mmHg. Digital rectal examination shows a nontender, smooth, firm, and enlarged prostate gland. No nodules are noted. Serum creatinine and prostate-specific antigen levels obtained from his annual physical examination are within normal limits. Results of urinalysis are within normal limits. Which of the following is the most appropriate next step?
   A. Administer saw palmetto
   B. Administer terazosin
   C. Administer tolterodine
   D. Refer for laser transurethral prostate ablation
   E. Refer for transurethral resection of the prostate

5. A 45-year-old man comes to the emergency department because he has had pain in the right flank that radiates to the right lower quadrant of the abdomen for the past five hours. He also has had nausea and vomiting during this time. He has not had fever or chills. Medical history includes no chronic disease conditions. Temperature is 37.0°C (98.6°F), pulse rate is 110/min, respirations are 20/min, and blood pressure is 140/90 mmHg. Physical examination shows tenderness to palpation of the costovertebral angle on the right. Urinalysis shows red blood cells of 20/hpf (N ≤ 2/hpf) and no white blood cells (N ≤ 2/hpf); results are negative for leukocyte esterase. Results of complete blood cell count and basic metabolic panel are within normal limits. Which of the following studies is the most appropriate next step in diagnosis?

A. Abdominal ultrasonography
B. Contrast-enhanced MRI of the abdomen
C. CT scan of the abdomen and pelvis
D. Intravenous pyeloureterography
E. X-ray studies of the kidneys, ureter, and bladder

6. A 15-year-old boy is brought to the emergency department by his parents because he has had pain and swelling of the right testicle for the past 10 hours. The patient also has had some nausea and vomiting, and he rates the pain as a 10 on a 10-point scale. Medical history includes asthma, for which he takes albuterol via metered dose inhaler as needed. Ultrasonography shows absent blood flow to the right testicle. Which of the following is the most appropriate definitive management?

A. Intravenous antibiotics
B. Manual derotation
C. Oral antibiotics
D. Surgical derotation
E. Urology consultation

7. A 68-year-old woman, gravida 6, para 6, comes to the clinic because she has had urinary incontinence during the past year. She says she leaks urine when laughing, coughing, or sneezing and needs to wear an absorbent pad in her underwear. The patient does not experience an urge to urinate prior to the episodes of incontinence. She has no history of trauma or injury. She is otherwise healthy, has an active lifestyle, and lives independently. The patient takes no medications. Medical history includes uncomplicated spontaneous vaginal deliveries for each of her six children. This patient is most likely experiencing which of the following types of incontinence?

A. Functional
B. Mixed

C. Overflow
D. Stress
E. Urge

8. A 45-year-old man comes to the emergency department because he has had painful and frequent urination for the past five days as well as fever for the past three days. He has not had abdominal pain, nausea and vomiting, or chills. Medical history includes no chronic disease conditions. Temperature is 39.2°C (102.5°F); all other vital signs are within normal limits. The patient appears well and is not in acute distress. Results of urinalysis are positive for nitrites and leukocyte esterase; white blood cells are 20/hpf (N = 2 to 5/hpf). Which of the following is the most appropriate oral treatment regimen for this patient?

A. Cephalexin for 14 days
B. Ciprofloxacin for 28 days
C. Clindamycin for 28 days
D. Levofloxacin for 10 days
E. Trimethoprim-sulfamethoxazole for 10 days

9. A 66-year-old woman comes to the office because she has had a fever to 38.3°C (100.9°F), chills, urinary urgency, dysuria, and nausea and vomiting during the past four days. Current temperature is 38.0°C (100.4°F), and pulse rate is 110/min. All other vital signs are within normal limits. On physical examination, costovertebral angle tenderness is noted. Urinalysis shows bacteriuria and numerous red blood cells and is positive for nitrites. Which of the following bacteria is most likely to be seen on culture of the urine?

A. *Enterococcus faecalis*
B. *Escherichia coli*
C. *Proteus mirabilis*
D. *Staphylococcus aureus*
E. *Streptococcus agalactiae*

10. A 64-year-old man comes to the office because he has had decreased libido and erectile dysfunction during the past few months since his medications for diabetes mellitus, depression, hypothyroidism, and hypertension were adjusted. Which of the following medications is most likely contributing to the symptoms in this patient?

A. Doxazosin
B. Enalapril
C. Insulin
D. Levothyroxine
E. Sertraline

11. A 55-year-old man who is of African descent comes to the primary care clinic with his interpreter from the immigration center. The patient has had a painless, slowly growing lesion on his penis for the past six months. Vital signs are within normal limits. Cardiac, pulmonary, and abdominal examinations show no abnormalities. Retraction of a slightly inflamed foreskin shows an irregular, centrally ulcerated, warty lesion that is shallow and 1 cm in diameter on the proximal dorsal glans penis. Scattered malodorous curdled debris is also noted. Firm, nontender inguinal lymphadenopathy is noted bilaterally. No edema is noted in the lower extremities. Which of the following is the most likely diagnosis?
A. Adenomatoid tumor
B. Chancroid lesion
C. Condylomata acuminata
D. Kaposi sarcoma
E. Squamous cell carcinoma

12. A 25-year-old man comes to the emergency department because he has had pain and swelling of the left testicle for the past two weeks. He says he regularly engages in unprotected anal intercourse. Medical history includes no chronic disease conditions. Vitals signs are within normal limits. Physical examination shows edema and tenderness to palpation of the left testicle as well as the epididymis. Results of urinalysis are positive for nitrites and leukocyte esterase; white blood cells are 20/hpf (N $\leq$ 2 to 5/hpf). Ultrasonography of the testis shows no abnormalities. Results of gonorrhea and chlamydia testing are pending, and the patient requests that he begin treatment immediately. Which of the following is the most appropriate treatment?
A. Acyclovir and trimethoprim-sulfamethoxazole
B. Ceftriaxone and doxycycline
C. Ceftriaxone and trimethoprim-sulfamethoxazole
D. Levofloxacin and trimethoprim-sulfamethoxazole
E. Metronidazole and doxycycline

13. A 60-year-old woman comes to the office because she has had urinary urgency for the past six months. She says she gets a strong, sudden urge to urinate and feels like she needs to pass urine many times during the day and night. The urgency is getting worse and is interfering with her office job. The patient does not leak urine. Medical history includes hypertension, for which she takes benazepril, and vitamin D deficiency, for which she takes a supplement. Results of chemical urinalysis are within normal limits. A malfunction in which of the following muscles is most likely responsible for the symptoms in this patient?
A. Detrusor
B. External oblique
C. Obturator internus
D. Piriformis
E. Transversus abdominis

14. A 58-year-old man comes to the clinic because his penis has been curving upwards when he has had an erection during the past six months. He says that the degree of bending has been getting more severe and now he has associated pain. It is becoming more difficult to have intercourse due to the bending. Physical examination of the flaccid penis shows a palpable nodule on the dorsal aspect of the mid shaft. Ultrasonography of the penis, which is required prior to scheduling an appointment with the local urologist, shows a localized plaque with calcification in the tunica albuginea on the dorsum of the penis. Which of the following is the most likely diagnosis?
A. Balanitis
B. Dupuytren contracture
C. Penile fracture
D. Peyronie disease
E. Phimosis

15. A 14-year-old boy is brought to the emergency department by his father because he had acute onset of testicular pain 90 minutes ago. The patient says the pain started in his left testis and is now present throughout his scrotum. The father says that the patient also has had fever, fatigue, and chills since this morning, and his cheeks have been significantly swollen for the past week. The patient had been previously healthy and has no known sick contacts. He has never been vaccinated and has no history of surgical procedures. Temperature is 38.7°C (101.6°F), pulse rate is 99/min, and respirations are 16/min. Physical examination shows mild, bilateral testicular enlargement and tenderness and erythema of the scrotum. The testicles are not high riding, and there is no penile discharge. The epididymis is not enlarged, and cremasteric reflex is positive. Which of the following is the most likely diagnosis?
A. *Chlamydia trachomatis*
B. Epididymitis
C. Hydrocele
D. Orchitis
E. Testicular torsion

    Answer Key for this chapter begins on p. 99

16. A 38-year-old woman, gravida 1, para 1, comes to the office because she has had the urgency to defecate as well as leakage of stool since she gave birth to her son three months ago. Prenatal course was normal, and the baby was delivered vaginally at term. At the time of delivery, the patient was told that she had a tear, and it took longer for delivery of the placenta than usual. Her son's birth weight was 8 lb 2 oz. Medical history includes Hashimoto thyroiditis, for which she takes levothyroxine. She used to smoke cigarettes but quit when she became pregnant. Which of the following findings is the most likely predisposing factor related to the symptoms in this patient?
    A. Age at delivery of first child
    B. History of Hashimoto thyroiditis
    C. Prolonged third stage of labor
    D. Smoking history
    E. Vaginal tear

17. A 12-month-old girl is brought to the emergency department by her mother because she has had a fever for the past two days. The most recent measurement taken at home three hours ago was 38.9°C (102.0°F). The mother says the patient also has been irritable and eating less during this time. She has not had a runny nose, cough, vomiting, or diarrhea. Medical history includes a urinary tract infection (UTI) with fever four months ago that was treated successfully with antibiotic therapy. Renal ultrasonography obtained at that time showed no abnormalities. Current temperature is 39.0°C (102.2°F). The patient is crying but does not appear to be toxic. Physical examination shows suprapubic tenderness. Results of chemical urinalysis are positive for leukocyte esterase and nitrites. Results of microscopic urinalysis show pyuria. If urine culture confirms another UTI, which of the following diagnostic tests is most appropriate to perform after treatment?
    A. CT urography
    B. Plain film x-ray study of the kidneys, ureter, and bladder
    C. Renal angiography
    D. Voiding cystourethrography

18. A 71-year-old man is referred to the urology clinic by his primary care provider because he is suspected of having bladder cancer. If this patient has this type of cancer, which of the following presenting symptoms is most likely?

A. Dysuria
B. Edema of the lower extremities
C. Flank pain
D. Painless hematuria
E. Urinary urgency

19. A 41-year-old woman comes to the office because she has had frequent urination with a burning sensation as well as urgency for the past three days. She has no history of similar symptoms. Temperature is 37.3°C (99.2°F), pulse rate is 82/min, and blood pressure is 118/70 mmHg. Physical examination shows suprapubic tenderness. Findings on urinalysis include the following:

Chemical:

Bilirubin	Negative
Glucose	Negative
Ketones	Negative
Leukocyte esterase	Positive
Protein	Trace

Microscopic:

Red blood cells	3–4/hpf (N = 0–5/hpf)
White blood cells	>100,00/hpf (N = 0–5/hpf)

Which of the following is the most likely diagnosis?
A. Cystitis
B. Interstitial nephritis
C. Pyelonephritis
D. Urge incontinence
E. Urolithiasis

20. A 55-year-old man who is uncircumcised comes to the emergency department because he has had penile pain and difficulty pulling his foreskin back for the past two days. Medical history includes no chronic disease conditions. Vitals signs are within normal limits. On physical examination, the foreskin is in the retracted position and cannot be reduced distally past the glans penis. Edema of the foreskin is noted. Attempts at manual repositioning fail. Injection of which of the following into the foreskin is most appropriate?
    A. Epinephrine
    B. Hyaluronidase
    C. Lidocaine
    D. Mannitol
    E. Solumedrol

Answers

1. **Answer: B** Radical prostatectomy is a procedure generally performed in patients with localized prostate cancer who are expected to live more than 10 years. Greater than 50% of men who undergo radical prostatectomy experience postoperative erectile dysfunction, option B.
The other common complication of radical prostatectomy is urinary incontinence and not fecal incontinence, option C. Anal fissuring, option A, and testicular injury, option D, are not common complications of radical prostatectomy. Inguinal hernia is a possible complication of this surgery, not ventral hernia (option E). **Task:** D2—Clinical Intervention

2. **Answer: E** Varicocele, option E, is a common and benign condition that is usually painless and causes scrotal edema. It is often described as having a "bag of worms" appearance. Varicocele is caused by varicosities in the pampiniform plexus and most commonly develops in boys between 10 and 15 years of age.
Epididymitis, option A, is inflammation of the epididymis and causes testicular pain, which this patient does not have. Orchitis, option B, is inflammation of the testicle and is also a painful condition. Testicular torsion, option C, is a cause of acute scrotal pain and is characterized by torsion of the spermatic cord. Patients with a testicular tumor, option D, typically have a palpable testicular mass. **Task:** A—History Taking and Performing Physical Examination

3. **Answer: B** Option B, drink plenty of fluids and void before and after sexual intercourse, is appropriate to recommend to this patient because both of these suggestions help to clear the urinary tract.
Emptying the bladder frequently and completely (option E) is appropriate advice, but recommending the patient limit fluid intake (options D and E) is inappropriate. All the other options are inappropriate recommendations to give this patient, since limiting fluids and holding urine before and after sexual intercourse will only worsen her symptoms and increase her risk for urinary tract infections in the future. **Task:** D1—Health Maintenance, Patient Education, and Disease Prevention

4. **Answer: B** Terazosin, option B, is an alpha-blocker and relaxes the muscles in the prostate and the opening of the bladder thus increasing the flow of urine.
Saw palmetto, option A, is a supplement to promote prostate health. Recent studies show that this drug is no better than a placebo for the treatment of benign prostate hypertrophy (BPH). Tolterodine, option C, is an anticholinergic that is used to treat overactive bladder (OAB). It is used for BPH when OAB symptoms are also present and is usually combined with an alpha-blocker or a 5-alpha reductase inhibitor. Referral for laser transurethral prostate ablation or transurethral resection of the prostate, options D and E, are invasive procedures and reserved for patients who fail pharmacotherapy. **Task:** D3—Pharmaceutical Therapeutics

5. **Answer: C** This patient has symptoms of nephrolithiasis, and the best study to determine the diagnosis is a CT scan of the abdomen and pelvis without contrast, option C. A CT scan using low-dose radiation is the preferred examination for most adults with similar symptoms. It has the highest diagnostic accuracy for renal and ureteral stones. It provides information on the stone size, location, and site of obstruction. This study is also useful in determining an alternate diagnosis.
Abdominal ultrasonography, option A, does not provide good visualization for all types of renal stones. Contrast-enhanced MRI of the abdomen, option B, is not the most appropriate next diagnostic tool for kidney stones. Intravenous pyeloureterography or plain x-ray studies (options D and E) could be used, but these will not give the specifics about the stones and are not the most appropriate next step in this setting. **Task:** B—Using Diagnostic and Laboratory Studies

6. **Answer: D** Although a provider may attempt to perform manual derotation (option B), definitive treatment of testicular torsion involves surgical derotation of the spermatic cord, option D, followed by bilateral testicular fixation with nonabsorbable sutures. If the affected testis is nonviable, orchiectomy of the affected testis and orchiopexy of the contralateral side are performed.
Intravenous antibiotics, option A, may be provided before, during, or after surgery, but it will not correct the testicular torsion in this patient. Oral antibiotics, option C, will not provide definitive treatment for testicular torsion. A urology consultation, option E, may be required for this patient, however surgical intervention will definitively manage the testicular torsion. **Task:** D2—Clinical Intervention

7. **Answer: D** Stress incontinence, option D, is most common in postmenopausal, multiparous women and is caused by weakness in the urinary sphincter. It is characterized by incontinence that coincides with laughing, coughing, or sneezing.
Functional incontinence, option A, refers to incontinence caused by an inability to access a toilet or urinal in a timely manner, often due to decreased mobility.

This is not the most likely diagnosis because the scenario specifically says that the patient is in good health, active, and lives independently. Mixed incontinence, option B, refers to incontinence that has elements of both stress and urge incontinence. Urge incontinence, option E, refers to incontinence that is immediately preceded by an urge to urinate. Because this patient does not experience urinary urgency, neither option B nor E are correct. Overflow incontinence, option C, is most common in men with bladder outlet obstruction and is not associated with Valsalva maneuvers. **Task:** A—History Taking and Performing Physical Examination

8. **Answer: B** This patient has signs and symptoms of prostatitis. Fluoroquinolone antibiotics are appropriate first-line therapy for acute and chronic bacterial prostatitis. Ciprofloxacin, option B, and levofloxacin, option D, have demonstrated cure rates of 73% to 75%. For those with acute prostatitis, oral ciprofloxacin 500 mg orally, twice daily for four to six weeks, or levofloxacin 500 mg orally, once daily for four to six weeks is appropriate for nonseptic patients.

Option A, cephalexin for 14 days, is primarily used to treat a simple urinary tract infection without signs and symptoms of acute prostatitis. Clindamycin for 28 days, option C, is not an appropriate regimen for the treatment of patients with urinary tract infection or acute prostatitis. Levofloxacin, option D, is an appropriate medication, however, the length of treatment is not appropriate. Trimethoprim-sulfamethoxazole for 10 days, option E, may be used to treat a simple urinary tract infection but not suspected acute prostatitis. **Task:** D3—Pharmaceutical Therapeutics

9. **Answer: B** Based on this patient's symptoms and the findings on physical examination and laboratory studies, this patient has pyelonephritis. The most common causative organisms that cause this condition are gram-negative bacteria, as noted on urine culture. Therefore, *Escherichia coli*, option B, is correct because it is a gram-negative bacterium.

Enterococcus faecalis, Staphylococcus aureus, and *Streptococcus agalactiae* (options A, D, and E) are all gram-positive bacteria and are unlikely to show up on a urine culture of this patient. *Proteus mirabilis*, option C, is a gram-negative bacterium, but it is a rare cause of urinary infections including pyelonephritis. **Task:** E—Applying Basic Scientific Concepts

10. **Answer: E** Erectile dysfunction has many risk factors including age and the presence of comorbid conditions such as diabetes mellitus, hypertension, dyslipidemia, obstructive sleep apnea, cardiovascular disease, cigarette smoking, alcohol/drug use, and obesity. Lifestyle modifications, reduction of risk factors, and medical

therapy including phosphodiesterase-5 inhibitors are the cornerstone of management. The most likely pharmaceutical cause of the low libido and erectile dysfunction in this patient is sertraline, option E, which is a selective serotonin reuptake inhibitor used to treat depression.

The alpha$_1$-blocker doxazosin (option A), which is used to treat hypertension, may actually improve sexual function. Enalapril, insulin, and levothyroxine (options B, C, and D), which are used to treat hypertension, diabetes mellitus, and hypothyroidism respectively, do not have erectile dysfunction listed as a potential adverse effect. **Task:** D3—Pharmaceutical Therapeutics

11. **Answer: E** This patient has signs and symptoms of squamous cell carcinoma of the penis, option E. This is the most common penile cancer (98%) and most commonly presents in uncircumcised males in the fifth decade of life. Penile cancers in males from the United States are extremely rare, but penile carcinoma in males of African descent may represent up to 10% to 20% of all malignant lesions.

Adenomatoid tumor, option A, is the most common tumor of the testicle and feels solid on palpation during physical examination. A chancroid lesion, option B, is a painful ulcer without surrounding inflammation. Lymphadenopathy rapidly becomes fluctuant in patients with this type of penile lesion. Condylomata acuminate, option C, presents as a grapelike cluster, which is not evident in this patient. Kaposi sarcoma, option D, is indicated by a painful, blue-purple papule on the penis. **Task:** A—History Taking and Performing Physical Examination

12. **Answer: B** This patient has symptoms of acute epididymitis, likely caused by a sexually transmitted infection. The 2020 CDC recommendations call for ceftriaxone 500 mg intramuscularly in a single dose, and if a chlamydial infection has not been excluded, then doxycycline 100 mg orally twice daily for seven days is added to the regimen. Therefore, option B is the most appropriate treatment.

Acyclovir is used to treat herpes virus infections, and trimethoprim-sulfamethoxazole is indicated for urinary tract infections and not sexually transmitted diseases. Therefore, options A, C, and D are incorrect. Metronidazole, option E, is an antibiotic used to treat bacterial and parasitic diseases but is not indicated for chlamydia or gonorrhea. **Task:** D3—Pharmaceutical Therapeutics

13. **Answer: A** The correct answer is detrusor, option A. Dysfunction in the detrusor muscle is characterized by dysuria and urinary frequency as well as suprapubic tenderness.

The external oblique muscle, option B, is located on the sides of the abdomen and is responsible for twisting of the trunk. The obturator internus muscle, option C, is a hip muscle that rotates the extended thigh and abducts the flexed thigh. The piriformis muscle, option D, is in the buttocks near the hip joint; it stabilizes the hip joint and is not related to bladder function. The transversus abdominis muscles, option E, are located on the lateral sides of the abdominal wall and provide thoracic and pelvic stability. **Task:** E—Applying Basic Scientific Concepts

14. **Answer: D** This patient has Peyronie disease, option D. Although usually diagnosed from the patient's history alone, ultrasonography is often able to delineate the anatomic pathology associated with this progressive condition.
Balanitis, option A, is infection and/or inflammation of the glans portion of the penis. Although serious, balanitis is confined to the glans and is not capable of producing alterations in the configuration of the shaft. Dupuytren contracture, option B, involves the palm of the hand and is the result of a sclerosing process similar to that described in this question. Since Dupuytren is unrelated to the penis, option B is incorrect. However, studies show that more than 20% of men with Dupuytren contracture also have a contracture of the tunica albuginea of the penis. Penile fracture, option C, is incorrect because a penile fracture is an acute rupture of the tunica albuginea, usually resulting from forceful bending during intercourse. A slower, more chronic problem is described in this patient. Phimosis, option E, is a condition whereby the foreskin is so tight it cannot be retracted off the glans penis. Phimosis does not result in a curved shaft of the penis. **Task:** C—Formulating Most Likely Diagnosis

15. **Answer: D** This patient has orchitis, option D, due to a mumps infection. Orchitis is a common finding, which occurs approximately 7 to 10 days after the onset of parotitis in children. The occurrence of mumps has decreased due to vaccinations.
Chlamydia trachomatis, option A, is typically spread by sexual transmission; there is no indication of this patient's sexual history in the scenario. Chlamydia is often asymptomatic but may present with penile discharge. Epididymitis, option B, is an inflammation of the epididymis that causes unilateral pain and edema and is most common in sexually active men. A hydrocele, option C, is a collection of fluid in the membranes surrounding the scrotum. It is usually painless and present in newborns. Testicular torsion, option E, is an emergency caused by the twisting of a testicle that presents as high riding. **Task:** A—History Taking and Performing Physical Examination

16. **Answer: E** The correct answer is vaginal tear, option E. Vaginal delivery with a tear may result in internal or external anal sphincter disruption, causing fecal incontinence (FI).
The patient's age at delivery of her first child, option A, is not a predisposing factor for FI. History of Hashimoto thyroiditis, option B, and smoking, option D, are not related to FI. Prolonged third stage of labor, option C, refers to the placenta delivery and is not associated with FI. **Task:** D1—Health Maintenance, Patient Education, and Disease Prevention

17. **Answer: D** The correct answer is voiding cystourethrography (VCUG), option D. Guidelines recommend that febrile infants with urinary tract infections (UTIs) should undergo renal and bladder ultrasonography to detect abnormal anatomic structures after a first UTI. VCUG should be performed after a second UTI to identify infants with very high-grade reflux because of the risk of renal scarring.
CT urography, plain film x-ray studies of the kidneys, ureter, and bladder, and renal angiography (options A, B, and C) are not optimal studies to identify vesicoureteral reflux. VCUG uses fluoroscopy and a contrast material that fills the bladder to show the organs in motion, making it more likely to detect reflux. The CT urography and plain film x-ray studies will not show motion. Renal angiography is used to study the blood vessels in the kidney. **Task:** B—Using Diagnostic and Laboratory Studies

18. **Answer: D** Bladder cancer is the sixth most common malignancy in the United States, is most common in males, and is associated with smoking and occupational exposures. Though dysuria, edema of the lower extremities, flank pain, and urinary urgency (options A, B, C, and E) can be symptoms of bladder cancer, painless gross hematuria (option D) is the most common presenting symptom. Any patient who has painless hematuria should be evaluated for bladder cancer. **Task:** A—History Taking and Performing Physical Examination

19. **Answer: A** Cystitis, option A, is the correct answer because this condition is characterized by dysuria and urinary frequency as well as suprapubic tenderness, all of which are present in this patient. Interstitial nephritis, option B, is a kidney disorder that affects the filtering capabilities of the kidneys. Patients with interstitial nephritis usually have hematuria, fever, and nausea. Patients with pyelonephritis, option C, usually have irritative voiding symptoms like cystitis (urgency, frequency, dysuria) but also have flank pain and fever. Physical examination of patients with this disorder shows costovertebral angle tenderness, and urinalysis shows pyuria. Urge incontinence, option D, is the urge

to urinate with leaking, which this patient does not have. Urolithiasis, option E, is defined as a stone in the urinary tract. The patient with this condition usually has severe pain on the side and/or back below the ribs; they will also have more blood in the urine. Pyuria is not a common finding unless there is a concomitant infection. **Task:** C—Formulating Most Likely Diagnosis

20. **Answer: B** This patient has symptoms of phimosis. One pharmacologic method for reducing foreskin edema includes the invasive injection of hyaluronidase, option B, into the edematous foreskin. Reduction of the glans penis can also be achieved through manual compression, ice packs, or wrapping the glans in compressive dressings. Reduction of the foreskin can also be achieved through making micro-punctures in the foreskin, thereby releasing edematous fluid. Epinephrine, option A, is a sympathomimetic, anti-arrhythmic, and inotropic pressor. It is not indicated for phimosis. Lidocaine, option C, is an antiarrhythmic used to treat arrhythmia as well as an anesthetic used to numb the skin. It is not indicated for the resolution of phimosis. Mannitol, option D, is a diuretic often used for cerebral edema and increased intraocular pressure. Solumedrol, option E, is a corticosteroid used for various corticosteroid-responsive conditions but not for the treatment of phimosis. **Task:** D3—Pharmaceutical Therapeutics

BIBLIOGRAPHY

Azmat, C., & Vaitla, P. (2020). Orchitis. *StatPearls [Internet]*.

Breyer, B. N., & McAninch, J. W. Disorders of the penis and male urethra. In: J. W. McAninch & T. F. Lue (Eds.), *Smith & Tanagho's General Urology* (19th ed.). McGraw-Hill.

Corbo, J., & Wang, J. (2019). Kidney and ureteral stones. *Emergency Medicine Clinics of North America, 37*(4), 637-648.

Elsamra, S. (2021). Evaluation of the urologic patient: history and physical examination. In A. Partin, R. Dmochowski, L. Kavoussi, & C. Peters (Eds.), *Campbell-Walsh-Wein Urology* (12h ed., pp. 1-13). Elsevier, Inc. e1.

Fayssoux, K. (2020). Bacterial infections of the urinary tract in women. *Conn's Current Therapy 2020*, (1st ed., pp 1136-1138).

Ferri, F. (2021). Prostate cancer. In F. Ferri (Ed.), *Ferri's clinical advisor 2021* (pp. 1166-1170). Elsevier, Inc.

Ferri, F. F. (2021). Testicular Torsion. In F. Ferri (Ed.), *Ferri's Clinical Advisor* (pp. 1349-1349). Elsevier, Inc.

Kristy McKiernan Borawski. *Sexually transmitted diseases*. Campbell-Walsh-Wein Urology, 58, pp. 1251-1272.e4.

Lobo, R., Gershenson, D., & Lentz, G. (2017). (7th ed.) *Comprehensive gynecology* (21, pp. 474-504). Elsevier.

Offenbacher, J., & Barbera., A. (2019). Penile emergencies. *Emergency Medicine Clinics of North America, 37*(4), 583-592.

Papadakis, M. A., & McPhee, S. J. (2020). *Current Medical Diagnosis & Treatment* (pp. 990-995). McGraw-Hill Education/Medical.

Papadakis, M., McPhee, S., & Rabow, M. (2019). *Current medical diagnosis & treatment 2020* (59th ed.). Cenveo Publisher Services.

Papadakis, M. A., McPhee, S. J., & Rabow, M. W. (2020). Chapter 23: Urologic disorders: *Current medical diagnosis & treatment 2020* (pp. 972-977). McGraw-Hill Education.

Porten, S. P. & Presti, J. C. Jr. Genital tumors. In: J. W. McAninch & T. F. Lue (Eds.), *Smith & Tanagho's general urology* (19th ed.). McGraw-Hill.

Powell, C. R. (2020). Prostatitis. *Conn's Current Therapy*, 1128-1130.

Rathore, B. (2021). Bladder cancer. In F. Ferri (Ed.), *Ferri's clinical advisor 2021* (pp. 247-250). Elsevier, Inc. e2.

Snyder, P. J., & Rosen, R. C. (2020). Overview of male sexual dysfunction. In T. Post (Ed.), *UpToDate*. Waltham, MA: UpToDate.

Subcommittee on Urinary Tract Infection, & Steering Committee on Quality Improvement and Management. (2011). Urinary tract infection: Clinical practice guideline for the diagnosis and management of the initial UTI in febrile infants and children 2 to 24 months. *Pediatrics, 128*(3), 595-610.

Subki, A. H., Fakeeh, M. M., Hindi, M. M., Nasr, A. M., Almaymuni, A. D., & Abduljabbar, H. S. (2019). Fecal and urinary incontinence associated with pregnancy and childbirth. *Mater Sociomed, 31*(3), 202-206.

Van Kirk, E., & Caraganis, A. (2021). Varicocele. In F. Ferri (Ed.), *Ferri's clinical advisor 2021*. Elsevier, Inc. 1437.e4-1437.e5.

Wein, A. J., & Rackley, R. R. (2006). Overactive bladder: a better understanding of pathophysiology, diagnosis and management. *The Journal of Urology, 175*(3 Pt 2), S5-10.

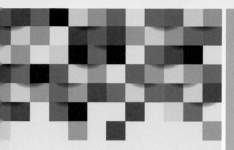
Questions

1. A 67-year-old woman comes to the clinic because she has been experiencing her second episode of herpes zoster within the past year. The first episode occurred nine months ago and was resolved after five weeks; this current episode began six days ago and was accompanied by worsening fatigue and night sweats. Physical examination shows pale skin, mucocutaneous petechiae, and enlarged nontender lymph nodes in the right axilla. Peripheral blood smear shows a mature cell line and the presence of smudge cells. Which of the following is the most likely diagnosis?
   A. Acute myeloid leukemia
   B. Chronic lymphocytic leukemia
   C. Hairy cell leukemia
   D. Non-Hodgkin lymphoma
   E. Small lymphocytic lymphoma

2. A 54-year-old man comes to the office because he has had worsening fatigue over the past two months. Medical history includes end-stage renal disease that is being treated with dialysis. Findings on laboratory studies of serum obtained one day ago during dialysis include the following:

Ferritin	121 ng/mL (N = 23–336 ng/mL)
Iron	30 μg/dL (N = 45–182 μg/dL)
Iron-binding capacity	259 μg/dL (N = 255–450 μg/dL)
Hemoglobin	9.7 g/dL (N = 12–18 g/dL)
Mean corpuscular volume	88 μm³ (N = 80–100 μm³)
Reticulocyte count	1.0% of red cells (N = 0.3–2.3% of red cells)

Based on these findings, which of the following is the most likely diagnosis?

A. Anemia of chronic disease
B. Folate deficiency
C. Iron deficiency anemia
D. Thalassemia
E. Vitamin B_{12} deficiency

3. A 70-year-old woman comes to the office because she has had an enlarging lump on the side of her neck that she first noticed two months ago while she was applying makeup. She says the lump is not painful, and she has not had a sore throat, cough, or cold during the past six months. Medical history includes hypertension and osteoarthritis, for which she takes hydrochlorothiazide and diclofenac, respectively. Vital signs are within normal limits. Physical examination shows a nontender, 3-cm anterior cervical lymph node on the right side; the node feels rubbery. Results of complete blood cell count are within normal limits, and a chest x-ray study shows no abnormalities. Which of the following is the most appropriate next step?
   A. Bronchoscopy
   B. Epstein-Barr virus antibody titer
   C. Excisional node biopsy
   D. Serum protein electrophoresis
   E. Throat culture

4. The parents of a newborn are informed that universal newborn screening has determined that their child has sickle cell disease. As part of parental education, they are told that it is necessary that their child have antibiotic prophylaxis administered from infancy until at least 5 years of age. This prophylaxis is directed at preventing infection with which of the following?
   A. Group B streptococcus
   B. *Staphylococcus aureus*
   C. *Staphylococcus saprophyticus*
   D. *Streptococcus pneumoniae*
   E. *Streptococcus pyogenes*

5. A 56-year-old woman is in the hospital awaiting transfusion of packed red blood cells for treatment of anemia secondary to bleeding from a gastric ulcer. Shortly after the transfusion begins, the patient notices that she has development of hives on her arms. Vital signs are within normal limits; physical examination shows no edema of the lips, tongue, or throat. Auscultation of the lungs shows no wheezing or stridor. Laboratory studies show no evidence of hemolysis. Which of the following is the most appropriate treatment?
   A. Acetaminophen
   B. Albuterol
   C. Diphenhydramine
   D. Epinephrine
   E. Furosemide

6. A patient with a recent diagnosis of hemochromatosis is scheduled to undergo phlebotomy for the first time and comes to the office to learn about the procedure. When educating this patient about the possible effects of phlebotomy in treating hemochromatosis, it is most appropriate to tell them which of the following?
   A. Arthropathy and hypogonadism are very responsive to treatment
   B. Insulin requirements and cardiac function are not often affected
   C. Malaise, changes in skin pigmentation, and abdominal pain are not likely to be relieved
   D. Reversal of hepatic fibrosis and regression of mild-to-moderate cirrhosis may occur
   E. Risk for hepatocellular carcinoma decreases in patients with cirrhosis

7. A 41-year-old man comes to the office because he has had extreme exhaustion, tachycardia, and palpitations for the past six weeks. Six months ago, he underwent gastric bypass surgery; since then, he has lost a total of 45 lb. His diet has been limited, and he says he has been craving ice chips. Laboratory findings include the following:

Serum	
Ferritin	9.9 ng/mL (N = >10–20 ng/mL)
Iron	22 μg/dL (N = 50–150 μg/dL)
Iron-binding capacity	458 μg/dL (N = 250–410 μg/dL)
Transferrin saturation	5.6% (N = 15–20%)
Hematocrit	29.6% (N = 42–52% for males)
Hemoglobin	7.8 g/dL (N = 14–18 g/dL for males)
Mean corpuscular hemoglobin	24 pg/cell (N = 27–33 pg/cell)
Mean corpuscular hemoglobin concentration	20.1 g/dL (N = 31–35 g/dL)
Mean corpuscular volume	71.5 μm³ (N = 80–96 μm³ for males)
Red cell distribution width	18% (N = 11–16%)

Which of the following nail findings is most likely in this patient?
   A. Koilonychia
   B. Lindsay nails
   C. Onychoschizia
   D. Terry nails
   E. Trachyonychia

8. A 56-year-old woman who is currently undergoing chemotherapy for treatment of breast cancer comes to the primary care clinic because she has had cough for the past two days. Temperature is 39.2°C (102.6°F), and the patient appears ill. Physical examination shows decreased breath sounds in the left lung base. Complete blood cell count shows leukopenia and an absolute neutrophil count of 900/mm³ (N = >1500/mm³). Which of the following is the most appropriate next step?
   A. Order an outpatient chest x-ray study
   B. Prescribe oral azithromycin
   C. Recommend at-home symptomatic treatment
   D. Repeat laboratory studies in three days
   E. Send the patient to the emergency department

9. A 25-year-old woman comes to the clinic to discuss the results of a commercial genetic testing service that she purchased on her own. The report she received says that she is heterozygous for the factor V Leiden gene mutation. Based on this information, this patient is at increased risk for which of the following conditions?
   A. Alzheimer disease
   B. Beta thalassemia
   C. Breast cancer
   D. Celiac disease
   E. Venous thromboembolism

10. A 55-year-old man comes to the office for follow-up to discuss results of recent laboratory studies that were obtained one week ago during routine physical examination. Laboratory studies show increased red blood cell count and elevated hemoglobin levels. When the patient is asked if he has any symptoms, he says that he has occasional headaches and itching after taking a hot bath. Polycythemia vera is suspected. The presence of which of the following on additional laboratory analysis will most likely confirm this diagnosis?
   A. Auer rods
   B. Bence Jones protein
   C. *JAK2* V617F mutation
   D. Philadelphia chromosome
   E. Reed-Sternberg cells

11. A 52-year-old woman comes to the office with her husband because she has had difficulty walking as well as a sharp sensation in her feet for the past three months. Her husband is concerned because she occasionally has confusion and difficulty with concentration. Medical history includes gastric bypass surgery one year ago. She has been successful with monitoring and following the prescribed diet and has lost 100 lb during the past year. Physical examination shows decreased sensation to vibration and decreased proprioception in the lower extremities. Based on these findings, this patient most likely has a deficiency in which of the following vitamins?
    A. Niacin
    B. Thiamine
    C. Vitamin A
    D. Vitamin B_{12}
    E. Vitamin D

12. A 58-year-old man comes to the office because he has had fatigue and night sweats for the past four months. He says he has felt feverish at times, but he has not taken his temperature. He is otherwise healthy. Medical history includes no chronic disease conditions, and he takes no medications. Temperature is 38.0°C (100.4°F), pulse rate is 90/min, respirations are 20/min, and blood pressure is 140/86 mmHg. On physical examination, the spleen is palpated 4 cm below the costal margin. Findings on complete blood cell count include the following:

Red blood cell count	3.8 million/mm³ (N = 4.4–6.3 million/mm³)
Hematocrit	37% (N = 41–53%)
Hemoglobin	13.1 g/dL (N = 14–18 g/dL)
White blood cell count	80,500/mm³ (N = 4000–9900/mm³)
Neutrophils	67% (N = 54–62%)
Bands	9% (N = 3–5%)
Eosinophils	3% (N = 1–3%)
Lymphocytes	7% (N = 25–33%)
Metamyelocytes	5% (N = 0%)
Monocytes	2% (N = 3–7%)
Myelocytes	3% (N = 0%)
Platelet count	280,000/mm³ (N = 150,000–450,000/mm³)

Cytogenic analysis shows the presence of the Philadelphia chromosome. Which of the following is the most likely diagnosis?
    A. Chronic myeloid leukemia
    B. Leukemoid reaction
    C. Multiple myeloma
    D. Polycythemia vera
    E. Primary myelofibrosis

13. A 44-year-old woman comes to the emergency department because she has had bruising on her lower extremities for the past week. She says she also has not been feeling like herself lately. She has no history of injury or trauma. Low-grade fever is noted, and the patient has slight confusion. Physical examination shows ecchymosis on the lower extremities. Laboratory studies show hemoglobin level of 7.0 g/dL (N = 12-16 g/dL), platelet count of 10,000/mm³ (N = 130,000–450,000/mm³), and serum creatinine level of 1.6 mg/dL (N = 0.7–1.3 mg/dL). Peripheral blood smear shows schistocytes and an elevated reticulocyte count. Which of the following is the most important initial treatment?
    A. Aspirin
    B. Fresh frozen plasma
    C. Intravenous heparin
    D. Intravenous immune globulin
    E. Plasma exchange

14. A 12-year-old girl is brought to the emergency department by her mother because she has had fatigue for the past three days. Ten days ago, the patient had nonproductive cough without a fever and was treated with amoxicillin therapy for seven days. The mother says the cough is still present, although slightly diminished, but now the patient seems weak and pale and has no energy. Medical history includes no chronic disease conditions. Current temperature is 37.0°C (98.6°F), pulse rate is 120/min, respirations are 18/min, and blood pressure is 100/60 mmHg. Physical examination shows pallor and a systolic flow murmur. The lungs are clear to auscultation. Laboratory findings include the following:

Red blood cell count	2.7 million/mm³ (N = 4.4–6.3 million/mm³)
Hematocrit	22.6% (N = 36–46%)
Hemoglobin	8.5 g/dL (N = 14–18 g/dL)
White blood cell count	7500/mm³ (N = 4000–9900/mm³)
Mean corpuscular volume	83 μm³ (N = 80–100 μm³)
Reticulocyte count	14.1% (N = 0.5–1.5%)
Serum	
Bilirubin, total	1.5 mg/dL (N = 0.1–1.0 mg/dL)
Bilirubin, indirect	1.2 mg/dL (N = 0.2–0.8 mg/dL)
Haptoglobin	18 mg/dL (N = 30–200 mg/dL)

Result of direct Coombs test is positive. Which of the following is the most likely diagnosis?
    A. Anemia of chronic disease
    B. Aplastic anemia
    C. Autoimmune hemolytic anemia
    D. Iron deficiency anemia
    E. Thalassemia minor

15. A 48-year-old man with a history of alcohol use comes to the clinic because he has had worsening fatigue over the past three to six months. He also says that his tongue has been sore during this time. Vital signs are within normal limits. On physical examination, the tongue is beefy red and smooth. Neurologic examination shows no focal deficits. Results of complete blood cell count and peripheral blood smear confirm megaloblastic anemia. Based on this finding, this patient most likely has a deficiency in which of the following vitamins?
A. A
B. B
C. C
D. D
E. K

16. A 63-year-old man comes to the office for follow-up to discuss the results of laboratory and x-ray studies that were obtained one week ago. At that time, the patient was evaluated because he had a two-month history of worsening back pain and fatigue. X-ray studies of the thoracic and lumbar spine show osteolytic lesions. Laboratory studies show anemia, hypercalcemia, and renal insufficiency. Which of the following additional tests is most likely to determine the diagnosis?
A. PET scan of the spine
B. Protein electrophoresis
C. Skeletal survey
D. Ultrasonography of the spine
E. Whole-body CT scan

17. A 70-year-old woman is undergoing transfusion of packed red blood cells after losing blood during abdominal surgery. Results of preoperative compatibility testing are negative for red blood cell alloantibodies. Eight minutes into the transfusion, the patient says that she is not feeling well. Which of the following findings in this patient is most likely to indicate an ABO incompatibility transfusion reaction?
A. Angioedema
B. Bradycardia
C. Elevated blood pressure
D. Fever
E. Skin rash

18. Universal screening of a male newborn who is African American shows that he is positive for sickle hemoglobin. Which of the following is the most appropriate initial step in treatment?
A. Ciprofloxacin
B. Glutamine
C. Hydroxyurea
D. Penicillin
E. Voxelotor

19. A 32-year-old woman has had menorrhagia with associated fatigue and exertional dyspnea during her daily workout for the past two months. Resting heart rate is 116/min. On physical examination, pale conjunctivae are noted. Which of the following findings are most likely on laboratory studies of serum?

	Hemoglobin	Mean corpuscular volume	Ferritin	Total iron-binding capacity
A.	Decreased	Decreased	Decreased	Increased
B.	Decreased	Decreased	Increased	Decreased
C.	Decreased	Increased	Increased	Increased
D.	Normal	Decreased	Increased	Decreased
E.	Normal	Increased	Decreased	Decreased

20. A 58-year-old man comes to the office because he has had painful, enlarging lymph nodes in the neck over the past two months. He says that he was prescribed antibiotics one month ago, and no significant improvement was noted. Since completing the course of antibiotics, he has had generalized itching, fatigue, occasional fevers, and dyspnea. He says that the pain in the lymph nodes worsens with alcohol consumption. Lymph node biopsy shows the presence of Reed-Sternberg cells. Which of the following symptoms in this patient is classified as a B symptom of this condition?
A. Alcohol-induced lymph node pain
B. Dyspnea
C. Fatigue
D. Generalized pruritus
E. Intermittent fever

21. A 14-year-old boy is brought to the clinic because when he had his wisdom teeth removed two weeks ago, his dentist had difficulty controlling bleeding throughout the procedure. The patient says that even minor trauma causes him to bruise and bleed excessively. Family medical history includes an uncle who also bleeds and bruises easily. Vital signs are within normal limits. Physical examination shows a large $(15 \times 10 \, cm)$ bruise on the patient's left anterior thigh that he says was caused by inadvertently walking into a piece of furniture two days ago. This patient is most likely to have a deficiency in which of the following clotting factors?
A. Factor V
B. Factor VII
C. Factor IX
D. Factor XI
E. Factor XII

22. A 53-year-old man comes to the clinic because he has had fatigue, lethargy, arthralgia, and abdominal pain for the past month. Medical history includes diabetes mellitus and cirrhosis. He has not been examined by his primary care provider recently and discontinued all previously prescribed medications over a year ago. Physical examination shows hyperpigmentation of the skin. Abdominal examination shows tenderness to palpation of the right upper quadrant that is associated with hepatomegaly and splenomegaly. Chest x-ray study shows cardiomegaly. Laboratory studies show serum ferritin level of 935 ng/mL (N = <300 ng/mL), fasting serum glucose level of 230 mg/dL (N = 60–109 mg/dL), and fasting serum transferrin saturation of 75% (N = 16–45%). Which of the following is the most appropriate management?

A. Aggressive photoprotection

B. Biweekly therapeutic phlebotomy

C. D-penicillamine

D. Intravenous glucocorticoids

E. Liver transplantation

Answer Key for this chapter begins on p. 108

Answers

1. **Answer: B** Chronic lymphocytic leukemia (CLL), option B, is characterized by lymphocytes on peripheral blood smear with the presence of smudge cells. Patients with CLL are at risk for recurrent infections, including herpes zoster.
Peripheral blood smear of acute myeloid leukemia, option A, would result in immature cells of the granulocyte cell line. Patients with hairy cell leukemia, option C, typically have pancytopenia and lack lymphadenopathy. Non-Hodgkin lymphoma, option D, is not characterized by lymphocytosis with smudge cells on a peripheral blood smear. Peripheral blood smear of a patient with small lymphocytic lymphoma, option E, would not show lymphocytosis in the peripheral blood. **Task:** C—Formulating Most Likely Diagnosis

2. **Answer: A** This patient has anemia of chronic disease, option A. This type of anemia is characterized by a normal mean corpuscular volume (MCV) level, decreased iron level, decreased iron-binding capacity, and normal or elevated ferritin level.
Folate deficiency and vitamin B_{12} deficiency (options B and E) are characterized as macrocytic anemias with MCV levels typically >100 μm^3. Iron deficiency anemia, option C, is associated with an MCV level <80 μm^3, decreased ferritin level, decreased iron level, and an elevated iron-binding capacity. Thalassemia, option D, is incorrect because similar to iron deficiency anemia, the MCV level is typically <80 μm^3. In addition, this condition is associated with an elevated reticulocyte count and the presence of target cells. **Task:** C—Formulating Most Likely Diagnosis

3. **Answer: C** In patients with non-Hodgkin lymphoma (NHL) as well as other lymphomas, painless lymphadenopathy is the most common presentation. Normal results on complete blood cell count and chest x-ray study are consistent with early NHL. Excisional node biopsy, option C, will confirm or rule out lymphoma. Bronchoscopy, option A, is performed to obtain a lung biopsy and is inappropriate for this patient. Epstein-Barr virus (EBV) antibody titer, option B, is used to diagnose EBV infection, which can cause a sore throat and lymphadenopathy. However, this patient's age is not consistent with EBV infection, she does not have a sore throat, and the adenopathy in EBV is usually in the posterior cervical chain. Serum protein electrophoresis, option D, is performed when multiple myeloma is the suspected diagnosis. Throat culture, option E, can determine if a bacterial throat infection is present, which could cause lymphadenopathy; however, the patient has not had a sore throat, and her history, her age, and the size of the node are not consistent with a throat infection. **Task:** B—Using Diagnostic and Laboratory Studies

4. **Answer: D** Patients with sickle cell anemia (SCA), especially children, have an increased risk of bacterial infections. The correct answer is *Streptococcus pneumonia*, option D, which is an encapsulated bacterium. This polysaccharide capsule makes it more difficult for the immune system to clear the infection.
The other options are not encapsulated bacteria. Group B streptococcus, option A, may cause serious infection in newborns but is not related to sickle cell disease. *Staphylococcus aureus*, option B, is a bacterium found on the skin that can also cause serious infections. *Staphylococcus saprophyticus*, option C, may cause urinary tract infections in young women. Finally, *Streptococcus pyogenes*, option E, most often causes streptococcal pharyngitis. **Task:** E—Applying Basic Scientific Concepts

5. **Answer: C** This patient is receiving a blood transfusion and has development of urticaria without other signs or symptoms to suggest a more serious allergic-type reaction or another type of transfusion reaction. An allergic reaction of mild severity, characterized by urticaria and sometimes flushing, is a common reaction to receiving a blood transfusion and can be treated with antihistamines such as diphenhydramine, option C.
Fever is another common reaction from a blood transfusion, but this patient is afebrile, so there is no indication for antipyretic therapy such as acetaminophen, option A. More severe allergic-type reactions, including anaphylaxis, are possible in patients receiving blood products. However, because this patient has no wheezing, there is no indication for albuterol, option B, or other medications used to treat more serious allergic reactions like epinephrine, option D. Furosemide, option E, is used to treat patients who develop a more serious transfusion reaction called transfusion-associated circulatory overload. **Task:** D3—Pharmaceutical Therapeutics

6. **Answer: D** When phlebotomy is used to treat patients with hemochromatosis, reversal of hepatic fibrosis and regression of mild-to-moderate cirrhosis may occur; therefore, option D is most appropriate to tell this patient.
Arthropathy and hypogonadism are very responsive; option A is incorrect because these two conditions are either less responsive or do not respond to phlebotomy at all. Options B and C are incorrect because certain clinical features, including insulin requirements, cardiac function, malaise, skin pigmentation, and abdominal

pain, are either ameliorated or improved with phlebotomy. Risk for hepatocellular carcinoma decreases in patients with cirrhosis; option E is incorrect because phlebotomy for treatment of hemochromatosis does not decrease the risk for hepatocellular carcinoma once cirrhosis develops. **Task: D1—Health Maintenance, Patient Education, and Disease Prevention**

7. **Answer: A** This patient has iron deficiency anemia, and the most likely nail finding is koilonychia, option A. Koilonychia is a spooning of the nail. There is the upward curving of the distal nail plate that results in a spoon-shaped nail that could hold a drop of water on the surface.

   Lindsay nails (option B), also called half-and-half nails, are a manifestation of chronic renal insufficiency and uremia. Lindsay nails are characterized by a red, pink, or brown horizontal distal band that occupies one-quarter to one-half of the total length of the nail. The proximal portion of a half-and-half nail usually has a dull, white, ground-glass appearance. Onychoschizia, option C, is caused by exposure to external factors such as wet work, chemicals, or trauma. Onychoschizia, also known as lamellar dystrophy, is characterized by lamellar splitting at the distal edge of the nail due to impairment of intercellular adhesive factors of the nail plate. Terry nails, option D, are a manifestation of cirrhosis and other systemic diseases. Terry nails are characterized by leukonychia that involves more than the proximal two-thirds of the nail plate, whereas the distal third appears red. Trachyonychia, option E, also called twenty-nail dystrophy, is characterized by a nail plate abnormality resulting in nail roughness, excessive longitudinal ridging, pitting, thickening of the cuticle, and distal brittleness. Trachyonychia predominantly affects children and may be idiopathic or associated with other skin diseases, most commonly psoriasis, lichen planus, alopecia areata, or atopic eczema. **Task: A—History Taking and Performing Physical Examination**

8. **Answer: E** This patient has neutropenic fever. Neutropenia is defined as an absolute neutrophil count of <1500/mm³. Chemotherapeutic agents are frequent causes of neutropenia. Fever in a patient who is neutropenic is a medical emergency and requires prompt evaluation in an emergency department setting. Therefore, option E is the correct answer.

   Because this patient requires emergent evaluation for the cause of fever and early administration of parenteral antibiotics, the other options are not appropriate and will delay proper care for this patient. **Task: D2—Clinical Intervention**

9. **Answer: E** Factor V Leiden mutation is the most common cause of inherited thrombophilia. Patients with this mutation, whether heterozygous or homozygous, are at increased risk for venous thromboembolism, option E.

   Alzheimer disease, option A, is associated with the *APOE* gene. Beta thalassemia, option B, is associated with the *HBB* gene. Breast cancer, option C, is associated with the *BRCA* genes. Celiac disease, option D, is associated with the *HLA* genes. **Task: D1—Health Maintenance, Patient Education, and Disease Prevention**

10. **Answer: C** Polycythemia vera is characterized by the increased production of red blood cells (erythrocytosis). The presence of *JAK2* V617F mutation, option C, is strongly associated with this diagnosis.

    The presence of Auer rods, option A, is associated with a diagnosis of acute myeloid leukemia. Bence Jones protein, option B, is associated with multiple myeloma. A Philadelphia chromosome, option D, is associated with chronic myeloid leukemia. The presence of Reed-Sternberg cells, option E, is associated with a diagnosis of Hodgkin lymphoma. **Task: B—Using Diagnostic and Laboratory Studies**

11. **Answer: D** Vitamin B_{12} deficiency, option D, leads to numbness and tingling of the hands and feet in a stocking-glove distribution, weakness, fatigue, and anemia. After gastric bypass surgery, vitamin B_{12} deficiency is secondary to the duodenum being bypassed and decreased production of intrinsic factor. Intrinsic factor is a carrier protein for vitamin B_{12} that enables it to be absorbed in the ileum.

    The absorption of niacin, thiamine, vitamin A, and vitamin D (options A, B, C, and E) is usually less affected by the gastric bypass procedure. Niacin is absorbed primarily in the small intestines. Symptoms associated with a niacin deficiency include pellagra, dermatitis, diarrhea, dementia, and death. Thiamine deficiency can lead to Beriberi and Wernicke-Korsakoff syndrome. Absorption of thiamine occurs in the small intestine. Vitamin A is absorbed in the lumen of the small intestine. Deficiencies cause night blindness and poor wound healing. Vitamin D is not affected by gastric bypass. Deficiencies in vitamin D can lead to complications with osteoporosis, hypocalcemia, or hyperparathyroidism. **Task: A—History Taking and Performing Physical Examination**

12. **Answer: A** The correct answer is chronic myeloid leukemia, option A, as this is a disorder characterized by overproduction of myeloid cells and a specific molecular abnormality represented by the presence of the Philadelphia chromosome, which is not found in any of the other diseases listed in the answer options.

    Leukemoid reaction, option B, is characterized by an increase in the white blood cell count, which can mimic leukemia. The reaction is caused by an infection or another disease and is not a sign of cancer. Also, the Philadelphia chromosome is not found in patients with this disorder. Multiple myeloma, option C, is a malignancy of plasma cells. Neutrophil counts in patients with this disorder are usually within normal limits. Polycythemia vera, option D, causes overproduction of all three hemopoietic cell lines but most prominently the red blood cells. Primary myelofibrosis, option E, is characterized by fibrosis of the bone marrow. The white blood cell count is variable (usually not higher than 50,000/mm³), but there are usually prominent abnormalities in the red blood cell line including nucleated red blood cells and teardrop forms. **Task:** C—Formulating Most Likely Diagnosis

13. **Answer: E** This patient has thrombotic thrombocytopenic purpura (TTP). Plasma exchange, option E, is the most important initial treatment for TTP and should be initiated promptly to improve response. Additional supportive treatment in conjunction with plasma exchange therapy includes antiplatelet agents, folate supplementation, packed red blood cells, and platelet transfusion.
Aspirin, option A, is incorrect because aspirin should not be used alone when treating TTP but rather in combination with another treatment such as plasma exchange. Although fresh frozen plasma, option B, is sometimes used as a supportive treatment, it is not considered the most important treatment for TTP. Intravenous heparin, option C, is used to treat conditions such as disseminated intravascular coagulation if there is thrombosis; however, this is not the most important treatment for TTP. Intravenous immune globulin, option D, is the most important treatment for idiopathic thrombocytopenic purpura rather than TTP. **Task:** D3—Pharmaceutical Therapeutics

14. **Answer: C** This patient has autoimmune hemolytic anemia, option C. After recovering from an infection, patients can produce antibodies that lyse the red blood cells (RBCs), resulting in a normocytic or macrocytic anemia. The reticulocyte count is elevated as the bone marrow releases young RBCs into the peripheral circulation. Hemolysis causes a decreased haptoglobin level. Only autoimmune hemolytic anemia would cause a positive direct Coombs test.
Anemia of chronic disease, option A, causes normocytic anemia, but patients will have a normal reticulocyte count and haptoglobin level. Aplastic anemia, option B, causes a deficiency of all blood cell types. Iron deficiency anemia, option D, causes microcytic anemia, but patients have a normal haptoglobin level. Thalassemia minor, option E, is a hereditary hemoglobinopathy that may cause mild anemia. Mean corpuscular volume is usually decreased, and reticulocytes are normal. Bilirubin and haptoglobin levels are usually normal as well in patients with thalassemia minor. **Task:** C—Formulating Most Likely Diagnosis

15. **Answer: B** This patient, who has a history of alcohol use, comes to the clinic because he has fatigue and glossitis. Laboratory studies then confirm megaloblastic anemia. This item tests the examinee's ability to recognize that this patient's presentation is consistent with a vitamin B deficiency, specifically B₉ or folic acid deficiency, which is option B.
Vitamin A deficiency, option A, can cause ocular manifestations. Vitamin C deficiency, option C, leads to the syndrome known as scurvy, which is a collagen-production disorder. Vitamin D deficiency, option D, can lead to rickets in children and osteomalacia in adults. Vitamin K deficiency, option E, can lead to easy bleeding from coagulation defects. **Task:** E—Applying Basic Scientific Concepts

16. **Answer: B** This patient has multiple myeloma. Protein electrophoresis, option B, will show the presence of a paraprotein spike, known as an M spike. The presence of an M protein spike is diagnostic for multiple myeloma.
PET scan of the spine, option A, is used to evaluate for suspected extramedullary disease outside of the spine and is not appropriate for confirming a diagnosis of multiple myeloma. A skeletal survey, option C, will show manifestations of multiple myelomas, such as pathologic fractures and osteolytic lesions, but this is not diagnostic for this disease. Option D, ultrasonography of the spine, is incorrect. This test is indicated for diagnosing spinal conditions such as a spinal tumor or abscess rather than multiple myeloma. Whole-body CT scan, option E, is incorrect. Similar to the skeletal survey, the whole-body CT scan is used for the detection of lytic lesions or pathologic fractures rather than for diagnostic purposes. **Task:** B—Using Diagnostic and Laboratory Studies

17. **Answer: D** This patient is experiencing early signs of an ABO incompatibility transfusion reaction. The correct answer is fever, option D. Stopping the transfusion at the first sign of incompatibility, usually fever, is critical for preventing serious sequelae. Most febrile reactions to transfusion are not caused by incompatibility, but it is initially inappropriate to exclude this as a possibility.
Angioedema and skin rash (i.e., urticaria), options A and E, are signs of an allergic reaction, not incompatibility. Bradycardia, option B, is incorrect because tachycardia occurs after fever in patients with ABO incompatibility transfusion reactions. Elevated blood pressure, option C, is incorrect because hypotension occurs later in the course of ABO incompatibility. **Task:** D2—Clinical Intervention

18. **Answer: D** Initiation of oral penicillin, option D, twice daily is appropriate prophylaxis against pneumococcal

disease in children with sickle cell disease from infancy to at least 5 years of age.

Ciprofloxacin, option A, is not an appropriate antibiotic choice in the prevention of pneumococcal disease in children with sickle cell disease. Option B, glutamine, is not an appropriate treatment because this drug is indicated for patients 5 years of age and older. Hydroxyurea, option C, should only be used in patients 9 months or older. Voxelotor, option E, is indicated for patients with sickle cell disease who are 12 years of age or older. **Task:** D3—Pharmaceutical Therapeutics

19. **Answer: A** In this patient with iron deficiency anemia, laboratory studies are most likely to show a decreased hemoglobin level, decreased mean corpuscular volume of <80 μm^3, decreased serum ferritin, and increased total iron-binding capacity (option A). Options B, C, D, and E are incorrect because they do not fit the expected laboratory pattern for a patient with iron deficiency anemia. **Task:** B—Using Diagnostic and Laboratory Studies

20. **Answer: E** This patient has Hodgkin lymphoma, and B symptoms of Hodgkin lymphoma consist of intermittent fever (option E), night sweats, and weight loss. The presence of B symptoms indicates disease advancement. Alcohol-induced lymph node pain, option A, is a distinct characteristic of Hodgkin lymphoma; however, this is not classified as a B symptom. Dyspnea, option B, often results from mediastinal adenopathy causing airway compression. Although fatigue, option C, may occur with Hodgkin lymphoma, it is not classified as a B symptom. Generalized pruritus, option D, may develop weeks to months before other clinical signs of lymphoma. **Task:** A—History Taking and Performing Physical Examination

21. **Answer: C** This question presents a scenario in which an adolescent has a history of easy bleeding and bruising throughout his life, with a recent dental procedure causing heavy bleeding. This is a common presentation of moderate hemophilia. Hemophilia is an inherited bleeding disorder usually affecting males that is caused by clotting factor deficiencies. The two most common types of hemophilia are hemophilia A, caused by factor VIII deficiency, and hemophilia B, caused by factor IX deficiency (option C). Deficiencies in factors V, VII, XI, and XII (options A, B, D, and E) exist but are exceedingly rare. **Task:** E—Applying Basic Scientific Concepts

22. **Answer: B** Biweekly therapeutic phlebotomy, option B, is the recommended treatment for this patient with hemochromatosis. Hereditary hemochromatosis is an excess of iron deposited in organs that leads to organ toxicity. The classic triad for hemochromatosis is skin hyperpigmentation due to a combination of iron deposition and melanin cutaneous deposition, diabetes mellitus, and cirrhosis. Cirrhosis may progress to hepatocellular carcinoma. Diabetes mellitus is caused by iron accumulation in the pancreatic beta cells. The mainstay of therapy for hemochromatosis is biweekly phlebotomy.

Aggressive photoprotection, option A, is used to treat dermatomyositis. D-penicillamine, option C, is used to treat patients with Wilson disease. Intravenous glucocorticoids and transplantation of the liver, options D and E, do not play a role in the treatment of hemochromatosis. **Task:** D2—Clinical Intervention

BIBLIOGRAPHY

Adamson, J. W., & Longo, D. L. (2018). Anemia and polycythemia. In J. Jameson, A. S. Fauci, D. L. Kasper, S. L. Hauser, D. L. Longo, & J. Loscalzo (Eds.), *Harrison's principles of internal medicine* (20th ed.). McGraw-Hill.

Amato, A. A., & Barohn, R. J. (2014). Peripheral neuropathy. In D. Kasper, A. Fauci, S. Hauser, D. Longo, J. Jameson, & J. Loscalzo (Eds.), *Harrison's principles of internal medicine* (19th ed.). New York, NY: McGraw-Hill.

Asiedu, D. (2021). Vitamin deficiency (hypovitaminosis). In F. Ferri (Ed.), *Ferri's clinical advisor 2021* (pp. 1453-1554). Philadelphia, PA: Elsevier, Inc.

Bartus, C. L., & Parker, S. R. (2011). Hodgkin lymphoma presenting as generalized pruritus in an adolescent. *Cutis, 87*(4), 169-172.

Byrd, J. C. (2020). Chronic Lymphocytic Leukemia. In L. Goldman & A. Schafer (Eds.), *Goldman-Cecil medicine* (26th ed). Elsevier.

Castillo, J. J., & Lacasce, A. S. (2021). Non-Hodgkin Lymphoma. In F. Ferri (Ed.), *Ferri's clinical adviser.* Elsevier.

Chitlur, M., Ozgonenel, B., & Kulkarni, R. (2020). Hemophilia and related conditions. In R. Kellerman & D. Rakel (Eds.), *Conn's Current Therapy 2020* (pp. 417-424). Philadelphia, PA: Elsevier, Inc.

Clinical Overview. (2019). *Iron deficiency anemia.* Elsevier Point of Care.

Clinical Overview. (2020). *Hemochromatosis.* Elsevier Point of Care.

Clinical Overview. (2020). *Sickle cell disease.* Elsevier Point of Care.

David, J. A. (Ed.), (2020). Hematologic disorders. In *Current Practice Guidelines in Primary Care 2020.* McGraw-Hill.

Domino, F. J., Baldor, R. A., Golding, J., & Stephens, M. B. (2019). *The 5-minute clinical consult 2020.* Lippincott Williams & Wilkins.

Epocrates [online]. (2013). San Francisco, CA: Epocrates, Inc. http://www.epocrates.com. Updated continuously.

Hardin, J. (2021). Thrombotic thrombocytopenic purpura. In K. J. Knoop, L. B. Stack, A. B. Storrow, & R. Thurman (Eds.), *The atlas of emergency medicine* (5th ed.). McGraw Hill.

Hauser, S. L., & Ropper, A. H. (2014). Diseases of the spinal cord. In D. Kasper, A. Fauci, S. Hauser, D. Longo, J. Jameson, & J. Loscalzo (Eds.), *Harrison's principles of internal medicine* (19th ed.). New York, NY: McGraw Hill.

Jacobson, C. A., & Longo, D. L. Hodgkin's lymphoma. In J. Jameson, A. S. Fauci, D. L. Kasper, et al. (Eds.), Hauser SL, D. L. Longo,

J. Loscalzo (Eds.) *Harrison's principles of internal medicine* (20th ed.). McGraw-Hill.

Konkle, B. A. (2018). Disorders of platelets and vessel wall. In J. Jameson, A. S. Fauci, D. L. Kasper, S. L. Hauser, D. L. Longo, & J. Loscalzo (Eds.), *Harrison's principles of internal medicine* (20th ed.). McGraw Hill.

Lopez, A., Cacoub, P., Macdougall, I. C., & Peyrin-Biroulet, L. (2016). Iron deficiency anaemia. *The Lancet, 387*(10021), 907-916. https://doi.org/10.1016/S0140-6736(15)60865-0.

Mair, S. M., & Weiss, G. (2009). New pharmacological concepts for the treatment of iron overload disorders. *Current Medicinal Chemistry, 16*(5), 576-590.

Murphy, M., Pasi, K. J., & Roy, N. (2021). Haematology. In A. Feather, D. Randall, & M. Waterhouse (Eds.), *Kumar and Clark's clinical medicine* (pp. 319-378). Philadelphia, PA: Elsevier, Inc.

Nester, T. (2020). Blood component therapy and transfusion reactions. In R. Kellerman & D. Rakel (Eds.), *Conn's Current Therapy 2020* (pp. 394-400). Elsevier, Inc.

Pietrangelo, A. (2004). Hereditary hemochromatosis—A new look at an old disease. *The New England Journal of Medicine, 350*(23), 2383-2397.

Rich, M. D., Phoebe. *Overview of nail disorders*. UpToDate. Updated: December 05, 2019.

Savage, W. (2018). Transfusion Reactions to Blood and Cell Therapy Products. In L. Silberstein, J. Anastasi, R. Hoffman, E. Benz, H. Heslop, J. Weitz, M. Salama, & S. Abutalib (Eds.) *Hematology: Basic principles and practice* (7th ed.). Elsevier.

Torres, R., & Rinder, H. (2016). Disorders of hemostasis: Thrombosis. In I. Benjamin (Ed.), *Andreoli and Carpenter's cecil essentials of medicine* (9th ed., pp. 564-573). Philadelphia, PA: Elsevier, Inc.

US Department of Health and Human Services, NIH. (2014). *Evidence-based management of sickle cell disease.*

Weng, T. C., Chang, C. H., Dong, Y. H., Chang, Y. C., & Chuang, L. M. (2015). Anaemia and related nutrient deficiencies after Roux-en-Y gastric bypass surgery: A systematic review and meta-analysis. *BMJ Open, 5*(7), e006964.

White, L., & Ybarra, M. (2014). Neutropenic fever. *Emergency Medicine Clinics of North America, 32*(3), 549-561.

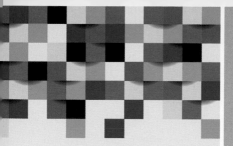

CHAPTER 8
Infectious Diseases

Questions

1. A 72-year-old woman comes to the clinic because she has had white patches on her tongue for the past two weeks. Medical history includes asthma, for which she takes maintenance therapy with fluticasone/salmeterol via inhaler. Vital signs are within normal limits. Physical examination shows white areas on the soft palate and tongue that scrape off with a tongue blade. Which of the following is the most likely diagnosis?
   A. Behçet disease
   B. Candidiasis
   C. Herpes simplex virus type 1
   D. Leukoplakia
   E. Streptococcal pharyngitis

2. A 20-year-old man comes to the emergency department because he has had yellowish discharge from his penis for the past four days. He says he recently had unprotected sex with a new partner. Vitals signs are within normal limits. Physical examination shows yellowish discharge from the penile meatus. Based on the 2020 CDC guidelines, the most appropriate treatment includes which of the following medication regimens?
   A. Ceftriaxone 1 g intramuscularly (IM) and azithromycin 250 mg orally (PO)
   B. Ceftriaxone 500 mg IM and doxycycline 100 mg orally twice daily for seven days
   C. Penicillin 1 g IM and metronidazole 500 mg orally twice daily for seven days
   D. Penicillin 250 mg IM and metronidazole 1 g PO
   E. Penicillin 500 mg IM and azithromycin 500 mg PO

3. A 6-year-old girl is brought to the office by her father because she has had an earache and bilateral swelling in her neck for the past day. She also has had fever, headache, fatigue, and inappetence for the past four days. The father says that the swelling in her neck started on the left side but then progressed to both sides. The patient's older brother came home from his first semester of college about three weeks ago and was sick during the time that he was home. Neither child has received any vaccinations. Physical examination shows edema and tenderness to palpation of both parotid glands. Which of the following is the most likely potential complication of this condition?
   A. Oophoritis
   B. Postherpetic neuralgia
   C. Reye syndrome
   D. Rheumatic fever
   E. Subacute sclerosing panencephalitis

4. A 26-year-old transgender man comes to the emergency department because he has had fever, headache, myalgia, nausea and vomiting, and abdominal discomfort since waking up this morning. He says he also has a rash on his palms and soles. The patient is an Appalachian trail through hiker and says that he successfully extracted a tick embedded in his right upper extremity three days ago. He has been otherwise healthy. Physical examination shows a petechial-like rash on the palms and soles. Which of the following tickborne illnesses is most likely?
   A. Babesiosis
   B. Ehrlichiosis
   C. Lyme disease
   D. Powassan virus
   E. Rocky Mountain spotted fever

5. A 27-year-old woman comes to the family medicine clinic three days after she underwent drainage of an abscess in her right axilla at a local urgent care facility. She currently has pain at the incision site that does not radiate and has had a low-grade fever and chills since this morning. The patient says she returned to the urgent care center yesterday to have the site packed with gauze and was informed that the site looked normal. She was not prescribed any medication from the urgent care facility but was instructed to return every two days for repacking. She has been alternating acetaminophen and ibuprofen for pain relief and fever, and her only other medication is a daily multivitamin. Medical history does not include any chronic disease conditions, and she has no history of surgery. Temperature is 38.3°C (100.9°F), pulse rate is 87/min, respirations are 16/min, and blood pressure is 121/74 mmHg. Oxygen saturation is 100%. Which of the following is the most appropriate oral medication to prescribe?

A. Cephalexin
B. Clindamycin
C. Linezolid
D. Metronidazole
E. Valacyclovir

6.

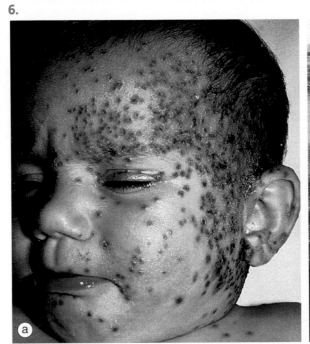
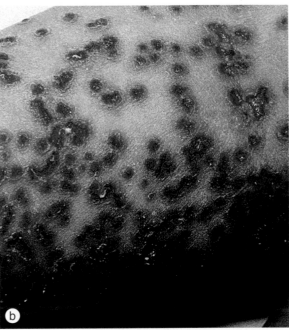

A 9-month-old male infant with a history of atopic dermatitis is brought to the clinic by his parents because he had sudden onset of rash and high fever three days ago. Temperature is 39.9°C (103.8°F). Findings on physical examination are shown in the photographs. Bedside Tzanck test shows multinucleated giant cells. Which of the following is the most likely diagnosis?

A. Eczema herpeticum
B. Keratosis pilaris
C. Molluscum contagiosum
D. Pityriasis rosea
E. Seborrheic dermatitis

7. A 50-year-old man comes to the emergency department because he has had cough, fever, and shortness of breath for the past week. He says he just received the results of a COVID-19 test, and it was positive. Medical history includes hypertension and type 2 diabetes mellitus, for which he takes hydrochlorothiazide and metformin. Temperature is 39.4°C (103.0°F), pulse rate is 90/min, respirations are 24/min, and blood pressure is 150/90 mmHg. Oxygen saturation is 88% on room air and is 84% with exertion. On physical examination, auscultation of the lungs shows bilateral rhonchi. Results of a chest x-ray study are pending, but the patient is admitted to the hospital based on his clinical presentation. Elevated levels on which of the following laboratory studies is most likely to be associated with a poor clinical outcome for this patient?

A. Basic metabolic panel
B. Complete blood cell count
C. D-dimer assay
D. Hepatic panel
E. Thyroid function studies

8. A 60-year-old man comes to the urgent care center because he sustained a laceration to his left hand while changing the oil in his car. Medical history includes hypertension that is well controlled and atrial fibrillation for which he takes anticoagulant therapy. Generalized wound care is applied to the wound, and multiple sutures are placed. Which of the following vaccinations is most appropriate to administer to this patient prior to discharge?
   A. Influenza vaccine
   B. Measles, mumps, and rubella vaccine
   C. Pneumococcal vaccine
   D. Recombinant zoster vaccine
   E. Tetanus toxoid-containing vaccine

9. A 36-year-old woman comes to the primary care clinic because she has had fever to 39.4°C (102.9°F), chills, nausea and vomiting, headache, and backache since she returned from a trip to Nigeria four days ago. The patient is a nurse, and she went to Nigeria on a medical mission trip for two weeks. The patient says she sustained multiple mosquito bites during her trip and was not prescribed prophylactic medication prior to her arrival in Africa. Based on these findings, which of the following parasites was most likely transmitted to this patient via mosquito bite?
   A. *Babesia*
   B. *Cryptosporidium*
   C. *Filarioidea*
   D. *Phthiraptera*
   E. *Plasmodium*

10. A 17-year-old girl is brought to the office because she has had fever, headache, and sore throat for the past week. She is a senior in high school and involved in jazz band and varsity soccer. Medical history includes irritable bowel syndrome. Temperature is 38.5°C (101.3°F). The patient does not appear to be in acute distress. On physical examination, posterior cervical lymphadenopathy is noted. Laboratory studies show elevated lymphocytes and mildly elevated results of liver function tests. Which of the following is the most appropriate next step?
   A. MRI of the abdomen
   B. Oral amoxicillin therapy
   C. Oral corticosteroid therapy
   D. Ultrasonography of the abdomen
   E. Observation

11. A 42-year-old man who has been HIV positive for the past four years comes to the emergency department because he has had cough productive of yellow sputum, loss of appetite, and subjective fever for the past three days. Medications include antiretroviral therapy; he takes no other medications. The patient's most recent CD4+ lymphocyte count was 400 cells/μL (N = 500–1000 cells/μL) six weeks ago. He smokes one half-pack of cigarettes daily. Temperature is 38.3°C (101.0°F), pulse rate is 110/min, respirations are 22/min, and blood pressure is 128/76 mmHg. Oxygen saturation is 92% on room air. The patient does not appear to be in acute respiratory distress. Physical examination shows dullness to percussion over the right lower lung. Auscultation of the lungs shows decreased breath sounds in the same area. STAT gram stain of sputum shows gram-positive diplococci. Chest x-ray study shows a localized infiltrate in the right lower lobe. Which of the following is the most likely cause of the findings in this patient?
   A. Human metapneumovirus
   B. Mycobacterium avium complex infection
   C. Pneumococcal pneumonia
   D. Pneumocystis pneumonia
   E. Pulmonary coccidioidomycosis

12. A 19-year-old woman comes to the clinic because she has had increasing vaginal discharge for the past three days. She says the discharge is yellowish green and malodorous, and she has associated mild vaginal pruritis. The patient does not have pelvic pain. She is sexually active with a new male partner. Vital signs are within normal limits. Physical examination shows no abdominal tenderness. Pelvic examination shows a frothy, yellow-green discharge. No cervical motion tenderness is noted. Result of pregnancy test is negative. Which of the following is the most appropriate next step?
   A. Fungal culture of vaginal secretions
   B. Human papillomavirus test
   C. Normal saline preparation of vaginal secretions
   D. Serologic testing for herpes simplex virus
   E. Urine dipstick test

13. A 7-year-old girl is brought to the office because she has had a severe sore throat for the past two weeks. According to the Jones Criteria, which of the following findings on physical examination is most likely to indicate that this patient has acute rheumatic fever?
   A. Carditis and chorea
   B. Carditis and prolonged PR interval
   C. Erythema marginatum and monoarthralgia
   D. Erythema marginatum and temperature ≥38.5°C (101.3°F)
   E. Temperature ≥38.5°C (101.3°F) and polyarthropathy

Answer Key for this chapter begins on p. 119

14. A 34-year-old woman comes to the office for follow-up six months after she underwent renal transplantation for treatment of congenital focal and segmental glomerulonephritis. She is prescribed mycophenolate for immune suppression to prevent rejection of the transplant. Trimethoprim-sulfamethoxazole is then prescribed three times weekly to prevent against pneumonia caused by which of the following agents?
    A. Cytomegalovirus
    B. *Haemophilus influenzae*
    C. *Mycoplasma pneumoniae*
    D. *Pneumocystis jirovecii*
    E. *Streptococcal pneumoniae*

15. A 41-year-old man is admitted to the hospital for treatment of acute progressive encephalopathy, facial numbness, rash, paresthesia, and inability to protect his airway due to dyspnea. The patient's partner says that he had a flulike illness about 10 days ago. The patient works as an air conditioning repairman and was recently working on a job site where there was a bat infestation in the home. Based on these findings, which of the following is the most likely suspected diagnosis?
    A. Anaplasmosis
    B. Babesia
    C. Lyme disease
    D. Malaria
    E. Rabies

16. A six-year-old girl is brought to the urgent care clinic by her mother because she has had fever, runny nose, mild sore throat, body aches, and fatigue for the past 24 hours. The mother says the patient seems more tired than usual and had development of a mild rash on her face that spread to her trunk three days ago. She also noted that the patient had swelling behind her ears last week that has since improved. Which of the following findings on laboratory studies is most likely to determine the diagnosis?
    A. Leukopenia
    B. Negative viral culture
    C. Positive for group A streptococcus infection
    D. Positive result of VDRL test
    E. Thrombocytosis

17. A patient comes to the clinic for follow-up of a PPD skin test that was done 48 hours ago. He has not had fever, night sweats, unexpected weight loss, or recent illness. Medical history includes no chronic disease conditions, and he takes no medications. The patient is HIV negative. He has a history of recreational use of intravenous drugs and only consumes alcoholic beverages socially. The patient has no history of recent travel outside the country and has never been incarcerated. Which of the following induration sizes is considered a positive test result for this patient?

A. ≥5 mm
B. ≥10 mm
C. ≥15 mm
D. ≥20 mm
E. ≥25 mm

18. A 72-year-old woman comes to the office because she has had a painful, burning sensation and itching on the right lower side of her chest for the past two days. This morning she noticed a rash in the area. She has not had fever or chills. She initiated therapy with acetaminophen for treatment of the pain one day ago. Medical history includes hypertension and Hashimoto thyroiditis. Current medications include enalapril and levothyroxine. Vital signs are within normal limits. Physical examination shows an erythematous maculopapular rash with a cluster of vesicles on the right lower chest. Which of the following is most appropriate to administer at this time?
    A. Acitretin
    B. Acyclovir
    C. Baloxavir marboxil
    D. Methicillin
    E. Penicillin G benzathine

19. A 45-year-old woman comes to the urgent care center because she had abrupt onset of fever, chills, body aches, sore throat, headaches, and nonproductive cough 12 hours ago. Medical history includes no chronic disease conditions. Temperature is 39.2°C (102.5°F); all other vital signs are within normal limits. Physical examination shows no abnormalities. Which of the following studies is the most appropriate next step in diagnosis?
    A. Chest x-ray study
    B. CT scan of the chest
    C. Heterophil antibody test
    D. Rapid molecular assays
    E. Rapid strep test

20. A 25-year-old woman comes to the emergency department because she has had whitish vaginal discharge that has the consistency of cottage cheese as well as vaginal itching for the past two days. She has not had abdominal pain, fever, or chills. Medical history includes type 2 diabetes mellitus. Current medications include metformin. Vital signs are within normal limits. Pelvic examination shows whitish, thick discharge in the vaginal vault and outside the cervix. No odor is noted. Which of the following is the most likely diagnosis?
    A. Bacterial vaginosis
    B. Candidiasis
    C. Chlamydia
    D. Gonorrhea
    E. Trichomoniasis

21. The mother of a 6-year-old boy calls the office to speak to the physician assistant because her son has had runny nose, fever, and decreased appetite for the past day. She says that he was exposed to two children with erythema infectiosum (fifth disease) at his school approximately one week ago. The mother wants to know how she can tell if her son also has this condition. It is most appropriate to tell the mother that if the patient has erythema infectiosum (fifth disease), he will have development of which of the following?
    A. Bright red rash on the cheeks
    B. Café au lait spots on the extremities
    C. Koplik spots inside the mouth
    D. Liquid-filled blisters on the trunk
    E. Pink colored conjunctivae

22. A 24-year-old man who is HIV positive comes to the clinic for routine physical examination. During the interview, he asks if he can receive the human papillomavirus vaccine. Which of the following is most appropriate to tell this patient regarding this immunization?
    A. He cannot receive the vaccination because he is immunocompromised
    B. He cannot receive the vaccination because he is too old
    C. He should receive one dose today and one in six months
    D. He should receive one dose today, one in two months, and one in six months
    E. He should receive the quadrivalent vaccine (4vHPV) rather than the bivalent vaccine (2vHPV) because it provides better coverage

23. An 8-year-old boy who lives in Western Pennsylvania is brought to the office by his parents because he has had aches and pains in his joints as well as a rash on his abdomen for the past four days. The parents say that they have no history of recent travel, but they spend a lot of time outdoors. The patient has sustained several tick bites during the past month. Temperature is 36.7°C (98.1°F), pulse rate is 70/min, respirations are 12/min, and blood pressure is 105/65 mmHg. The patient appears healthy. Physical examination of the rash shows an 8-cm well-demarcated red area with central clearing along the lower left abdomen. The abdomen is soft and nontender to palpation. No other abnormalities are noted. Which of the following is the most likely diagnosis?
    A. Ehrlichiosis
    B. Histoplasmosis
    C. Lyme disease

D. Rheumatoid arthritis
E. Rocky Mountain spotted fever

24. A 38-year-old man comes to the primary care clinic because he has had a rash on his penis for the past four weeks. He says that he has had recent sexual intercourse with multiple female partners and does not use condoms. Physical examination shows a shallow, nontender lesion on the glans penis with associated inguinal lymphadenopathy. Results of laboratory studies are pending. This patient most likely has which of the following sexually transmitted infections?
    A. Chlamydia
    B. Gonorrhea
    C. Hepatitis C
    D. HIV
    E. Syphilis

25. A 10-month-old female infant is brought to the emergency department by her mother because she has had a rash on her chest, abdomen, and back for the past 24 hours. Three days ago, the patient had development of a high fever with associated irritability and decreased appetite. The mother says that the fever has now resolved. Temperature is 36.6°C (97.8°F). The child appears alert and nontoxic. Physical examination shows scattered pink macules, 3 to 4 mm in size, located predominantly on the trunk. Which of the following is most appropriate to tell the mother regarding the progression of this disorder?
    A. This condition is self-limited
    B. This condition will resolve with a short course of antibiotics
    C. The fever will reoccur after resolution of the rash
    D. The rash will begin to fade in two weeks
    E. Treat this condition symptomatically with aspirin

26. A 24-year-old woman who is at 10 weeks' gestation with her first child comes to the clinic because she has had fever, chills, myalgia, and swollen lymph nodes for the past two days. During the interview, the patient says that her husband was out of town for several days last week, and she had to take care of their two cats and dog. Physical examination shows edema of several bilateral cervical lymph nodes that are nontender and 1 to 2 cm in size. Which of the following is the most likely diagnosis?
    A. Cytomegalovirus infection
    B. Epstein-Barr virus infection
    C. HIV infection
    D. *Toxoplasma gondii* infection
    E. Zika virus infection

27. A 25-year-old man comes to the emergency department because he has had four skin infections during the past six weeks at various locations and stages in healing. Vital signs are within normal limits. Physical examination shows multiple areas of pustules on erythematous bases on both the arms and legs. Methicillin-resistant *Staphylococcus aureus* (MRSA) infection is suspected. A history of which of the following most likely increases this patient's risk of recurrent MRSA infection?
    A. Intravenous drug use
    B. Playing team sports
    C. Red ant bites
    D. Scratches from a cat
    E. Working out at a gym

28. A 4-year-old girl is brought to the office by her mother because she has had persistent nocturnal perirectal itching for the past three weeks. The mother says that the patient has had normal bowel habits during this time, and she has not had pruritus anywhere else on her body. Vital signs are within normal limits. The patient appears healthy. Physical examination of the skin shows no involvement of webbed spaces or flexure surfaces. Redness and excoriations are noted in the perianal area. No other abnormalities are noted. Which of the following is the most likely causative organism?
    A. *Enterobius vermicularis*
    B. *Giardia duodenalis*
    C. *Pediculus capitis*
    D. *Sarcoptes scabiei*
    E. *Treponema pallidum*

29. A 24-year-old woman who is at 26 weeks' gestation comes to the clinic because she has had purulent vaginal discharge for the past two weeks. Temperature is 38.2°C (100.8°F). On pelvic examination, cervicitis with mild endocervical bleeding is noted. Results of urinalysis are positive for chlamydial infection. Which of the following is the most appropriate oral treatment?
    A. Azithromycin 1 g as a single dose
    B. Ciprofloxacin 500 mg twice daily for three days
    C. Doxycycline 100 mg twice daily for seven days
    D. Erythromycin estolate 500 mg four times daily for seven days
    E. Trimethoprim-sulfamethoxazole 80 mg/400 mg twice daily for 10 days

30. An 8-month-old male infant is brought to the travel medicine clinic by his father because they are travelling to Europe within the next month and the father wants to make sure the patient has all appropriate immunizations. The patient has been healthy and is up to date with all recommended childhood immunizations. According to the CDC guidelines, it is most appropriate to administer which of the following vaccines at this time?
    A. Human papillomavirus
    B. Measles, mumps, rubella
    C. Meningococcal
    D. Meningococcal B
    E. Yellow fever

Answers

1. **Answer: B** Inhaled corticosteroids are a common cause of thrush, or oropharyngeal candidiasis, option B. Behçet disease, option A, is an autoimmune disease that includes oral ulcerations that typically occur during childhood. The blisters associated with herpes simplex virus type 1, option C, are most commonly found on the lips and not on the tongue. Leukoplakia, option D, consists of firm, adherent plaques that do not scrape off with use of a tongue blade and are precancerous. Patients with streptococcal pharyngitis, option E, typically have fever and acute onset of sore throat. **Task:** A—History Taking and Performing Physical Examination

2. **Answer: B** The 2020 CDC recommendations indicate that gonococcal infections be treated with a single dose of ceftriaxone 500 mg intramuscularly and doxycycline 100 mg orally twice daily for seven days, option B. Ceftriaxone effectively treats the gonorrhea, and doxycycline treats chlamydia and is typically added to the regimen since these two infections tend to occur simultaneously.
Option A is incorrect now that azithromycin in conjunction with ceftriaxone is no longer recommended. Penicillin and metronidazole, options C and D, at any dose are not indicated for the treatment of suspected gonococcal urethritis. Penicillin and azithromycin, option E, are not indicated for suspected gonococcal urethritis. **Task:** D3—Pharmaceutical Therapeutics

3. **Answer: A** This patient has signs and symptoms of mumps, a viral infection that is preventable by vaccination. It previously was a disease of childhood. However, it currently has been seen in unvaccinated individuals as well as vaccinated adults, which suggests that the protection from the vaccine may wane over time. Typically, the disease is self-limiting. However, it can cause complications such as oophoritis in female patients, option A. Other potential complications include orchitis, meningitis, encephalitis, and deafness.
Postherpetic neuralgia, option B, is a complication of herpes zoster virus and is characterized by significant nerve pain after the rash from the virus subsides. Reye syndrome, option C, is a complication of the varicella-zoster virus, which is also known as chickenpox. Rheumatic fever, option D, is a potential complication of streptococcal pharyngitis. Subacute sclerosing panencephalitis, option E, is a fatal complication that can occur seven to 10 years after a natural infection with measles. **Task:** C—Formulating Most Likely Diagnosis

4. **Answer: E** This patient most likely has Rocky Mountain spotted fever, option E, which is a tickborne infection that often presents clinically as a febrile illness associated with a petechial-like rash in 90% of cases. Rocky Mountain spotted fever is caused by the bacterium *Rickettsia rickettsii*, which is transmitted via the bite of an infected tick. Many tick bites go unrecognized by hosts and as a result many patients do not report a known recent tick bite in their clinical history. It is most prevalent in the south Atlantic and south central regions of the United States, and it has the highest incidence rate in the summer months.
Babesiosis, option A, is an illness that causes fever, hemolytic anemia, and acute renal failure. Ehrlichiosis, option B, causes fever, malaise, and fatigue, and includes transaminitis, leukopenia, and thrombocytopenia. More severe disease can progress to meningoencephalitis, acute renal failure, respiratory failure, hepatitis, and myocarditis. Lyme disease, option C, is also a tickborne illness that causes a localized skin reaction called erythema migrans. Disseminated Lyme disease can cause neurologic, cardiac, rheumatologic, and genitourinary symptoms. Powassan virus, option D, includes clinical signs of recent tick bite, fever with nonspecific malaise, and an eventual transition to encephalitis. Most cases of this virus occur in the Northeast and Great Lakes region. The case fatality rate for Powassan virus is approximately 50%. **Task:** A—History Taking and Performing Physical Examination

5. **Answer: B** This patient is suspected of having an infection with methicillin-resistant *Staphylococcus aureus* (MRSA), and the most appropriate oral antibiotic for suspected MRSA infections is clindamycin, option B. Cephalexin, option A, is used only when there is low suspicion of MRSA or confirmed susceptibility. Linezolid, option C, is FDA-approved for MRSA treatment, however, it is expensive, and treatment may extend longer than two to three weeks, making it a less optimal treatment option for this patient. Metronidazole, option D, is an antibiotic used to treat various bacterial and parasitic infections; however, it does not provide adequate treatment for MRSA. Valacyclovir, option E, is an antiviral medication that is used to treat herpes virus infections and is not indicated in the treatment of MRSA infection. **Task:** D3—Pharmaceutical Therapeutics

6. **Answer: A** Eczema herpeticum, option A, is the primary cutaneous manifestation of herpes simplex virus in patients with atopic dermatitis. The rash is characterized by clustered, 2- to 3-mm vesicles. Tzanck test showing multinucleated giant cells supports the diagnosis.

Keratosis pilaris, option B, is characterized by horny follicular papules on the extremities and cheeks. Molluscum contagiosum, option C, is incorrect because these lesions are small, contain pink dome-shaped lesions, and usually occur singularly or in small groups. Pityriasis rosea, option D, is characterized by 3- to 5-mm scaly pink patches, and in many cases features a large herald patch. Option E, seborrheic dermatitis, is a rash that is characterized by symmetric, red scaling patches on hair-bearing and intertriginous areas. **Task:** C—Formulating Most Likely Diagnosis

7. **Answer: C** Elevated levels on D-dimer assay, option C, are most likely to be associated with a poor clinical outcome for this patient with COVID-19. An increased concentration at the time of hospital admission and throughout the hospital stay is associated with a thromboembolic event and death, and a concentration four times above normal is associated with approximately five-fold higher odds of critical illness than a normal D-dimer concentration.
Basic metabolic panel, option A, will provide information on electrolytes, which are not as necessarily associated with poor clinical outcomes as elevated levels on D-dimer assay are in patients with COVID-19. Complete blood cell count, hepatic panel, or thyroid function studies (options B, D, and E) are not specifically associated with poor clinical outcomes in patients with COVID-19 infection. **Task:** B—Using Diagnostic and Laboratory Studies

8. **Answer: E** Tetanus toxoid-containing vaccine, option E, is most appropriate to administer to this patient prior to discharge because of the mechanism of injury and the nature of the wound. Tetanus is an acute, noncommunicable, toxin-mediated disease caused by *Clostridium tetani*. Without prevention or appropriate treatment, the disease is potentially fatal. *Clostridium tetani* spores are found in soil and various animal feces. Spores are very resilient and can survive for years despite adverse conditions, as well as cleaning agents. *Clostridium tetani* enters through open areas of skin, lacerations, punctures, animal bites, burns, and surgical sites.
The rest of the options are not the correct vaccine for the prevention of *Clostridium tetani*. Influenza vaccine, option A, is a vaccine that is recommended seasonally, which contains a combination of influenza A and B variants in order to prevent complications from severe cases of influenza. Measles, mumps, and rubella vaccine, option B, is a live virus vaccine that aims to prevent infection with measles, mumps, or rubella. This vaccine is administered to children as well as other qualified adults who have not been immunized previously in childhood. Pneumococcal vaccines, option C, are offered at various stages of adulthood for the prevention of pneumococcal disease. Recombinant zoster vaccine, option D, is a vaccine used to prevent herpes zoster in adults 50 years of age and older. **Task:** D1—Health Maintenance, Patient Education, and Disease Prevention

9. **Answer: E** Based on the findings in this patient and her most recent trip to Africa, she most likely has malaria, which is a systemic febrile illness transmitted by a bite from an infected *Anopheles* mosquito most often occurring in endemic parts of the world. The infection itself is caused by one of five *Plasmodium* species, option E, transmitted by the vector mosquito. Malaria is usually suspected in any individual who presents with a febrile illness and who has recently traveled to an endemic country, although alternative diagnoses must also remain in the differential with travel history in mind.
Babesia, option A, includes a group of organisms that are transmitted to humans by the bite of the *Ixodes ricinus* family of ticks. Babesiosis, Lyme disease, anaplasmosis, *Borrelia miyamotoi* infection, ehrlichiosis, and Powassan virus are all similar organisms transmitted by this family of ticks. *Cryptosporidium*, option B, is an organism found in contaminated food, contaminated water, and farm animals that causes a diarrheal infection which is usually self-limited in healthy hosts, although it can be severe in immunocompromised hosts. *Filarioidea*, option C, includes a group of vector-borne parasitic worms that are endemic to Africa, India, Southeast Asia, Central and South America, as well as the South Pacific Islands. Once inside a human host, adult worms can live inside the lymphatic system, spreading their larva to blood, subcutaneous tissue, and other organs. Chronic infections can cause lymphatic filariasis, also known as elephantiasis. *Phthiraptera* species, option D, is a group of organisms that cause common head lice infections. **Task:** E—Applying Basic Scientific Concepts

10. **Answer: D** This patient has symptoms that are suggestive of Epstein-Barr virus. Ultrasonography of the abdomen, option D, is indicated in any person who plays contact sports to rule out splenomegaly caused by Epstein-Barr virus.
MRI of the abdomen, option A, is not appropriate first-line imaging to evaluate for splenomegaly. Oral amoxicillin therapy, option B, is incorrect because most patients with Epstein-Barr virus treated with penicillins develop a generalized, pruritic exanthem during the course of treatment. Oral corticosteroid therapy, option C, is only indicated in severe disease involving encroachment of the airway, cytopenias, or liver failure. Observation, option E, is not appropriate management because this patient plays a contact sport and is at risk for splenic rupture if splenomegaly is present. **Task:** D2—Clinical Intervention

11. **Answer: C** The correct answer is pneumococcal pneumonia, option C, which is the most common cause of pneumonia in patients with HIV infection even with relatively high CD4+ lymphocyte counts. This disease is more common in patients with HIV who smoke and who use injectable drugs. Chest x-ray study usually shows a localized infiltrate, and gram stain shows gram-positive diplococci.
Human metapneumovirus, option A, causes a viral pneumonia. Chest x-ray study findings are most often bilateral. Mycobacterium avium complex infection, option B, is a multisystem disease that usually does not develop until the CD4+ lymphocyte count is less than 50 cells/µL. Pneumocystis pneumonia, option D, usually does not occur until the CD4+ lymphocyte count is less than 200 cells/µL. Chest x-ray study of patients with this condition shows ground-glass opacities. Pulmonary coccidioidomycosis, option E, is a fungal infection endemic in the Southwestern United States. There are acute and chronic forms of this infection, and findings on chest x-ray study are usually multifocal. **Task:** C—Formulating Most Likely Diagnosis

12. **Answer: C** The correct answer is normal saline preparation of vaginal secretions, option C. The three most common causes of vaginitis are bacterial vaginosis, trichomoniasis, and yeast infections. This patient's presentation is suggestive of trichomoniasis infection, but the other causes are also possible. The most common method for confirming trichomoniasis infection is observing motile organisms on normal saline preparation of vaginal secretions.
Fungal culture of vaginal secretions, option A, is unlikely to distinguish between yeast that is part of the normal vaginal flora and yeast causing infection. Human papillomavirus test, option B, is incorrect because the most common symptom of this disorder is genital warts and not vaginal discharge. Serologic testing for herpes simplex virus, option D, is incorrect because this virus usually presents with vesicles on the genitalia. Diagnosis is clinical or with a polymerase chain reaction test from a scraping of the vesicles. Option E, urine dipstick test, is not correct because the patient's chief symptom is vaginal discharge, which is confirmed on pelvic examination. Therefore, a urinary cause is unlikely. **Task:** B—Using Diagnostic and Laboratory Studies

13. **Answer: A** There is no definitive test for acute rheumatic fever, and diagnosis relies on fulfilling either two major or one major and two minor criteria, as outlined in the revised Jones Criteria for Diagnosis of Rheumatic Fever. Carditis and chorea, option A, are two major criteria that meet the requirements for this disorder.
Carditis and prolonged PR interval, erythema marginatum and monoarthralgia, and erythema marginatum

and temperature ≥38.5°C (101.3°F) (options B, C, and D) only include one major and one minor Jones criteria each. Temperature ≥38.5°C (101.3°F) and polyarthropathy, option E, includes only two minor criteria. **Task:** A—History Taking and Performing Physical Examination

14. **Answer: D** *Pneumocystis jirovecii*, option D, is an opportunistic infection that occurs in immunocompromised patients including those with HIV infection and those who have undergone transplantation. Trimethoprim-sulfamethoxazole (TMP-SMZ) is the most effective antibiotic to prevent this disease.
Cytomegalovirus, option A, is a viral cause of infection in patients after transplantation, but TMP-SMZ is not protective against this pathogen. *Haemophilus influenzae, Mycoplasma pneumoniae*, and *Streptococcal pneumoniae* (options B, C, and E) are common causes of community-acquired pneumonia, but TMP-SMZ three times weekly is not indicated for prevention or treatment of these infections. **Task:** D3—Pharmaceutical Therapeutics

15. **Answer: E** This patient has most likely been bitten by a bat and is demonstrating symptoms of rabies, option E. This is a zoonotic disease caused by an RNA virus belonging to the *Rhabdoviridae* family, genus *Lyssavirus*, which causes acute progressive encephalomyelitis, hypersalivation, neurologic disturbances, emotional lability, and issues with temperature regulation. If left untreated after exposure, rabies almost always leads to death within 10 days of symptom onset due to multisystem organ failure, paralysis, and coma. Bat bites can be very superficial and can go unnoticed because of lack of dermatologic symptoms. Because of this, any human encounter with a bat requires evaluation by a clinician to determine if postexposure prophylactic treatment should be administered.
Options A and B are transmitted by the *Ixodes* tick. Anaplasmosis, option A, often presents with peripheral neuropathy. Babesia, option B, is an illness that causes symptoms and clinical signs including fever, hemolytic anemia, and acute renal failure. Option C, Lyme disease, is also a tickborne illness that causes a localized skin reaction called erythema migrans. Disseminated Lyme disease can cause neurologic, cardiac, rheumatologic, and genitourinary symptoms. Malaria, option D, is most often diagnosed in people who recently traveled to endemic areas. Malaria is a systemic febrile illness caused by an infection from one of the *Plasmodium* species that is transmitted by the bite of an *Anopheles* mosquito. **Task:** A—History Taking and Performing Physical Examination

16. **Answer: A** This patient has signs and symptoms of rubella; and leukopenia, option A, is a common laboratory finding in patients with this condition.

A positive viral culture, and not a negative viral culture (option B), would be expected in this patient because rubella is caused by a togavirus. Being positive for group A streptococcus infection, option C, will help confirm a diagnosis of scarlet fever and not rubella. A positive result on VDRL test, option D, is indicative of a diagnosis of syphilis. Thrombocytopenia, and not thrombocytosis (option E), is an expected finding in patients with rubella. **Task:** B—Using Diagnostic and Laboratory

17. **Answer: B** Because of his history of intravenous drug use, a positive PPD skin test for this patient is ≥10 mm of induration, option B. Other positive PPD criteria for ≥10 mm include: recent arrival (<5 years) from high-prevalence countries; resident/employee of high-risk congregate settings; mycobacteriology laboratory personnel; comorbid conditions; children less than 4 years of age; and infants, children, and adolescents exposed to high-risk categories.

An induration of ≥5 mm, option A, is considered a positive PPD test for patients who are HIV positive, who have had recent contact with someone with tuberculosis, who have fibrotic changes on x-ray studies, or who have undergone organ transplantation. An induration of ≥15 mm, option C, is considered a positive PPD skin test for people with no known risk factors for the disease. Options D and E are not classifications on the tuberculin skin test. **Task:** B—Using Diagnostic and Laboratory Studies

18. **Answer: B** This patient has signs and symptoms of herpes zoster infection. The correct answer is acyclovir, option B, which is an antiviral drug that is most effective at slowing the growth and spread of the condition if administered in the first 72 hours after the rash appears.

Acitretin, option A, is an oral retinoid used for treatment of psoriasis and not herpes zoster. Baloxavir marboxil, option C, is an antiviral drug used to treat influenza virus. Methicillin, option D, is an antibiotic used to treat bacterial skin infections caused by *Staphylococcus aureus*. Penicillin G benzathine, option E, is an antibiotic used to treat bacterial skin infections such as erysipelas. **Task Category**: D3—Pharmaceutical Therapeutics

19. **Answer: D** Influenza can be difficult to diagnose by clinical signs and symptoms alone, which can be similar to those of other infectious agents. The correct answer is option D, rapid molecular assays. Nucleic acid amplification tests such as this are preferred when diagnosing influenza.

Chest x-ray study and CT scan of the chest, options A and B, are not indicated because there are no findings on physical examination that warrant these imaging studies. Also, in most cases there are no findings on chest x-ray study even in symptomatic patients.

Heterophil antibody test, option C, would not be positive with 12 hours of symptoms. Rapid strep test, option E, is not indicated because based on the presenting symptoms, this patient has a low risk for streptococcal pharyngitis. **Task:** B—Using Diagnostic and Laboratory Studies

20. **Answer: B** Based on physical examination, this patient most likely has vaginal candidiasis, option B, because she has vaginal discharge that is thick, white, and looks like cottage cheese. These are the classic signs of this disorder.

Bacterial vaginosis, option A, usually presents with thin, homogeneous, fishy-smelling gray discharge. Patients with chlamydia, option C, often have a yellowish vaginal discharge and dysuria. Gonorrhea, option D, is indicated by white, yellow, or green discharge. Trichomoniasis, option E, includes a greenish-yellow, purulent malodorous discharge. **Task:** A—History Taking and Performing Physical Examination

21. **Answer: A** The correct answer is bright red rash on the cheeks, option A, which gives the appearance of a slapped cheek. This is the typical sign of erythema infectiosum (fifth disease).

Café au lait spots on the extremities, option B, may be an indication that a child has neurofibromatosis, which is a genetic disorder and not infectious. Koplik spots, option C, are white spots on the buccal mucosa found in patients with measles. Liquid-filled blisters on the trunk, option D, is a typical sign of chickenpox in childhood. Pink colored conjunctivae, or pink eye (option E), is most often caused by adenovirus and coronavirus and is not an indication of erythema infectiosum (fifth disease). **Task:** A—History Taking and Performing Physical Examination

22. **Answer: D** Patients who are 15 to 26 years of age should receive the three-dose series of the human papillomavirus vaccine. Therefore, this patient should receive one dose today, one in two months, and one in six months (option D).

He cannot receive the vaccination because he is immunocompromised, option A, is incorrect because immunocompromised patients can and should receive this vaccination. As stated previously, this vaccination can be administered to patients up to 26 years of age. Therefore, option B, he cannot receive the vaccination because he is too old, is incorrect. Receiving one dose of the vaccine today and again at six months, option C, is the appropriate immunization regimen for patients who are 11 to 14 years of age. Also, all immunocompromised patients, whether 11 to 14 or 15 to 26 years of age, should receive the three-dose series. He should receive the quadrivalent vaccine (4vHPV) rather than the bivalent vaccine (2vHPV) because it provides better coverage, option E, is incorrect. A choice between these two types of vaccines is not necessary, because the nonavalent vaccine (9vHPV) is currently available in the United States and protects the body against infection with nine different types of human papillomavirus. **Task:** D1—Health Maintenance, Patient Education, and Disease Prevention

23. **Answer: C** Lyme disease, option C, is endemic to the Eastern United States and is common in patients spending time outdoors with antecedent or probable tick bites. It is characterized by a spreading "bull's-eye" rash with central clearing, as noted in this patient. Ehrlichiosis, option A, occurs most often within a week of the bite of the lone star tick and is characterized by fever, severe headaches, malaise, myalgia, and chills. Histoplasmosis, option B, is a lung infection that is caused by inhalation of *Histoplasma capsulatum* fungal spores. Rheumatoid arthritis, option D, is an autoimmune disease that includes inflammatory arthritis, which this patient does not have. Rocky Mountain spotted fever, option E, is common in the Western United States and southern states from Oklahoma to North Carolina, and is characterized by fever and headache followed by a petechial rash starting on the wrists and ankles. **Task:** A—History Taking and Performing Physical Examination

24. **Answer: E** This patient has syphilis, option E, which is a sexually or congenitally transmitted infection caused by *Treponema pallidum*. Syphilis can have varying symptoms depending on the stage of the disease progression, defined separately as primary, secondary, and tertiary (or late) stages. In the primary stage of the disease process, the patient often has a genital lesion that is consistent with a chancre, as in the case of this patient. The treatment of choice for all stages of syphilis is parenteral penicillin G, with the route of administration dependent on the stage of the disease process. Individuals with known exposure to an individual with syphilis should be treated prophylactically based on CDC guidelines and specifics related to exposure.

The other options are not typically associated with genital rashes or specific lesions. Chlamydia, option A, is asymptomatic in approximately 40% to 60% of men. When symptomatic, it consists of urethritis and is associated with a mucoid urethral discharge. Gonorrhea, option B, includes clinical manifestations of mucopurulent urethritis or cervicitis within a week of exposure. In men, approximately 30% of gonorrhea urethral infections are asymptomatic. Hepatitis C, option C, is contracted by means of direct unprotected contact with the blood of a person with hepatitis C. HIV, option D, is a transmissible retrovirus that attacks CD4+ cells and causes immunodeficiency. HIV is primarily transmitted via blood and other body fluids. **Task:** A—History Taking and Performing Physical Examination

25. **Answer: A** This patient has roseola, and it is most appropriate to tell the patient's mother that this condition is self-limited, option A. Roseola is a benign, self-limited infection commonly caused by human herpesvirus 6 (HHV6). This condition typically resolves within three days after the onset of the rash. Roseola will not resolve with a short course of antibiotics, option B, because roseola is a viral condition commonly caused by HHV6 and treated symptomatically with antipyretics and oral hydration. Telling the mother that the fever will reoccur after the resolution of the rash, option C, is incorrect because this condition typically resolves within three days after onset of the rash without recurrence of fever. Telling the mother that the rash will begin to fade in two weeks, option D, is incorrect because the rash associated with roseola usually resolves within three days of onset. Treating this condition symptomatically with aspirin, option E, is incorrect because aspirin is contraindicated in infants due to the risk of Reye syndrome. Acetaminophen or ibuprofen are the best choices for symptomatic management. **Task:** D2—Clinical Intervention

26. **Answer: D** This patient's history of taking care of her cats (i.e., cleaning a litter box) as well as the findings on physical examination are consistent with *Toxoplasma gondii* infection, option D. Toxoplasmosis is caused by a protozoan parasite that infects cats as the definitive host. Cats shed oocysts in feces that then can infect birds and mammals. Infection in humans can occur with ingestion of a single cyst and can occur with emptying a litter box or ingesting infected meat. It is most commonly asymptomatic and self-limited but can cause nonspecific symptoms such as fever, chills, headache, myalgia, pharyngitis, abdominal pain, and maculopapular rash. Pregnant women who are infected can transmit the infection to the fetus and cause congenital toxoplasmosis; therefore, this should be in the differential in all pregnant women who present with these symptoms.

Cytomegalovirus infection, option A, can cause a mononucleosis syndrome including fever, chills, myalgia, and headache but does not typically have the exudative pharyngitis and cervical lymphadenopathy seen in mononucleosis caused by Epstein-Barr virus (EBV). EBV infection, option B, causes infectious mononucleosis that includes posterior cervical lymphadenopathy, but it will typically include pharyngitis and tonsillitis with exudate and fatigue as well as atypical lymphocytes seen on complete blood cell count. Acute symptomatic HIV infection, option C, includes fever, fatigue, nontender lymphadenopathy of the axillary, cervical, and occipital nodes, sore throat without exudate, mucocutaneous ulcers, generalized rash, headache, and gastrointestinal symptoms. Zika virus infection, option E, includes low-grade fever, pruritic rash, nonpurulent conjunctivitis, and arthralgia. This infection is transmitted via mosquitoes. **Task: A—** History Taking and Performing Physical Examination

27. **Answer: A** One of the biggest risk factors for recurrent abscesses caused by MRSA infection include intravenous drug use, option A. Other risk factors include shaving of legs, axillae, and pubic hair and colonization or prior infection with MRSA.

Playing team sports, option B, may increase the patient's risk for staphylococcal infections because of the shared locker/showers but not as much as intravenous drug use. Red ant bites, option C, does not increase a patient's risk for recurrent MRSA infections. Scratches from a cat, option D, will not increase a patient's risk of recurrent MRSA infections unless the patient continually scratches the involved location. Working out at a gym, option E, may increase a patient's risk of MRSA but not as much as intravenous drug use. **Task:** D1—Health Maintenance, Patient Education, and Disease Prevention

28. **Answer: A** Pinworm infestation is a common cause of perirectal itching. This condition is caused by *Enterobius vermicularis*, option A.

Giardia duodenalis, option B, causes giardiasis, which is a common cause of diarrhea. This patient does not have this symptom. *Pediculus capitis*, option C, causes lice infestation of the hair, which is not consistent with this patient's presentation. *Sarcoptes scabiei*, option D, is the mite that causes scabies. As there are no other areas of rash or pruritus, scabies is not the most likely diagnosis in this patient. *Treponema pallidum*, option E, is the bacteria that causes syphilis, which is not consistent with this patient's presentation. **Task:** E— Applying Basic Scientific Concepts

29. **Answer: A** This pregnant patient has a chlamydial infection of the cervix. Azithromycin 1 g as a single dose, option A, is recommended by the CDC and is generally considered safe and effective during pregnancy and lactation.

Ciprofloxacin 500 mg twice daily for three days, option B, is not preferred over azithromycin, which is considered first-line therapy. Doxycycline 100 mg twice daily for seven days, option C, is not recommended in patients who are pregnant, because tetracyclines may affect tooth development and cause discoloration of the teeth in the infant. Erythromycin estolate 500 mg four times daily for seven days, option D, is contraindicated in pregnancy because of the risk of drug-induced hepatotoxicity. However, erythromycin and erythromycin ethylsuccinate are approved alternatives to azithromycin for treatment of chlamydia in pregnancy. Trimethoprim-sulfamethoxazole 80 mg/400 mg twice daily for 10 days, option E, is not effective for the treatment of chlamydial infection. **Task:** D3—Pharmaceutical Therapeutics

30. **Answer: B** The measles, mumps, rubella vaccine, option B, is commonly administered to children 12 to 18 months of age, but when a child is travelling internationally it is recommended for infants over 6 months of age. Human papillomavirus, meningococcal, and meningococcal B vaccines (options A, C and D) are administered to adolescents. Yellow fever vaccine, option E, would be indicated if the family were travelling to Africa or other areas with endemic yellow fever. **Task:** D1—Health Maintenance, Patient Education, and Disease Prevention

BIBLIOGRAPHY

Albrecht, M. A. (2020). Mumps. In T. Post (Ed.), *UpToDate*. Waltham, MA: UpToDate.

Benner, D. (2021). Chlamydia Genital Infections. In F. Ferri (Ed.), *Ferri's clinical adviser*. Elsevier.

Bennett, J. E., Dolin, R., & Blaser, M. J. (2019). *Mandell, Douglas, and Bennett's principles and practice of infectious diseases*. Elsevier.

Borawski, K. M. (2021). Sexually Transmitted Diseases. In A. Partin, R. Dmochowski, L. Kavoussi, C. Peters, & A. Wein (Eds.), *Campbell-Walsh-Wein urology* (12th ed.) Elsevier.

Breyre, A., & Frazee, B. W. (2018). Skin and soft tissue infections in the emergency department. *Emergency Medicine Clinics of North America*, *36*(4), 723-750.

CDC: Malaria: malaria diagnostic tests: Malaria diagnosis (U.S.)—Microscopy. CDC website. Last Reviewed February 19, 2020.

CDC: Malaria: Treatment of malaria: Guidelines for clinicians (United States). Part 2: General Approach to Treatment and Treatment of Uncomplicated Malaria. CDC website. Updated November 15, 2018.

CDC: Rocky mountain spotted fever: Clinical and laboratory diagnosis. CDC website. Updated October 26, 2018.

CDC: Rocky mountain spotted fever: Signs and symptoms. CDC website. Updated February 19, 2019.

Centers for Disease Control and Prevention. (2015). *Sexually transmitted diseases treatment guidelines*.

Clinical Overview: Lyme Disease. In *Elsevier Point of Care*. Updated June 18, 2020. Elsevier.

Cohen, B. A. (January 1, 2013). *Pediatric dermatology* (4th ed.), chapter 3, pp. 68-103. Saunders.

Elsevier Point of Care. *Influenza*, Updated September 9, 2020. Copyright Elsevier BV.

Flint, P. Throat disorders. *Goldman-Cecil Medicine*, *401*, 2565-2571.e1.

Greenlee, G. E. Rabies. Merck manuals professional edition website. Updated January 2019.

Hankins, D. G., & Rosekrans, J. A. (2004). Overview, prevention, and treatment of rabies. *Mayo Clinic Proceedings*, *79*(5), 671-676.

Havers, F. P., Moro, P. L., Hunter, P., Hariri, S., & Bernstein, H. (2014). Use of tetanus toxoid, reduced diphtheria toxoid, and acellular pertussis vaccines: updated recommendations of the advisory committee on immunization practices—United States, 2019. Morbidity and Mortality Weekly Report Jackson AC: Rabies. *Handbook of clinical neurology*, *123*, 601-618.

James, W. Parasitic infestations, stings and bites. *Andrews' Diseases of the Skin*, *20*, 421-452.e3.

James, W. D., Elston, D., Treat, J. R., Rosenbach, M. A., & Neuhaus, I. M. (2020). *Andrew's diseases of the skin* (13th ed.), pp. 362-420. Elsevier.

Kent, M. E., & Romanelli, F. (2008). Reexamining syphilis: an update on epidemiology, clinical manifestations, and management. *The Annals of Pharmacotherapy*, *42*, 226-236.

Knox, M. A., Coutinho, B., Takedai, T., & Brown, S. R. (2020). Skin diseases in infants & children. In J. E. South-Paul, S. C. Matheny, & E. L. Lewis (Eds.), *Current diagnosis & treatment: Family medicine, 5e*. McGraw-Hill.

Kristy McKiernan Borawski. Sexually transmitted diseases. *Campbell-Walsh-Wein Urology*, *58*, 1251-1272.

Kroger, A. T., Pickering, L. K., Mawle, A., Hinman, A. R., & Orenstein, W. A. (2020). Immunization. In J. Bennett, R. Dolin, & M. Blaser (Eds.) *Mandell, Douglas and Bennett's principles and practice of infectious diseases*. (9th ed). Elsevier.

Lee, S. G., Fralick, M., & Sholzberg, M. (2020). Coagulopathy associated with COVID-1. *Canadian Medical Association Journal*, *192*(21), E583-E583.

Malone, M. A. & Jain, V. Vulvovaginitis. *Conn's current therapy 2020*, pp. 1181-1185.

Manning, S. E., Rupprecht, C. E., Fishbein, D., Hanlon, C. A., Lumlertdacha, B., Guerra, M., et al. (2008). Human rabies prevention—United States, 2008: recommendations of the Advisory Committee on Immunization Practices. *MMWR. Recommendations and Reports: Morbidity and Mortality Weekly Report. Recommendations and Reports/Centers for Disease Control*, *57*(RR-3), 1-28.

Papadakis, M., McPhee, S., & Rabow, M. (2019). *Current medical diagnosis & treatment 2020* (59th Ed.). Cenveo Publisher Services.

Petersen, E., & Mandelbrot, L. (2020). Toxoplasmosis and pregnancy. In T. Post (Ed.), *UpToDate*. Waltham, MA: UpToDate.

Puligandla, P. S. & Laberge, J. M. (2012). Infections and Diseases of the Lungs, Pleura, and Mediastinum. In A. G. Coran, A. Caldamone, N. S. Adzick, T. M. Krummel, J. M. Laberge, & R. Shamberger (Eds.) *Pediatric Surgery* (7 ed.). Elsevier.

Rubella. *Epocrates*. Updated June 30, 2020.

Stevens, D. L., Byrant, A. E., & Hagman, M. M. *Goldman–Cecil Medicine*, *274*, 1871-1878.

Yen, L. M., & Thwaites, C. L. (2019). Tetanus. *Lancet*, *393*(10181), 1657-1668.

Answer Key for this chapter begins on p. 119

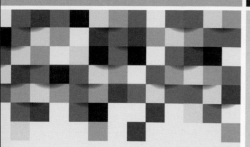

CHAPTER 9
Musculoskeletal System

Questions

1. A 42-year-old woman who is otherwise healthy comes to the office because she has had pain in her right shoulder, especially with overhead movements, and occasionally at night during the past week. She says she has been a house painter for the past five years and is always painting walls and ceilings. She rates the pain as a 5 on a 10-point scale but rates it as a 1 when the arm is at rest by her side. The patient has not stopped working because she needs the money, but the pain is preventing her from working efficiently. She has been applying ice to the right shoulder but has not taken any medications to help relieve the pain. Physical examination shows no muscular atrophy. No weakness of the right arm is noted. Which of the following is the most appropriate initial management?
   A. Oral nonsteroidal anti-inflammatory drugs (NSAIDs) for one week followed by surgical intervention
   B. Oral NSAIDs with physical therapy for one month
   C. Physical therapy for one week followed by subacromial corticosteroid injection
   D. Subacromial corticosteroid injection followed by surgical intervention one month later
   E. Surgical intervention followed by physical therapy for two months

2. A 20-year-old man comes to the emergency department because he had pain in the right knee immediately after he twisted his knee during a soccer match. He says he went to kick the ball with his left foot and twisted his right knee, which was planted. Medical history includes no chronic disease conditions. Vital signs are within normal limits. Physical examination shows pain with active range of motion of the right knee. Minimal edema and tenderness to palpation of the knee are noted. Which of the following studies of the knee is most likely to definitively detect the suspected injury in this patient?

A. Arthroscopy
B. Bone scan
C. CT scan
D. Ultrasonography
E. X-ray studies

3. A 45-year-old man comes to the office because he has had gradual onset of fever, dull pain, and diffuse body shakes over the past two days since he underwent vertebral surgery. Physical examination shows a small, warm, erythematous area around the incision site. Exquisite tenderness to palpation of the area is noted. Which of the following is the most likely causative agent?
   A. Gram-negative bacilli
   B. Group A *Streptococcus*
   C. *Pseudomonas aeruginosa*
   D. *Staphylococcus aureus*
   E. *Streptococcus equisimilis*

4. A 38-year-old man comes to the office because he has had lower back pain for the past three weeks. He cannot identify a precipitating incident, but he thinks the pain may be related to the weightlifting he started doing at the gym four weeks ago. He describes the pain as aching across the central lower back with intermittent radiation to the left buttock. No leg pain is present. The patient's symptoms are worse with activity and improve with rest. He has not had weakness or loss of sensation in the lower extremity, fever, or change in bladder or bowel control. Vital signs are within normal limits. Physical examination shows tenderness on forward flexion and on returning to the erect position. No other abnormalities are noted. Which of the following is the most likely cause of the lower back pain in this patient?
   A. Ankylosing spondylitis
   B. Lumbar compression fracture
   C. Lumbar disk herniation
   D. Muscle strain
   E. Spinal stenosis

5.

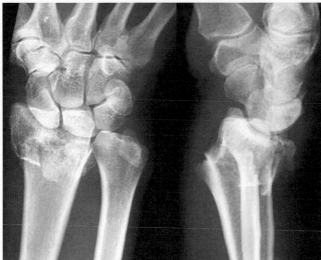

A 65-year-old woman is brought to the urgent care by her husband immediately after she fell on her outstretched right hand. Physical examination shows edema and tenderness to palpation over the distal radius. X-ray studies of the wrist are shown. This patient has most likely sustained which of the following types of fracture?
A. Colles
B. Galeazzi
C. Nightstick
D. Smith
E. Torus

6. A 20-year-old man who is a pitcher on his college's baseball team comes to the campus clinic because he has had pain and stiffness in the medial aspect of the elbow for the past month. Which of the following physical examination maneuvers is most likely to cause discomfort in this patient?
A. Applying resistance distal to the proximal interphalangeal joint when the patient extends the third digit of the hand
B. Applying resistance when the patient makes a fist, pronates the forearm, and radially deviates and extends the wrist
C. Applying valgus stress to the elbow while passively flexing the elbow with the forearm held in pronation
D. Passively pronating the patient's forearm, flexing the wrist, and extending the elbow
E. Passively supinating the patient's forearm and extending the elbow and wrist

7. A 32-year-old woman comes to the urgent care clinic because she has had a throbbing pain in the lateral aspect of her right ankle since she injured the ankle while jogging one hour ago. She says she stepped on a stone and her ankle rotated outward. The pain does not radiate, and the patient rates the pain as a 6 on a 10-point scale. Physical examination shows stable weight bearing, mild localized edema on the lateral aspect of the ankle, and tenderness to palpation anterior to and inferior to the lateral malleolus; no ecchymosis is noted. Strength, range of motion, pulses, and sensation are intact. Which of the following ligaments is most likely injured?
A. Anterior talofibular
B. Calcaneofibular
C. Inferior transverse
D. Medial deltoid
E. Tibiofibular

8. A 7-year-old girl is brought to the clinic by her mother because she has had knee pain for the past seven weeks. She has no history of injury to the knee. The mother says that the patient has had high fevers to 39.4°C (103.0°F) accompanied by a pink rash off and on over the past two weeks. The patient was also treated for uveitis by an ophthalmologist three months ago. Current physical examination shows mild erythema and edema of the knee. Which of the following is the most appropriate first-line treatment?
A. Allopurinol
B. Hydroxychloroquine
C. Methotrexate
D. Nonsteroidal anti-inflammatory drugs
E. Sulfasalazine

9. A 44-year-old man comes to the clinic because he has had intense, worsening pain in the left leg for the past 24 hours. Twenty-four hours ago, he was examined in the emergency department after he was involved in a motorcycle collision. At that time, an x-ray study showed an intact left tibia and fibula. He was discharged to home with advice to rest and elevate the affected leg and to take hydrocodone/acetaminophen as needed for pain. Currently, he says that his leg feels even tighter than it did when he was in the emergency department. On physical examination, full range of motion of the affected leg is noted at the knee. However, more intense pain is elicited over the gastrocnemius when the leg is extended and the foot flexed and extended. Edema, erythema, and tenderness to palpation of the gastrocnemius are noted. Pulses are decreased in the affected leg. Which of the following is the most appropriate intervention?
A. Application of a splint
B. Fasciotomy
C. Nonsteroidal anti-inflammatory drugs as needed
D. Physical therapy
E. Rest, ice, compression, and elevation

10.

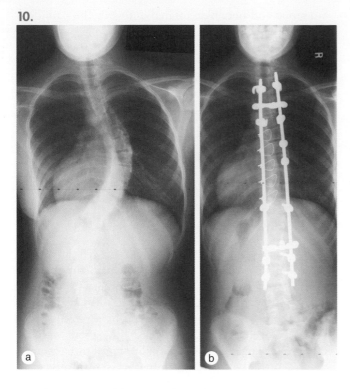

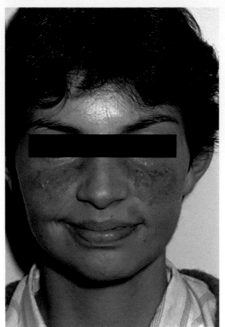

A 14-year-old girl is brought to the office by her mother for routine follow-up of scoliosis. X-ray study of the spine (image A) shows a 68-degree right thoracic curve and a 53-degree left lumbar scoliosis. This finding confirms that this patient's curve is progressing despite the use of a brace. Instrumented posterior spinal fusion is performed, and postoperative x-ray study is shown (image B). Which of the following postoperative recommendations regarding physical activity is most appropriate to tell this patient and her parents?

A. Activity will be limited for six to nine months because she will need to wear a body cast
B. Bending, lifting, and twisting can be done seven days postoperatively
C. She can participate in noncontact sports three months postoperatively
D. She will need to wait six months before returning to routine activities
E. She will need to work with a physical therapist to mobilize within 24 hours after surgery

11.

A 27-year-old woman comes to the clinic because she has had fatigue, joint pain, and a rash on her face for the past three months. She says she feels tired all the time and has achiness in most of her joints. Temperature is 38.0°C (100.4°F). A photograph of the rash is shown. Which of the following laboratory studies is most likely to determine the diagnosis?

A. Antineutrophil cytoplasmic antibody test
B. Antinuclear antibody test
C. Cyclic citrullinated peptide antibody test
D. HLA-B27 antibody test
E. Rheumatoid factor assay

12. A 68-year-old woman comes to the office because she has had pain in her right shoulder for the past three months. She has no history of recent trauma or falls. The patient says she plays tennis but had to stop playing six weeks ago because of increasing pain. The pain is aggravated by overhead movements and is worse at night. She has been taking ibuprofen, which has only provided slight relief of pain. Medical history does not include shoulder problems, and she has no history of chronic disease conditions. Physical examination shows significant tenderness over the superior and anterior shoulder. Passive range of motion of the shoulder shows no abnormalities; however, inability to actively raise the right arm over the head is noted. An MRI shows small, partial-thickness tears of the subscapularis and teres minor tendons. Which of the following is the most appropriate initial step in management?

A. Electrical muscle stimulation
B. Injection of platelet-rich plasma into the shoulder
C. Intramuscular dry needling
D. Physical therapy to strengthen the muscles
E. Surgical referral

13. A 38-year-old man comes to the clinic because he has had worsening pain in the right groin over the past year. He has no history of injury or trauma. Vital signs are within normal limits. Physical examination shows pain with passive internal rotation of the hip. X-ray study of the right hip shows subchondral collapse, flattening of the femoral head, and loss of joint space. Chronic use of which of the following types of medication is the most likely cause?
    A. Beta-blockers
    B. Corticosteroids
    C. Opioids
    D. Statins
    E. Sulfonylureas

14. A 42-year-old woman comes to the emergency department because she has had severe lower back pain for the past two days. She says she was referred to the emergency department by her primary care provider who was concerned that she may have cauda equina syndrome. If this patient has this condition, which of the following findings on physical examination is most likely?
    A. Decreased anal tone
    B. Fever
    C. Hyperreflexia in the lower extremities
    D. Pelvic instability
    E. Positive straight-leg raising test

15. A 45-year-old man is brought to the emergency department wearing a cervical collar 45 minutes after he was involved in a motor vehicle collision. He was the passenger in the vehicle and was wearing his seat belt. He says he has numbness and weakness in his arms and legs. The patient is alert and oriented to person, place, and time. Temperature is 36.6°C (97.8°F), pulse rate is 118/min, and blood pressure is 146/82 mmHg. CT scan, including sagittal reconstruction, shows translational displacement of C6-C7 in the axial plane. Which of the following is the most likely diagnosis?
    A. Burst fracture
    B. Compression fracture
    C. Distraction injury
    D. Extension injury
    E. Fracture-dislocation

16. A 62-year-old woman comes to the office because she has had gradual onset of pain in the left knee over the past six months. She says the pain has recently increased, especially when she walks up and down stairs. The patient has no history of recent trauma to the knee, and she has not had any locking or giving way of the knee. She says she took glucosamine for the pain but stopped taking it because it did not provide relief. Medical history includes no chronic disease conditions, and she takes no medications. Body mass index is 25 kg/m² (N = 18.5−24.9 kg/m²). Vital signs are within normal limits. Physical examination of the left knee shows decreased extension with standing and slight varus deformity. No edema or tenderness to palpation of the joint is noted. Tests of the ligaments show no abnormalities. Plain film x-ray studies of the knee show narrowing of the joint space. Which of the following drugs is most likely to be effective in improving this patient's symptoms?
    A. Acetaminophen
    B. Calcium carbonate
    C. Colchicine
    D. Methotrexate
    E. Naproxen

17. A 3-month-old female infant is brought to the office by her parents because they are concerned that her skull is misshapen. The patient is twin A of an uncomplicated vaginal delivery, and she has reached all developmental milestones since birth. However, the parents say that the patient's head commonly tilts to the left and the skull appears to be flattened on the left side. On physical examination, the patient becomes fussy when placed in the prone position. Which of the following is the most appropriate management?
    A. Inject botulinum toxin into the strap muscles of the neck
    B. Prescribe oral corticosteroid therapy
    C. Recommend watchful waiting
    D. Refer for physical therapy
    E. Refer for surgical correction of the head tilt

18. A 45-year-old man who works as a painter has had aching and tenderness over the anterior aspect of the right shoulder for the past several weeks. He says the pain is exacerbated with referred pain to the upper arm when he raises his right arm overhead. On physical examination with the patient's arm flexed at 90 degrees, the palm facing the ground, and the arm stabilized against the thorax, tenderness is noted when the patient is asked to supinate the forearm, externally rotate the humerus, and flex the elbow against resistance. Which of the following is the most likely diagnosis?
    A. Adhesive capsulitis
    B. Biceps tendonitis
    C. Cervical spondylosis
    D. Glenohumeral osteoarthritis
    E. Rotator cuff tendonitis

    Answer Key for this chapter begins on p. 135

19. A 42-year-old woman comes to the office because she has had chronic fatigue, pain in the neck, shoulders, and lower back, chronic headaches, and irritable bowel symptoms during the past several years. Pulse rate is 96/min, respirations are 18/min, and blood pressure is 115/80 mmHg. On physical examination, tenderness is noted on palpation of the trigger points around the occiput, lateral epicondyle of the elbows, gluteal area, and medial fat pads of the knees. On laboratory studies of serum, erythrocyte sedimentation rate, C-reactive protein level and antinuclear antibody level are within normal limits. Which of the following is the most likely diagnosis?
    A. Fibromyalgia
    B. Osteoporosis
    C. Polymyalgia rheumatica
    D. Rheumatoid arthritis
    E. Systemic lupus erythematosus

20. A 14-year-old boy is brought to the office by his mother because he has had worsening pain in the right knee over the past two weeks. His mother says that he recently grew several inches, and they had to buy new soccer shorts and cleats. He says the pain has limited him from running and jumping in practice, and he has pain when he climbs the stairs at home or walks up the hill to the soccer field. The patient has no history of injury to the knee. Which of the following findings on physical examination is most likely?
    A. Catching sensation with the patient standing on the right leg flexed 20 degrees while internally and externally rotating the knee
    B. Increased translation with the patient lying supine with the knee flexed 90 degrees and the proximal tibia pulled anteriorly
    C. Marked tenderness, localized erythema, and edema anterior to the patella and patellar tendon
    D. Right tibia sagging below the level of the left tibia with the patient lying supine with the hip flexed to 45 degrees and the knee flexed to 90 degrees
    E. Tenderness and bony prominence of the tibial tubercle that increases with extending the knee against resistance

21. A 45-year-old man comes to the clinic because he is concerned about his strong family history of Paget disease of bone. He is currently asymptomatic but wonders if there is a test that could indicate whether or not he has this disease. It is most appropriate to tell the patient that an elevation in which of the following

serum laboratory values is most indicative of Paget disease?
    A. Alkaline phosphatase
    B. Ammonia
    C. Blood urea nitrogen
    D. Troponin I
    E. Uric acid

22. A 48-year-old woman who is right-hand dominant comes to the office because she has had pain as well as a burning sensation in her right hand, particularly in her thumb, index, and long fingers, for the past six weeks. She says she has tried taking acetaminophen and using a hand brace, but they did not provide relief; her symptoms are continuing to worsen, particularly at night. Medical history includes type 2 diabetes mellitus and hypertension for which she takes metformin and enalapril, respectively. On physical examination, direct application of pressure over the volar surface of the wrist elicits numbness and tingling. Which of the following additional symptoms and signs is most likely to indicate that surgery is necessary at this time?
    A. Inability to grasp or pinch objects as she did in the past
    B. Inability to identify different textures with the hand
    C. Pain that radiates proximally to the forearm
    D. Pain with making a fist
    E. Tingling sensation in the palm

23. A 22-year-old woman is brought to the emergency department by ambulance and local law enforcement immediately after she jumped out of a second-floor window in an attempt to evade the police. She says she landed on her feet and immediately felt pain in her right heel. Vital signs are within normal limits. Physical examination shows no obvious deformity, but significant edema and tenderness to the entire right foot are noted. No pain or tenderness to palpation are noted in the right leg or hip. X-ray studies of the right and left feet and ankles show a fracture of the right calcaneus. X-ray studies of which of the following areas of the body is most appropriate to order next?
    A. Cervical spine and scapula
    B. Lumbar and thoracic spine
    C. Sacral spine and pelvis
    D. Femur and hip
    E. Tibia and fibula

24. A 28-year-old man comes to the primary care clinic because he has a six-year history of episodic stiffness in his lower back and hips as well as a mild, aching pain that does not radiate. He says the symptoms are worse in the morning, improve with movement, and have responded to therapy with ibuprofen in the past. The patient's father also had similar symptoms. Vital signs are within normal limits. On physical examination, mild tenderness is noted on palpation of the lumbar spine and sacroiliac joint. Extension of the lumbar spine is decreased by 15 degrees. No edema is noted in the lower extremities, and strength, pulses, and sensation are intact, bilaterally. In addition to x-ray studies, which of the following studies is most likely to determine a diagnosis?
    A. CT scan of the lumbar spine
    B. Erythrocyte sedimentation rate
    C. HLA-B27 antigen test
    D. Indium white blood cell scan
    E. Rheumatoid factor assay

25. A 45-year-old man who has obesity comes to the urgent care clinic because he had sudden onset of pain over the base of the big toe on his right foot six hours ago. He has no history of recent trauma and has never had similar symptoms. Temperature is 37.2°C (99.0°F), pulse rate is 88/min, respirations are 16/min, and blood pressure is 130/80 mmHg. The patient appears uncomfortable. Physical examination of the first metatarsophalangeal joint on the right shows edema, redness, warmth, and tenderness to palpation. Further evaluation will most likely show an elevation of which of the following serum values?
    A. Antinuclear antibody
    B. Phosphate
    C. Procalcitonin
    D. Rheumatoid factor
    E. Uric acid

26. A 45-year-old man comes to the clinic because he has had a low-grade fever, malaise, headache, and diffuse nonspecific abdominal pain for the past two weeks. Medical history includes hypertension, renal insufficiency, and chronic hepatitis B. Medications include captopril and interferon. Blood pressure is elevated. Laboratory studies show worsening renal function. Polyarteritis nodosa is suspected. If this diagnosis is confirmed, a history of which of the following conditions is most likely in this patient?
    A. Chronic splenomegaly
    B. Diffuse arthritis
    C. Mastoid infections
    D. Pulmonary congestion
    E. Recurrent uveitis

27. A 40-year-old woman comes to the primary care clinic because she has had slowly worsening photosensitivity, a sensation of grit under her eyelids, thick strands of inner canthi secretions associated with dry mouth, and difficulty swallowing dry food over the past four months. Medical history includes mild anxiety and depression following the loss of a child eight months ago. Physical examination shows intact vision and dry conjunctiva. Oral mucosa is sticky and erythematous. Filiform papillae atrophy is noted on the dorsal tongue. The parotid glands are enlarged bilaterally, and cloudy saliva is expressed with palpation. It is most appropriate to recommend consultation with which of the following types of specialists at this time?
    A. Allergy
    B. Endocrinology
    C. Ophthalmology
    D. Otolaryngology
    E. Rheumatology

28. A 25-year-old man is brought to the emergency department on a backboard and wearing a cervical collar immediately after he was shot in the neck and back. Vital signs are within normal limits. The patient is angry that he was shot and says that he needs to use the bathroom before he has an accident. Physical examination shows loss of motor function and significantly diminished sensation to light touch and vibration on the right side and loss of sensation to pinprick and temperature on the left. Based on these findings, which of the following is the most likely diagnosis?
    A. Anterior cord syndrome
    B. Brown-Séquard syndrome
    C. Cauda equina syndrome
    D. Central cord syndrome
    E. Horner syndrome

29. A 15-year-old girl is brought to the clinic by her mother because she has had intermittent pain in the right hip, groin, thigh, and knee for the past five to six months. The patient says that the pain worsens with long periods of walking or short periods of a high-intensity activity such as running. The patient walks with a limp. On physical examination, internal rotation is limited. Which of the following findings is most likely on anteroposterior and frog-leg lateral x-ray studies of the right hip?
    A. Crossover sign
    B. Displacement of the right femoral head
    C. Flattening of the femoral head epiphysis
    D. Ossification of the proximal femoral epiphysis
    E. Thin sclerotic line that crosses the femoral neck

 Answer Key for this chapter begins on p. 135

30. A 37-year-old man comes to the clinic because he has had recurrent pain and weakness in his left shoulder during the past four months. He says he also has had loss of active range of motion in the shoulder. The patient has participated in competitive bodybuilding for several years, and he says his current symptoms are affecting his training, although he has no desire to stop resistance training. Medical history includes several episodes of bursitis of the left shoulder that were treated with nonsteroidal anti-inflammatory drugs, rest, and injection of corticosteroids as well as physical therapy; he says his symptoms have been relieved by this regimen, but then they always return. The two most recent episodes included septic bursitis that was successfully treated with intravenous antibiotics. Vital signs are within normal limits, and the shoulder appears normal on physical examination. Which of the following is the most appropriate next step?
    A. Administer intravenous antibiotics
    B. Recommend the patient refrain from bodybuilding
    C. Recommend the patient try physical therapy again
    D. Refer the patient to an orthopedic surgeon
    E. Repeat injection of corticosteroids

31. A 37-year-old woman comes to the clinic because she has had a thickening of the skin on her face, hands, and neck over the past six months. She has not had itching or pain in the involved areas but says that both of her hands swell intermittently. Medical history includes Raynaud phenomenon and esophageal motility disorder. Vital signs are within normal limits. Physical examination shows fibrotic skin changes, and telangiectasias are noted on both hands without vesicles, patches, or pustules. Mild finger curling is noted with shiny skin of the distal fingers. Which of the following is the most likely diagnosis?
    A. Dyshidrotic eczema
    B. Folliculitis
    C. Hand, foot, and mouth disease
    D. Lichen simplex chronicus
    E. Scleroderma

32. A 59-year-old woman comes to the office because she has had lower back pain for the past year. She has no history of injury to the spine or recent falls. The patient says she also feels like she has lost some height over the past few years. She does not exercise and drinks one to two glasses of wine every night with dinner. Physical examination shows tenderness to palpation of the lumbar spine. X-ray studies show no abnormalities. Osteoporosis is suspected, and pharmacotherapy is being considered. Which of the following best

describes the sequelae of the pharmacologic management of this disease?
    A. Decreased osteoclastic activity
    B. Decreased reabsorption of calcium from the renal tubules
    C. Decreased vitamin D absorption from the gastrointestinal tract
    D. Increased calcitriol secretion from the kidneys
    E. Stimulation of parathyroid hormone secretion

33. A two-day-old female newborn is brought to the clinic by her parents for routine well-child examination. The patient was born via caesarean delivery at 39 weeks' gestation because she was in the breech position. On physical examination, a clunk is felt as the left femoral head dislocates and pops out of the socket or acetabulum when the hip is adducted and gentle force is applied to the knee. Which of the following is the name of this test?
    A. Barlow test
    B. Flexion, adduction, and internal rotation test
    C. Ortolani test
    D. Thomas test
    E. Trendelenburg test

34. A 58-year-old woman comes to the office because she has had a slowly enlarging mass on her left wrist for the past six months. On physical examination, a 3-mm mass is noted on the dorsal aspect of the left wrist. The mass is nontender, mobile, and transilluminates with a penlight. The left upper extremity is neurovascularly intact. Which of the following is the most appropriate management?
    A. Arthroscopic decompression of the cyst
    B. Closed rupture of the cyst with a heavy object
    C. Injection of a sclerosing agent into the cyst
    D. Open excision of the cyst
    E. Observation

35. A 75-year-old woman comes to the clinic because she has had worsening pain in the upper back over the past six months. She says the pain is constant and dull and does not radiate. Acetaminophen provides relief. She has no history of trauma or injury. Physical examination shows an exaggeration of the normal thoracic kyphosis. Based on this finding, this patient most likely has a history of which of the following conditions?
    A. Cirrhosis
    B. Emphysema
    C. Gout
    D. Osteoporosis
    E. Rheumatoid arthritis

36. A 58-year-old woman comes to the office because she has had worsening pain in the left knee over the past four days. She is not able to bend her knee when she sits down, gets in the car, or walks up stairs. The patient has no history of injury to the knee. Medical history includes arthritis and diabetes mellitus. Temperature is 38.8°C (101.8°F), and pulse rate is 112/min. Physical examination of the knee shows edema and erythema, and the knee is warm to touch. Which of the following is the most appropriate next step to determine the diagnosis?
    A. Blood culture
    B. Culture of synovial fluid
    C. Measurement of C-reactive protein level
    D. Ultrasonography of the knee
    E. X-ray study of the knee

37. A 45-year-old man who works in construction comes to the emergency department because he has a two-day history of sharp pain in the lower back that radiates all the way down the posterior aspect of his right leg to his foot. He has no history of recent trauma, and he has not had any changes in bowel or bladder control or movement. The patient does not have any numbness in the groin area. Medical history includes no chronic disease conditions. Vital signs are within normal limits. Which of the following is the most likely diagnosis?
    A. Acute sciatica
    B. Cauda equina syndrome
    C. Lumbosacral strain
    D. Scoliosis
    E. Spinal fracture

38. A 32-year-old woman comes to the office because she has had pain in the dorsal radial aspect of the wrist for the past three months. She says that the pain increases when she is feeding her 7-month-old baby. The patient has no history of trauma to the wrist, and x-ray studies show no abnormalities. Result of which of the following physical examination tests is most likely to be positive in this patient?
    A. Empty can
    B. Finkelstein
    C. Phalen
    D. Speed
    E. Yergason

39.

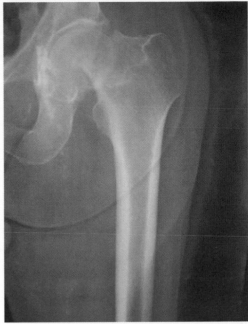

A 75-year-old woman with a history of osteoporosis comes to the emergency department because she has had pain in her left hip since she sustained a mechanical ground-level fall at her home 30 minutes ago. Initial physical examination shows that the left leg is shorter than the right and is externally rotated. An x-ray study of the left hip is shown. Which of the following is the most appropriate definitive management of the left hip?
    A. Arthroplasty
    B. Hip spica cast
    C. Open reduction and internal fixation
    D. Pelvic binding
    E. Traction splinting

40. A 22-year-old woman who plays racquetball comes to the emergency department because she has had constant, dull pain in the lateral aspect of the right elbow for the past week. She says the pain radiates to her forearm, and she rates the pain as 5 on a 10-point scale. On physical examination, the lateral elbow is tender to palpation, and tenderness is exacerbated with wrist extension against resistance while the elbow is extended. Grip strength and range of motion are within normal limits. Pulses and sensations are intact. Which of the following findings is most likely on MRI of the arm?
    A. Collateral ligament rupture
    B. Extensor carpi radialis brevis tear
    C. Flexor pronator hyperdensity
    D. Humeral epicondyle calcification
    E. Normal findings

    Answer Key for this chapter begins on p. 135

41. A 41-year-old man who is a housepainter comes to the preoperative clinic for physical examination prior to undergoing surgery for treatment of thoracic outlet syndrome. He has a six-month history of episodic numbness in the medial aspect of the left hand and little finger. He says the symptoms occasionally wake him up at night. Based on these symptoms and the diagnosis, which of the following findings is most likely on physical examination?
   A. Atrophy of the thenar eminence
   B. Bruit with internal arm rotation
   C. Diminished unilateral radial pulse
   D. Edema below the elbow
   E. Symmetrical grip strength

42.

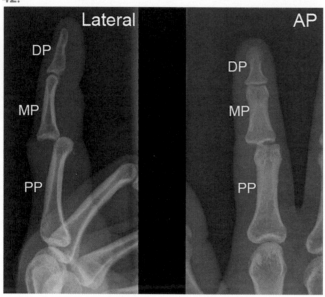

A 15-year-old boy comes to the emergency department because he has had swelling and pain in his index finger since he jammed the finger during basketball practice earlier in the day. X-ray study of the finger is shown. Which of the following is the most appropriate management?

A. Apply a dorsal aluminum foam splint
B. Apply ice and use nonsteroidal anti-inflammatory drugs as needed for pain
C. Buddy tape the index and middle fingers
D. Perform digital blockade and closed reduction
E. Refer for open reduction

43. A 36-year-old woman is brought to the emergency department by ambulance after she sustained an injury to her right arm while having a tonic-clonic seizure 45 minutes ago. Medical history includes a seizure disorder that was diagnosed five years ago, for which she takes phenytoin. The patient is holding her right arm in adduction and internal rotation. On physical examination, the right arm is neurovascularly intact with no obvious ecchymosis, edema, or visible elevation of the clavicle relative to the acromion. No crepitus is noted on palpation of the proximal humerus, clavicle, or medial and lateral epicondyle. Active and passive external rotation of the right arm is limited. Which of the following is the most likely diagnosis?
   A. Acromioclavicular joint separation
   B. Clavicle fracture
   C. Posterior shoulder dislocation
   D. Proximal humerus fracture
   E. Radial head subluxation

44. A 58-year-old woman comes to the office because she has had worsening back pain over the past eight weeks. She says the pain improves with sitting. Medical history includes osteoarthritis in the lumbar spine. Spinal stenosis is suspected. Which of the following findings on history and physical examination is most likely to support this diagnosis?
   A. Intermittent edema of both feet
   B. Pain that worsens with back extension
   C. Radiculopathy of the upper extremities
   D. Recurrent cervical muscle spasms
   E. Recurrent neck pain

Answers

1. **Answer: B** This patient has rotator cuff tendinitis due to repetitive overhead activity as a house painter, increased pain with overhead movement, and the resolution of pain at rest. The lack of atrophy and lack of weakness of the arm indicates that there is no severe tear of the rotator cuff. Therefore, oral nonsteroidal anti-inflammatory drugs (NSAIDs) with physical therapy for one month, option B, is correct because it is the most conservative management.

   Options A, D, and E are not appropriate initial steps in management because they include surgical intervention, which is not appropriate at this stage. Surgical intervention would only be appropriate if the patient had a tear of the rotator cuff. Option C is incorrect because injection of corticosteroids into the subacromial space is too invasive of a procedure at this early stage. If NSAIDs and physical therapy do not relieve this patient's symptoms, then injection of corticosteroids can be considered. **Task**: D2—Clinical Intervention

2. **Answer: A** This patient most likely has a soft-tissue injury to the right knee as a result of a twisting injury. Arthroscopy, option A, is the definitive study for diagnosing soft-tissue injuries of the knee because there is direct visualization of the joint.

   Bone scan, option B, is a nuclear medicine radiological scan best suited to diagnose bone disease and not ligamentous/soft-tissue injuries. CT scan of the knee, option C, is used to evaluate severely injured patients when a fracture is suspected and plain x-ray studies show no abnormalities. Ultrasonography, option D, is incorrect because this study does not provide direct visualization of the bones and soft tissue in the joint. X-ray studies of the knee, option E, do not visualize soft-tissue structures of the knee. **Task**: B—Using Diagnostic and Laboratory Studies

3. **Answer: D** This patient has signs and symptoms of acute vertebral osteomyelitis, and the most common causative organism of this condition is *Staphylococcus aureus*, option D. Acute osteomyelitis evolves over several days to weeks and can progress to a chronic infection. The pathogenesis of osteomyelitis is multifactorial and develops when there is a large inoculation of organisms, the presence of bone damage, and/or the presence of hardware or other foreign material. Factors that may influence the course of infection include the infecting organism, immune status, and bone vascularity.

   Gram-negative bacilli, option A, are related to primary infections of the urinary tract, abdomen, and respiratory tract. Group A *Streptococcus*, option B, is a gram-positive coccus causing an infection involving the respiratory tract and soft tissues. *Pseudomonas aeruginosa*, option C, is a gram-negative bacillus. *Pseudomonas aeruginosa* is the most serious pathogen causing ventilator-associated pneumonia and burn wounds, and it is the most important pathogen in patients with cystic fibrosis. *Streptococcus equisimilis*, option E, is associated primarily with horses, suppurative lymphadenitis, and respiratory infections. **Task**: E—Applying Basic Scientific Concepts

4. **Answer: D** The correct answer is muscle strain, option D, because this patient's pain is across the back without localization and does not extend below the knee, which is typical of a muscle strain. Also, the pain refers to the buttocks, worsens with activity, and is relieved by rest, which are all typical symptoms of muscle strain.

   Ankylosing spondylitis, option A, is incorrect because the onset of this condition is usually during the late teens or early 20s. This type of back pain includes stiffness that is worse in the morning and improves with activity. Lumbar compression fracture, option B, is incorrect because most compression fractures occur at the bottom of the thoracic spine and the first vertebra of the lumbar spine, which would result in pain higher than this patient describes. Also, this condition is more common in older adults with osteoporosis. Lumbar disk herniation (option C), when symptomatic, causes nerve root compression manifested as radicular pain down the back of the leg to the calf or foot. Spinal stenosis, option E, usually affects adults over 50 years of age. The pain associated with this condition worsens with extension. There often are unilateral or bilateral leg symptoms that are worse after walking for several minutes and relieved by sitting (neurogenic claudication). **Task**: A—History Taking and Performing Physical Examination

5. **Answer: A** This patient has sustained a Colles fracture, option A, of the distal radius with dorsal displacement and angulation, as shown in the x-ray studies. A Colles fracture is the most common fracture of the wrist.

   Galeazzi fracture, option B, is a fracture of the distal radius with radioulnar subluxation caused by a direct blow or fall on an outstretched hand. Patients with this type of fracture have edema and tenderness to palpation at the distal ulna and tenderness to palpation over the radioulnar joint. Nightstick fracture, option C, is a fracture of the proximal third of the ulna caused by a direct blow to the arm usually when held above the head in a defensive position to guard against a head injury. Smith fracture, option D, is a fracture of the distal radius with volar angulation. Physical examination shows tenderness to palpation over the distal radius and a characteristic "garden spade" deformity with a volar displacement of the hand. Torus fracture, option E, is also called a buckle fracture. It is a fracture of the distal radius with buckling of the cortex noted in x-ray studies. **Task**: B—Using Diagnostic and Laboratory Studies

6. **Answer: E** If this patient has pain over the medial epicondyle of the humerus when the examiner passively supinates the forearm and extends the elbow and wrist, option E, this is a positive sign of medial epicondylitis. This condition is often called golfer's elbow and is also common in athletes who perform repetitive overhead motion.
   The maneuvers described in options A, B, and D are tests that are performed when evaluating a patient with lateral epicondylitis, or tennis elbow. Applying valgus stress to the elbow while passively flexing the elbow with the forearm held in pronation, option C, is a maneuver that is used to evaluate plica impingement of the elbow. **Task**: A—History Taking and Performing Physical Examination

7. **Answer: A** Anterior talofibular ligament, option A, is correct because this ligament is most commonly injured with a simple inversion mechanism of injury. The mild symptoms and stable physical examination findings also indicate this type of ligament injury.
   Calcaneofibular ligament, option B, is the second most common ligament injury and is associated with joint instability on examination, which this patient does not have. Inferior transverse ligament, option C, is a less common ligament injury and is associated with an additional rotation of the foot or leg. The medial deltoid ligament, option D, is a rare eversion injury that is associated with significant edema and tenderness to palpation on examination. Tibiofibular ligament, option E, is commonly injured with external rotation of the ankle. **Task**: C—Formulating Most Likely Diagnosis

8. **Answer: D** This patient has signs and symptoms of pauciarticular juvenile rheumatoid arthritis (JRA), which accounts for 75% of all pediatric connective tissue diseases. Diagnosis is based on clinical signs and symptoms. In 33% to 50% of patients with JRA, onset is in a single joint, usually the knee. Age of onset is less than 16 years of age. Appropriate first-line therapy includes conventional nonsteroidal anti-inflammatory drugs (NSAIDs), option D. Conventional NSAIDs inhibit both cyclooxygenase (COX)-1 and COX-2. COX-2 produces prostaglandins involved in the inflammatory process.
   Allopurinol, option A, is used to treat patients with gout and not JRA. Hydroxychloroquine, option B, is a disease-modifying antirheumatic drug (DMARD) that has failed to demonstrate efficacy in the treatment of JRA. Adverse reactions to hydroxychloroquine include irreversible retinopathy and hemolysis. Methotrexate, option C, is currently the most frequently used DMARD for patients with JRA, but it is not a first-line treatment. Methotrexate is effective in the treatment of polyarticular and pauciarticular JRA; however, patients with systemic onset may not respond to this therapy. Sulfasalazine, option E, is used in chronic JRA to suppress disease activity. However, severe adverse drug reactions keep this drug from being considered first-line therapy, including hypersensitivity reactions, high fevers, rash, elevated liver transaminases, leukopenia, hypogammaglobulinemia, and gastrointestinal problems. **Task**: D3—Pharmaceutical Therapeutics

9. **Answer: B** This patient has acute compartment syndrome. He has worsening leg pain and swelling after an initial medical evaluation showed normal findings and he was sent home with symptomatic care for the injury and pain. Acute compartment syndrome typically follows an acute injury, and the pain is often described as more severe than what would be expected from the injury. Due to blood and fluid accumulating in the affected muscle area, which is unable to escape because of the tight fascia surrounding the muscle, pressure causes intense pain. Such pressure can lead to irreversible neurovascular damage to the limb. Acute compartment syndrome is a medical emergency that requires prompt surgical intervention to relieve the pressure and restore blood flow by a procedure called fasciotomy, option B.
   Application of a splint, option A, is an appropriate treatment when a limb or joint needs stabilization to promote healing and prevent reinjury. There is no evidence of fracture in this patient. Nonsteroidal anti-inflammatory drugs as needed, option C, will relieve pain and inflammation but will not correct the dangerously increased pressure of the muscle compartment. Physical therapy, option D, is often an appropriate first-line therapy for chronic exertional compartment syndrome but is not appropriate for acute compartment syndrome because its effects are not immediate. Rest, ice, compression, and elevation, option E, is the initial treatment recommended for limb injury with the expectation that the injury will be mitigated and eventually healed. This is not an appropriate intervention for this patient. **Task**: D2—Clinical Intervention

10. **Answer: E** This patient and her parents should be told that she will need to mobilize within 24 hours after surgery, option E. Mobilization one day after surgery is necessary for this patient because early ambulation prevents physical deconditioning, postoperative ileus, and postoperative deep venous thrombosis.

Activity will be limited for six to nine months because she will need to wear a body cast, option A, is incorrect because typically no braces or casts are used postoperatively, and movement is crucial to recovery in patients who have undergone spinal fusion. Bending, lifting, and twisting can be done seven days postoperatively, option B, is not an appropriate recommendation because this patient should avoid these types of activities for up to six months. Telling this patient that she can participate in noncontact sports three months postoperatively, option C, is also incorrect because she needs to wait at least six months before returning to noncontact sports. Option D, she will need to wait six months before returning to routine activities, is also an inappropriate recommendation because a slow return to routine activities should be started immediately to ensure a successful recovery. **Task**: D1—Health Maintenance, Patient Education, and Disease Prevention

11. **Answer: B** This patient has joint pain, arthralgia, a low-grade fever, and a malar rash, which are findings suggestive of systemic lupus erythematosus (SLE). This item tests the examinee's ability to diagnose this condition and then to recall that antinuclear antibody testing, option B, is most likely to determine a diagnosis of SLE.
Antineutrophil cytoplasmic antibody testing, option A, is used in the diagnosis of vasculitis and glomerulonephritis. Cyclic citrullinated peptide antibody test and rheumatoid factor assay, options C and E, are used to support a diagnosis of rheumatoid arthritis. HLA-B27 antibody test, option D, is used to support a diagnosis of ankylosing spondylitis. **Task**: B—Using Diagnostic and Laboratory Studies

12. **Answer: D** This patient has an atraumatic, degenerative rotator cuff tear. The correct answer is physical therapy to strengthen the muscles, option D. This is a first-line intervention and is effective in approximately 70% of cases.
Electrical muscle stimulation, option A, is not first-line therapy, although it has been used for the treatment of weakness in the rotator cuff. Injection of platelet-rich plasma into the shoulder, option B, is not appropriate first-line therapy. However, it has been used for some patients with rotator cuff disease. Intramuscular dry needling, option C, is not appropriate first-line therapy, as it is used to treat weakness in the rotator cuff. Surgical referral, option E, is only indicated if conservative measures such as physical therapy fail. **Task**: D2—Clinical Intervention

13. **Answer: B** This patient is a young male with a history of worsening nontraumatic groin pain, and x-ray findings show avascular necrosis of the femoral head. Avascular necrosis of the femoral head is most commonly associated with chronic corticosteroid use, option B.

The other options are not known to commonly cause avascular necrosis. Chronic use of beta-blockers, option A, can lead to rebound tachycardia if abruptly stopped. Chronic use of opioids, option C, can lead to physical dependence and requires judicious use and careful monitoring. Statins, option D, can cause myalgia and, rarely, rhabdomyolysis. Long-term use of sulfonylureas, option E, is not classically associated with adverse effects. **Task**: D1—Health Maintenance, Patient Education, and Disease Prevention

14. **Answer: A** Cauda equina syndrome is a neurosurgical emergency caused by compression of the cauda equina nerve roots, most commonly due to a large central disk herniation or prolapse. This leads to decreased sensation of the perineum, impaired bladder function, and impaired bowel function due to decreased anal tone (option A).
Fever, option B, with back pain can indicate an infectious cause. Decreased reflexes, not hyperreflexia (option C), may occur in patients with cauda equina syndrome. Pelvic instability, option D, is associated with traumatic injuries to the bony pelvis. A positive straight-leg raising test, option E, is used to evaluate for sciatica and is not useful in the diagnosis of cauda equina syndrome. **Task**: A—History Taking and Performing Physical Examination

15. **Answer: E** The defining feature of a fracture-dislocation, option E, is translational displacement in the axial plane. These injuries are typically severe and cause neurologic damage, which is evident in this patient by the numbness and weakness in his arms and legs.
Burst fracture, option A, is incorrect because the key feature of this injury is posterior vertebral body cortex fracture with retropulsion of bone into the canal and widening of the interpedicular distance. Compression fractures, option B, are characterized by loss of vertebral height anteriorly, which is not evident on this patient's CT scan. Distraction injury, option C, is defined by lengthening of the posterior spine that extends into the middle portion or potentially all the way through the anterior-most portion of the spine. Extension injury, option D, is identified by anterior spinal lengthening and most commonly occurs in the thoracic spine. **Task**: C—Formulating Most Likely Diagnosis

16. **Answer: E** This patient has osteoarthritis, and nonsteroidal anti-inflammatory drugs such as naproxen, option E, are effective treatments for this condition. Their toxicity can limit use, but this patient has no contraindications.
Acetaminophen, option A, is incorrect. Its impact on pain is usually minimal, and it is no longer recommended as first-line therapy for patients with osteoarthritis. Calcium carbonate, option B, is a calcium

 Answer Key for this chapter begins on p. 135

supplement. Patients with osteoarthritis have the same indications for supplementation as those without osteoarthritis. This drug is usually recommended for patients with osteoporosis and not osteoarthritis. Colchicine, option C, is an effective treatment for gouty arthritis. A few studies have shown some improvement in osteoarthritis with this drug, but it is not yet accepted as an appropriate first-line treatment. Methotrexate, option D, is usually the first-line treatment for rheumatoid arthritis and is not used in treating osteoarthritis. **Task:** D3—Pharmaceutical Therapeutics

17. **Answer: D** This patient has torticollis, and physical therapy, option D, is the most appropriate next step in management. Home therapy programs are also used as a treatment adjunct.

Injection of botulinum toxin into the strap muscles of the neck, option A, is performed by a specialist and is only appropriate if the patient fails at-home physical therapy. Prescribing oral corticosteroid therapy, option B, is not an appropriate treatment option for torticollis in an infant. Watchful waiting, option C, is not indicated for torticollis; the earlier the intervention, the better the chances are of the patient recovering from this condition. Referral for surgical correction of the head tilt, option E, is appropriate only if the patient fails physical therapy and botulinum toxin injections. **Task:** D2—Clinical Intervention

18. **Answer: B** Biceps tendonitis, option B, is associated with a positive finding on the physical examination maneuver described in the stem, which is also called the Yergason test. The bicep muscle has two tendons at the shoulder. Tendonitis occurs most frequently in the long head of the biceps tendon. Inflammation is a response from micro tears in the tendon associated with frequent pulling, lifting, or reaching and overuse injuries. The physical examination maneuver is performed with the patient's arm pronated and flexed at the elbow 90 degrees. The patient attempts to supinate the arm against resisted isometric force. Pain localized to the long bicep tendon indicates a positive Yergason test.

Adhesive capsulitis, option A, is more common in female patients from 40 to 50 years of age with a history of diabetes mellitus. X-ray studies typically show no abnormalities. Physical examination shows a limitation of both active and passive glenohumeral motion. Cervical spondylosis, option C, is caused by degenerative changes that start from the intervertebral disks associated with osteophyte formation. Typically, this occurs in middle age with symptoms such as neck pain, stiffness, and neurologic deficits. Glenohumeral osteoarthritis, option D, is associated with acute flares centered in the anterior shoulder, but symptoms are more gradual over the course of several years. Typically, the patient is greater than 60 years of age and has loss of active and passive range of motion. X-ray studies show decreased joint space and sclerosis. Rotator cuff tendonitis, option E, is indicated by a positive Speed test and/or positive Yergason test. However, examination findings include weakness with focal muscle testing and positive drop-arm sign. **Task:** A— History Taking and Performing Physical Examination

19. **Answer: A** This patient has signs and symptoms suggestive of fibromyalgia, option A. The American College of Rheumatology 1990 criteria for the classification of fibromyalgia is a history of widespread pain and in 11 out of 18 tender points. Additional laboratory and imaging studies help rule out other etiologies but are often negative in patients with fibromyalgia. Osteoporosis, option B, is not associated with diffuse pain and is not associated with irritable bowel disease or chronic headaches. Patients with a history of osteoporosis will usually have a loss of height and an increased risk of fracture. Polymyalgia rheumatica, option C, is an inflammatory rheumatic condition characterized clinically by aching and morning stiffness of the shoulders, hip girdle, and neck. It can be associated with giant cell arteritis. Laboratory findings in patients with polymyalgia rheumatica include elevated erythrocyte sedimentation rate (ESR) and C-reactive protein (CRP) level. Rheumatoid arthritis, option D, typically presents with joint pain, edema of the peripheral joints rather than the lower back, and increased morning stiffness. ESR and CRP are typically elevated in patients with rheumatoid arthritis. Patients with systemic lupus erythematosus, option E, present with variable clinical features ranging from constitutional symptoms, myalgia, arthralgia, and skin involvement. The antinuclear antibody test is positive in all patients with systemic lupus erythematosus. **Task:** C—Formulating Most Likely Diagnosis

20. **Answer: E** This patient has Osgood-Schlatter disease, which is a common cause of knee pain in children who are active in sports. This causes pain and edema of the tibial tubercle that increases with the pulling of the tendon with activation of the quadriceps, option E. Patients can develop a persistent bony prominence that lasts into adulthood.

The maneuver described in option A describes a positive Thessaly test, which is consistent with a meniscus tear. A positive anterior drawer test, which is the maneuver described in option B, is consistent with a tear of the anterior cruciate ligament. Edema, tenderness, and erythema over the patella and patellar tendon, option C, is consistent with prepatellar or infrapatellar bursitis. The findings described in option D indicate a positive Godfrey test, which is consistent with a tear of the posterior cruciate ligament. **Task:** A—History Taking and Performing Physical Examination

21. **Answer: A** Paget disease causes disordered bone remodeling and results in bone of poor quality that is susceptible to deformation and fracture. The ongoing bone remodeling causes an elevation in serum alkaline phosphatase, option A, which is the correct answer.
An elevated ammonia level, option B, is indicative of advanced liver disease. Elevation in the blood urea nitrogen level, option C, is a likely laboratory finding in patients with kidney disease. Troponin I levels that are elevated, option D, is indicative of myocardial ischemia. Uric acid levels, option E, are increased in patients who have gout. **Task**: B—Using Diagnostic and Laboratory Studies

22. **Answer: A** This patient has carpal tunnel syndrome (CTS). The correct answer is option A, inability to grasp or pinch objects as she did in the past. The indications for surgery are (1) thenar muscle weakness or atrophy and (2) symptoms persisting for more than three months despite conservative treatment. The inability to grip, grasp, or pinch due to weakness of the thenar muscles is a strong indicator of severe CTS. The inability to identify different textures with the hand, option B, is incorrect. The inability to identify textures by rubbing them between the thumb and index finger may occur with CTS but is not an indication for surgery without further conservative treatment. Pain that radiates proximally to the forearm, option C, is a common finding with CTS but not an indication for surgery without conservative treatment. Pain with making a fist, option D, and tingling sensation in the palm, option E, are incorrect. Both may occur in patients with CTS but are not indicators for surgery without further conservative treatment. **Task**: D2—Clinical Intervention

23. **Answer: B** If the vertical forces of this patient's fall were significant enough to cause a calcaneal fracture, x-ray studies of the thoracic and lumbar spine, option B, should also be obtained. With calcaneal fractures resulting from a fall from an elevated height, there is a high incidence of associated axial spine fractures, such as the thoracic and lumbar spine.
Cervical spine and scapula injuries, option A, are not commonly associated with this mechanism of injury. Sacral spine and pelvis injuries, option C, may occur; however, they are less likely based on the mechanism of injury. Injury to the femur and hip or the tibia and fibula, options D and E, are less likely as there is no pain or tenderness to palpation of the leg or hip. **Task**: E—Applying Basic Scientific Concepts

24. **Answer: C** This patient is suspected of having ankylosing spondylitis. HLA-B27 antigen test, option C, is correct because the inflammatory aspect of this patient's presentation places ankylosing spondylitis high in the differential diagnosis. In the primary care

setting, this diagnosis can be found in up to 16% of patients between 18 and 45 years of age who have had back pain for more than three months. Ninety percent of patients with ankylosing spondylosis are positive for HLA-B27.
CT scan of the lumbar spine, option A, is not indicated in the evaluation of this patient. An MRI is more appropriate because of its ability to identify earlier changes. Erythrocyte sedimentation rate, option B, is a nonspecific inflammatory marker. Indium white blood cell scan, option D, is used for diagnosing infections. Rheumatoid factor assay, option E, is used to evaluate the symptoms of rheumatoid arthritis, of which this patient does not have. **Task**: B—Using Diagnostic and Laboratory Studies

25. **Answer: E** This patient is having an acute episode of gout. The correct answer is uric acid, option E. A single uric acid determination during an episode of acute gout is elevated in approximately 75% of cases.
An elevation in antinuclear antibody level, option A, is incorrect. This laboratory value is used to evaluate people with autoimmune diseases such as systemic lupus erythematosus. It is not helpful in the diagnosis of gout. An elevated serum phosphate level, option B, most often indicates the presence of a kidney disorder and not gout. Serum procalcitonin levels, option C, are significantly lower in patients with acute gout than in patients with a bacterial infection such as cellulitis. Rheumatoid factor, option D, is helpful in diagnosing rheumatoid arthritis but is not helpful in diagnosing gout. **Task**: B—Using Diagnostic and Laboratory Studies

26. **Answer: B** Diffuse arthritis, option B, is correct because arthralgia, myalgia, and arthritis are present in up to 64% of patients with polyarteritis nodosa.
Option A, chronic splenomegaly, and option E, recurrent uveitis, are incorrect because this disorder does not commonly affect the spleen or eye. Mastoid infections, option C, is incorrect because the mastoid system is not affected by polyarteritis nodosa. Pulmonary congestion, option D, is incorrect because polyarteritis nodosa vasculitis does not involve the pulmonary or bronchial arteries. The pulmonary system is one of the only major systems not affected by this condition. **Task**: A—History Taking and Performing Physical Examination

27. **Answer: E** Rheumatology, option E, is correct because this patient has the common symptoms of Sjögren syndrome. A rheumatologist is indicated for this autoimmune disease, which is most common in middle-aged females with impaired function of the salivary and lacrimal glands. Up to two-thirds of patients with primary Sjögren syndrome present with bilateral enlargement of the salivary glands. Poor coping with a

stressful life event prior to the onset of symptoms has also been found to be common in patients with this condition.

This patient has an autoimmune disease, therefore consultation with specialists in allergy, endocrinology, ophthalmology, and otolaryngology (options A through D) are incorrect because the rheumatologist is best suited to evaluate an autoimmune disease. **Task**: D2—Clinical Intervention

28. **Answer: B** This patient has Brown-Séquard syndrome (option B), or hemisection of the spinal cord, which usually results from penetrating trauma but may also be seen after lateral mass fractures of the cervical spine. Patients with this lesion have ipsilateral loss of position and vibration sense and motor paralysis, but they also have contralateral loss of pain and temperature sensation distal to the level of injury.

Anterior cord syndrome, option A, is characterized by paralysis and hypoalgesia below the level of injury, with preservation of posterior column functions including position, touch, and vibratory sensations. Cauda equina syndrome, option C, is characterized by perineal or bilateral leg pain, bowel or bladder dysfunction, perianal anesthesia, diminished rectal sphincter tone, and lower extremity weakness. Central cord syndrome, option D, is characterized by loss of motion and sensation in both of the arms and hands. Horner syndrome, option E, results from damage to the cervical sympathetic chain and is characterized by ipsilateral ptosis, miosis, and anhidrosis. **Task**: A—History Taking and Performing Physical Examination

29. **Answer: B** This patient is suspected of having a slipped capital femoral epiphysis (SCFE) based on her symptoms and the findings on physical examination. X-ray studies of the hip are most likely to show displacement of the right femoral head, option B.

The crossover sign, option A, is noted in anteroposterior x-ray studies when the anterior acetabular wall lies anterior to the posterior acetabular wall in the superior portion of the joint. This sign can be found in patients with femoroacetabular impingement. Flattening of the femoral head epiphysis, option C, also known as coxa plana, is a finding associated with many skeletal disorders but not with SCFE. Ossification of the proximal femoral epiphysis, option D, is a late finding in patients with developmental dysplasia of the hip. A thin sclerotic line that crosses the femoral neck, option E, also called the "sagging rope" sign, is seen in Legg-Calvé-Perthes disease. **Task**: B—Using Diagnostic and Laboratory Studies

30. **Answer: D** This patient has recurrent septic and aseptic bursitis, and the most appropriate next step is referral to an orthopedic surgeon for surgical removal of the bursa, option D.

The patient's current presentation does not describe signs of an infection, which would include erythema, edema, tenderness, and warmth, which makes administration of intravenous antibiotics, option A, incorrect. Recommending the patient refrain from bodybuilding, option B, is not appropriate especially since he has no desire to quit. The patient has failed physical therapy in the past; therefore, option C is incorrect. Repeat injection of corticosteroids, option E, is incorrect because this therapy failed in the past as well. **Task**: D2—Clinical Intervention

31. **Answer: E** This patient has signs and symptoms of scleroderma, option E. This condition consists of fibrosis of the face, neck, and distal extremities. A history of Raynaud phenomenon is typically present in patients with scleroderma along with esophageal motility disorder, sclerodactyly, and telangiectasias.

Dyshidrotic eczema, option A, presents with fluid-filled vesicles on the palms and fingers and is associated with intense itching. Folliculitis, option B, presents with small pustules and papules with itching in areas where hair grows. Hand, foot, and mouth disease, option C, is a self-limited viral illness that most commonly affects children. The rash is present on the palms of the hands, feet, and around the mouth. Lichen simplex chronicus, option D, consists of well-circumscribed areas of thickened skin due to recurrent friction (i.e., scratching or rubbing) of the skin. **Task**: A—History Taking and Performing Physical Examination

32. **Answer: A** Bisphosphonates are recommended for initial pharmacotherapeutic treatment in a patient with osteoporosis after lifestyle modification and supplementation with vitamin D and calcium. Bisphosphonates are recommended for 5 to 10 years with reevaluation by DEXA scan every two years or based on fracture history.

Bisphosphonates promote bone formation by inhibiting the activity of osteoclasts, option A. Options B, C, and E are incorrect because drugs of the bisphosphonate class have no activity on the resorption of calcium or vitamin D from the renal tubules and gastrointestinal tract, respectively, and they have no activity on the release of parathyroid hormone. Note that parathyroid hormone increases osteoclastic activity, thereby promoting calcium and phosphate release from bone. Also, decreasing vitamin D and calcium levels will worsen the bone loss seen in patients with osteoporosis. While increased renal calcitriol secretion will increase calcium absorption from the gastrointestinal tract and thus indirectly decrease bone loss, its release from the kidneys (option D) is not influenced by the administration of bisphosphonate medications. **Task**: E—Applying Basic Scientific Concepts

33. **Answer: A** This patient has developmental dysplasia of the hip based on the positive findings on the Barlow test, option A, in which the femoral head dislocates from the acetabulum when the hip is adducted and gentle force is applied to the knee.

    The flexion, adduction, and internal rotation (FADIR) test, option B, is performed by bringing the hip into maximal FADIR and is the most sensitive indicator of femoroacetabular impingement, a condition in which extra bone grows along the bones that form the hip joint. After performing the Barlow test, the femoral head needs to be placed back into the acetabulum. If there is a clunk heard as the femoral head is put back into place, this is considered a positive Ortolani test, option C. The Thomas test, option D, is used to measure the flexibility of the hip flexors and is done with the patient lying down. This test is performed on a patient who is at an age where they can follow instructions. The Trendelenburg test, option E, can be done to assess developmental dysplasia of the hip in a patient who can stand on their own. **Task:** A—History Taking and Performing Physical Examination

34. **Answer: E** This patient has a ganglion cyst, and observation, option E, is the correct answer. A ganglion cyst is a benign mass that primarily causes a cosmetic deformity. Conservative management is the first-line treatment unless there is evidence of neurovascular compromise.

    Arthroscopic decompression of the cyst, option A, is only recommended if there is significant vascular compromise. Closed rupture of the cyst with a heavy object, option B, is incorrect because of possible complications such as a distal radial fracture or injury to surrounding structures. Injection of a sclerosing agent into the cyst, option C, is not considered primary treatment because of a reported failure rate of over 90%. Open excision of the cyst, option D, is recommended only if the ganglion cyst causes paresthesia, muscle weakness, or vascular compromise. **Task:** D2—Clinical Intervention

35. **Answer: D** This patient has a Dowager hump, a type of hyperkyphosis, and this condition is most commonly related to postmenopausal osteoporosis, option D.

    Cirrhosis, option A, can cause characteristic skin changes such as jaundice and spider angiomas, but it is not associated with kyphosis. Physical findings in a patient with emphysema, option B, include barrel chest appearance and not hyperkyphosis. Gout, option C, can cause tophaceous joint depositions but is not associated with a Dowager hump. Rheumatoid arthritis, option E, can cause the development of rheumatoid nodules but is not associated with kyphosis. **Task:** A—History Taking and Performing Physical Examination

36. **Answer: B** Septic arthritis is most commonly caused by a bacterial infection spread by hematogenous seeding. *Staphylococcus aureus* is the most common bacterial cause. This is more likely to occur in patients with a history of arthritis and can cause joint destruction if not treated appropriately with joint drainage and antibiotic therapy. The definitive diagnosis comes from aspiration, analysis, and culture of synovial fluid from the affected joint, option B.

    Blood culture, ultrasonography of the knee, and x-ray study of the knee (options A, D, and E) are all part of the workup of septic arthritis; however, they will not definitively confirm the diagnosis. C-reactive protein (CRP), option C, is an acute phase reactant that will likely be elevated in this patient. However, an elevated CRP will not differentiate an infectious versus a noninfectious cause of inflammation, thus it will not help to determine the diagnosis. **Task:** B—Using Diagnostic and Laboratory Studies

37. **Answer: A** Acute sciatica, option A, refers to the neuralgia following the sciatic nerve down the leg along its distribution. Sciatica usually occurs unilaterally. Pain is described as sharp or aching, and it typically radiates from the buttock down the leg posteriorly, laterally, or anteriorly depending on the level of nerve root compression. Sciatica is usually caused by disk herniation at the L4 to L5 and L5 to S1 level, less commonly at the L3 to L4 level.

    Cauda equina syndrome, option B, is characterized by perineal or bilateral leg pain, bowel or bladder dysfunction, perianal anesthesia, diminished rectal sphincter tone, and lower extremity weakness. Lumbosacral strain, option C, includes lower back pain that is usually unilateral and tender to palpation without radiating sharp pain. Scoliosis, option D, is a curvature of the spine resulting in lower back pain and muscle spasms, but it is not characterized by unilateral neuralgia. Spinal fracture, option E, is unlikely since this patient has no history of trauma or medical conditions that would lead to a fracture. **Task:** A—History Taking and Performing Physical Examination

38. **Answer: B** This patient has de Quervain tenosynovitis most likely caused by the repetitive movement of feeding her child with a spoon. De Quervain tenosynovitis is the most common tenosynovitis affecting the dorsal tendons of the wrist. It usually occurs between 30 and 50 years of age with a female to male ratio of 10:1. De Quervain tenosynovitis is related to an inflammation of the tendon sheath of the extensor pollicis brevis and abductor pollicis longus. Finkelstein test, option B, is performed with the hand in a fist, the thumb tucked under the fingers, and the hand in passive ulnar deviation. Intense pain in the area of the radial styloid process constitutes a positive result.

    Answer Key for this chapter begins on p. 135

The empty can test, option A is used to assess for injury to the supraspinatus muscle or tendon. It is performed by having the patient place a straight arm in about 90 degrees of abduction and 30 degrees of forward flexion, and then internally rotating the arm completely (i.e., thumb pointing down). The patient then resists the clinician's attempts to depress the arm. The Phalen test, option C, is positive in a patient with carpal tunnel injury. The Phalen maneuver is performed by placing the backs of the hands against each other to provide hyperflexion of the wrist; the elbows remain flexed. A positive Phalen sign is defined as pain and/or paresthesia in the median-innervated fingers with one minute of wrist flexion. The Speed test, option D, is used to assess biceps tendon instability or tendonitis. It is considered positive if pain is reported in the bicipital groove with weakness. A speed test is performed with the patient's arm extended in full supination with the shoulder flexed. In this position, the patient is instructed to elevate the arm against a resisted isometric force. The Yergason test, option E, is used to evaluate for biceps tendonitis. This test is performed with the patient's arm pronated and flexed at the elbow to 90 degrees. The patient then attempts to supinate the arm against a resisted isometric force. Pain localized to the long biceps tendon indicates a positive test. **Task**: A—History Taking and Performing Physical Examination

39. **Answer: A** This patient has a hip fracture based on risk factors (age, gender, history of osteoporosis), mechanism of injury, physical examination findings, and findings on an x-ray study. The correct answer is arthroplasty, option A, which is the most appropriate treatment for a hip fracture in an elderly patient.
A hip spica cast, option B, is used most commonly in children who undergo surgery for hip dysplasia. Open reduction and internal fixation, option C, is a surgical option reserved for younger patients. Pelvic binding, option D, is used to stabilize an open-book pelvic fracture, which is not evident in the x-ray study provided. Traction splinting, option E, is generally used to treat fractures of the femoral shaft. **Task**: D2—Clinical Intervention

40. **Answer: E** Normal findings, option E, is correct because this is the most common finding on MRI of the arm when evaluating a patient with suspected lateral epicondylitis.
Collateral ligament rupture, option A, is incorrect because this is the most common finding on imaging of an elbow dislocation. Extensor carpi radialis brevis tear, option B, is incorrect. The extensor carpi radialis brevis is the most common site of injury for this presentation, but such a tear would not be noted on MRI. Option C, flexor-pronator hyperdensity, is incorrect because the common flexor-pronator is involved in

medial epicondylitis and this presentation is of lateral epicondylitis. Humeral epicondyle calcification, option D, is incorrect because this finding is a rare (<10%) soft-tissue finding on MRI. **Task**: B—Using Diagnostic and Laboratory Studies

41. **Answer: E** Option E, symmetrical grip strength, is correct because motor deficits are indicative of chronic severe compression. This patient presents with only periodic positional nerve compression over a six-month period, so grip strength is likely to be symmetrical.
Atrophy of the thenar eminence, option A, is incorrect because the thenar eminence is at the base of the thumb and is not in the ulnar nerve distribution where this patient has symptoms. Bruit with internal arm rotation, option B, is incorrect because if the patient has arterial thoracic outlet syndrome, arm abduction will elicit a subclavian bruit. Diminished unilateral radial pulse, option C, is incorrect because this is a sign of arterial thoracic outlet syndrome. If present, it would only be found with arm abduction with the head rotated to the contralateral side. This patient is presenting with neural symptoms. Edema below the elbow, option D, is incorrect because unilateral edema is associated with thoracic outlet syndrome due to venous compression. **Task**: A—History Taking and Performing Physical Examination

42. **Answer: D** This patient has a type II dorsal dislocation of the proximal interphalangeal (PIP) joint. The correct answer is D, perform digital blockade and closed reduction. Appropriate initial management includes closed reduction after administering a digital block and then splinting the finger.
Apply a dorsal aluminum foam splint, option A, should only be done after closed reduction has been performed successfully. Apply ice and use nonsteroidal anti-inflammatory drugs as needed for pain, option B, may be used at home after reduction of the joint has occurred. Buddy tape the index and middle fingers, option C, is incorrect because the joint first needs to be reduced. Following reduction, buddy taping is not recommended as it does not provide the stability to retain the stability of the joint. Refer for open reduction, option E, is not indicated as initial management of a closed dislocation of the PIP joint. **Task**: D2—Clinical Intervention

43. **Answer: C** This patient has sustained a posterior shoulder dislocation, option C. Posterior dislocations often occur following electrocution or seizure. Patients will present with the arm held in adduction and internally rotated with the inability to externally rotate the affected extremity actively or passively. In standard anteroposterior (AP) x-ray views, the humerus can

appear to be reduced; however, adding axillary views will confirm the diagnosis.

An acromioclavicular joint separation, option A, is associated with tenderness and edema over the acromioclavicular joint. On physical examination, there is a visible elevation of the clavicle relative to the acromion. Clavicle fracture, option B, is incorrect. Similar to proximal humeral fractures, clavicle fractures will result in limited range of motion with associated edema, ecchymosis, and pain in the clavicular area. Additionally, physical examination may show crepitation and pain on palpation of the fracture site. Proximal humeral fractures, option D, result in significant edema of the upper arm, bruising, and pain with range of motion of the shoulder. AP and lateral x-ray studies of the shoulder will confirm the presence of a fracture. Patients with a radial head subluxation, option E, present with the affected arm in extension and pronation rather than in adduction and internal rotation, as seen with this patient. This condition typically occurs in children between the ages of six months and five years of age. **Task**: A—History Taking and Performing Physical Examination

44. **Answer: B** A common finding in patients with spinal stenosis is pain that worsens with the extension of the back, option B.

Intermittent edema of both feet, option A, is often associated with hypertension or cardiac conditions. Radiculopathy of the upper extremities, option C, is often associated with trauma. Recurrent cervical muscle spasms and recurrent neck pain, options D and E, may be due to chronic injury or the patient's lifestyle (exercise and sleeping patterns). **Task**: A—History Taking and Performing Physical Examination

BIBLIOGRAPHY

Agabegi, S. S., & Agabegi, E. D. (2012). *Step-up to medicine* (3rd ed.). Philadelphia, PA: Lippincott Williams and Wilkins.

American Academy of Orthopedic Surgeons. (2009). *Compartment syndrome*.

Argoff, C., & McCleane, G. (2009). *Pain management secrets* (3rd ed.). Philadelphia, PA: Mosby Inc.

Binder, A. I. (2007). Cervical spondylosis and neck pain. *BMJ, 334*(7592), 527-531.

Brennan, D. What is juvenile rheumatoid arthritis? *WebMD Medical Reference*. Published May 19, 2019.

Carrascosa, M. F., Fernández-Ayala, M., Salcines-Caviedes, J. R., & Fernández-Sampedro, M. (2017). Acute osteomyelitis: It is still here. *Journal of Global Infectious Diseases, 9*(3), 126-127.

Chumley, H. S. Ankylosing spondylitis. In R. P. Usatine, M. A. Smith, E. J. Mayeaux, Jr., & H. S. Chumley (Eds.), *The color atlas and synopsis of family medicine* (3th ed.). McGraw-Hill.

Domino, F. J., Baldor, R. A., Golding, J., & Stephens, M. B. (2019). *The 5-minute clinical consult 2020*. Lippincott Williams & Wilkins.

Ebraheim, N. A., Thomas, B. J., Fu, F. H., Muller, B., Vyas, D., Niesen, M., et al. (2019). Orthopedic surgery. In F. Brunicardi, D. K. Andersen, T. R. Billiar, D. L. Dunn, L. S. Kao, & J. G. Hunter (Eds.), *Schwartz's principles of surgery* (11th ed.). McGraw-Hill.

Epocrates [Online]. (2013). San Francisco, CA: Epocrates, Inc. http://www.epocrates.com. Updated continuously.

Fitzgerald, P. A. (2022). Osteoporosis. In M. A. Papadakis, S. J. McPhee, M. W. Rabow, & K. R. McQuaid (Eds.), *Current medical diagnosis & treatment 2022*. McGraw Hill.

Franko, O. I. (2020). *Dislocation reduction of the PIP and DIP joints*. https://www.clinicalkey.com/#!/content/medical_procedure/19-s2.0-mp_EM-067. Elsevier.

Gilek-Seibert, K. (2021). Systemic lupus erythematosus. In F. Ferri (Ed.), *Ferri's clinical advisor 2021* (pp. 1332-1337.e3). Elsevier, Inc.

Goldenberg, D. L., & Sexton, D. J. (2020). Septic arthritis in adults. In T. Post (Ed.). *UpToDate*.

Hart, R. G., Rittenberry, T. J., & Uehara, D. T. (1999). *Handbook of orthopedic emergencies*. Lippincott- Raven Publishers.

Ilowite, N. T. (2002). Current treatment of juvenile rheumatoid arthritis. *Pediatrics, 109*(1), 109-115.

Kaji, A. H., & Hockberger, R. S. Spinal injuries. In Rosen's emergency medicine: Concepts and clinical practice (Chapter 36, pp. 345-371.e2).

Kalb, R. L., & Fowler, G. C. Fracture care. In Pfenninger and Fowler's procedures for primary care (Chapter 178, pp. 1193-1211).

Kienstra, A. J., & Macias, C. G. (2020). Osgood-Schlatter disease (tibial tuberosity avulsion). In T. Post (Ed.). *UpToDate*.

Knee injury (other than dislocation or fracture) Elsevier Point of Care. Updated July 29, 2020. Elsevier.

Kolmodin, J., & Gurd, D. Scoliosis. In R. P. Usatine, C. Sabella, M. Smith, E. J. Mayeaux, Jr. H. S. Chumley, & E. Appachi (Eds.), *The color atlas of pediatrics*. McGraw-Hill.

Langford, C. A., & Fauci, A. S. The vasculitis syndromes. In J. Jameson, A. S. Fauci, D. L. Kasper, S. L. Hauser, D. L. Longo, & J. Loscalzo (Eds.), *Harrison's principles of internal medicine* (20th ed.), McGraw-Hill.

Long, B., Koyfman, A., & Gottlieb, M. (2020). Evaluation and management of cauda equina syndrome in the emergency department. *American Journal of Emergency Medicine, 38*(1), 143-148.

Luke, A., & Ma, C. Ankle injuries. In M. A. Papadakis, S. J. McPhee, & M. W. Rabow (Eds.), *Current medical diagnosis & treatment 2021*. McGraw-Hill.

Magee, D. J. (2014). *Orthopedic physical assessment* (Chapter 6, pp. 388-428).

Magee, D. J. (2014). Thoracic (dorsal) spine. *Orthopedic physical assessment* (pp. 508-549) (6th ed.). Philadelphia, PA: Elsevier, Inc.

Magee, D. J. (2014). *Orthopedic physical assessment* (6th ed., Chapter 9). Elsevier.

McMahon, P. J., Kaplan, L. D., & Popkin, C. A. (2014). Chapter 3: Sports medicine. In H. B. Skinner & P. J. McMahon (Eds.), *Current diagnosis & treatment in orthopedics* (5th ed.). McGraw-Hill.

Moutsopoulos, H. M. Sjögren's syndrome. In J. Jameson, A. S. Fauci, D. L. Kasper, S. L. Hauser, D. L. Longo, & J. Loscalzo (Eds.), *Harrison's principles of internal medicine* (20th ed.), McGraw-Hill.

Pallin, D. J. (2018). Knee and lower leg. In R. M. Walls (Ed.), *Rosen's emergency medicine: Concepts and clinical practice* (9th ed., pp. 614-633.e2). Elsevier.

Papadakis, M. A., & McPhee, S. J. (2020). *Current medical diagnosis & treatment 2020*. McGraw-Hill.

Rhodes, J. T., Tagawa, A., Niswander, C., Coomer, W., Erickson, M. A., & De, S. Orthopedics. (2020). In W. W. Hay Jr., M. J. Levin, M. J. Abzug, & M. Bunik (Eds.), *Current diagnosis & treatment: Pediatrics* (25th ed.). McGraw-Hill.

Roof, A., Jinguji, T., White, K., Goldberg, M., & Imrie, M. (2015). Developmental dysplasia of the hip. In D. K. Stevenson, R. S. Cohen, & P. Sunshine (Eds.), *Neonatology: Clinical practice and procedures*. McGraw-Hill.

Rossignol, M. (1998). *De Quervain's tenosynovitis*, Editions MultiMondes. *ProQuest Ebook Central*.

Sharma, G., & Shah, S. K. Arteries. (2020). In G. M. Doherty (Ed.), *Current diagnosis & treatment: Surgery* (15th ed.), McGraw-Hill.

Shirakbari, A., & Feldmeier, M. Orthopaedics: Non-traumatic disorders. (2014). In C. Stone, R. L. Humphries, D. Drigalla, & M. Stephan (Eds.), *CURRENT diagnosis & treatment: Pediatric emergency medicine*. McGraw-Hill.

Silverstein, J., Moeller, J., & Hutchinson, M. (2016). Common issues in orthopedics. In R. Rakel & D. Rakel (Eds.), *Textbook of family medicine* (9th ed., pp. 648-683.e2). Elsevier, Inc.

Simons, S. M., & Dixon, J. B. (2020). *Physical examination of the shoulder*. UpToDate.

Simons, S. M., & Dixon, J. B. *Biceps tendinopathy and tendon rupture*. UpToDate.

Stefans, V. A. (2019). History and physical examination of the pediatric rehabilitation patient. In R. Mitra (Ed.), *Principles of rehabilitation medicine*. McGraw-Hill.

Tubbs, R. J., Savitt, D. L., & Suner, S. (2016). Extremity conditions. In K. J. Knoop, L. B. Stack, A. B. Storrow, & R. Thurman (Eds.), *The Atlas of emergency medicine* (4th ed.). McGraw-Hill.

Tucci, J. (2021). Paget disease of bone. In F. Ferri (Ed.), *Ferri's clinical advisor 2021* (pp. 1030-1030.e3). Elsevier, Inc.

Weinlein, J. (2017). Fractures and dislocations of the hip. In F. Azar, J. Beaty, & S. Canale (Eds.), *Campbell's operative orthopedics* (13th ed., pp. 2817-2864.e9). Elsevier, Inc.

Wessels, M. R. *Group C and group G streptococcal infection*. Literature review current through: October 2020. This topic last updated: August 18, 2020.

Williams, K. D. *Campbell's operative orthopaedics* (14th ed., Chapter 41, pp. 1756-1823). Elsevier.

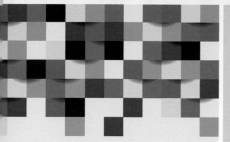

CHAPTER 10
Neurologic System

Questions

1. A 20-year-old woman comes to the clinic because she has had infrequent episodes of a sudden, brief loss of consciousness during the past three years. She says she has recovered completely after each episode without intervention. Medical history is otherwise unremarkable. Family medical history includes similar episodes in her mother. Physical examination shows no abnormalities. Based on this information, which of the following is the most common etiology of the syncopal episodes in this patient?
   A. Cardiac
   B. Glycemic
   C. Hypoxic
   D. Neural
   E. Orthostatic

2. A 46-year-old man comes to the office because he has had recurrent episodes of unilateral headache lasting for 20 minutes associated with redness and tearing of the ipsilateral eye during the past three months. He describes the pain as sharp and stabbing. Vital signs are within normal limits. Neurologic examination shows no focal deficits. Which of the following is the most likely diagnosis?
   A. Acute frontal sinusitis
   B. Cluster headache
   C. Meningioma
   D. Migraine
   E. Tension headache

3. A 19-year-old man is admitted to the ICU after being struck by a car while riding his motorcycle. Currently, the patient is comatose, on mechanical ventilation, and being monitored by neurology and neurosurgical services. When a painful stimulus is applied by pressing strongly on the supraorbital ridges during physical examination, the patient adducts the shoulders, flexes the elbows, wrists, and fingers, and internally rotates the legs and ankles. This reflex is characteristic of a lesion in which of the following areas of the central nervous system?

   A. Above the brainstem
   B. Cerebellum
   C. Midbrain
   D. Pontine and medullary regions
   E. Upper cervical spinal cord

4. A 78-year-old woman with a history of aortic stenosis is admitted to the hospital to undergo aortic valve replacement. The medical team is concerned about the patient's risk for development of delirium while hospitalized because she has a history of mild cognitive impairment and delirium during a previous hospitalization. Which of the following measures is most likely to decrease the risk of delirium developing in this patient?
   A. Attaching a device to the patient that alerts staff when she changes position
   B. Encouraging early mobility and physical activity
   C. Not allowing any family members to be present
   D. Using benzodiazepine sleep aids
   E. Using blackout curtains to disrupt circadian sleep patterns

5. A 17-year-old girl is brought to the emergency department after she fell and hit her head during a volleyball game one hour ago. At the time of the incident, she lost consciousness for approximately two minutes and was unable to continue playing for the remainder of the game. Currently, she says she has a headache. The patient identifies her parents and can state her full name and date of birth; however, she does not remember hitting her head or playing the volleyball game. Concussion is suspected, and the parents are advised that the patient may have headaches, nausea, irritability, clumsiness, and visual disturbances during the next few days to weeks. Prior to discharging the patient, which of the following studies is most appropriate to rule out intracranial bleeding?
   A. Bone scan of the head
   B. CT scan of the head
   C. Electroencephalography
   D. MRI of the brain
   E. X-ray study of the skull

6. A 31-year-old man comes to the office because he has had numbness, paresthesia, and pain in the thumb, index, and long fingers of both hands for the past six months. He says the symptoms are worse at night and after strenuous activity. The patient has been taking nonsteroidal anti-inflammatory drugs for several weeks, but they have not provided relief. Which of the following physical examination maneuvers is most likely to confirm a diagnosis?
   A. Brachioradialis reflex testing
   B. Handgrip test
   C. Neer test
   D. Phalen test
   E. Range of motion testing of the wrist

7. A 14-year-old girl is brought to the neurology clinic by her mother for follow-up of tonic-clonic seizure disorder. The seizures have been well controlled with anticonvulsant medication. The mother says that the patient's gums have been painful and bleeding more than usual. On physical examination, gingival hyperplasia is noted. No other abnormalities are noted. Which of the following anticonvulsant medications is this patient most likely taking?
   A. Gabapentin
   B. Lacosamide
   C. Levetiracetam
   D. Oxcarbazepine
   E. Phenytoin

8. A 64-year-old man comes to the clinic for routine follow-up examination. He says he has new onset of a slight decrease in sensation in his feet. He has a 20-year history of type 2 diabetes mellitus treated with metformin. Physical examination shows intact skin and sensation. Pedal pulses are 2+ and symmetrical. Which of the following is the most appropriate next step for early detection and prevention of future complications of this patient's condition?
   A. Arterial Doppler ultrasonography and use of off-loading shoe inserts
   B. Doppler waveforms and custom-molded shoes
   C. Home foot inspections and hemoglobin A_{1c} target of <7.5%
   D. Monofilament examinations and oral nortriptyline therapy
   E. Nerve conduction studies and hemoglobin A_{1c} target of <6.5%

9. A 28-year-old woman is brought to the office by her mother because she had sudden onset of blurry vision in her right eye as well as pain when moving the eye 30 minutes ago. She says she could not see the red color on the stop signs and stop light on her way to the office. The patient also has had weakness on walking during the past several months. She says she used to be able to walk two miles to her job without any issues; now after walking less than a few blocks, she notices that her right leg drags behind her. The weakness starts to resolve after 15 to 30 minutes of rest and completely resolves after an hour. MRI shows demyelinating lesions in the central nervous system. Results of lumbar puncture are positive for oligoclonal bands of IgG. Electromyography shows no abnormalities. Which of the following is the most likely diagnosis?
   A. Amyotrophic lateral sclerosis
   B. Duchenne muscular dystrophy
   C. Fibromyalgia
   D. Guillain-Barré syndrome
   E. Multiple sclerosis

10. A 50-year-old woman comes to the primary care clinic for follow-up to review the results of an outpatient CT scan of the head that was obtained after she was involved in a motor vehicle collision. Medical history shows neurofibromatosis type 2 and multiple cranial imaging studies for a variety of unrelated reasons. Vital signs are within normal limits. Physical examination shows no abnormalities, and neurologic examination shows no focal deficits. The CT scan report indicates a small densely enhanced lesion that is extra-axial and originates from the dura. Once a metastatic process has been excluded, which of the following is the most likely diagnosis?
   A. Ganglioglioma
   B. Glioblastoma
   C. Lymphoma
   D. Meningioma
   E. Xanthoastrocytoma

11. A 52-year-old woman comes to the office because she has had tremor in her hands bilaterally for the past six months. She has not had issues with handwriting, and she has no history of falls or rigidity. The patient says that caffeine tends to worsen the tremor. Medical history includes no chronic disease conditions. Vital signs are within normal limits. Physical examination shows fine tremor in both hands at rest. No noticeable bradykinesia or gait disorder with ambulation is noted. Which of the following medications is the most appropriate initial therapy?
   A. Carbidopa/levodopa
   B. Gabapentin
   C. Methylphenidate
   D. Propranolol
   E. Ropinirole

12. A 38-year-old man comes to the office because he has had abnormal jerking movements and worsening behavioral outbursts over the past several months. Family medical history includes development of similar symptoms in multiple family members in their upper 30s. Vital signs are within normal limits. Mini Mental Status Examination score is 20/30. The patient is alert but answers questions slowly and incompletely with halting speech. During the physical examination, verbal outbursts and repeated jerking movements of the arms and head are noted. The remainder of the examination shows no abnormalities. Which of the following is the most likely diagnosis?
    A. Alzheimer dementia
    B. Huntington disease
    C. Lyme disease
    D. Multiple sclerosis
    E. Parkinson disease

13. A 54-year-old man comes to the clinic for routine physical examination. He says he is concerned about having a spontaneous intracranial hemorrhage similar to what his friend recently experienced. Medical history includes hypertension and type 2 diabetes mellitus, for which he takes metoprolol and metformin, respectively. He has a 34-year history of cigarette smoking. Body mass index is 33 kg/m² (N = 18.5–24.9 kg/m²). Which of the following is the most appropriate advice to give the patient to help decrease his risk of intracranial hemorrhage?
    A. Control blood pressure
    B. Initiate an aerobic exercise routine
    C. Maintain an ideal body weight
    D. Manage diabetes mellitus
    E. Quit smoking cigarettes

14. A 56-year-old man comes to the clinic because he has had persistent pain in his right lower leg since he underwent surgery to treat a fracture of the right fibula nine months ago. He says the distal leg and foot feel cooler than the left leg, and he says the pain includes a burning sensation. Vital signs are within normal limits. The patient is alert. Physical examination shows well-healed surgical scars on the right distal femur; no redness or obvious deformity is noted. Pulses are intact in the legs, bilaterally. Increased sensation to light touch and pinprick is noted over the distal right leg. The right leg feels cooler to touch than the left leg. X-ray studies of the leg show intact hardware and anatomic alignment. Arterial and venous studies of the legs show no abnormalities. Which of the following is the most likely diagnosis?
    A. Arterial occlusive disease
    B. Autonomic neuropathy

C. Complex regional pain syndrome
D. Occult fracture
E. Pretibial myxedema

15. A 19-year-old woman who is a college student comes to the office because she has had worsening headache, fever, and neck stiffness over the past 24 hours. She says that another resident in her dormitory had similar symptoms a few days ago. Medical history includes no chronic disease conditions. The patient immigrated to the United States at 13 years of age and is unsure of which vaccinations she has received. Temperature is 38.9°C (102.0°F). Physical examination shows nuchal rigidity. Analysis of cerebrospinal fluid shows elevated leukocytes (predominantly neutrophils), elevated protein level, and decreased glucose level. A gram stain shows gram-negative diplococci. Which of the following is the most likely causative agent?
    A. *Cryptococcus neoformans*
    B. Herpes simplex virus
    C. *Neisseria meningitidis*
    D. *Staphylococcus aureus*
    E. *Streptococcus pneumoniae*

16. A 37-year-old woman comes to the clinic three days after she was examined in the emergency department after being physically abused and assaulted by her husband. Immediately after the trauma, she had neck pain. A CT scan of the cervical spine at that time showed no abnormalities, and she was subsequently discharged to home with prescriptions for a nonsteroidal anti-inflammatory drug and a muscle relaxer. She says she has been taking both medications as prescribed, but the neck pain has worsened and is now focused in the lower part of her neck. The patient also has noticed that when she looks up or tilts her head to the right, she experiences an intense shooting pain down her right lateral and dorsal forearm and into her thumb and index finger. Vital signs are within normal limits. On physical examination, range of motion of the cervical spine is limited by 25% in all directions. The shooting pain into the right upper extremity is easily reproduced by extending and bending the neck to the right lateral side. Sensation and motor function in the upper extremities is intact, bilaterally. However, deep tendon reflexes of the biceps and triceps are decreased in the right upper extremity. Which of the following is the most likely diagnosis?
    A. Acute cervical disk protrusion
    B. Cervical radiculopathy
    C. Cervical spondylosis
    D. Complex regional pain syndrome
    E. Subluxed cervical facet joints

 Answer Key for this chapter begins on p. 151

17. A 23-year-old woman is brought to the emergency department by her roommate because she had a seizure two hours ago that lasted two minutes. During the examination, the patient has another seizure that continues for more than five minutes despite administration of 100% oxygen via nasal cannula and an intravenous bolus of dextrose. Which of the following is the most appropriate medication to administer to this patient?
A. Gabapentin
B. Lorazepam
C. Phenobarbital
D. Propofol
E. Valproic acid

18. A 9-year-old boy is brought to the emergency department by his parents because he had sudden onset of headache and seizure one hour ago. The parents say the seizure began with jerking of the right upper extremity and progressed to a generalized tonic-clonic seizure. The patient is now postictal and is not actively seizing. He is awake and responds to voices but is not able to intelligibly answer questions. On physical examination, strength and tone in the right upper extremity are diminished. CT scan of the head shows a large area of hemorrhage in the left temporal lobe. Which of the following is the most likely underlying cause of the symptoms in this patient?
A. Arteriovenous malformation
B. Atherosclerotic cardiovascular disease
C. Cavernous sinus thrombosis
D. Saccular aneurysm
E. Von Willebrand disease

19. A 3-year-old girl is brought to the clinic for annual well-child examination. The patient was born premature at 31 weeks' gestation. She has been delayed in meeting motor milestones, cannot yet walk independently, and has muscle spasticity in the lower extremities. These symptoms have been static and have not worsened since birth. She has met all cognitive, speech, and social milestones. The patient is otherwise healthy, eats a varied diet, and has no history of recent illnesses or injuries. On physical examination, Ortolani and Barlow signs are negative. Which of the following is the most likely diagnosis?
A. Cerebral palsy
B. Guillain-Barré syndrome
C. Hip dysplasia
D. Legg-Calvé-Perthes disease
E. Muscular dystrophy

20. After appropriate workup, Alzheimer disease is diagnosed in a 76-year-old man. During evaluation to discuss treatment options, the patient and his spouse agree to initiate pharmaceutical therapy at this time. Although only modestly effective, which of the following agents has been shown to decrease the rate of cognitive decline, presumably by increasing levels of intracerebral acetylcholine?

A. Carbidopa/levodopa
B. Donepezil
C. Fluoxetine
D. Memantine
E. Olanzapine

21. A 48-year-old man comes to the office because he has had intermittent episodes of persistent tight, viselike headache for the past month. He has not had fever, photophobia, phonophobia, sinus pressure, rhinorrhea, nasal congestion, or nausea. He says he has been staying hydrated and sleeping regularly. Ibuprofen and acetaminophen provide relief of the headache. Medical history includes no chronic disease conditions or surgical procedures. The patient says that he has been under more stress than usual because he received a promotion at work two months ago, and his workload and responsibilities have dramatically increased. Vital signs are within normal limits, and physical examination shows no abnormalities. Based on these findings, the headache in this patient is most likely to be located in which of the following areas of the head?
A. Back of the head
B. Behind the eyes
C. Frontal area
D. One side of the head
E. Temporal area

22. A 28-year-old woman comes to the office because she has had slowly worsening generalized muscle weakness and double vision over the past two months. She has no history of similar symptoms. Medical history includes no chronic disease conditions, and she takes no medications. Physical examination shows ptosis and rapid fatigue with repeated handgrip testing. Which of the following is the most likely cause of the symptoms in this patient?
A. Degeneration of cells in the anterior horn
B. Delayed breakdown of acetylcholine
C. Destruction of acetylcholine receptors
D. Disrupted axonal transmission
E. Inhibition of acetylcholine release

23. An 8-year-old girl is brought to the pediatric clinic by her mother to discuss treatment options for recently diagnosed Tourette disorder. The mother says that the patient spontaneously hops and repeatedly makes barking sounds for a few seconds, and this behavior is interfering with classroom participation at school. Physical examination shows no new abnormalities. After educating the mother about the specifics of this disorder, it is most appropriate to recommend which of the following?
A. Deep brain stimulation
B. Dopamine antagonists
C. Electroconvulsive therapy
D. Habit reversal training
E. Psychostimulants

24. A 32-year-old man is brought to the emergency department by a friend who says the patient has had fever, malaise, night sweats, and anorexia for the past three days, but his condition has worsened over the past 24 hours, and he is now disoriented and lethargic. Medical history includes heroin addiction and HIV infection. The friend says that the patient has not taken his HIV-related medications for several months. Temperature is 39.1°C (102.4°F), pulse rate is 92/min, respirations are 16/min, and blood pressure is 78/50 mmHg. On physical examination, the patient is unable to be aroused but retracts the extremities in response to painful stimuli. The left eye is rotated medially, but pupillary reflexes are intact. Laboratory studies show a mildly increased white blood cell count, and complete metabolic profile is within normal limits. CD4+ lymphocyte count is 8 cells/μL (N = 359–1725 cells/μL), and viral load is 120,000 copies/mL (N = 0 copies/mL). Examination of the cerebrospinal fluid shows a mildly increased opening pressure; protein and glucose concentrations are within normal limits. Results of gram, acid-fast, and India ink staining are negative. CT scan of the head shows no abnormalities. Which of the following is the most likely diagnosis?
A. Cryptococcus meningitis
B. Cytomegalovirus encephalitis
C. Progressive multifocal leukoencephalopathy
D. Toxoplasmic encephalitis
E. Tuberculous meningitis

25. A 71-year-old man comes to the emergency department because he had sudden onset of left-sided facial droop and weakness two hours ago. Pulse rate is 90/min, and blood pressure is 160/95 mmHg. Physical examination confirms the presenting symptoms. Noncontrast CT scan of the head shows no abnormalities. Which of the following is the most appropriate pharmacologic intervention?
A. Alteplase
B. Aspirin
C. Atorvastatin
D. Heparin
E. Rivaroxaban

26. A 32-year-old woman comes to the emergency department because she had sudden onset of diplopia three hours ago. Medical history includes no chronic disease conditions. Vital signs are within normal limits. Physical examination shows inability to fix the gaze to the left lateral side. These findings are most consistent with an abnormality in which of the following cranial nerves?
A. Abducens
B. Oculomotor
C. Optic
D. Trigeminal
E. Trochlear

27. An 18-year-old woman comes to the urgent care clinic because she woke up this morning with weakness in her feet and knees such that it was difficult to push the gas pedal of her car and to walk into the building. She is a freshman at the local university and is away from home for the first time in her life. Three days ago, the patient was evaluated in the student health clinic because she had vomiting, diarrhea, and intense headache that began shortly after eating homemade pickles. While at the clinic, she says she obtained a refill for oral contraceptive pills and also received a university-mandated meningococcal vaccine. Current vital signs are within normal limits. Physical examination shows decreased strength in dorsiflexion and plantarflexion of the ankles and extension and flexion of the knees. Achilles and patella deep tendon reflexes are absent bilaterally but are 2+ in the upper extremities. Sensation and pulses in the bilateral lower extremities are within normal limits. Which of the following is the most likely diagnosis?
A. Botulism
B. Conversion disorder
C. Guillain-Barré syndrome
D. Multiple sclerosis
E. Myasthenia gravis

28. A 26-year-old woman comes to the clinic because she has had unilateral headaches that are located behind her left eye and are accompanied by photophobia, phonophobia, and nausea. She says she has had this type of headache approximately once a month during the past three years. Family medical history includes similar headaches in her mother and sister. Which of the following treatments is most appropriate for this condition?
A. Gabapentin
B. Oxycodone
C. Oxygen
D. Tizanidine
E. Sumatriptan

29. A 61-year-old man with a recent diagnosis of lung cancer comes to the clinic because he has had morning headaches and nausea during the past two months. He says these symptoms usually resolve after two to three hours. The headaches are located across the top of his head and feel like "pressure." He does not have associated aura, photophobia, or visual changes. Vital signs are within normal limits, and neurologic examination shows no focal deficits. Contrast-enhanced MRI of the brain shows a homogeneously enhancing mass with surrounding edema at the grey-white junction. Which of the following is the most likely diagnosis?
A. Arteriovenous malformation
B. Epidural hematoma
C. Intracranial abscess
D. Meningioma
E. Metastatic tumor

30. A 67-year-old woman comes to the urgent care clinic because she had onset of a diffuse, sharp headache and disorientation while driving 24 hours ago. She says she had to pull over to the side of the road to take a nap. The patient remembers waking up in the car with the door open and vomit on the ground. She is not certain of how long she was asleep. The patient continued to be disoriented and confused the rest of the day, but this resolved shortly after she woke up this morning. She says she has some irritability and a mild stiff neck, but she currently does not have pain or other symptoms. Pulse rate is 82/min, respirations are 16/min, and blood pressure is 160/92 mmHg; she is afebrile. Physical examination shows a regular heart rate and rhythm. The lungs are clear to auscultation. Abdominal examination shows no abnormalities, and neurologic examination shows no focal deficits. Funduscopic examination shows no abnormalities. These findings most likely increase this patient's risk of which of the following conditions?
    A. Cerebral aneurysm
    B. Cluster headache syndrome
    C. Delirium tremens withdrawal
    D. Malignant hypertension sequelae
    E. Transient ischemic attack

31. A 78-year-old man comes to the primary care clinic because he has had worsening weakness, impairment in gait, and a decrease in manual dexterity over the past three years which have become even worse over the past six months. He says he also has had increased stiffness and has been afraid that he might fall. The patient works as a carpenter and has not been examined by a primary care clinician for the past 30 years. Family medical history includes similar symptoms in his father as he aged, but the patient does not believe a diagnosis was ever established. Physical examination shows bradykinesia, a shuffling, short-stepped gait, hypophonia, decreased facial expression, and a resting tremor in the right upper extremity. Which of the following is the most appropriate initial treatment?
    A. Benztropine
    B. Bromocriptine
    C. Cabergoline
    D. Carbidopa/levodopa
    E. Memantine

32. A 16-year-old girl comes to the primary care office because she has had headache, dizziness, vertigo, nausea, fatigue, and sensitivity to noise and light for the past month. She also has had worsening difficulty with attention and concentration in the classroom. The patient is a soccer player and says that her symptoms began after she collided heads with another player during a game. After the injury, the patient fell to the ground, hit her head on the ground, and lost consciousness. The high school athletic trainer evaluated her after the injury by asking her a series of concussion questions. She says that she felt well immediately afterward and did not seek further medical attention. Neurologic examination shows no deficits. The Patient Health Questionnaire-9 score is 4. Which of the following is the most appropriate next step in management?
    A. Noncontrast CT scan of the head
    B. Referral for physical therapy
    C. Referral to a neurologist
    D. Referral to a psychiatrist
    E. Watchful waiting

33. A 93-year-old woman comes to the emergency department after she struck her head on her coffee table when she fell 90 minutes ago. She says she did not lose consciousness. The patient lives independently. Medical history includes coronary artery disease, atrial fibrillation, hypertension, hyperlipidemia, and previous stroke. Current medications include warfarin, atorvastatin, metoprolol, amlodipine, aspirin, and losartan. CT scan of the head is most likely to show which of the following?
    A. Hydrocephalus
    B. Intracranial abscesses
    C. Intracranial hemorrhage
    D. Intracranial mass
    E. Ischemic stroke

34. A 46-year-old man is brought to the emergency department by ambulance after his coworkers witnessed him convulsing 15 minutes ago. A CT scan of the head is immediately obtained and shows an intracranial hemorrhage without an identifiable source of bleeding. Arteriovenous malformation (AVM) is suspected, and arteriography is planned. Which of the following types of AVM is most likely to be noted on arteriography of this patient?
    A. Arachnoid
    B. Brainstem
    C. Cerebellar
    D. External carotid
    E. Frontal

Answers

1. **Answer: D** Neural, option D, is correct because neurally mediated syncope (e.g., vasovagal or reflex syncope) is the most common cause of syncope. The incidence of syncope is higher in women than men, in younger age groups, and in patients who have a first-degree relative with similar history.

   Cardiac, option A, is incorrect because cardiovascular structural changes or arrhythmias are the second most common cause of syncope. Older patients are also more commonly affected when the etiology of syncope is cardiac. Options B and C, glycemic and hypoxic, are incorrect because they are not major classifications of syncope. Orthostatic, option E, is incorrect because orthostatic hypotension is not as common as neural mediated or cardiac syncope, and it is more prevalent in the aging population. **Task:** D1—Health Maintenance, Patient Education, and Disease Prevention

2. **Answer: B** Cluster headache, option B, is the most likely diagnosis because this type of headache is unilateral, lasts 20 minutes, and is associated with redness and tearing of the ipsilateral eye. Acute frontal sinusitis, option A, includes headache that is associated with nasal discharge and pressure, both of which this patient does not have. Meningioma, option C, may or may not cause headache, but if this were the most likely diagnosis the patient would have neurologic deficits. Migraine, option D, is more common in females and is not associated with redness and tearing of the ipsilateral eye. Tension headaches, option E, are bilateral and characterized by throbbing and aching, which are not present in this patient. **Task:** A—History Taking and Performing Physical Examination

3. **Answer: A** This patient has unfortunately suffered a traumatic brain injury resulting in coma to the extent of posturing following application of a painful stimulus. Decorticate posturing is characterized by flexion of the upper extremities with extension and internal rotation of the lower extremities. This type of reflexive posturing, as noted in this patient, occurs with lesions above the brainstem (option A). Specifically, the lesion is above the mesencephalon up to the level of the diencephalon (thalamus).

   Traumatic brain injury involving the cerebellum is uncommon, option B. Despite the role of the cerebellum in coordinating movement, posturing in response to a painful stimulus is not observed in cerebellar lesions. Rather, cerebellar lesions typically result in loss of coordinated movement, dysmetria, adiadochokinesia, intention tremor, ataxic gait, hypotonia, ataxic dysarthria, and nystagmus. The mesencephalon is considered the midbrain, option C. A lesion to the midbrain results in decerebrate posturing, which is characterized by internal rotation of the shoulders and forearms, extension of the elbows and wrists, and extension of the legs. Decerebrate posturing resulting from brain dysfunction descending to the level of the midbrain is generally considered more severe than that observed with decorticate posturing. Patients with lesions to the pons and medulla oblongata regions, option D, are flaccid and typically have no response to painful stimuli, which is not characteristic of this patient. Lesions of the upper cervical spinal cord (option E) between C1 and C4 typically result in death due to interruption of descending input to the C4 cord that gives rise to the phrenic nerves. A cord lesion below C4 and into the levels of the brachial plexus results in various degrees of quadriplegia. Spinal cord lesions below T1 and into the lumbar region result in paraplegia. **Task:** E—Applying Basic Scientific Concepts

4. **Answer: B** Encouraging early mobility and physical activity after the procedure, option B, will decrease the risk of delirium in this patient. Studies show that the primary intervention to prevent the development of delirium is to provide the patient with the opportunity to receive physical therapy and occupational therapy, and to allow them to perform primary mobility at the first possible chance.

   Attaching an alert device to the patient, option A, is incorrect because it will be noisy and prevent movement, which are counterproductive to preventing delirium. A quiet environment and movement are recommended after surgery. Not allowing family members to visit, option C, is incorrect because the presence of familiar people and support are helpful in preventing delirium. The use of benzodiazepines, option D, is incorrect because this class of drugs causes sedation which can increase confusion and lead to delirium. Using blackout curtains, option E, will increase the likelihood of delirium. It is important that patients know day from night. If possible, the patient's bed should be placed close to the window so she can notice the change in the morning and night; if not, changes should be made in room lighting based on the time of day. **Task:** D2—Clinical Intervention

5. **Answer: B** CT scan of the head, option B, is the most appropriate imaging study to rule out intracranial bleeding in this patient. The CT scan will provide images fast and will also show organ and skeletal structures.

   Bone scan of the head, option A, helps diagnose bone pathology but will not help identify an intracranial bleed. Electroencephalography, option C, is used to test electrical activity in the brain and will not show evidence of an intracranial bleed. An MRI of the brain, option D, will indicate a brain bleed, but the study takes longer than the preferred imaging study of a CT scan. X-ray study of the skull, option E, will help identify the presence of intracranial bleeding, but it is not definitive nor does it provide an adequate level of detail. **Task:** B—Using Diagnostic and Laboratory Studies

6. **Answer: D** Option D, Phalen test, is the correct answer. The patient has the classic manifestations of carpal tunnel syndrome, which results from the compression of the median nerve as it passes through the bones of the wrist. The Phalen test exerts further pressure on these structures, which exacerbates symptoms and supports the diagnosis of carpal tunnel syndrome.
Brachioradialis reflex testing, option A, is incorrect because this tests the radial nerve; carpal tunnel syndrome involves compression of the median nerve. Further, the brachioradialis is proximal to the site of nerve compression and is unlikely to be abnormal. Handgrip test, option B, does not directly evaluate the structures of the carpal tunnel. Handgrip testing may be painful for a patient with carpal tunnel syndrome, but numerous other conditions could also result in that finding. Neer test, option C, is a test of shoulder impingement and therefore is not an appropriate maneuver for diagnosing carpal tunnel syndrome. Range of motion testing of the wrist, option E, is not a specific test for carpal tunnel compression. As with handgrip testing, there may be pain or limitation of wrist range of motion in patients with carpal tunnel syndrome, but numerous other conditions could also cause that finding. **Task:** A—History Taking and Performing Physical Examination

7. **Answer: E** This patient has most likely been taking phenytoin, option E, for treatment of her seizure disorder. This medication is highly metabolized in the liver; therefore, close serum concentrations and therapeutic ranges need to be monitored. If phenytoin reaches toxic concentrations, it can induce seizures, confusion, nausea and vomiting, gait ataxia, tremors, and anorexia. One of the more common adverse effects of phenytoin is that it may cause gingival hyperplasia, as in this patient. Patients should have regular dental screenings and cleanings and report phenytoin use to their dental providers.
Gabapentin, lacosamide, levetiracetam, and oxcarbazepine (options A through D) are all therapies that can be used to treat and manage seizure disorders. However, they do not have gingival hyperplasia as a possible adverse effect. **Task:** D3—Pharmaceutical Therapeutics

8. **Answer: C** Home foot inspections and hemoglobin A_{1c} target of less than 7.5%, option C, is correct because a patient's own foot inspections is one of the most important fundamental self-care practices for patients with diabetes mellitus. Also, hemoglobin A_{1c} target of less than 7.5% is the recommendation for older adults. The most common complication of type 2 diabetes mellitus in older adults is neuropathy, and it occurs in up to 50% of these patients. Optimal glucose control significantly decreases the incidence of end-organ disease such as peripheral neuropathy.
Arterial Doppler ultrasonography and use of offloading shoe inserts, option A, is incorrect because an arterial Doppler study is not indicated when normal pulses are present. Also, offloading shoe inserts are used to help ulcers heal. Doppler waveforms and custom-molded shoes, option B, is incorrect because Doppler waveforms are used to evaluate arterial disease and healing potential. Molded shoes are used in the presence of foot deformities, which this patient does not have. Monofilament examinations and oral nortriptyline therapy, option D, is incorrect because oral nortriptyline therapy is used to treat pain in patients with diabetic neuropathy. Nerve conduction studies and hemoglobin A_{1c} target of less than 6.5%, option E, is incorrect because nerve conduction studies are not helpful in this clinical situation, and a hemoglobin A_{1c} target of less than 6.5% is recommended during pregnancy. **Task:** D1—Health Maintenance, Patient Education, and Disease Prevention

9. **Answer: E** This patient has multiple sclerosis (MS), option E. Optic neuritis is a common presenting symptom in patients with MS. In addition, there are demyelinating lesions of the central nervous center (CNS) on MRI as well as oligoclonal bands of IgG on lumbar puncture; these are typical findings in 80 to 90% of patients with MS.
Amyotrophic lateral sclerosis, option A, is incorrect because electromyography will show some abnormalities, and MRI may be abnormal but will not show demyelinating lesions in the CNS. Duchenne muscular dystrophy, option B, is incorrect because this is an X-linked recessive disease that is almost always found in males and is less likely in a 28-year-old woman. Fibromyalgia, option C, is incorrect because MRI and lumbar puncture typically show no abnormalities in patients with this diagnosis. MRI of patients with Guillain-Barré syndrome, option D, is most likely to show no abnormalities. **Task:** C—Formulating Most Likely Diagnosis

10. **Answer: D** Meningioma, option D, is correct because it is the primary brain tumor that is most commonly diagnosed in up to 35% of cases. Incidental findings on imaging studies are increasingly common. The lesion arises from the dura, is extra-axial, and is densely

enhanced. Meningiomas occur in women more than men, and incidence increases with age. Meningiomas are commonly associated with history of prior cranial irradiation and in patients with neurofibromatosis, type 2. A dural metastasis is the most significant differential diagnosis that must be ruled out.
Ganglioglioma, option A, is incorrect because it is uncommon and most often occurs in younger adults. Glioblastoma, option B, is incorrect because this is an infiltrative tumor that is ring-enhancing with central necrosis on imaging and usually occurs symptomatically in the sixth or seventh decade. Lymphoma, option C, is incorrect because this is found in less than 3% of primary brain tumors and is densely enhanced. Xanthoastrocytoma, option E, is incorrect because, like option A, it is also an uncommon glioma that occurs in younger adults. **Task:** C—Formulating Most Likely Diagnosis

11. **Answer: D** Essential tremor occurs frequently and is differentiated from Parkinson disease on a clinical basis as a tremor without other neurologic abnormalities. Parkinson tremor tends to be asymmetric and is associated with decreased facial expression, slowness of movement, and shuffling gait. Treatment for essential tremor is most often initiated with propranolol therapy, option D. Carbidopa/levodopa and ropinirole, options A and E, are primarily used to treat patients with Parkinson disease. Gabapentin, option B, is a second-line agent for treatment of essential tremor. Methylphenidate, option C, is a stimulant that may exacerbate tremor and should be avoided. **Task:** D3—Pharmaceutical Therapeutics

12. **Answer: B** Huntington disease, option B, is an autosomal dominant disease with characteristic onset in the late 30s. Typically, it presents with movements of chorea as well as behavioral outbursts and progresses to death on average within 17 years from onset.
Alzheimer dementia, option A, tends to present later in life and does not include associated abnormal body movements. Lyme disease, option C, may include central nervous system symptoms but is not an inherited disease and is not associated with the decrease in cognition. Multiple sclerosis, option D, may also present at this age but typically includes vision changes and numbness. Parkinson disease, option E, also tends to present later in life and typically includes asymmetric tremor, which this patient does not have. **Task:** C—Formulating Most Likely Diagnosis

13. **Answer: A** Control blood pressure, option A, is correct because hypertension is usually the etiology of spontaneous intracranial hemorrhage.
Initiating an aerobic exercise routine, maintaining an ideal body weight, managing diabetes mellitus, and quitting smoking (options B through E) are incorrect.

Although it is important for this patient to do these things, these measures do not have as much influence in decreasing his risk for spontaneous intracranial hemorrhage as controlling his hypertension. **Task:** D1—Health Maintenance, Patient Education, and Disease Prevention

14. **Answer: C** This patient has complex regional pain syndrome, option C. The Budapest clinical diagnostic criteria for complex regional pain syndrome include:
1. Continuing pain that is disproportionate to any inciting event.
2. Patient must report one symptom in three of the four following categories:
   a. Vasomotor: temperature asymmetry and/or skin color changes and or skin color asymmetry
   b. Sensory: hyperesthesia and/or allodynia
   c. Motor/trophic: Decreased range of motion and/or motor dysfunction (weakness, tremor, dystonia) and/or trophic changes (hair, nail, and/or skin)
   d. Sudomotor/edema: Edema and/or sweating changes and/or sweating asymmetry
3. Patient must exhibit one sign at the time of evaluation in two or more of the following categories:
   a. Vasomotor: Temperature asymmetry and/or skin color changes and/or asymmetry
   b. Sensory: Hyperalgesia to pinprick and/or allodynia

This patient's clinical presentation meets these criteria because he has consistent pain without an inciting event, temperature asymmetry, and hyperalgesia to pinprick. Arterial occlusive disease, option A, is characterized by coolness of the involved leg with diminished pulses and abnormal arterial vascular studies with diminished perfusion. Autonomic neuropathy, option B, occurs with abnormalities in blood pressure and pulse rate, sweating, and abnormalities in bowel/bladder emptying. Occult fracture, option D, is unlikely because the x-rays show intact hardware and anatomic alignment. Pretibial myxedema, option E, occurs bilaterally and in the setting of thyroid disease. **Task:** C—Formulating Most Likely Diagnosis

15. **Answer: C** Option C, *Neisseria meningitidis*, is the correct answer. This patient has the classic manifestations of meningitis, and the cerebrospinal fluid (CSF) analysis suggests bacterial meningitis. *Neisseria meningitidis* is a common cause of meningitis and is the only pathogen listed that is a gram-negative diplococcus. *Cryptococcus neoformans*, option A, is incorrect because the laboratory tests indicate the presence of bacteria rather than this fungal pathogen (diagnosed with antigen testing or, historically, the India ink stain). Additionally, cryptococcal meningitis is most common in patients with advanced HIV infection or other significant immunocompromised conditions. Herpes simplex virus, option B, causes increased

lymphocytes (rather than neutrophils). CSF does not show a decreased glucose level, and gram stain is not positive with this virus. *Staphylococcus aureus*, option D, is a gram-positive diplococcus and is also a rare cause of meningitis. *Streptococcus aureus*, option E, is a common cause of meningitis but is incorrect because it is a gram-positive diplococcus. **Task: E—Applying Basic Scientific Concepts**

16. **Answer: B** Cervical radiculopathy, option B, is the correct answer based on an absence of radiographic lesions and radiating neurologic symptoms consistent with the C6 and C7 dermatomes and myotomes. The timing is also consistent with continued inflammation following a traumatic event. As for management, in addition to nonsteroidal anti-inflammatory drugs (NSAIDs) and muscle relaxants, this patient may benefit at this stage from use of a soft cervical collar, a tricyclic antidepressant as a sleep aid, and, although controversial, a short course of oral corticosteroids if the pain is severe. MRI or CT myelography, physical therapy, electromagnetic testing, and/or adding acetaminophen are all plausible choices in management. Acute cervical disk protrusion, option A, is a plausible choice. However, the CT scan does not indicate an actual herniation with spinal nerve impingement as the cause of the radiculopathy. If the symptoms persist, a closer look with MRI or CT myelography would be indicated. Cervical spondylosis, option C, results from chronic disk degeneration with herniation, secondary calcification, and osteophytic outgrowths. The condition generally occurs after the age of 50 with pain and stiffness in the neck and radicular pain in the arms. However, unlike the patient in the scenario, cervical spondylosis is also characterized by an upper motor neuron deficit in the lower extremities. Complex regional pain syndrome, option D, is characterized by pain that follows an injury but spreads beyond the site of trauma. The pain also does not conform to a particular peripheral nerve, is greater than would be expected given the extent of the injury, and may progress with time. The spinal nature or origin of this patient's symptoms makes this option an incorrect choice. The CT scan of the patient's cervical spine obtained in the emergency department at the time of the trauma showed no abnormalities. This finding does not support a diagnosis of subluxed cervical facet joints, choice E, as the correct answer. However, it is important to note that subluxation is a well-recognized complication of motor vehicle collisions. **Task: A—History Taking and Performing Physical Examination**

17. **Answer: B** This patient is in status epilepticus. After administering oxygen and dextrose, a benzodiazepine such as lorazepam, option B, is most appropriate to administer to help stop the convulsions.

Gabapentin, option A, is an oral medication that is used in the outpatient setting for partial seizures; it is not indicated for this patient. Phenobarbital, propofol, and valproic acid, options C, D, and E, are second- and third-line medications that can be administered for treatment of status epilepticus if there is no improvement with benzodiazepine therapy. **Task: D3—Pharmaceutical Therapeutics**

18. **Answer: A** This patient has typical manifestations of an arteriovenous malformation, option A, which results from the flow of blood from an artery directly into a thin-walled vein without passing through a capillary bed. Arteriovenous malformations are more common in children and often manifest with hemorrhage. Atherosclerotic cardiovascular disease, option B, is an important cause of stroke but is unlikely to cause hemorrhage and is not likely to affect children. Hemorrhages due to cavernous sinus thrombosis, option C, are typically in the anterior brain rather than the distribution of the middle cerebral artery. Cavernous sinus thrombosis may cause hemorrhage, but this is rare, and the patient will often have cranial nerve (especially ocular) palsies. Option D, saccular aneurysm, includes hemorrhages that are typically in the Circle of Willis or posterior circulation. Option E, von Willebrand disease, very rarely causes major hemorrhages. Other bleeding diatheses like hemophilia can cause intracranial hemorrhages, though hemarthroses and gastrointestinal bleeding are more common. **Task: C—Formulating Most Likely Diagnosis**

19. **Answer: A** Cerebral palsy, option A, is a disorder that causes motor dysfunction and neurologic impairment that is not progressive and is caused by an insult to the developing brain. This patient has findings consistent with diplegic cerebral palsy due to spasticity involving the lower extremities, which is common in premature infants and does not affect intelligence. Guillain-Barré syndrome, option B, classically causes an acute ascending paralysis related to an antecedent viral infection. Hip dysplasia, option C, can be a cause of delayed walking in children but is associated with positive Ortolani and Barlow signs. Option D, Legg-Calvé-Perthes disease, is avascular necrosis of the hip in children and classically presents with a limp in already ambulatory children. Muscular dystrophy, option E, is a progressive cause of motor dysfunction in children; therefore, this is not the most likely diagnosis since this patient's condition has been static since birth. **Task: A—History Taking and Performing Physical Examination**

20. **Answer: B** Unfortunately, pharmaceutical treatment of dementia, whether from Alzheimer disease, frontotemporal dementia, dementia with Lewy bodies, or normal pressure hydrocephalus, offers no cure. At

best in early stages of the disease, drug therapy provides a deceleration in the rate of cognitive decline. Progressive loss of memory and other higher cortical functions are believed to be due to a decrease in the level of the neurotransmitter acetylcholine in the cerebral cortex. To counteract the neurotransmitter loss, donepezil (option B) is believed to increase intracerebral acetylcholine levels by inhibiting the degrading enzyme acetylcholinesterase.

Carbidopa/levodopa, option A, is an effective drug used in the treatment of Parkinson disease. While parkinsonism is a feature of dementia with Lewy bodies, carbidopa/levodopa works on dopaminergic systems in the brain to control tremor without having an effect on cognition. Depression is a treatable condition that commonly develops in patients with dementia. Mostly all selective serotonin reuptake inhibitors (SSRIs) such as fluoxetine, option C, are effective in addressing this comorbidity. As the name of the drug class implies, the action of SSRIs is to focus on increasing serotonin levels in the cortex, rather than acetylcholine. SSRIs have not been approved to specifically treat cognitive decline. Memantine, option D, is also FDA-approved to treat Alzheimer disease but works to block overexcited N-methyl-D-aspartate (NMDA) channels. Olanzapine, option E, is an atypical antipsychotic frequently used in patients with dementia for control of agitation. Although olanzapine's exact mechanism of action is unknown, it antagonizes receptors for dopamine, serotonin, and other neurotransmitters. **Task: D3**—Pharmaceutical Therapeutics

21. **Answer: A** This patient is most likely having a tension headache due to increased levels of stress. The viselike description of the headache provided by the patient is indicative of a tension headache, and the most likely location of this type of headache is at the back of the head, option A.

A headache that is localized behind the eyes, option B, is usually noted in patients with migraine or sinus headaches. Patients with cluster headaches most often have pain localized in the frontal area, option C. Pain that is localized to one side of the head, option D, is indicative of migraine. Pain that is localized in the temporal area, option E, is noted in patients with giant cell arteritis. **Task: A**—History Taking and Performing Physical Examination

22. **Answer: C** Option C, destruction of acetylcholine receptors, is the correct answer. This patient has the classic manifestations of myasthenia gravis, which usually results from immune-mediated damage. Its symptoms include muscle weakness, most notably of the ocular and facial muscles, and fatiguability.

Degeneration of cells in the anterior horn, option A, is incorrect because the patient does not have the typical symptoms of amyotrophic lateral sclerosis, which include mixed upper and lower motor neuron defects. Delayed breakdown of acetylcholine, option B, causes increased rather than decreased muscle contractility. This is why acetylcholinesterase inhibitors are used in the treatment of patients with myasthenia gravis. Disrupted axonal transmission, option D, is incorrect because there is no indication in the patient's history of delayed or absent transmission of nerve impulses. Inhibition of acetylcholine release, option E, is incorrect because the patient experiences fatiguing with repeated handgrips. Inhibition of acetylcholine release is the cause of Lambert-Eaton syndrome, which is a paraneoplastic disorder most commonly seen in patients with small cell lung cancer. In Lambert-Eaton syndrome, repeated use of a muscle increases the amount of acetylcholine released through increased presynaptic calcium influx due to the multiple depolarizations. **Task: E**—Applying Basic Scientific Concepts

23. **Answer: D** Habit reversal training, option D, has shown to be an effective treatment for patients with Tourette disorder. Support, education, and cognitive-behavioral interventions are appropriate initial treatment of Tourette disorder.

Deep brain stimulation, option A, is used for medically intractable tics in adults. Dopamine antagonists, option B, may be considered if the patient does not respond to cognitive-behavioral interventions. Electroconvulsive therapy, option C, remains experimental in the treatment of Tourette disorder. Psychostimulants, option E, may be considered if the patient does not respond to cognitive-behavioral interventions. **Task: D2**—Clinical Intervention

24. **Answer: B** This patient is obviously critically ill. His symptoms, especially with the accompanying sixth cranial nerve palsy, indicate disease involving the central nervous system such as meningitis or encephalitis. The CD4+ lymphocyte count, which is less than 200 cells/μL, confirms that the patient has AIDS and an increased risk of opportunistic infections. Options A, B, D, and E are all opportunistic infections of the central nervous system in patients with AIDS.

Patients with HIV with CD4+ lymphocyte counts less than 50 to 100 cells/μL are at risk for cytomegalovirus (CMV) encephalitis (option B), the correct answer. This patient's symptoms, particularly the cranial nerve palsy, are consistent with CMV infection of the central nervous system. Furthermore, the results of the cerebrospinal fluid (CSF) study are consistent with a viral etiology over a metabolically active organism. Meningitis resulting from infection with *Cryptococcus neoformans*, option A, is characterized by a markedly increased opening pressure on lumbar puncture and decreased glucose and elevated protein levels in CSF. An India ink preparation shows the encapsulated organism in approximately 75% of HIV-infected patients.

Option C, progressive multifocal leukoencephalopathy (PML), is a rare disorder seen in immunocompromised individuals, including those with AIDS. PML is a demyelinating disorder caused by human polyomavirus 2, commonly referred to as the John Cunningham virus. Although viral in origin, the disease is diagnosed by the presence on noncontrast CT scan of multifocal, hypodense lesions of the central nervous system white matter without mass effect. Toxoplasmosis, choice D, is the most common opportunistic infection of the central nervous system in patients with AIDS who are not receiving prophylactic therapies. Signs and symptoms of toxoplasmosis of the central nervous system are consistent with the findings in this patient. However, multiple lesions on CT scan of the head described as "ring enhancing" are pathognomonic for the infection. On analysis of CSF, tuberculous meningitis (option E) is characterized by elevated protein and decreased glucose levels along with possibly visualizing the organism in an acid-fast preparation. **Task:** C—Formulating Most Likely Diagnosis

25. **Answer: A** This patient has the classic manifestations of a stroke and imaging studies that support an ischemic, rather than hemorrhagic, stroke. The patient is within 4.5 hours of symptom onset, and vital signs are not a contraindication to thrombolytic therapy. Alteplase, option A, is the preferred agent for thrombolysis.
Aspirin, option B, does not have a role in the acute treatment of an ischemic stroke. Instead, aspirin is used for secondary prevention to decrease the risk of subsequent strokes. Atorvastatin, option C, does not have a role in the acute treatment of an ischemic stroke. Like aspirin, high-intensity statins are helpful in secondary prevention of stroke. Heparin, option D, does not have a role in the acute treatment of most strokes except for some cases of cardioembolic stroke. Rivaroxaban, option E, does not have a role in the acute treatment of an ischemic stroke. It is frequently used to decrease the risk of embolic stroke in patients with atrial fibrillation, and it also has a role in the treatment of venous thromboembolism. **Task:** D3—Pharmaceutical Therapeutics

26. **Answer: A** The lateral rectus muscle is responsible for lateral movement of the eye. This has innervation by cranial nerve VI, which is the abducens, option A.
The oculomotor nerve, option B, which is cranial nerve III, innervates the muscles that allow visual tracking and gaze fixation. The optic nerve, option C, carries sensory visual information from the retina to the vision center of the brain. The trigeminal nerve, option D, carries sensory information from the face to the brain. The superior oblique muscle is responsible for movement of the eyeball medially, and that is innervated by the trochlear nerve, option E, which is cranial nerve IV. **Task:** E—Applying Basic Scientific Concepts

27. **Answer: C** This question describes a young woman presenting with sudden onset of muscle weakness. It is important to note that she received a vaccination three days prior to the onset of symptoms. As with all vaccinations, a serious adverse effect is option C, Guillain-Barré syndrome (GBS). GBS is characterized as an ascending demyelinating disorder that typically reaches maximal weakness two weeks after the inciting event. In addition to vaccinations being associated with Guillain-Barré syndrome, over two-thirds of the inciting events include acute respiratory or gastrointestinal infection.
Botulism, option A, is a concern given this patient's recent ingestion of homemade pickles. However, symptoms associated with botulism include blurred vision, dry mouth, nausea, unreactive or delayed reactive pupils, urinary retention, and constipation. This disorder is also characterized by a descending flaccid paralysis beginning in the head and neck. Areflexia also accompanies GBS. While conversion disorder, option B, is plausible given her new life situation, this patient would be highly unlikely to recreate an absence of deep tendon reflexes in a somatic symptom disorder. Multiple sclerosis, option D, is an inflammatory demyelinating disease of the central nervous system (CNS) with an abrupt or chronic onset. While this is a plausible choice, the CNS lesions result in reflexes that are hypertonic, which is consistent with an upper motor neuron disease. Myasthenia gravis, option E, is a neuromuscular disease of the peripheral nervous system characterized by the presence of autoantibodies directed against the acetylcholine receptor. The disease results in skeletal muscle weakness but with normal deep tendon reflexes. Unlike this patient, the weakness of myasthenia gravis is primarily associated with muscles innervated by the cranial nerves and in the muscle groups of the proximal limbs. **Task:** A—History Taking and Performing Physical Examination

28. **Answer: E** This patient has the classic symptoms of migraine, which include unilateral headaches associated with nausea and photophobia/phonophobia. Migraine also has a familial component, as is the case with this patient. Sumatriptan, option E, is a medication used to abort acute migraine and is the appropriate treatment for this patient.
Gabapentin, option A, is an anticonvulsant medication used in the treatment of numerous conditions including neuropathic pain, but it is not generally used for the treatment of migraine. Oxycodone, option B, is an opioid that is not recommended in the treatment of migraine. Option C, oxygen, can be used to treat cluster. Tizanidine, option D, is a skeletal muscle relaxant used to treat tension-type headaches. **Task:** D3—Pharmaceutical Therapeutics

29. **Answer: E** Metastatic brain tumors, option E, are the most common brain tumors diagnosed in the United States. This is the most likely diagnosis in a patient with known cancer and a tumor identified on imaging.

The other answer choices, options A through D, are types of space-occupying lesions that are not related to malignancy. Therefore, they are not the most likely diagnosis based on this patient scenario. **Task: C—Formulating Most Likely Diagnosis**

30. **Answer: A** Cerebral aneurysm, option A, is correct because this patient's presentation is highly suspect of a cerebral aneurysm herald bleed that has devastating consequences for the patient if missed by the provider. Risk factors include female sex, older age, smoking history, hypertension, heavy alcohol use, and non-white race. The main characteristics of this disorder are new onset severe headache associated with nausea and vomiting and change in mental status which, if regained, may be associated with irritability or confusion. A stiff neck may also be present. These symptoms may appear hours or a few days before the significant subarachnoid hemorrhage.

Cluster headache syndrome, option B, is characterized by severe recurrent unilateral headaches and associated ipsilateral eye symptoms. Delirium tremens withdrawal, option C, often includes anxiety, hallucinations, autonomic hyperactivity, and a headache that is different from this patient's headache. Malignant hypertension sequelae, option D, is associated with significant ocular findings and no changes in mental status. Transient ischemic attack, option E, includes findings such as unilateral weakness or speech and vision changes, which are not present in this patient. **Task: D1—Health Maintenance, Patient Education, and Disease Prevention**

31. **Answer: D** This patient has signs and symptoms of Parkinson disease, which is defined as a progressive neurodegenerative movement disorder characterized by classic physical traits, including bradykinesia, decreased manual dexterity, muscular rigidity, resting tremor that decreases when intentional movements are pursued, postural instability, gait impairment, hypophonia, stone face, autonomic dysfunction, and cognitive related impairment. The diagnosis is made based on the patient's history and physical examination findings. The most appropriate initial treatment for motor symptoms is dopamine precursors and dopamine receptor agonists, such as carbidopa/levodopa, option D.

Benztropine, option A, is used as adjunct therapy to carbidopa/levodopa as a method of treating worsening tremors or additional adverse effects of medications used to treat Parkinson disease. Bromocriptine and cabergoline, options B and C, are dopamine receptor agonists that are used to treat hyperprolactinemia. They also can be used as an adjunct therapy to carbidopa/levodopa when control of motor symptoms is difficult in patients with Parkinson disease. Memantine, option E, is a memory-enhancing medication that is used to treat Alzheimer dementia and dementia associated with advanced Parkinson disease. **Task: D3—Pharmaceutical Therapeutics**

32. **Answer: C** This patient has postconcussion syndrome, which is described as a group of symptoms that occur in the weeks to months after a mild traumatic brain injury, also known as a concussion. Referral to a neurologist, option C, specifically one that specializes in traumatic brain injuries and concussions, is the most appropriate next step in management. The constellation of symptoms associated with postconcussion syndrome includes headache, dizziness, nausea, fatigue, photophobia, or sensitivity to noise. Additional symptoms include difficulty with short-term memory and attention, as well as psychological and mood-related symptoms including emotional lability, anxiety, and depression. Many of these symptoms persist for a period of time beyond the expected period of recovery from a mild traumatic brain injury.

Noncontrast CT scan of the head, option A, may be necessary but it is not the most appropriate next step, and the neurologist can determine if it is needed after consultation. Referral for physical therapy, option B, is not indicated at this time since the patient is neurologically intact; however, the neurologist may recommend this therapy after consultation. Referral to a psychiatrist, option D, is not indicated as the Patient Health Questionnaire-9 score of 4 is low and is not suggestive of depression as the primary diagnosis. Watchful waiting, option E, is not the most appropriate next step since this patient's symptoms have been ongoing for more than four weeks and further examination is indicated. **Task: D2—Clinical Intervention**

33. **Answer: C** A CT scan of this patient is most likely to show intracranial hemorrhage, option C. Falls and associated head injuries are common reasons for geriatric patients to come to the emergency department. It is also well documented that aging individuals are more likely to be taking antiplatelet or anticoagulant therapy for treatment or prophylactic management of common medical comorbidities, such as cardiovascular disease or cerebrovascular disease. With any head injury, there is always potential intracranial hemorrhage related to trauma. Many studies suggest that there is an increased risk of intracranial hemorrhage while on antiplatelet, warfarin, or other direct oral anticoagulants.

Options A, B, D, and E are incorrect because the mechanism of this patient's injury suggests a traumatic cause. Hydrocephalus, option A, is often a progressive condition that is related to increased intracranial pressure and poor drainage of cerebrospinal fluid from the ventricles. Intracranial abscesses, option B, are often associated with systemic infection. Intracranial mass, option D, is benign or malignant, can be easily excluded on brain imaging, and is unlikely to be the primary issue based on the mechanism of injury. Ischemic stroke, option E, seems much less likely in this scenario because the patient is taking appropriate medical therapy for prevention of future stroke with warfarin and aspirin. **Task:** C—Formulating Most Likely Diagnosis

34. **Answer: E** This patient most likely has a frontal arteriovenous malformation (AVM), option E, because seizures are most commonly noted in patients with this type of AVM.

An AVM cannot exist in the arachnoid membrane surrounding the brain, option A, because it lacks blood vessels. Obstructive hydrocephalus is most commonly seen in patients with brainstem or cerebellar AVMs (options B and C). Headaches are more commonly seen with external carotid AVMs, option D. **Task:** B—Using Diagnostic and Laboratory Studies

BIBLIOGRAPHY

Ali, A. Complex regional pain syndrome. (2018). *Rutherford's Vascular Surgery and Endovascular Therapy* (9th ed.), Chapter 192, 2488-2500. Elsevier.

Alter, S. M., Solano, J. J., Engstrom, G. , & Shih, R. D. (2020). Traumatic intracranial hemorrhage in geriatric patients on warfarin, direct oral anticoagulants, or no anticoagulation: a prospective study. *Annals of Emergency Medicine,* 76(4). S37-S37, 2020.

American Academy of Pediatric Dentistry Reference Manual. (2016\2017). Guidelines on periodontal diseases of children and adolescents. *Pediatric Dentistry,* 38, 388-396.

Bloch, M. H., &, Leckman, J. F. Tourette syndrome, tic disorders, and obsessive–compulsive disorder in children and adolescents. In: M. H. Ebert, J. F. Leckman, & I. L. Petrakis (Eds.), *Current diagnosis & treatment: Psychiatry* (3rd ed.), McGraw-Hill.

Clinical Overview: Myasthenia gravis. (2022). In *Elsevier Point of Care.* Elsevier.

Cree, B. C., & Hauser, S. L. Multiple sclerosis. In: J. Jameson, A. S. Fauci, D. L. Kasper, S. L. Hauser, D. L. Longo & J. Loscalzo (Eds.), *Harrison's principles of internal medicine* (20th ed.), McGraw-Hill.

Daroff, R. B. (2016). Headache and other craniofacial pain: *Bradley's Neurology in clinical practice* (pp. 1686-1719) (7th ed.). Philadelphia, PA: Elsevier.

DeAngelis L. M., & Wen P. Y. Primary and metastatic tumors of the nervous system. In: J. Jameson, A. S. Fauci, D. L. Kasper, S. L. Hauser, D. L. Longo, & J. Loscalzo (Eds.), *Harrison's principles of internal medicine* (20th ed). McGraw-Hill.

Dexter, D. T., & Jenner, P. (2013). Parkinson disease: From pathology to molecular disease mechanisms. *Free Radical Biology & Medicine,* 62, 132-144.

Donahue, S. Nuclear and fascicular disorders of eye movement. *Ophthalmology,* 9.15, 930-934.e1.

Douglas, V. C., & Aminoff, M. J. Stroke. In: M. A. Papadakis, S. J. McPhee, & M. W. Rabow (Eds.), *Current medical diagnosis & treatment 2021.* McGraw-Hill.

Douglas, V. C., & Aminoff, M. J. Stroke. In: M. A. Papadakis, S. J. McPhee, & M. W. Rabow (Eds.), *Current medical diagnosis & treatment 2021.* McGraw-Hill.

Freeman R. (2018). Syncope. In: J. Jameson, A. S. Fauci, D. L. Kasper, S. L. Hauser, D. L. Longo, & J. Loscalzo (Eds.), *Harrison's Principles of Internal Medicine,* (20th ed). McGraw-Hill.

Goldman, L., Schafer, A. I., & Nath, A. (2020). Meningitis: Bacterial, viral, and other: *Goldman-Cecil medicine* (pp. 2442-2458) (26th ed.). Philadelphia, PA: Elsevier.

Hoffman, J. (2018). Diagnosis, pathophysiology, and management of cluster headache. *Lancet Neurology,* 17(1), 75-83.

Inouye, S. K., Westendorp, R. G., & Saczynski, J. S. (2014). Delirium in elderly people. *Lancet,* 383(9920), 911-922.

Kalia, L. V., & Lang, A. E. (2015). Parkinson's disease. *The Lancet,* 386(9996), 896-91.

Kasper D., & Fauci A., & Hauser S., & Longo D., & Jameson J., & Loscalzo J. (Eds.). (2014). *Harrison's Principles of Internal Medicine,* (19th ed.) McGraw-Hill.

Lucas, S. (2011). Headache management in concussion and mild traumatic brain injury. *PM R,* 3, S406-S412.

Masharani, U. Diabetes mellitus. In: M. A. Papadakis, S. J. McPhee, M. W. Rabow (Eds.), *Current medical diagnosis & treatment 2021.* McGraw-Hill.

Merrell, R. (2020). Brain tumors. In R. Kellerman & D. Rakel (Eds.), *Conn's current therapy 2020* (pp. 686-690). Philadelphia, PA: Elsevier, Inc.

Nunneley, C. Essential tremor, *Ferri's clinical advisor 2021,* 546-547. e1. Elsevier.

Ossig, C., & Reichmann, H. (2015). Treatment strategies in early and advanced Parkinson disease. *Neurologic Clinics,* 33(1), 19-37.

Papadakis, M., McPhee, S., & Rabow, M. (2019). *Current medical diagnosis & treatment 2020* (59th Ed.). Cenveo Publisher Services.

Papadakis, M. A., McPhee, S. J., & Rabow, M. W. (2020). Chapter 24: Nervous system: *Current medical diagnosis & treatment 2020.* New York: McGraw-Hill Education.

Pasternak, J. (2021). Diseases affecting the brain. *Stoelting's anesthesia and co-existing disease,* (8th ed). Chapter 13, pp. 265-303. Elsevier.

Powers, W. J., Rabinstein, A. A., Ackerson, T., Adeoye, O. M., Bambakidis, N. C., Becker, K., et al. (2018). 2018 Guidelines for the early management of patients with acute ischemic stroke: a guideline for healthcare professionals from the American Heart Association/American Stroke Association. *Stroke,* 49(3), e46-e110.

Sawyer, J., & Spence, D. (2017). Cerebral palsy. In F. Azar, J. Beaty, & S. Canale (Eds.), *Campbell's operative orthopedics* (13th ed.). Philadelphia, PA: Elsevier, Inc. 1249-1303.

Simon, R. P. Aminoff, M. J. & Greenberg, D. A. (2018). *Clinical neurology* (10th ed., pp. 50-51, 245-246, 254, 306, 309-310).

Smits, M., Houston, G. C., Dippel, D. W., Wielopolski, P. A., Vernooij, M. W., Koudstaal, P. J., et al. (2011). Microstructural brain injury in post-concussion syndrome after minor head injury. *Neuroradiology,* 53(8), 553-563.

Status Epilepticus. *Epocrates.* https://online.epocrates.com/diseases/46442/Status-epilepticus/Treatment-Options. Updated October 2020.

Stilman, N., & Masdeu, J. C. (1985). Incidence of seizures with phenytoin toxicity. *Neurology, 35*, 1769-1772.

Tungare, S., & Paranjpe, A. G. (2020). Drug induced gingival overgrowth. [Updated 2020 Oct 5]: *StatPearls [Internet]*. Treasure Island (FL): StatPearls Publishing.

Turcato, G., Zaboli, A., Zannoni, M., Ricci, G., Zorzi, E., Ciccariello, L., et al. Risk factors associated with intracranial bleeding and neurosurgery in patients with mild traumatic brain injury who are receiving direct oral anticoagulants. *American Journal of Emergency Medicine*.

Walling, A. (2020). Migraine Headache. In R. Kellerman & D. Rakel (Eds.), *Conn's current therapy 2020* (pp. 702-706). Philadelphia, PA: Elsevier, Inc.

Williams, D. T., & Kim, H. T. (2018). Wrist and forearm: In: *Rosen's emergency medicine: concepts and clinical practice* (pp. 508-529) (9th ed.). Philadelphia, PA: Elsevier.

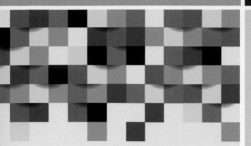

CHAPTER 11
Psychiatry and Behavioral Science

Questions

1. A 22-year-old man is brought to the emergency department by a friend because he has been unconscious for the past 15 minutes. Medical history includes recent admission to an outpatient drug treatment program. Temperature is 34.0°C (93.2°F), and respirations are 6/min and shallow. On physical examination, pupillary constriction is noted, bilaterally. A response is elicited with a sternal rub. Administration of naloxone therapy is planned. Which of the following effects is most likely to occur with the administration of this medication?
   A. Projectile vomiting
   B. Pulmonary vasoconstriction
   C. Renal insufficiency
   D. Sinus tachycardia
   E. Withdrawal symptoms

2. A 43-year-old woman comes to the clinic because she has had persistent lack of enjoyment in daily activities, fatigue, changes in appetite, and unintentional weight gain during the past three months. She has not had similar symptoms in the past. Medical history includes tubal ligation. The patient smokes one pack of cigarettes daily and would like to quit. Physical examination shows no abnormalities. Which of the following medications is most appropriate to treat this patient's symptoms as well as help her to quit smoking cigarettes?
   A. Bupropion
   B. Buspirone
   C. Olanzapine
   D. Sertraline
   E. Venlafaxine

3. A 12-year-old boy is placed in the county juvenile detention center by the courts after he is caught burglarizing three homes in his neighborhood. During the court proceeding, testimony is given that over the past year, the boy bludgeoned several of the neighbor's cats and small dogs, sexually assaulted a 10-year-old neighbor girl, set fire to a neighbor's shed, and was usually truant from school. This type of behavior is typical of which of the following personality disorders?
   A. Antisocial personality disorder
   B. Attention-deficit/hyperactivity disorder
   C. Borderline personality disorder
   D. Conduct disorder
   E. Schizoid personality disorder

4. A 43-year-old man is brought to the emergency department by family members who say that he has had a lack of continuity in thoughts, actions, memories, surroundings, and ideas since experiencing the trauma of seeing his family killed four months ago. Vital signs are within normal limits. Physical examination shows no abnormalities. However, during the interview, the patient says that he cannot remember the incident in which his family members were killed. This patient is most likely experiencing symptoms of which of the following disorders?
   A. Dissociative disorder
   B. Generalized anxiety disorder
   C. Major depressive disorder
   D. Schizoaffective disorder
   E. Schizophrenia

5. A 21-year-old woman is brought to the clinic by her mother because she is concerned about her daughter's decreasing weight. The patient is majoring in dance at a local university and says that there is an emphasis in her program on maintaining body appearance. The patient says that she does not have a problem with her weight and insists that it is important to stay fit in order to succeed at school. To maintain her high level of fitness, she says her daily workout routine lasts six hours. During the interview, the patient admits to dieting throughout her high school years, but the mother insists that the degree of the patient's dieting over the past two years has become extreme. Body mass index is 15.2 kg/m² (N = 18.5–24.9 kg/m²). Vital signs are within normal limits. Physical examination shows a gaunt appearance, healthy dentition, and significant paucity of subcutaneous fat. Laboratory studies show decreased hemoglobin and red blood cell indices. Serum urea nitrogen and creatinine levels are decreased. Thyroid-stimulating hormone, glucose, electrolytes, albumin, liver transaminases, and cholesterol levels are within normal limits. Electrocardiography shows normal sinus rhythm. Which of the following is the most likely diagnosis?
   A. Anorexia nervosa
   B. Avoidant/restrictive food intake disorder
   C. Bulimia nervosa
   D. Pica
   E. Rumination disorder

6. A 58-year-old man comes to the emergency department because he has had severe back pain for the past five days. He has no history of recent falls or injury, loss of control of bowel or bladder function, paresthesia, pallor, or radicular symptoms. He requests oxycodone for analgesia because acetaminophen and ibuprofen have not provided relief. The patient's medical record indicates that he has been evaluated at this emergency department multiple times this year for similar symptoms. Medical history includes multiple orthopedic injuries for which he required surgery. Physical examination shows multiple scars from the previous surgeries. No clear neuromuscular impairment is noted. It is most appropriate to refer this patient for physical therapy for treatment of the back pain and to also refer this patient to which of the following outpatient services?
   A. Alcoholics Anonymous
   B. Neurosurgery
   C. Opioid addiction counseling
   D. Orthopedic surgery

7. A 24-year-old woman comes to the office for follow-up two months after she was evaluated in the emergency department because she had been having frequent episodes of fear associated with chest pain, palpitations, nausea, and dizziness. She says that every day for the past two months she has been fearful that she will have another episode of these symptoms again. Current vital signs are within normal limits. The patient appears healthy and is alert and oriented. On physical examination, the pupils are equal, round, and reactive to light and accommodation. Cardiac auscultation shows a regular rhythm without murmur or ectopy. The lungs are clear to auscultation. Reflexes and coordination are intact. Results of laboratory studies including complete blood cell count, complete metabolic panel, and thyroid function studies are within normal limits. Based on these findings, which of the following is the most likely diagnosis?
   A. Adjustment disorder
   B. Bipolar disorder
   C. Conversion disorder
   D. Panic disorder
   E. Schizoaffective disorder

8. A 3-year-old boy is brought to the clinic by his mother as a new patient for routine well-child examination. The mother says that the previous primary care physician, who evaluated the patient at 2 years of age, was concerned about delayed development. The physician suggested at that time that they wait and see if the patient develops appropriately over the next year. The patient's health has been good, and immunizations are up-to-date. The mother is concerned because the patient has not started talking and shows no affection toward her, although he will hold her hand and be led when walking. At home, he spends hours quietly tugging at fibers in the carpet and does not interact with his two older siblings. Oftentimes, when in a new environment like a restaurant, the patient will start shouting and can only be consoled by offering him the salt and pepper shakers, the contents of which he promptly shakes onto the table or floor. He is in the 90th percentile for height and the 50th percentile for weight. Vital signs are within normal limits. Physical examination shows no abnormalities. This patient's behavior and development are most likely associated with which of the following disorders?
   A. Attention-deficit/hyperactivity disorder
   B. Autism spectrum disorder
   C. Childhood-onset fluency disorder
   D. Intellectual development disorder
   E. Prader-Willi syndrome

    Answer Key for this chapter begins on p. 166

9. A 27-year-old woman who is at 20 weeks' gestation comes to the office to discuss treatment options for major depressive disorder. The patient is currently taking sertraline 50 mg daily and doing well with this therapy. However, she wants to know what changes need to be made to her treatment regimen either for the remainder of her pregnancy or in the postpartum period. Which of the following is the most appropriate recommendation?
   A. Continue with the current medication regimen but stop once breastfeeding begins
   B. Discontinue sertraline now and begin cognitive behavioral therapy
   C. Increase the dose of sertraline in the postpartum period
   D. Increase the dose of sertraline in the third trimester
   E. Switch now to paroxetine 40 mg daily

10. A 38-year-old man comes to the emergency department because he has multiple injuries consistent with trauma. He says he tripped over his dog at home and fell down the stairs 30 minutes ago. The patient lives at home with his husband. Physical examination shows multiple bruises all over the body in various stages of healing, one of which appears to be handprint shaped. In addition to treating the patient's injuries, which of the following is another important concern to address?
   A. Depression with suicidal ideation
   B. Dissociative identity disorder
   C. Factitious disorder
   D. Intimate partner violence
   E. Substance use disorder

11. A 16-year-old boy is brought to the pediatrician's office by his mother because he has had changes in his behavior since his parents' divorce two months ago. The mother says the patient has been tearful, has started skipping school, and has had four episodes of fighting with his classmates. During the interview, the patient says he has not had harmful ideations. Medical history is unremarkable, and physical examination shows no abnormalities. Which of the following is the most appropriate intervention at this time?
   A. Anger management therapy
   B. Behavior modification therapy
   C. Oral fluoxetine therapy
   D. Oral lorazepam therapy
   E. Supportive psychotherapy

12. A 21-year-old man who is homeless is admitted to the behavioral health crisis center under police guard. Earlier in the day, the patient met his parents at a local convenience store. He has had worsening mental illness over the past three years, and it was the parents' goal for the meeting to convince him to voluntarily enter a psychiatric facility. During the meeting, the patient became increasingly agitated and started shouting that his father was Satan and was only there "to get him." The patient then pulled out a knife and stabbed his father in the head, killing him instantly. He ran from the store but was captured by police and taken to the crisis center. Vital signs are within normal limits, and the results of serum drug screen are negative. The patient is unable to provide a history because he displays diminished emotional expression at one time and then begins to converse with an imaginary individual at other times. After the patient is stabilized at the crisis center, he is discharged to the county jail. Which of the following medications is most appropriate to initiate at the time of discharge?
   A. Frovatriptan
   B. Lorazepam
   C. Memantine
   D. Olanzapine
   E. Pregabalin

13. A 32-year-old woman comes to the office because she has had difficulty sleeping, eating, and caring for her two children since her husband passed away suddenly six weeks ago. She does not have thoughts of harming herself or others, but she says she has intense pangs of grief and loneliness and cries frequently. According to the *Diagnostic and Statistical Manual of Mental Disorders*, 5th edition (DSM-5), this patient is most likely to meet the diagnostic criteria for complex bereavement disorder at which of the following timeframes?
   A. At any time if the patient believes her symptoms are causing impairment in daily function
   B. At any time if the patient develops thoughts of harming herself or others
   C. The patient meets the criteria at this time
   D. When the patient's symptoms persist for three months
   E. When the patient's symptoms persist for longer than six months

14. A 62-year-old woman returns to the office for follow-up of cellulitis. She says that treatment was successful, and the cellulitis has resolved. She now wants to discuss other symptoms that she has had for the past two years, which include decreased energy, increased need for sleep, difficulty concentrating, and feeling sad for no reason. The patient says her symptoms got worse after retiring from her job, and she wants to know if there is a medication she can take to relieve her symptoms. She does not drink alcoholic beverages or use illicit drugs. Vital signs are within normal limits, and physical examination shows no abnormalities. In addition to complete blood cell count, which of the following laboratory studies is most appropriate to order?
    A. Measurement of serum ferritin level
    B. Measurement of serum phosphate level
    C. Measurement of serum thyroid-stimulating hormone level
    D. Rheumatoid factor assay
    E. Tissue transglutaminase antibody test

15. A 64-year-old woman comes to the office for routine annual physical examination. Medical history includes coronary artery disease and myocardial infarction four months ago. During the interview, the patient says that she is still smoking one pack of cigarettes per day despite being urged to quit. The patient says that she is worried about quitting and has little confidence in her abilities to be successful. In addition to advising the patient about the benefits of quitting smoking, which of the following is the most appropriate next step?
    A. Advise the patient to quit cold turkey
    B. Arrange for a follow-up visit two months after the patient has quit smoking
    C. Assess the patient's readiness to quit
    D. Begin replacement therapy with nicotine patches
    E. Recommend the patient begin smoking e-cigarettes to decrease cravings

16. A 7-year-old girl is brought to the clinic by her grandfather for routine physical examination. The grandfather is the patient's only guardian, and she lives with no other siblings or family members. Weight is below the 5th percentile. The patient appears withdrawn and lethargic. Pulse rate is 130/min. Physical examination shows pale skin and a swollen tongue. If child abuse is suspected in this patient, which of the following additional findings is most likely to confirm this diagnosis?
    A. History of occasional bed wetting
    B. Laboratory findings of anemia
    C. Multiple bruises in various healing stages on the anterior lower extremities

D. Shyness that causes anxiety when the patient is asked to participate in school
E. X-ray studies showing a single radial fracture

17. A 21-year-old male college student is brought to the emergency department by his mother because he has had recent changes in his behavior, such as worsening distraction, talking excessively, and not sleeping at night. The mother says that the patient has been working day and night on a book that will provide evidence that the 2020 Presidential election was a fraud. After a thorough physical examination and laboratory studies, a manic episode of bipolar disorder is diagnosed, and treatment is discussed. In addition to recommending treatment with a mood stabilizer, which of the following is most likely to improve treatment adherence and decrease the risk of relapse?
    A. Adding an antidepressant to the treatment regimen
    B. Beginning a second mood stabilizer if there is no improvement in one week
    C. Discouraging the patient from participating in treatment decisions
    D. Initiating cognitive behavioral therapy
    E. Limiting family involvement in care and treatment

18. A 30-year-old man comes to the clinic because he has had episodes in which he unintentionally falls asleep during the day during the past four years. Physical examination shows no abnormalities. A daytime sleep study confirms abrupt REM sleep transitions, and narcolepsy is diagnosed. Treatment with dextroamphetamine is planned. In addition to measuring pulse rate and blood pressure, which of the following baseline evaluations is most appropriate?
    A. Cardiac
    B. Hepatic
    C. Neurologic
    D. Pulmonary
    E. Renal

19. A 40-year-old man who is a veteran comes to the office because he has had flashbacks, irritability, and inability to concentrate at work since he returned from overseas duty three months ago. Medical history includes traumatic brain injury while in the service. Pulse rate is 105/min. The patient appears restless. Physical examination shows a slight tremor of the hands. Which of the following is the most appropriate first-line treatment for this patient?
    A. Cognitive restructuring and reframing therapy
    B. Electroconvulsive therapy
    C. Fluoxetine therapy
    D. Mirtazapine therapy
    E. Prolonged exposure therapy

20. A 16-year-old girl is brought to the pediatric clinic by her mother because she is concerned about changes in the patient's behavior. During the past few months, the mother says that the patient has had frequent episodes of overeating, she has heard the patient vomiting shortly after dinner, and she found over-the-counter laxatives in the patient's bedroom. During the interview, the patient says she is anxious about being overweight and cannot stop thinking about it. She does not have harmful ideations. Vital signs are within normal limits. The patient appears neatly dressed, is wearing detailed makeup, is appropriately proportioned, and does not appear to be in acute distress. Results of a basic metabolic panel are within normal limits. Which of the following therapeutic regimens is most appropriate at this time?
    A. Gastroenterology consultation and therapy with sertraline
    B. Liver function studies and therapy with lorazepam
    C. Nutritional consultation and therapy with lorazepam
    D. Nutritional consultation and therapy with phentermine
    E. Psychotherapy and therapy with fluoxetine

21. A 33-year-old man comes to the office with his wife because she says he has spent a significant amount of time over the past two years gambling at a local casino. Although the patient's gambling has resulted in the loss of all equity in their house and high balances on several credit cards, he is adamant that he does not need help for an addiction. After he was fired from his job last week, his wife insisted that he be evaluated. After careful history taking, physical examination, and laboratory studies, no organic cause of this patient's behavior is determined. Which of the following statements made by the patient or observed during history taking is most likely to confirm a diagnosis of gambling disorder?
    A. He admits to having aggressive impulses that have resulted in assaults to others
    B. He expresses inflated self-esteem and grandiosity toward his abilities as a gambler
    C. He has a decreased need for sleep, with three hours usually enabling him to feel rested
    D. He says he develops significant physical tension before he arrives at and enters the casino
    E. He says he frequently returns to the casino the following day to get even with his losses

22. An 82-year-old woman is brought to the clinic by her caregiver for routine physical examination. The patient has dementia and is reliant on the caregiver in order to remain in her home. The patient and caregiver have no new complaints. A 12-lb weight loss is noted since the patient's most recent visit six months ago. Vital signs are within normal limits. Physical examination shows several small areas of ecchymosis on the arms and back that resemble bruises in various stages of healing. Physical abuse of the patient is suspected. Which of the following additional factors is most likely to increase the likelihood that this caregiver is abusing this patient?
    A. The caregiver also maintains a part-time job outside the patient's home
    B. The caregiver has only a high school-level education
    C. The caregiver is an employee of a home-health agency
    D. The caregiver is financially better off than the patient
    E. The caregiver is a relative who resides with the patient

23. A 24-year-old man comes to the clinic because he has had insomnia for the past two years. During the interview, he says that he feels stressed and anxious at his job and frequently thinks about how to improve his work performance. He feels fearful of making mistakes; therefore, he constantly rechecks his work and corrects the work of others. Which of the following is the most appropriate first-line treatment for this patient?
    A. Cognitive processing therapy
    B. Electroconvulsive therapy
    C. Exposure and response therapy
    D. Mirtazapine therapy
    E. Venlafaxine therapy

24. A 19-year-old woman comes to the emergency department because she has had worsening depression, anxiety, and thoughts of self-harm over the past three weeks. Medical history includes bulimia, prior suicide attempts, and alcohol use disorder. She also has a history of self-injurious behavior, is impulsive, and has extremely unstable relationships. Physical examination shows multiple areas of cutting on both upper extremities. The patient is admitted to the inpatient behavioral health unit for further management. During the patient's interaction with medical staff, she has rapid fluctuations in mood, from periods of confidence to despair. Which of the following personality disorders is most likely?
    A. Avoidant
    B. Borderline
    C. Histrionic
    D. Narcissistic
    E. Obsessive-compulsive

25. A 4-year-old boy is brought to the clinic by his parents because he has had inattentive, hyperactive, and impulsive behavior at home as well as at school during the past nine months. Medical history includes asthma and multiple food allergies. Immunizations are up-to-date. Height and weight are appropriate for his age. During the physical examination, the patient is fidgety and unable to sit still. Based on these findings, which of the following is the most appropriate initial treatment to recommend?
A. Elimination diet
B. Methylphenidate therapy
C. Neurofeedback therapy
D. Omega-3 fatty acid supplementation
E. Parent behavior training program

26. A 20-year-old woman comes to the clinic because she has had increasing worry and concern about her ability to remain in college as well as an increase in muscle tension and tightness in her shoulders and neck. She says she also has fatigue, which she attributes to an inability to get a good night's sleep. These symptoms have been intensifying over the past eight months. The patient intends to apply to a physician assistant school next year, but despite maintaining a 3.8 GPA, she feels constantly restless, as if she is on the edge of academic failure. She is otherwise healthy, takes no medications, and does not smoke cigarettes or use illicit drugs. Vital signs are within normal limits, and physical examination shows no abnormalities. Therapy with which of the following drugs is most appropriate to initiate in this patient?
A. Aripiprazole
B. Methylphenidate
C. Modafinil
D. Olanzapine
E. Venlafaxine

27. A 22-year-old man is brought to the emergency department by the police after he sustained a laceration to his left arm while being arrested for breaking and entering into his neighbor's garage. According to the patient, the patient's mother, and the police officer, the patient has a history of multiple arrests for minor infractions, impulsive behavior, fighting, quitting jobs, and not showing responsibility for his finances. The patient's mother says that this behavior started in his early teens. He has no history of suicidal ideations. Based on these findings, this patient most likely has which of the following personality disorders?
A. Antisocial
B. Borderline
C. Dependent
D. Narcissistic
E. Schizotypal

28. A 45-year-old man is brought to the emergency department by ambulance after he was found lying alongside the road 15 minutes ago. This is the third time over the past month that this patient has been brought to the emergency department due to similar circumstances. Review of the patient's medical records from a recent treatment program shows a 20-year history of alcohol use disorder, worsening resting tremors, awkward stance, unsteady gait, and frequent blackouts. Therapy with benzodiazepines was recently initiated. Oxygen saturation is 96% on room air; all other vital signs are within normal limits. Physical examination shows responsiveness to painful stimuli with posturing. Laboratory findings include the following:

Serum	
Alanine aminotransferase	60 U/L (N = 8–20 U/L)
Alkaline phosphatase	140 U/L (N = 20–70 U/L)
Aspartate aminotransferase	80 U/L (N = 8–20 U/L)
Blood alcohol level	0.30 g/dL

Which of the following findings most likely indicates that this is a medical emergency?
A. Alanine aminotransferase level
B. Blood alcohol concentration
C. Combination of alcohol and benzodiazepines
D. History of frequent blackouts
E. History of worsening stance and gait

 Answer Key for this chapter begins on p. 166

Answers

1. **Answer: E** This patient has overdosed on opiates. Withdrawal symptoms, option E, is correct because naloxone may induce acute withdrawal symptoms in a patient with opiate dependence.

   Projectile vomiting, pulmonary vasoconstriction, renal insufficiency, and sinus tachycardia (options A through D) are all incorrect because they are not commonly associated with the adverse effect profile of naloxone when the opiate effects are reversed. **Task:** D3—Pharmaceutical Therapeutics

2. **Answer: A** This patient has symptoms of depression and is a current smoker who wishes to quit. She has had a tubal ligation, so the risk of pregnancy is decreased. Bupropion, option A, has been proven effective to treat depression and to help with smoking cessation.

   Buspirone, option B, is used to treat anxiety and is not an appropriate treatment for this patient. Olanzapine, option C, is an appropriate treatment for refractory depression, which this patient does not have, and it is not appropriate to use for smoking cessation. Sertraline, option D, is used to treat depression but not smoking cessation. Venlafaxine, option E, is used to treat depression and anxiety, but it will not help with smoking cessation. **Task:** D3—Pharmaceutical Therapeutics

3. **Answer: D** The behaviors displayed by this patient are consistent with the diagnostic criteria for conduct disorder (option D). This disorder, when occurring in childhood or adolescence, is characterized by a repetitive and persistent pattern of behavior in which the rights of others or societal norms are violated. Broad categories of anomalous behavior include aggression toward people and animals, destruction of property, deceitfulness or theft, and serious violations of rules. Antisocial personality disorder, option A, is the persistence of conduct disorder into adulthood. While the diagnostic criteria for an antisocial personality disorder are similar to those of conduct disorder, a distinguishing characteristic is that the patient must be at least 18 years of age to receive the diagnosis. Attention-deficit/hyperactivity disorder (ADHD), option B, is characterized by inattention, hyperactivity, and impulsivity. The criminality and disregard for the rights of others displayed by this patient are not consistent with behaviors observed in ADHD. Borderline personality disorder, option C, is a common condition that affects up to 2% of the general population. Symptoms of this disorder may appear as early as the teen years to early 20s, with many cases not becoming evident until after 30 years of age. This disorder is best

   characterized as the individual having a tumultuous life with unstable moods and relationships, suicidal ideations, and often displaying self-injurious behavior, such as cutting. The term schizoid personality disorder, option E, is used to define adult individuals who demonstrate a detachment from social relationships and blunting of emotions in interpersonal situations. The person is generally described as aloof or a loner. While this patient may possess these characteristics, people with schizoid personality disorder are able to function in society without destructive behavior or violence. **Task:** A—History Taking and Performing Physical Examination

4. **Answer: A** This patient is experiencing symptoms of dissociative disorder, option A. Features of this disorder include a disturbance in identity, memory, perception, and consciousness. This disorder tends to develop after a patient experiences severe emotional or physical trauma.

   Generalized anxiety disorder and major depressive disorder, options B and C, often coexist with dissociative disorders but are not characterized by the symptoms described in this patient. Schizoaffective disorder, option D, is characterized by psychosis in the absence of mania or depression and by mood episodes (manic or depressed) with psychotic features. Schizophrenia, option E, is characterized by disorders of perceptions, cognition, and behavior with insidious onset, which this patient is not exhibiting. **Task:** A—History Taking and Performing Physical Examination

5. **Answer: A** The patient is exhibiting signs and symptoms consistent with anorexia nervosa, option A. In the patient's history, there are several indications of a reduced caloric intake, personal and professional pressure to be thin, and an excessive exercise schedule. Her body mass index places her in the severe category of anorexia. While anemia and decreased serum urea nitrogen and creatinine levels are common in anorexia, serum albumin is surprisingly within normal limits.

   Avoidant/restrictive food intake disorder, option B, is a condition that begins during infancy or early childhood. The disorder is characterized primarily by a lack of interest in eating or a distaste for certain food odors, textures, temperature, and/or colors. Although a decreased weight is characteristic of avoidant/restrictive food intake disorder, the patient's history makes this option incorrect. Bulimia nervosa, option C, is characterized by binge eating until the individual becomes painfully full. Purging through forced vomiting, use of laxatives or enemas, and excessive exercise typically follows the binge. Problems with dentition due to frequent exposure to stomach acid may begin as soon as six months after the onset of purging. Interestingly, individuals with bulimia nervosa usually maintain a relatively normal weight, rather than becoming underweight. These characteristics do not correlate with this patient scenario. Pica, option D, is a condition whereby individuals crave substances that are not considered food, such as ice, soil, soap or detergent, hair, and chalk. Pica can occur at any age but is usually observed in children, pregnant women, and individuals with mental disorders. Rumination disorder, option E, is characterized by regurgitating food already chewed and swallowed, rechewing it, and then either swallowing it again or spitting it out. The disorder can occur at any age and can lead to inadequate nutrition and the patient being underweight. This patient's history is inconsistent with this condition. **Task:** C—Formulating Most Likely Diagnosis

6. **Answer: C** This patient should be referred for opioid addiction counseling, option C, because he has signs and symptoms of opioid use disorder. He says that he has pain that cannot be relieved by medications other than an opioid, and he has a history of recurrent visits for similar requests. Another symptom of this drug-seeking behavior is emotional instability if a request for a specific medication is not met. This patient most likely developed an addiction to opioids while recovering from frequent orthopedic surgical procedures. Abuse and addiction to opioids have grown to become a significant global public health problem. Opiate use disorder is a chronic, relapsing condition that is influenced by psychosocial, socioeconomic, pharmacologic, genetic, behavioral, and environmental factors. It is characterized by recurrent self-administration of opiate medications, resulting in tolerance, dependence, and withdrawal.
Referral to Alcoholics Anonymous, option A, is not appropriate because this patient does not have symptoms or signs of alcohol use disorder. Referral to neurosurgery or orthopedic surgery, options B and D, are incorrect because this patient has no clinical signs or symptoms that warrant the need for surgical consultation. **Task:** D1—Health Maintenance, Patient Education, and Disease Prevention

7. **Answer: D** This patient is having symptoms of panic disorder, option D, which typically includes unexpected panic attacks followed by at least one month of anticipatory anxiety about having another attack.
Adjustment disorder, option A, is diagnosed when a stressful event happens in close proximity to the onset of similar symptoms as the ones in this patient. Bipolar disorder, option B, is unlikely without clear evidence of a period of mania. Conversion disorder, option C, includes symptoms of motor or sensory dysfunction such as paralysis, blindness, numbness, or the inability

to speak. Schizoaffective disorder, option E, is characterized by psychosis in the absence of mania or depression and by mood episodes (manic or depressed) with psychotic features, which are not present in this patient. **Task:** C—Formulating Most Likely Diagnosis

8. **Answer: B** This patient is exhibiting several patterns of behavior pathognomonic for option B, autism spectrum disorder (ASD). The two major characteristics of ASD are impairments in communication and social interaction and restricted, repetitive patterns of behavior, interests, or activities. Although this patient is only 3 years of age, he fits each of these descriptors.
Option A, attention-deficit/hyperactivity disorder (ADHD), is characterized by inattention, hyperactivity, and impulsivity. The CDC estimates that approximately 10% of children from 4 to 17 years of age have received a diagnosis of ADHD. While possible, making a diagnosis of ADHD in a 3-year-old is atypical. Childhood-onset fluency disorder, option C, includes what was previously described as stuttering. As stated, the child has yet to begin speaking, which makes this disorder an incorrect option. Intellectual development disorder, option D, presents in childhood as significantly below-average intellectual and adaptive functioning. Conditions that fall under this broad disorder include Down syndrome, fetal alcohol syndrome, phenylketonuria, and inborn errors of metabolism, such as Lesch-Nyhan syndrome. While some of this patient's behaviors fit into one or more of these conditions, when viewed collectively, his behaviors are all consistent with ASD. Prader-Willi syndrome, option E, is a genetic disorder usually caused by a partial deletion of chromosome 15. Common symptoms include behavior problems, intellectual disability, short stature, and constant hunger leading to obesity. As the growth chart figures denote, this patient is tall and slender. **Task:** A—History Taking and Performing Physical Examination

9. **Answer: D** Increasing the dose of sertraline in the third trimester, option D, is appropriate management because dose adjustments are frequently needed to maintain therapeutic effect in the later stages of pregnancy, due to lower serum drug concentrations.
Continuing with the current medication regimen but stopping once breastfeeding begins, option A, is incorrect because experts recommend continuing medication used during pregnancy through breastfeeding, as it may minimize adverse manifestations in the infant. Discontinue sertraline now and begin cognitive behavioral therapy, option B, is incorrect because discontinuing or decreasing medication during pregnancy can lead to prenatal relapse or postpartum depression. Increasing the dose of sertraline in the postpartum period, option C, is incorrect because serum drug

concentrations return to prepregnancy levels after delivery. Therefore, a decrease, not an increase, in medication may be necessary in the postpartum period. Paroxetine, option E, has been reported to cause cardiovascular malformations. Therefore, switching to this drug now is contraindicated in this patient. **Task:** D3—Pharmaceutical Therapeutics

10. **Answer: D** This patient has signs of intimate partner violence, option D, which is defined by the CDC as physical, psychological, or sexual actions or threats from one partner to another. It has been documented that approximately one in four men and approximately one in three women will experience intimate partner violence in their lifetime. Many patients may not be willing to disclose information regarding the circumstances of injuries, especially if social, economic, physical, or emotional safety might be compromised. Historical clues that should raise suspicion for intimate partner violence include a vague or changing history, a history that is inconsistent with the injuries, and a history of similar injuries.

    The pattern of injuries noted in this patient are concerning for injuries inflicted on the patient by another person. Depression with suicidal ideation and factitious disorder, options A and C, are considered when there is a concern for self-inflicted harm. Dissociative identity disorder, option B, is not applicable to this patient and is a rare condition in which there are two very distinct identities with developed memories within one person. Substance use disorder, option E, is only considered when there are traumas associated with drug and alcohol use. **Task:** A—History Taking and Performing Physical Examination

11. **Answer: E** Supportive psychotherapy, option E, is correct because this is the initial standard of care for new onset of an adjustment disorder.

    Options A and B, anger management therapy and behavior modification therapy, are incorrect because supportive psychotherapy will treat the root cause of this adolescent's behavior. Therapy with oral fluoxetine or lorazepam, options C and D, are incorrect because these drugs are used judiciously as adjuncts to supportive psychotherapy, especially if anxiety and depression are also present in this patient and unresponsive to psychotherapy alone. **Task:** D2—Clinical Intervention

12. **Answer: D** This patient is exhibiting many of the diagnostic criteria of schizophrenia including delusions (particularly that of persecution), hallucinations, and the negative symptom of diminished emotional expression. Other criteria include disorganized or incoherent speech, disorganized or catatonic behavior, and avolition. There are several pharmaceutical options to treat schizophrenia. Of the choices, olanzapine (option D), is the only medication indicated for the treatment of schizophrenia.

    While the incorrect options are excellent drugs for treating their respective conditions, none have been approved for the treatment of schizophrenia. Frovatriptan, option A, is indicated for the treatment of migraine and acts by activating vascular serotonin receptors to produce vasoconstriction. Lorazepam, option B, is a benzodiazepine indicated for the treatment of seizure disorder and anxiety. Memantine, option C, is indicated in the treatment of Alzheimer disease. Although its mechanism of action is unknown, pregabalin (option E) is indicated for the treatment of neuropathy/neuralgia. **Task:** D3—Pharmaceutical Therapeutics

13. **Answer: E** According to the *Diagnostic and Statistical Manual of Mental Disorders*, 5th edition criteria, complex bereavement disorder is diagnosed when grieving symptoms become chronically disabling and distressing for six months or longer after the death of a loved one. Therefore, option E is correct. The timeframes in the other options are incorrect. **Task:** A—History Taking and Performing Physical Examination

14. **Answer: C** This patient has symptoms of dysthymia, and there is no laboratory study that can confirm this diagnosis. However, this patient's symptoms, and the symptoms of most patients with depression, could possibly be caused by hypothyroidism or anemia. Therefore, measurement of complete blood cell count and thyroid-stimulating hormone level, option C, are appropriate to order when considering a diagnosis of depression.

    Measurement of serum ferritin level, option A, is incorrect because this is a marker for iron stores in the body. While measuring ferritin is included in the workup for anemia, anemia proper is diagnosed via complete blood cell count. Measurement of serum phosphate level, option B, may be abnormal in renal disease and certain nutritional disorders. It will not be helpful in this patient presenting with symptoms of depression. Rheumatoid factor assay, option D, is a test to support a diagnosis of rheumatoid arthritis. Tissue transglutaminase antibody test, option E, helps to diagnose celiac disease, which usually presents with gastrointestinal symptoms or anemia. **Task:** B—Using Diagnostic and Laboratory Studies

15. **Answer: C** Assessing the patient's readiness to quit, option C, is the correct answer. All current smokers should be advised of the benefits of smoking cessation and then assessed for their readiness to quit.

    Advising the patient to quit cold turkey, option A, is incorrect. The use of pharmacotherapy and behavior support is found to increase successful tobacco cessation compared with using minimal/no pharmacotherapy intervention. Arranging for follow-up two months after the patient has quit smoking, option B, is incorrect. It is recommended that patients follow up within three to seven days after their scheduled quit date and at least monthly for three months thereafter.

Although replacement therapy with nicotine patches, option D, is used for smoking cessation, this option is only good if the patient is ready to quit. Recommend the patient begin smoking e-cigarettes to decrease cravings, option E, is incorrect. The use of e-cigarettes is not recommended due to an increased risk of lung disease. **Task:** D2—Clinical Intervention

16. **Answer: B** This patient is underweight and withdrawn and lethargic. Her pale skin, swollen tongue, and rapid pulse rate are consistent with iron deficiency anemia. Laboratory findings of anemia, option B, is correct because many children who suffer abuse or neglect may be underweight, withdrawn, have impaired attention span, and have anemia; these findings are related to malnutrition, which is a form of neglect.

History of occasional bed wetting, option A, is not indicative of abuse. Bed wetting can be a sign of stress but is generally considered a part of normal development in this age group. Multiple bruises in various healing stages on the anterior lower extremities, option C, is incorrect because bruising is common in children at this age. Bruising on the back, flank, and neck are less common and more concerning for child abuse. Shyness that causes anxiety when the patient is asked to participate at school, option D, is normal and is a common finding in children of this age. It is not an indication of abuse or neglect. X-ray studies showing a single radial fracture, option E, is incorrect because fractures of the upper extremities are common in young, active children. Child abuse should be suspected in a child with multiple fractures at various stages of healing. **Task:** A—History Taking and Performing Physical Examination

17. **Answer: D** Cognitive behavioral therapy, option D, used in conjunction with mood stabilizers, decreases relapse, improves function, and increases treatment adherence.

Adding an antidepressant to the treatment regimen, option A, will increase the risk of triggering manic episodes, thereby increasing the risk of relapse. Beginning a second mood stabilizer if there is no improvement in one week, option B, is incorrect. A patient is considered a nonresponder if there is no response to treatment within two weeks, after which time a medication adjustment should be considered. Discouraging the patient from participating in treatment decisions, option C, is incorrect. Patients should be encouraged to participate in treatment decisions. Evidence shows that individualized treatment based on the patient's

beliefs, values, and expectations improves adherence and quality of life. Limiting family involvement in care, option E, is incorrect. Close collaboration with family helps providers identify and manage stressful periods where the risk of relapse is increased, allowing for timely intervention. **Task:** D1—Health Maintenance, Patient Education, and Disease Prevention

18. **Answer: A** A baseline cardiac evaluation, option A, is indicated when prescribing a stimulant such as dextroamphetamine because of its cardiovascular side effect profile.

Hepatic, neurologic, pulmonary, and renal evaluations (options B through D) are not indicated when initiating dextroamphetamine, because these systems are not commonly affected by this medication. **Task:** D2—Clinical Intervention

19. **Answer: E** This patient has post-traumatic stress disorder (PTSD). To date, cognitive behavioral therapy (CBT), including prolonged exposure therapy (option E) and cognitive processing, have the greatest empirical support among psychotherapy approaches in the treatment of PTSD.

Cognitive restructuring and reframing therapy, option A, is a form of CBT used in patients with negative thinking patterns called cognitive distortions. Electroconvulsive therapy, option B, is a form of therapy used to treat major depressive disorder and not PTSD. Drug therapy with fluoxetine or mirtazapine, options C and D, is not preferred over CBT for the treatment of PTSD. Sertraline and paroxetine are the only FDA-approved medications for PTSD. Other medications, including fluoxetine and mirtazapine, have been used off-label for the treatment of PTSD. **Task:** D3—Pharmaceutical Therapeutics

20. **Answer: E** This patient has bulimia nervosa. Psychotherapy and therapy with fluoxetine, option E, is correct because these combined therapies are most appropriate for treating patients with classic bulimia nervosa. Psychotherapy is the mainstay of treatment, and fluoxetine is the medication with the most favorable results.

Options A through D are incorrect. First, gastroenterology consultation (option A) is not indicated, liver function studies (option B) are nonspecific, and nutritional consultation (options C and D) will not help the root cause of this patient's condition. Sertraline therapy (option A) is used to treat depression, but it has not been found to be useful in treating bulimia. Lorazepam (options B and C) is used to treat anxiety, but anxiety in this patient is a symptom and not the root cause of the bulimia nervosa. Phentermine (option D) is an appetite suppressant, which is not indicated for this patient or this disorder. **Task:** D2—Clinical Intervention

21. **Answer: E** Option E describes a need to gamble again in order to chase one's losses. This characteristic is typical of a gambling disorder. Other criteria include the following behaviors over a 12-month period: the need to gamble with increasing amounts of money to achieve the desired level of excitement, becoming irritable or restless when attempting to cut down or stop gambling, being preoccupied with gambling and with ways to obtain money to continue, concealing the extent of gambling involvement, incurring the loss of relationships and/or career due to gambling, and having to rely on others to provide financial resources to cover responsibilities (e.g., mortgage, car payment). Episodes of aggressive impulses leading to assaults or destruction of property, option A, are consistent with intermittent explosive disorder. The lifetime prevalence of this disorder is estimated at 5% to 7% of the general population. Inflated self-esteem, grandiosity, and a decreased need for sleep (options B and C) are diagnostic criteria for mania. Mania by itself can occur. However, it most often cycles over months with depressive episodes as a bipolar disorder. These are incorrect choices, because they are not criteria for a gambling addiction, and because the behavior of this patient has persisted for over two years without cycling. Developing tension leading up to the act, option D, and pleasurable anticipation of acting on the impulse is consistent with impulse-control disorders. These disorders include pedophilia, eating disorders, substance-related disorders, kleptomania, intermittent explosive disorder, and pyromania. **Task:** A—History Taking and Performing Physical Examination

22. **Answer: E** Studies have shown that risk factors for caregiver-inflicted elder abuse, whether physical, mental, neglectful, sexual, or financial, include a feeling by the caregiver of being overwhelmed or resentful, a history of substance abuse, a history of abusing others, dependence on the older person for housing or finances, a history of mental health problems, unemployment, a criminal history, or sharing a living situation with the older person. Furthermore, lower income or poverty appear to be associated with abusive individuals. Therefore, option E is correct, and options A and D are incorrect.

Level of education of the caregiver, option B, is not included as a risk factor for those who abuse the elderly. Although anyone can be an abuser, abuse from a caretaker who is employed by a home-health agency, option C, is most often associated with neglect and inadequate training of the paid individual. **Task:** D1—Health Maintenance, Patient Education, and Disease Prevention

23. **Answer: C** This patient has obsessive-compulsive disorder (OCD). Both pharmacotherapy and psychotherapy are considered first-line treatment for OCD, either alone or in combination. The most effective behavioral treatment for OCD is exposure and response therapy, option C, where the individual learns alternative responses to anxiety-provoking stimuli or situations.

Cognitive processing therapy, option A, is a form of cognitive behavioral therapy used in the treatment of patients with post-traumatic stress disorder. Electroconvulsive therapy, option B, is a form of therapy used in the treatment of major depressive disorder. Mirtazapine and venlafaxine, options D and E, are second-line agents if a patient is not responsive to a selective serotonin reuptake inhibitor. **Task:** D3—Pharmaceutical Therapeutics

24. **Answer: B** This patient has borderline personality disorder, option B, which can be diagnosed in childhood, teenage years, or adulthood. It is well differentiated by classic clinical symptoms, including severe fear of abandonment, labile mood, instability in interpersonal relationships and self-image, as well as a significant lack of impulse control.

The patient is not showing signs of the alternative personality types listed in the other options. Avoidant personality disorder, option A, is classified by symptoms of social discomfort, feelings of inadequacy, and lack of desire for intimacy. Histrionic personality disorder, option C, is classified by attention-seeking behavior, dramatic conversation, and rapidly changing emotions. Narcissistic personality disorder, option D, is classified by lack of empathy for others, a need for excessive admiration, troubled relationships, and an inflated sense of importance. Obsessive-compulsive personality disorder, option E, is classified by a need for control as well as a devotion to lists, rules, and perfectionism that interferes with interpersonal relationships and sometimes with the efficiency of time. **Task:** A—History Taking and Performing Physical Examination

25. **Answer: E** This preschool-aged patient has attention-deficit/hyperactivity disorder (ADHD). Recommending a parent behavior training program, option E, is the most appropriate initial treatment. According to the American Academy of Child and Adolescent Psychology, behavioral interventions are recommended for at least eight weeks before starting a pharmacologic agent if behavior management fails.

An elimination diet, option A, is not considered appropriate first-line treatment for preschool-aged patients with ADHD. Diets eliminating artificial food dyes and allergens may be effective in some children, but studies focusing on preschoolers are limited. Methylphenidate, option B, is a psychostimulant, which is not recommended as treatment before a trial of behavioral therapy. Neurofeedback therapy, option C, is incorrect because its efficacy is not conclusive in preschoolers. Omega-3 fatty acid supplementation, option D, in the treatment of ADHD has shown mixed results, and preschool-aged children were not included in the studies. **Task: D2—Clinical Intervention**

26. **Answer: E** This patient is exhibiting signs of generalized anxiety disorder (GAD). These include apprehensive expectations, difficulty in controlling worry, restlessness, muscle tension, and sleep disturbance occurring more days than not for at least six months. Other symptoms that complete the criteria for GAD include difficulty concentrating, irritability, difficulty controlling worry, and impairment in social, occupational, or other important areas of functioning. The correct answer is venlafaxine, option E. In addition to venlafaxine, other selective serotonin reuptake inhibitors have specific indications for the treatment of GAD including escitalopram, duloxetine, and paroxetine. Cautious use of benzodiazepines and psychotherapy are also options in the treatment of GAD.

Options A and D, aripiprazole and olanzapine, are both indicated for the treatment of schizophrenia and bipolar disorder. Aripiprazole is also indicated in the treatment of a major depressive disorder. Neither drug is indicated for anxiety-related disorders. Methylphenidate, option B, is indicated for the treatment of attention-deficit/hyperactivity disorder. It is likely that using a central nervous system stimulant such as methylphenidate would only serve to exacerbate this patient's symptoms. Modafinil, option C, is indicated for narcolepsy, obstructive sleep apnea, shift-work sleep disorder, and fatigue associated with multiple sclerosis. Although the patient reports sleep-related issues, the etiology is specifically anxiety-related rather than those indicated for use of modafinil. **Task: D3—Pharmaceutical Therapeutics**

27. **Answer: A** This patient has antisocial personality disorder, option A. The criteria for this disorder include three or more traits such as ignoring the law, acting impulsively, being easily provoked or aggressive, and not showing financial responsibility. All of these traits are noted in this patient's history and current behavior. Also, the individual must be 18 years of age or older to be diagnosed with this disorder, as in this patient's case.

Borderline personality disorder, option B, is often associated with suicidal behavior, which this patient does not have. Dependent personality disorder, option C, is associated more with passivity. Narcissistic personality disorder, option D, is not commonly associated with the type of aggression that is present in this patient. Schizotypal personality disorder, option E, is associated with odd speech and eccentric behaviors, which are not present in this patient. **Task: A—History Taking and Performing Physical Examination**

28. **Answer: B** Blood alcohol concentration, option B, is correct because concentrations between 0.30 and 0.40 g/dL can result in death.

An increased alanine aminotransferase level, option A, does not place the patient in immediate danger. The combination of alcohol and benzodiazepines, option C, increases the risk for overdose in this patient, but the medical emergency is his increased blood alcohol level. History of frequent blackouts, option D, and history of worsening stance and gait, option E, are effects of long-term alcohol use but do not constitute a medical emergency. **Task: D2—Clinical Intervention**

BIBLIOGRAPHY

American Psychiatric Association. (2013). Borderline personality disorder: In: *Diagnostic and statistical manual of mental disorders* (5th ed., pp. 663-666). American Psychiatric Association.

American Psychiatric Association. (2013). Opioid-related disorders: In: *Diagnostic and statistical manual of mental disorders* (5th ed., pp. 540-549). American Psychiatric Association.

Antisocial Personality Disorder (ASPD). (n.d.). Retrieved March 29, 2021, from Merckmanuals.com.

Bachem, R. (2018). Adjustment disorders: A diagnosis whose time has come. *Journal of Affective Disorders, 227,* 243-253.

Barlow, D. H., & Durand, V. M. (2015). *Abnormal psychology: An integrative approach* (7th ed.).

Barua, R. S., Rigotti, N. A., Benowitz, N. L., Cummings, K. M., Jazayeri, M.-A., Morris, P. B., et. al. (2018). 2018 ACC Expert Consensus Decision Pathway on Tobacco Cessation Treatment: A report of the American College of Cardiology Task Force on Clinical Expert Consensus Documents. *Journal of the American College of Cardiology, 72*(25), 3332-3365.

Bernstein, D., & Shelov, S. P. (2003). *Pediatrics for medical students* (2nd ed., pp. 105-111). Lippincott Williams and Wilkins.

Boelen, P. A., Lenferink, L. I., & Smid, G. E. (2019). Further evaluation of the factor structure, prevalence, and concurrent validity of DSM-5 criteria for persistent complex bereavement disorder and ICD-11 criteria for prolonged grief disorder. *Psychiatry Research, 273,* 206-210.

Bruneau, J., Ahamad, K., Goyer, M. È., Poulin, G., Selby, P., Fischer. B., et. al. (2018). Management of opioid use disorders: A national clinical practice guideline. *Canadian Medical Association Journal, 190,* E247-E257.

Chand, S. P., & Arif, H. (2021). Depression [Updated November 18, 2020]: *StatPearls [Internet].* StatPearls Publishing. Available from: https://www.ncbi.nlm.nih.gov/books/NBK430847/.

Clinical Overview: Major depressive disorder in pregnancy. (2020). In *Elsevier Point of Care.* Elsevier.

Compton, W. M. (2016). Relationship between nonmedical prescription-opioid use and heroin use. *New England Journal of Medicine, 374,* 154-163.

Answer Key for this chapter begins on p. 166

D'Avanzato, C. (2021, January 1). *Ferri's clinical advisor 2021* (pp. 1143-1144). Elsevier.

DeBattista, C. (2021). Psychiatric adjustment disorders. In M. A. Papadakis, S. J. McPhee, & M. W. Rabow (Eds.), *Current medical diagnosis & treatment*. McGraw-Hill.

Domino, F. J., Baldor, R. A., Golding, J., & Stephens, M. B. (2019). *The 5-minute clinical consult 2020*. Lippincott Williams & Wilkins.

Epocrates [online]. (2013). *Epocrates, Inc.* http://www.epocrates. com. Updated continuously.

Ferguson, J. E., 2nd. (2010). Why doesn't SOMEBODY do something? *American Journal of Obstetrics and Gynecology, 202*(6), 635-664.

Go, J. Naloxone. (2018). In: K. R. Olson, I. B. Anderson, N. L. Benowitz, P. D. Blanc, R. F. Clark, T. E. Kearney, S. Y. Kim-Katz, & A. B. Wu (Eds.), *Poisoning & drug overdose* (7th ed.). McGraw-Hill.

Gardner, D. G., & Shoback, D. (2018). *Greenspan's basic & clinical endocrinology* (10th ed., pp. 152). McGraw-Hill Education.

Houts, A., Sheets, K., Okonkwo, N., Kerzner, L. J. (2021). Detecting, assessing, & responding to elder mistreatment. In: L. C. Walter, A. Chang, P. Chen, G. Harper, J. Rivera, R. Conant, D. Lo, & M. Yukawa (Eds.), *Current diagnosis & treatment geriatrics* (3rd ed.). McGraw-Hill.

Kalia, R., & Walling, A. (2020, January 1) *Conn's current therapy 2020* (pp. 796-799). Elsevier.

Kosten, T. R., & Haile, C. N. (2018). Opioid-related disorders. In: J. Jameson, A. S. Fauci, D. L. Kasper, S. L. Hauser, D. L. Longo, & J. Loscalzo (Eds.), *Harrison's principles of internal medicine* (20th ed.). McGraw-Hill.

Li, L. (2020). Mood disorders. In F. R. Amthor, A. B. Theibert, D. G. Standaert, & E. D. Roberson (Eds.), *Essentials of modern neuroscience*. McGraw-Hill.

Lyness, J. (2020). Psychiatric disorders in medical practice. *Goldman-Cecil Medicine, 369*, 2305-2315.

Lyness, J. Psychiatric disorders in medical practice. *Goldman-Cecil Medicine*, 369, 2305-2315.

Miller, B. J. (2020). Schizophrenia. *Conn's current therapy* (pp. 806-809). Elsevier.

Munir, K. M., Friedman, S. L., & Leonard, E. L. (2019). Intellectual disability (intellectual developmental disorder). In: M. H. Ebert, J. F. Leckman, I. L. Petrakis (Eds.). *Current diagnosis & treatment: Psychiatry* (3rd ed.). McGraw-Hill.

Papadakis, M. A., McPhee, S. J., & Bernstein, J. (Eds.). (2020). In: *Quick medical diagnosis & treatment 2020*. McGraw-Hill.

Orchowski, L. M. (2021). Dissociative disorders. *Ferri's clinical advisor 2021* (pp. 479.e2). Elsevier.

Smith R. C., & Osborn G. G., & Dwamena F. C., & D'Mello D, & Freilich L, & Laird-Fick H. S.(Eds.). (2019). Other disorders and issues in primary care. In: *Essentials of psychiatry in primary care: Behavioral health in the medical setting*. McGraw-Hill.

Rigotti, N. A., & Kalkhoran, S. (2019). Tobacco use. In M. D. Feldman, J. F. Christensen, J. M. Satterfield, & R. Laponis (Eds.), *Behavioral medicine: A guide for clinical practice* (5th ed.). McGraw-Hill.

Saltzman, L., Fanslow, J., McMahon, P., & Shelley, G. A. (2002). Intimate partner violence surveillance: Uniform definitions and recommended data elements, version 1.0, Atlanta.

Saunders, K. H., & Igel, L. I. (2021). Bulimia nervosa. In M. A. Papadakis, S. J. McPhee, & M. W. Rabow (Eds.), *Current medical diagnosis & treatment*. McGraw-Hill.

Schuckit, M. A. (2018). Alcohol and alcohol use disorders. In: J. Jameson, A. S. Fauci, D. L. Kasper, S. L. Hauser, D. L. Longo, & J. Loscalzo (Eds.), *Harrison's principles of internal medicine* (20th ed.). McGraw-Hill.

Tandon, M., & Pergjika, A. (2017). Attention deficit hyperactivity disorder in preschool age children. *Child and Adolescent Psychiatric Clinics of North America, 26*(3), 523-538.

Wehler, C. (2020). Panic disorder. *Conn's current therapy* (pp. 800-802). Elsevier.

Wu, V., Huff, H., & Bhandari, M. (2010). Pattern of physical injury associated with intimate partner violence in women presenting to the emergency department: A systematic review and meta-analysis. *Trauma Violence Abuse, 11*, 71-82.

Zanarini, M. C., Vujanovic, A. A., Parachini, E. A., Boulanger, J. L., Frankenburg, F. R., & Hennen, J. (2003). A screening measure for BPD: The McLean Screening Instrument for Borderline Personality Disorder (MSI-BPD). *Journal of Personality Disorders, 17*(6), 568-573.

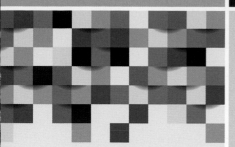

CHAPTER 12
Pulmonary System

Questions

1. A 45-year-old White woman comes to the clinic for routine annual physical examination. Medical history includes well-controlled type 2 diabetes mellitus and obesity with a body mass index of 34 kg/m² (N = 18.5-24.9 kg/m²). The patient says that her partner has told her that she snores at night, and she wonders if she may have obstructive sleep apnea. Which of the following findings in this patient most likely increases her risk of this condition?
   A. Age less than 50 years
   B. Caucasian race
   C. Female sex
   D. Obesity
   E. Type 2 diabetes mellitus

2. A 19-year-old woman who is a college student comes to the student health clinic because she has had fever, chills, hacking, nonproductive cough, wheezing, malaise, and generalized body aches for the past two days. She has not had rhinitis, diarrhea, or a change in taste or smell. The patient lives in a dormitory on campus and says several women on her floor have similar symptoms. A few of the women were examined at a local urgent care clinic and were prescribed antibiotic therapy. Temperature is 38.6°C (101.4°F), and respirations are 12/min. Pulse rate and blood pressure are within normal limits. Oxygen saturation is 96% on room air. Physical examination shows faint wheezes scattered in the midlung fields, bilaterally. Results of rapid influenza and COVID-19 tests are negative. Which of the following is the most likely diagnosis?
   A. Bronchitis
   B. Croup
   C. Pleurisy
   D. Pneumococcal pneumonia
   E. Pneumonitis

3. A 62-year-old man is brought to the emergency department by ambulance because he had sudden onset of coughing up copious amounts of blood 30 minutes ago. He also has had worsening dyspnea at rest and fatigue over the past week. Medical history includes chronic obstructive pulmonary disease, stroke, and heart failure; the patient takes several medications and uses supplemental oxygen. Temperature is 37.1°C (98.8°F), pulse rate is 104/min, respirations are 24/min, and blood pressure is 98/68 mmHg in both arms. Oxygen saturation is 86% via a portable oxygen concentrator. Physical examination shows jugular venous distension, poor air flow but audible breath sounds in all fields on inspiration, and an S_4 heart sound. Hepatomegaly with tenderness to palpation, an abdominal fluid wave, and 3+ bilateral dependent edema are also noted. Electrocardiography shows right-axis deviation. Chest x-ray study shows no active infiltrate, but significant cardiomegaly is noted. In addition to right heart failure, which of the following pathophysiologic processes is most likely present in this patient?
   A. Cardiac tamponade
   B. Esophageal varices
   C. Portal vein thrombosis
   D. Pulmonary hypertension
   E. Tension pneumothorax

4. A 4-year-old boy is brought to the urgent care clinic because he has had a runny nose and cough for the past four days. This morning, he woke up with a fever and worsening cough. Medical history includes no chronic disease conditions or asthma, and immunizations are up-to-date. Temperature is 38.3°C (101.0°F), and respirations are 50/min (N = 22–34/min in pediatric patients). On physical examination, edema of the nasal turbinates is noted; examination of the ears and throat shows no abnormalities. Tachypnea, intercostal retractions, and wheezing in the lower lungs are also noted. Which of the following findings on chest x-ray study is most likely to indicate that this patient has viral pneumonia rather than pneumococcal bacterial pneumonia?
   A. Air bronchograms
   B. Bilateral interstitial infiltrates
   C. Lobar consolidation
   D. Pleural effusion
   E. Well-defined, rounded opacities

5. A 62-year-old woman comes to the office because she has had dyspnea on exertion during the past six months. She has a 40–pack-year history of cigarette smoking. On physical examination, pectus carinatum is noted. Auscultation of the lungs shows diminished breath sounds in the lungs, bilaterally. Chest x-ray study shows hyperinflation with flattening of the diaphragm bilaterally. These findings are most consistent with which of the following diagnoses?
   A. Chronic bronchitis
   B. Emphysema
   C. Polymyositis
   D. Pulmonary embolism
   E. Sarcoidosis

6. A 2-year-old girl is brought to the emergency department by her mother because she had sudden onset of barking cough with labored breathing 30 minutes ago. The patient has had symptoms of an upper respiratory tract infection for the past two days. Physical examination shows a barking cough and inspiratory stridor. X-ray studies of the neck and chest show narrowing of the upper trachea and subglottis. Which of the following is the most appropriate treatment?
   A. Administration of antitoxin
   B. Administration of dexamethasone
   C. Initiation of albuterol as needed
   D. Initiation of empiric antibiotics
   E. Placement in droplet isolation

7. A 31-year-old woman comes to the emergency department because she has had shortness of breath and fatigue for the past three months. She says the fatigue is profound and interferes with her ability to work full-time. Two weeks ago, she had sudden eruption of painful red nodules on both lower extremities. Current temperature is 37.2°C (99.9°F). Physical examination shows diminished lung sounds. Chest x-ray study shows bilateral hilar lymphadenopathy with pulmonary infiltrates. The presence of which of the following on laboratory studies is most likely to determine the diagnosis?
   A. Acid-fast bacilli
   B. Beryllium lymphocyte proliferation
   C. Fungus isolation on silver stain
   D. Malignant cells on mediastinal biopsy
   E. Noncaseating granulomas

8. A 62-year-old woman comes to the clinic for routine physical examination. Medical history includes hypertension, emphysema, and obstructive sleep apnea. Medications include metoprolol and ipratropium bromide. She has a 42–pack-year history of cigarette smoking. Physical examination shows no abnormalities. Chest x-ray study of the lungs shows multiple diffuse nodules of various sizes that appear solid with smooth margins. Which of the following is the most likely diagnosis?
   A. Histoplasmosis nodules
   B. Metastasis
   C. Rheumatoid nodules
   D. Septic emboli
   E. Wegener granulomatosis

9. A 25-year-old man comes to the emergency department immediately after he was stabbed in his right upper back. He says he has extreme shortness of breath. Pulse rate is 110/min, respirations are 24/min and labored, and blood pressure is 80/50 mmHg; he is afebrile. Oxygen saturation is 90% on room air. Physical examination shows tracheal deviation to the left and distended neck veins. Lung sounds are absent on the right and present on the left. Heart sounds are muffled but present. The abdomen is soft and nontender. No distention is noted, and active bowel sounds are noted. Which of the following is the most appropriate immediate next step?
   A. Chest x-ray study
   B. CT scan of the chest
   C. Focused assessment with sonography for trauma (FAST) examination of the chest
   D. Needle decompression of the chest
   E. Tube thoracostomy of the chest

10. A 72-year-old man who is HIV positive is brought to the emergency department by his daughter because he has had altered mental status for the past six hours. He also has had fever to 38.8°C (101.8°F), chills, headache, and fatigue during the past three days. He has been taking acetaminophen for treatment of the headache and fever. Medical history includes no other chronic disease conditions. Oxygen saturation is 88% on room air. Result of rapid influenza test is positive for influenza B virus, and the patient is admitted to the hospital. Which of the following guidelines should be followed by the health care team during this patient's hospitalization?
   A. Implement airborne precautions by placing the patient in a negative-pressure room
   B. Place personal protective equipment that was used when caring for the patient on a hook outside the patient's door to be reused the next time he requires care
   C. Place the patient on droplet precautions until 24 hours after the respiratory symptoms and fever resolve
   D. Use alcohol-based hand rubs to clean hands that are visibly soiled after interactions with the patient
   E. Wear a gown and gloves for all interactions and use disposable or dedicated patient-care equipment when available

11. A 48-year-old woman with a history of hypertension and asthma comes to the office because she has had wheezing, chest tightness, coughing, and shortness of breath that have been worsening over the past two days despite treatment with inhalational albuterol and fluticasone propionate-salmeterol. She has not had any recent exposure to allergens or travel, and she has not had fever, chills, or chest pain. Vital signs are within normal limits. On physical examination, auscultation of the lungs shows inspiratory and expiratory wheezing. Chest x-ray study shows no abnormalities. Recent addition of which of the following medications to this patient's regimen is most likely to have caused this exacerbation of asthma?
A. Amlodipine
B. Losartan
C. Metoprolol
D. Montelukast
E. Nedocromil

12. A 76-year-old man with chronic obstructive pulmonary disease (COPD) is admitted to the hospital because he has had an acute exacerbation with increasing dyspnea over the past two weeks. Temperature is 37.3°C (99.2°F), pulse rate is 110/min, respirations are 28/min, and blood pressure is 130/84 mmHg. Oxygen saturation is 88% on room air. On physical examination, a barrel-shaped chest is noted, as well as significant jugular venous distention. Auscultation of the chest shows inspiratory crackles. Peripheral edema is noted. Chest x-ray study shows hyperinflated lungs and mild cardiomegaly. Which of the following conditions has most likely developed in this patient as a consequence of COPD?
A. Bronchiectasis
B. Cor pulmonale
C. Lung cancer
D. Peripheral artery disease
E. Pulmonary fibrosis

13. A 36-year-old man comes to the office for a preemployment physical examination. He says he is starting a new job in three weeks, and they require that he undergo PPD skin testing. The patient receives the skin test at the end of the physical examination, and he returns 60 hours later with 8 mm of induration. Which of the following findings on history taking is most likely to indicate that this is a positive PPD skin test in this patient?
A. He is an immigrant who has lived in the United States for seven years
B. He is currently working at a correctional facility
C. He is healthy and has no risk factors for tuberculosis
D. He is taking adalimumab for treatment of severe Crohn disease
E. He is taking insulin lispro and insulin glargine for treatment of uncontrolled diabetes mellitus

14.

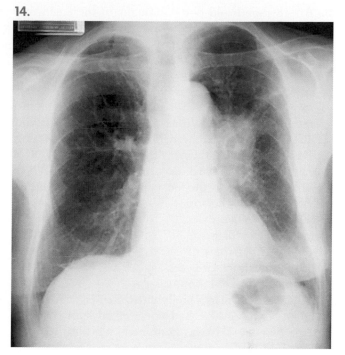

A 56-year-old man comes to the office because he has had unintentional weight loss of 15 lb and a cough during the past three months. He has a 25−pack-year history of cigarette smoking. Temperature is 36.9°C (98.4°F), pulse rate is 86/min, respirations are 20/min, and blood pressure is 118/74 mmHg. The patient is alert and oriented. On physical examination, cardiac auscultation shows a regular rhythm. Auscultation of the lungs shows diminished breath sounds bilaterally without rhonchi or wheezing. No edema is noted. Chest x-ray study is shown. Which of the following is the most likely diagnosis?
A. Adenocarcinoma
B. Carcinoid tumor
C. Pulmonary embolism
D. Sarcoidosis
E. Small-cell carcinoma

15. A 34-year-old woman who is pregnant comes to the emergency department because she has had worsening shortness of breath and nonproductive cough for the past two days. She also has had right-sided chest pain that worsens with deep inspiration. Pulse rate is 110/min, respirations are 20/min, and blood pressure is 138/78 mmHg. Oxygen saturation is 90% room air. On physical examination, the lungs are clear to auscultation. Examination of the lower extremities shows 1+ pitting edema, no calf tenderness, and 2/4 palpable pedal pulses. CT scan of the chest shows a moderate-sized pulmonary embolism. Which of the following is the most appropriate treatment for this patient?
A. Clopidogrel
B. Dabigatran
C. Enoxaparin
D. Rivaroxaban
E. Warfarin

    Answer Key for this chapter begins on p. 181

16. An 18-month-old boy is brought to the emergency department by his parents because he has had a runny nose, sneezing, cough, fever, and decreased appetite for the past four days. The parents say that he has been otherwise healthy and only has had one ear infection since birth. Vital signs are within normal limits except for a temperature of 39.1°C (102.3°F). Oxygen saturation is 98% on room air. On physical examination, auscultation of the chest shows expiratory wheezing. Result of a rapid influenza test is negative, and result of rapid respiratory syncytial virus test is positive. Which of the following is the most appropriate treatment?
    A. Antibiotic therapy
    B. Antipyretics
    C. Bronchodilators
    D. Corticosteroids
    E. No treatment is necessary

17. A 72-year-old man is brought to the emergency department because he has had worsening dyspnea over the past two days. He was examined by his primary care provider five days ago because he had a cough and fever; pneumonia was diagnosed, and he was treated with antibiotic therapy. He says his symptoms persisted despite treatment and then recently became worse. He smokes one-half pack of cigarettes daily. Temperature is 38.3°C (101.0°F), pulse rate is 120/min, respirations are 28/min, and blood pressure is 120/70 mmHg. Oxygen saturation is 86% on room air. The patient appears ill and has shortness of breath. Physical examination of the lungs shows diminished breath sounds. Cardiac examination shows tachycardia with a regular rhythm. Acute respiratory distress syndrome is suspected. Which of the following findings on chest x-ray study is most likely to support this diagnosis?
    A. Bilateral diffuse alveolar opacities
    B. Enlargement of the heart
    C. Large pleural effusion causing tracheal deviation
    D. Multiple lung nodules
    E. Symmetric hilar and mediastinal lymphadenopathy

18. A 25-year-old man with cystic fibrosis comes to the clinic for routine follow-up three weeks after long-term azithromycin therapy was initiated for treatment of *Pseudomonas aeruginosa* infection. Physical examination shows that pulmonary systems are back to functioning at baseline. Results of complete blood cell count, basic metabolic panel, and liver function studies are within normal limits. Electrocardiography shows no acute changes. Long-term use of azithromycin increases this patient's risk of developing which of the following conditions?
    A. Aplastic anemia
    B. *Clostridium difficile* infection
    C. Hepatic toxicity
    D. Prolonged QT interval
    E. Renal insufficiency

19. A 7-year-old girl is brought to the emergency department by her parents because she has had fever to 39.3°C (102.8°F) and sore throat for the past 24 hours despite initiating therapy with children's ibuprofen and acetaminophen. The parents say that she was examined by her pediatrician yesterday, and result of rapid strep test was negative. She has not received any immunizations. The patient appears to be sitting in a tripod position, with her hands on her knees and her head and neck pushing anteriorly. She has excessive drooling and stridor and appears to be toxic. X-ray study of the lateral neck shows a thumb sign. After admitting the patient to the hospital, which of the following medications are most appropriate to administer?
    A. Intravenous ceftriaxone and dexamethasone
    B. Intravenous ciprofloxacin and micafungin
    C. Intravenous clindamycin and oral oseltamivir
    D. Intravenous vancomycin and fluconazole
    E. Oral ivermectin and prednisone

20. A 43-year-old woman comes to the office one week after she was discharged from the hospital for treatment of worsening cough, hemoptysis, and wheezing over the past six months. During the past six months, she was treated for pneumonia twice, but her symptoms did not resolve. Recently, she has had intermittent episodes of facial flushing and diarrhea that worsen when she is stressed. Chest x-ray study obtained from the hospital one week ago showed no evidence of pneumonia. Current temperature is 36.7°C (98.1°F), pulse rate is 88/min, respirations are 18/min, and blood pressure is 140/84 mmHg. On physical examination, auscultation of the lungs shows focal wheezing in the left upper lobe. No rhonchi or crackles are noted. Laboratory studies show elevated urinary 5-hydroxyindoleacetic acid levels and elevated serum chromogranin A levels. Serum follicle-stimulating hormone and luteinizing hormone levels are within normal limits. Which of the following is the most likely diagnosis?
    A. Asthma
    B. Carcinoid tumor
    C. Menopause
    D. Pheochromocytoma
    E. Pulmonary foreign body

21. Occupational inhalation of asbestos fibers, silica dust, or coal mining dust is most likely to cause disease in which of the following parts of the thoracic cavity?
    A. Trachea
    B. Thymus gland region
    C. Mainstem bronchus
    D. Middle mediastinum
    E. Lung interstitium

22. A 62-year-old woman comes to the medical clinic because she has had fatigue, fever, chills, and cough productive of yellow-tinged sputum for the past week. Medical history includes hypertension and type 2 diabetes mellitus, for which she takes ramipril and glipizide, respectively. She has a 40–pack-year history of cigarette smoking. Temperature is 38.3°C (101.0°F), pulse rate is 84/min, respirations are 22/min, and blood pressure is 148/88 mmHg. Oxygen saturation is 96%. On physical examination, no murmur is noted on cardiac auscultation. Auscultation of the lungs shows crackles in the left posterior lobe on inspiration as well as dullness to percussion. Complete blood cell count is within normal limits. Chest x-ray study shows left lower pneumonia with evidence of moderate pleural effusion. Which of the following is the most appropriate next step?
   A. Antibiotic therapy
   B. Deoxyribonuclease injection
   C. Elective pleurodesis
   D. Needle aspiration
   E. Tube thoracostomy

23. A 65-year-old man comes to the clinic because he has had recurrent episodes of cough lasting for four months during the past three years. The cough is productive of white mucus and is accompanied by chest congestion and wheezing. Medical history includes obesity. He has a 35–pack-year history of cigarette smoking. Vital signs are within normal limits. On physical examination, the skin appears blue over the fingers and chest. Bibasilar breath sounds are decreased. Minimal pitting edema is noted. Chest x-ray study shows no acute consolidation or lesions. Which of the following is the most likely diagnosis?
   A. Chronic bronchitis
   B. Coccidiomycosis
   C. Diastolic congestive heart failure
   D. Pulmonary embolism
   E. Sarcoidosis

24. A 2-year-old boy is brought to the emergency department because he had an episode of gagging while eating a sandwich and fruit one hour ago. The gagging was followed by coughing, which persisted. He has no difficulty breathing, nor has he turned blue. Medical history does not include recent upper respiratory tract infection or fever. Temperature is 37.2°C (99.0°F). On physical examination, no stridor or cyanosis is noted. Auscultation of the chest shows localized wheezing on the right. A frontal chest x-ray study in expiration shows air trapped in the right lung and a mediastinal shift to the left. Which of the following is the most appropriate next step?
   A. Arterial blood gas analysis
   B. Bronchoscopy

C. Contrast esophagography
D. Thoracotomy
E. Upper gastrointestinal series

25. A 32-year-old man who has AIDS comes to the clinic to discuss the results of recent testing for pneumocystis pneumonia. Sputum culture, as well as chest x-ray study, confirm the diagnosis. Outpatient therapy with oral trimethoprim-sulfamethoxazole is planned. It is most appropriate to stop this drug at the first sign of which of the following adverse effects?
   A. Esophageal reflux
   B. New hyperglycemia
   C. Rash
   D. Unresponsive hypokalemia
   E. Worsening hypernatremia

26. A 62-year-old man comes to the clinic because he has had gradual onset of dyspnea while walking and climbing the stairs in his home over the past week. Medical history includes hypertension, for which he takes hydrochlorothiazide. Vital signs are within normal limits. On physical examination, auscultation of the chest shows some mild rhonchi, bilaterally. Chest x-ray study shows low lung volumes with diffuse reticular opacities and honeycombing. High-resolution CT scan shows subpleural fibrotic changes, traction bronchiectasis, and honeycomb cyst in the lower lobes. These findings are most consistent with which of the following diseases?
   A. Acute interstitial pneumonia
   B. Cryptogenic organizing pneumonia
   C. Idiopathic pulmonary fibrosis
   D. Sarcoidosis
   E. Tuberculosis

27. A 4-year-old girl is brought to the emergency department by her parents because she has had worsening fatigue, loss of appetite, and cough over the past two weeks. The cough was initially only at night but is now occurring in fits throughout the day. The parents say that sometimes after a coughing fit, the patient vomits. The family is from overseas and has been visiting the United States for the past six weeks. The patient has not received any immunizations. During the interview, the patient had a series of consecutive coughs followed by a deep, high-pitched inspiration. Which of the following medications is the most appropriate first-line treatment?
   A. Azithromycin
   B. Clindamycin
   C. Neomycin
   D. Streptomycin
   E. Vancomycin

                                                                    Answer Key for this chapter begins on p. 181

28. A 74-year-old man is brought to the emergency department by his daughter because he has had fever, productive cough, and shortness of breath for the past three days. Medical history includes congestive heart failure and stroke. Temperature is 39.2°C (102.6°F), pulse rate is 127/min, respirations are 32/min, and blood pressure is 104/62 mmHg. Oxygen saturation is 92% on room air. The patient is pleasant but has to take fast, shallow breaths as well as numerous deep breaths while answering questions. On physical examination, auscultation of the lungs shows crackles in the left lower lobe; when the patient is asked to say E, it sounds like A in that same area. Results of laboratory studies are within normal limits. Chest x-ray study shows left lower lobe pneumonia without pleural effusion. Which of the following is the most appropriate next step in management?
   A. Admit to the hospital and administer intravenous ceftriaxone and azithromycin
   B. Admit to the ICU and administer intravenous vancomycin, meropenem, and levofloxacin
   C. Discharge to home and prescribe amoxicillin-clavulanic acid
   D. Discharge to home and prescribe fluconazole
   E. Discharge to home and recommend conservative management

29. A 2-hour-old male infant who was born at 31 weeks' gestation has sudden development of respiratory distress with noticeable tachypnea and cyanosis. On physical examination, expiratory grunting, nasal flaring, and chest wall retractions are noted. Auscultation of the lungs shows scattered rhonchi bilaterally and poor air exchange despite vigorous respiratory effort. Chest x-ray study shows diffuse bilateral atelectasis. Which of the following is the most likely cause?
   A. G6PD deficiency
   B. Meconium aspiration
   C. Rh incompatibility
   D. Spontaneous pneumothorax
   E. Surfactant deficiency

30.

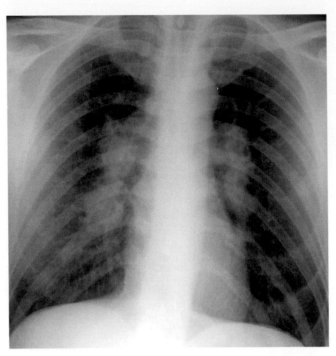

A 42-year-old Black woman comes to the office because she has had worsening shortness of breath and fatigue, as well as enlarging cervical lymph nodes over the past six months. She has no history of cigarette smoking. Vital signs are within normal limits. On physical examination, 2-cm lymph nodes are noted throughout the cervical chain. A chest x-ray study is shown. Elevated levels of which of the following laboratory values is most likely to confirm the suspected diagnosis?
   A. Angiotensin-converting enzyme
   B. Carcinoembryonic antigen
   C. D-dimer
   D. Neutrophil
   E. Potassium

31. A 23-year-old man comes to the emergency department because he had sudden onset of right-sided chest pain and shortness of breath while he was watching a movie at home 20 minutes ago. He is otherwise healthy and has no history of recent injury or illness. The patient appears tall and thin. Cardiovascular examination shows no abnormalities. Auscultation of the lungs shows diminished breath sounds and hyperresonance to percussion on the right side. The pain is not reproducible with palpation of the chest wall. Electrocardiography shows normal sinus rhythm without ST-segment or T wave changes. Which of the following is the most likely diagnosis?
    A. Costochondritis
    B. Myocardial infarction
    C. Pneumonia
    D. Pneumothorax
    E. Unstable angina

32. A 47-year-old man with lung cancer comes to the clinic to undergo scheduled chemotherapy with cisplatin and docetaxel. He has a history of nausea and vomiting with previous treatments. Based on this information, which of the following intravenous medications is most appropriate to administer at this time?
    A. Chlorpromazine
    B. Ondansetron
    C. Promethazine
    D. Metoclopramide
    E. Trimethobenzamide

33. A 55-year-old man comes to the office in late fall because he has had cough for the past week. The patient had a runny nose, nasal congestion, and sore throat for three days, and then these symptoms resolved; since then, he has had a lingering, productive cough in his chest. He has not had fever, chills, body aches, dyspnea, hemoptysis, chest pain, leg swelling, or palpitations. Temperature is 36.8°C (98.2°F), pulse rate is 82/min, and respirations are 16/min. Oxygen saturation is 99% on room air. Physical examination shows an occasional cough and mild rhonchi that clear after coughing. Which of the following is most appropriate to tell this patient about this condition?
    A. It is bacterial and will resolve after taking antibiotics for five days
    B. It is chronic and will require treatment with daily corticosteroids
    C. It is seasonal and will require treatment with antihistamines until winter
    D. It is self-limiting and will resolve within one to three weeks with conservative care
    E. It is severe and requires immediate transfer to the emergency department

34. A 2-year-old girl is brought to the emergency department by her parents late at night because she had sudden onset of a harsh, barking cough and seemed to be having difficulty breathing. The parents say that she has had cold symptoms for the past two days. Temperature is 38.0°C (100.4°F); oxygen saturation is 98% on room air. Physical examination shows mild tachypnea with some intercostal retractions. Which of the following findings on x-ray study is most likely to confirm the suspected diagnosis?
    A. Egg-on-a-string sign
    B. Football sign
    C. Sail sign
    D. Steeple sign
    E. Thumb sign

35. A 63-year-old man comes to the primary care office because he had sudden onset of shortness of breath that began earlier in the day. He says he has had worsening shortness of breath over the past year, but it has never been this severe. The patient works long hours in a sedentary job and smokes about two packs of cigarettes per shift. He has maintained this routine for the past three decades. The patient has not been examined by a medical provider in 20 years but says he is otherwise healthy and takes no medications. Pulse rate is 104/min, respirations are labored and 28/min, and blood pressure is 185/105 mmHg. Oxygen saturation is 86%. The patient appears thin, is using accessory muscles of respiration, and appears to be experiencing air hunger. On physical examination, the anteroposterior diameter of the chest approximates the lateral diameter. Auscultation of the chest shows diminished breath sounds on the left and absence of breath sounds on the right. No peripheral edema is noted. Which of the following is the most likely ongoing pathophysiologic process causing acute respiratory distress in this patient?
    A. Activation of factor V Leiden
    B. Bronchiectasis
    C. Mucus plugging
    D. Pulmonary embolism
    E. Rupture of emphysematous bullae

36. A 46-year-old woman comes to the clinic because she has had fever, nasal congestion, and cough for the past two days. Medical history includes no chronic disease conditions. Temperature is 39.0°C (102.2°F); all other vital signs are within normal limits. The patient does not appear to be in distress. On physical examination, the lungs are clear to auscultation. Chest x-ray study shows well-inflated lungs without consolidation. Rapid influenza test is positive for influenza A. Which of the following is the most appropriate treatment?
    A. Azithromycin
    B. Doxycycline
    C. Oseltamivir
    D. Remdesivir
    E. Valacyclovir

37. A 33-year-old woman comes to the emergency department because she had sudden onset of significant shortness of breath 30 minutes ago. She works for a ride-sharing service and developed the symptom while transporting a passenger. Medical history includes protein C deficiency, and examination at the emergency department three years ago for similar symptoms resulted in her being discharged with a prescription for 10 days of an antianxiety medication. Currently, her only medication is a triphasic oral contraceptive. Pulse rate is 108/min, respirations are 30/min, and blood pressure is 145/95 mmHg; she is afebrile. Oxygen saturation is 88% on room air. Physical examination shows tachypnea and tachycardia. Auscultation of the chest shows no abnormalities, and no peripheral edema is noted. Which of the following laboratory studies is most appropriate to obtain prior to imaging studies?
    A. Brain natriuretic peptide level
    B. C-reactive protein level
    C. D-dimer assay
    D. Lactate level
    E. Troponin T level

38. A 2-year-old girl is brought to the office by her mother because she has had cough and fever to 38.2°C (100.8°F) for the past two days. The mother says that the patient had a runny nose and congestion two days prior to onset of the fever. Today, the patient had two episodes in which she vomited after coughing, and the mother can hear some chest congestion when the patient breathes. Current temperature is 38.1°C (100.5°F), pulse rate is 122/min, and respirations are 36/min. Oxygen saturation is 96%. The patient does not appear to be toxic and is not in distress. On physical examination, auscultation of the lungs shows diffuse bilateral wheezing; occasional nonproductive cough is noted. Chest x-ray study shows bilateral diffuse interstitial infiltrates. Which of the following is the most likely diagnosis?
    A. Acute bronchiolitis
    B. Bacterial pneumonia
    C. Croup
    D. Upper respiratory tract infection
    E. Viral pneumonia

39. A 72-year-old woman comes to the clinic because she has had pain in her ribs since she fell at home this morning. Medical history includes a 55−pack-year history of cigarette smoking and chronic obstructive pulmonary disease. She says that her most recent physical examination was 10 years ago. Family medical history includes the death of her mother 20 years ago due to lung cancer. Chest x-ray study does not show a rib fracture but shows a solitary pulmonary nodule that is 23 mm in diameter. Which of the following studies of the chest is the most appropriate next step?
    A. CT scan
    B. MRI
    C. PET scan
    D. Repeat x-ray study
    E. Ultrasonography

40. A 35-year-old man comes to the emergency department because he has had productive cough, fever to 38.9°C (102.0°F), and shortness of breath for the past four days. Medical history includes hypertension, for which he takes metoprolol. Current temperature is 38.4°C (101.2°F), pulse rate is 90/min, respirations are 24/min, and blood pressure is 140/98 mmHg. Oxygen saturation is 99% on room air. On physical examination, auscultation of the chest shows bilateral rhonchi. Chest x-ray study shows an infiltrate in the right lower lobe. Which of the following is the most appropriate antibiotic to use when treating this patient?
    A. Amoxicillin
    B. Azithromycin
    C. Cefalexin
    D. Doxycycline
    E. Metronidazole

41. A 12-year-old boy is brought to the clinic by his mother because he has had wheezing and shortness of breath at least once daily for the past month. His mother says that he uses his albuterol metered-dose inhaler at least once daily and wakes up at night with symptoms at least once a week. The patient has been unable to participate in physical education classes at his school because of these symptoms. Which of the following classifications most accurately describes the severity of asthma in this patient?
    A. Intermittent
    B. Mild persistent
    C. Moderate persistent
    D. Severe persistent

Answers

1. **Answer: D** Other than the snoring, this patient's obesity, option D, is a risk factor for obstructive sleep apnea (OSA).

An age greater than 50 years, not less than 50 (option A), is a risk factor for OSA. Caucasian race, option B, is not a risk factor for OSA. African American and Asian patients are at increased risk of OSA. Females (option C) are not at increased risk of sleep apnea. Estrogen and progesterone are thought to have a protective effect against development of OSA. There is no relationship between type 2 diabetes mellitus (option E) and the development of OSA. **Task:** D1—Health Maintenance, Patient Education, and Disease Prevention

2. **Answer: A** This patient has an acute infection of the lower respiratory tract. The acute nature of onset and absence of phlegm production, crackles in the lung parenchyma, and respiratory distress indicates a viral-mediated inflammatory infection of the bronchiolar tree.

Bronchitis, option A, is characterized as a self-limiting viral respiratory infection localized to the bronchi and proximal to the alveoli. In addition to the symptoms described in this question, patients frequently have chest tightness and, occasionally, shortness of breath. Antibiotics are not indicated. Supportive therapies such as humidified air, fluids, and rest are the best treatment. Medications such as acetaminophen for fever, an albuterol inhaler to dilate the bronchi, a corticosteroid inhaler to decrease airway inflammation, and/or a codeine-containing syrup to suppress cough are routinely beneficial.

The etiology of croup (option B), also known as laryngotracheobronchitis, is almost always viral. The condition is relatively common in children between the ages of 6 months and 3 years. It is rare in children as old as 15 years of age. Croup is characterized by a barking cough, stridor, hoarseness, and dyspnea that worsens at night. The absence of these symptoms, along with the age of the patient, makes this an incorrect option. Pleurisy, option C, is an inflammatory process involving the visceral and parietal pleura. The condition causes sharp chest pain that worsens with deep inspiration and lessens when patients hold their breath. The etiology of pleurisy includes lung infections, autoimmune disorders (rheumatoid arthritis, lupus), sickle cell disease, lung cancer, pulmonary embolism, and certain medications. Pleurisy may be accompanied by effusion, atelectasis, and/or empyema. The absence of chest pain on inspiration makes this choice an incorrect option. The respiratory elements of the presenting symptoms in this patient are not consistent with pneumococcal pneumonia, option D. Infection with this bacterium involves the lung parenchyma resulting in crackles and shortness of breath. Incidentally, it is commonplace for universities to require vaccination against pneumococcal pneumonia for students living in dormitories. Pneumonitis, option E, includes general inflammation of the lung parenchyma at the alveolar level. Causes include radiation therapy, pulmonary fibrosis, inhalation of noxious chemicals (e.g., herbicides, fluorocarbons), and some chemotherapy agents. The acute nature of this patient's presenting symptoms and the absence of aberrant exposure make this an incorrect option. **Task:** C—Formulating Most Likely Diagnosis

3. **Answer: D** This patient is clearly having an exacerbation of symptoms related to profound right heart failure. There are many processes that can result in right heart failure, including chronic obstructive pulmonary disease (COPD). Of the available options, the one that links this patient's medical history, presenting signs and symptoms, and right heart failure is pulmonary hypertension, option D. COPD is a cause of pulmonary hypertension, and pulmonary hypertension is the cause of right heart failure in this patient. Furthermore, the sudden onset of hemoptysis is an ominous observation, indicating that the bleeding is most likely originating from the rupture of a branch of the pulmonary artery.

Cardiac tamponade, option A, may result in the patient's presenting complaints of tachycardia, hypotension, jugular venous distension, and hypoxemia. However, other cardinal features of cardiac tamponade, such as an enlarged pericardial shadow on chest x-ray study, electrical alternans and a low-voltage QRS on electrocardiography, and muffled heart sounds are not described in the scenario. Esophageal varices (option B), if present due to cirrhosis, would most likely present with venous congestion, hepatomegaly, and ascites as exhibited by the patient. However, varices are not directly linked to right heart failure.

Portal vein thrombosis, option C, is incorrect since this patient's condition is not related to right heart failure. Also, most individuals with this disorder actually have no symptoms. Symptoms that may exist include ascites, splenomegaly, and profuse esophageal bleeding from varices. It is also noteworthy that this patient has profuse hemoptysis and not hematemesis. Tension pneumothorax, option E, typically presents with poor oxygenation and hypotension. However, audible breath sounds are heard in all lung fields, and there is no indication of trauma to the chest, which is the usual etiology of developing a tension pneumothorax. Note that simple pneumothoraces often occur in patients with emphysematous COPD but without hypotension and the patient's other presenting symptoms. **Task:** E—Applying Basic Scientific Concepts

4. **Answer: B** Guidelines do not recommend a chest x-ray study for a pediatric patient with possible pneumonia if he/she appears well since the child will be treated as an outpatient, and a chest x-ray study will not change the treatment. This child is tachypneic; hospitalization is probably being considered, and the chest x-ray study will be helpful in making that determination. The correct answer is bilateral interstitial infiltrates, option B, because there is a correlation between interstitial infiltrates and viral pneumonia. Most often, these infiltrate bilaterally.

Air bronchograms, option A, is incorrect. An air bronchogram is a tubular outline of an airway made visible by the filling of the surrounding alveoli with fluid or inflammatory exudates. One of the causes of an air bronchogram is consolidation, as found in bacterial pneumonia. Lobar consolidation, option C, is a classic finding in the chest x-ray study of patients with bacterial pneumonia. Pleural effusion, option D, found on chest x-ray study, usually indicates a bacterial etiology. Well-defined, round opacities, option E, is only noted on chest x-ray studies of pediatric patients who have regions of infected consolidation consistent with bacterial pneumonia. **Task:** B—Using Diagnostic and Laboratory Studies

5. **Answer: B** Emphysema, option B, characteristically causes shortness of breath, a barrel-chested appearance, and flattening of the diaphragm shown in the chest x-ray study.

A smoking history with recurrent productive cough lasting three months or more over the past two years is consistent with a diagnosis of chronic bronchitis, option A. Polymyositis, option C, is characterized by progressive muscle weakness and elevations in creatine phosphokinase and muscle enzyme levels. Patients with pulmonary embolism, option D, tend to have chest pain and acute shortness of breath, possibly with hemoptysis. Sarcoidosis, option E, has an insidious onset with hilar adenopathy and shortness of breath as classic findings. **Task:** C—Formulating Most Likely Diagnosis

6. **Answer: B** This patient has symptoms of croup, and appropriate treatment consists of administration of dexamethasone, option B. Croup is a common childhood respiratory condition characterized by the sudden onset of a seal-like barking cough accompanied by stridor, voice hoarseness, and respiratory distress. The symptoms are a result of upper airway obstruction due to generalized inflammation of the airways resulting from a viral infection. Management of croup consists of administration of corticosteroids such as dexamethasone and nebulized epinephrine.

Administration of antitoxin, option A, is incorrect because antitoxin is used for the treatment of conditions such as diphtheria and botulism rather than croup. Initiation of albuterol as needed, option C, is incorrect. The mainstay treatment for croup is the administration of corticosteroids and nebulized epinephrine. Initiation of empiric antibiotics, option D, is incorrect. Croup is most commonly caused by parainfluenza virus. As a result, administering antibiotics is not appropriate for treatment of this condition. Placing the patient in droplet isolation, option E, is incorrect because this is not required for treating croup. Droplet isolation precautions are required for conditions transmitted through respiratory droplets such as diphtheria, pertussis, and influenza. **Task:** D3—Pharmaceutical Therapeutics

7. **Answer: E** The presence of noncaseating granulomas, option E, is the correct answer. Sarcoidosis is a chronic granulomatous disorder of unknown etiology that commonly affects the lungs, skin, and eyes. It is characterized by the formation of noncaseating granulomas in the lungs and other organs.

The presence of acid-fast bacilli, option A, is seen in patients with tuberculosis. The presence of beryllium lymphocyte proliferation, option B, indicates berylliosis. The presence of fungus isolation on silver stain, option C, is seen in patients with suspected histoplasmosis. Finally, the presence of malignant cells on mediastinal biopsy, option D, indicates lymphoma or lung cancer. **Task:** B—Using Diagnostic and Laboratory Studies

8. **Answer: B** The most common etiology of multiple nodules is infection-related or metastasis, option B. The diffuse distribution, size variation, and smooth margins of the nodules are most common in metastasis. Histoplasmosis nodules, option A, are related to previous infection, are calcified, and are similar in size. Rheumatoid nodules, option C, are located peripherally and have cavitations. Septic emboli, option D, are located peripherally and have different levels of cavitations. In patients with Wegener granulomatosis, option E, nodular infiltrates appear cavitary on x-ray study. **Task:** E—Applying Basic Scientific Concepts

9. **Answer: D** This patient has most likely sustained a tension pneumothorax, which is a diagnosis that can be made clinically. Needle decompression of the chest, option D, is the most appropriate next step. It is performed using a 14-gauge angiocatheter introduced in the second intercostal space in the mid clavicular line, a site that may be identified by carrying the line from the sternomanubrial junction to the mid clavicular line and inserting the needle perpendicular to the chest wall. After needle decompression, it is appropriate to place a definitive chest tube, option E.

A chest x-ray study and CT scan of the chest, options A and B, are not necessary. Time should not be spent getting these studies if the diagnosis can be made clinically. Focused assessment with sonography for trauma (FAST) examination of the chest, option C, could be used to determine the diagnosis, but it is likely to delay care and is not likely to offer more information than any other imaging study, especially since the diagnosis can be made clinically. **Task:** D2—Clinical Intervention

10. **Answer: C** Influenza B virus is transmitted by droplet nuclei in the respiratory tract. Therefore, placing the patient on droplet precautions until 24 hours after the resolution of respiratory symptoms and fever, option C, is the most appropriate precaution to take.

    Implementing airborne precautions by placing the patient in a negative-pressure room, option A is incorrect because the CDC guidelines indicate that only droplet precautions, in addition to standard precautions, are needed for patients infected with influenza B virus. Placing personal protective equipment that was used when caring for the patient on a hook outside the patient's door to be reused the next time he requires care, option B, is incorrect because all personal protective equipment should be removed and discarded before leaving the patient's room. Using alcohol-based hand rubs to clean hands that are visibly soiled after interactions with the patient, option D, is incorrect. According to the CDC recommendations, all health care workers must wash their hands with soap and water if their hands are visibly soiled. Wear a gown and gloves for all interactions and use disposable or dedicated patient-care equipment when available, option E, is incorrect because influenza B virus is not transmitted by contact. **Task:** D1—Health Maintenance, Patient Education, and Disease Prevention

11. **Answer: C** Metoprolol, option C, is the correct answer because it is a beta-blocker that is given to treat hypertension but can cause bronchospasms which can worsen asthma symptoms, as in this patient.

    Amlodipine, option A, is a calcium channel blocker used to treat hypertension that is safe for use in patients with asthma. Losartan, option B, is an angiotensin II receptor blocker that is used to treat hypertension but will not affect asthma. Montelukast, option D, is incorrect because this is a leukotriene inhibitor that can be given to help reduce asthma symptoms. Finally, nedocromil, option E, is a medication that can be used for long-term control to prevent asthma symptoms. **Task:** D3—Pharmaceutical Therapeutics

12. **Answer: B** The correct answer is cor pulmonale, option B. Increased pulmonary vascular resistance that develops in late-stage chronic obstructive pulmonary disease (COPD) leads to hypertrophy and dilatation of the right ventricle and right-sided heart failure. The physical examination findings of jugular venous distension and peripheral edema are consistent with cor pulmonale.

    Bronchiectasis, option A, is a dilation of the airways of the lung. Lung cancer, option C, does not develop as a consequence of COPD, although both conditions can result from cigarette smoking. Peripheral artery disease, option D, occurs when narrowed arteries decrease blood flow to the limbs resulting in muscle pain and cramping. Idiopathic pulmonary fibrosis, option E, is a scarring disease of the lungs, usually of unknown cause. **Task:** C—Formulating Most Likely Diagnosis

13. **Answer: D** The PPD skin test is considered positive with 8 mm of induration if this patient is taking adalimumab for treatment of severe Crohn disease, option D. According to CDC guidelines for tuberculosis, patients who are immunosuppressed such as those taking tumor necrosis factor alpha-inhibitors are considered to have a positive PPD skin test if the induration is 5 mm or more.

    If this patient is an immigrant who has lived in the United States for seven years (option A) and is healthy and has no risk factors for tuberculosis (option C), the PPD skin test would only be positive if this patient had induration of 15 mm or more. If he were living in the United States as an immigrant for less than five years, the induration would have to be 10 mm or greater to be positive. If this patient were currently working at a correctional facility (option B) or if he were taking insulin lispro and insulin glargine for treatment of uncontrolled diabetes mellitus (option E), the induration would have to be 10 mm or more to be considered positive. **Task:** B—Using Diagnostic and Laboratory Studies

14. **Answer: E** This chest x-ray study shows a left hilar mass, which is diagnostic of small-cell carcinoma of the lung, option E.

    Adenocarcinoma of the lung, option A, most often includes a peripheral lung nodule shown on chest x-ray study. Carcinoid tumors, option B, most commonly include a nodule that is 3 cm in size on chest x-ray study. Pulmonary embolism, option C, is rarely seen on chest x-ray study; patients with this condition have shortness of breath and chest pain. Sarcoidosis, option D, is typically associated with diffuse nodular opacities that are 1 to 5 mm with irregular borders in the upper and middle lung zones. **Task:** C—Formulating Most Likely Diagnosis

15. **Answer: C** Enoxaparin, option C, is a category B medication, which implies that controlled studies have not shown an increased risk of fetal abnormalities.

    Clopidogrel, option A, is not a standard treatment for pulmonary embolism. Dabigatran and rivaroxaban,

Answer Key for this chapter begins on p. 181

options B and D, and are incorrect because both medications are category C medications. In this case, use during pregnancy is indicated when the benefit outweighs the risk. Warfarin, option E, is contraindicated during pregnancy due to teratogenic effects. **Task:** D3—Pharmaceutical Therapeutics

16. **Answer: B** Most children and adults with respiratory syncytial virus (RSV) infection require no more than the usual care given to ensure comfort, fever control, and adequate fluid intake. Therefore, antipyretics, option B, is the most appropriate treatment.

    Preemptive administration of antibiotics, option A, to children with RSV infection has not been associated with an improved outcome. Bronchodilators and corticosteroids, options C and D, continue to be unnecessarily used; multiple studies and meta-analyses have shown that neither bronchodilators nor corticosteroids are effective treatment for RSV infection and are not recommended. Although treatment for RSV is minimal and requires only antipyretics, no treatment, option E, is inappropriate because it will not address the patient's fever or ensure that this patient is comfortable. **Task:** D2—Clinical Intervention

17. **Answer: A** The correct answer is bilateral diffuse alveolar opacities, option A. The diagnosis of acute respiratory distress syndrome (ARDS) cannot be made via chest x-ray study alone, but interstitial edema occurs with loss of aerated lung tissue that involves a large portion of the lungs and suggests ARDS.

    Enlargement of the heart, option B, is not associated with ARDS. However, it is associated with cardiogenic pulmonary edema, and the findings on chest x-ray study are similar to ARDS. Large pleural effusion causing tracheal deviation, option C, is incorrect because pleural effusions rarely occur in patients with ARDS. Multiple lung nodules, option D, is incorrect. This finding on chest x-ray study is indicative of metastatic cancer and not ARDS. Symmetric hilar and mediastinal lymphadenopathy, option E, is a chest x-ray finding that is typical of patients with sarcoidosis. **Task:** B—Using Diagnostic and Laboratory Studies

18. **Answer: B** Azithromycin is a commonly used treatment in culture-proven persistent *Pseudomonas aeruginosa* infection in patients with cystic fibrosis. *Clostridium difficile* infection, option B, is a known adverse effect of azithromycin therapy. The risk of this infection is further increased when azithromycin is prescribed long-term, such as in this patient's case. Aplastic anemia, option A, is incorrect because long-term use of azithromycin does not cause this condition. Hepatic toxicity, option C, is incorrect because azithromycin does not cause this level of liver involvement. Prolonged QT interval, option D, is incorrect

because azithromycin does not cause this condition. However, azithromycin should be used with caution or avoided if a patient has this as a preexisting condition. Renal insufficiency, option E, is incorrect because azithromycin does not cause this condition. However, this drug should not be used is patients with severe renal insufficiency as a preexisting condition. **Task:** D3—Pharmaceutical Therapeutics

19. **Answer: A** This patient has acute epiglottitis, which is most often caused by *Haemophilus influenzae*. With childhood immunizations against *H. influenzae*, this has become a less common cause. Since this patient has not received any childhood immunizations, this is most likely the cause of her symptoms. Intravenous ceftriaxone and dexamethasone, option A, are appropriate drugs to administer. Ceftriaxone is a third-generation cephalosporin that is effective in treating *H. influenzae*, and dexamethasone is a corticosteroid that will help to decrease the inflammation and edema of the epiglottis.

    Intravenous ciprofloxacin and micafungin, option B, are incorrect because ciprofloxacin is not used to treat *H. influenzae*, and micafungin is an antifungal, for which there is no indication in this patient. Intravenous clindamycin and oral oseltamivir, option C, are incorrect because even though clindamycin can be used to treat epiglottitis, oseltamivir is an antiviral, which is not appropriate to treat *H. influenzae*. Intravenous vancomycin and fluconazole, option D, are not appropriate treatments because even though vancomycin can be used, it should be used in conjunction with a third-generation cephalosporin. Also, fluconazole is an antifungal medication. Oral ivermectin and prednisone, option E, are incorrect because this patient needs intravenous intervention; in addition, ivermectin is an antiparasitic drug for which there is no indication. **Task:** D3—Pharmaceutical Therapeutics

20. **Answer: B** This patient has a carcinoid tumor, option B, which are neuroendocrine neoplasms with malignant potential and commonly present with the triad of symptoms: episodic flushing, secretory diarrhea, and bronchospasm/wheezing. Diagnostic test results include elevated 24-hour urinary 5-hydroxyindoleacetic acid (5-HIAA) level and elevated serum chromogranin A level. If the carcinoid tumor has pulmonary involvement, additional symptoms include hemoptysis, cough, focal wheezing, and recurrent pneumonia.

    Like carcinoid tumors, asthma (option A) presents with wheezing. However, patients with asthma do not have diarrhea and flushing. In addition, the 24-hour urinary 5-HIAA and serum chromogranin A levels would be within normal limits. Symptoms of menopause, option C, often include flushing, but follicle-stimulating hormone and luteinizing hormone levels would be elevated in patients with menopause.

Pheochromocytoma, option D, is associated with bouts of palpitations, diaphoresis, pallor, and paroxysmal hypertension. In this case, pheochromocytoma is less likely because the patient does not have increased blood pressure. The incidence of a pulmonary foreign body, option E, is increased in children, older individuals, or individuals with a psychiatric disability. Symptoms include stridor, wheezing, and pneumonia. **Task:** C—Formulating Most Likely Diagnosis

21. **Answer: E** The correct answer is lung interstitium, option E. After many years of breathing in chemical or fine mineral dust, the lung tissue gets inflamed, causing interstitial lung disease. The tissues that surround the air passages become thick and stiff from scarring.
    Options A and C, the trachea and mainstem bronchus, are incorrect because it is the tissue surrounding these passages that is affected rather than the air passages. Thymus gland region, option B, is incorrect because the thymus gland is located behind the sternum and between the lungs. After puberty, the thymus gland starts to shrink and is replaced by fat. Middle mediastinum, option D, is incorrect because this structural area contains the heart and its protective sheath, the pericardium. It also contains the tracheal bifurcation and the left and right main bronchi. **Task:** E—Applying Basic Scientific Concepts

22. **Answer: A** Antibiotic therapy, option A, is correct because uncomplicated parapneumonic effusions quickly resolve when pneumonia is treated with an antibiotic.
    Deoxyribonuclease injection, option B, could be a consideration in complicated parapneumonic effusion. Elective pleurodesis, option C, is used for recurrent pleural effusion. Needle aspiration, option D, and tube thoracostomy, option E, are incorrect because uncomplicated parapneumonic effusions do not need to be drained. **Task:** D2—Clinical Intervention

23. **Answer: A** This patient has the classic "blue bloater" signs with the appearance of blue skin with obesity along with recurrent episodes of cough with mucus production and wheezing, all of which are symptoms of chronic bronchitis, option A.
    Coccidiomycosis, option B, is a fungal infection common in desert regions that tends to form cavitary lesions notable on imaging studies of the lungs. Diastolic congestive heart failure, option C, includes symptoms such as edema and shortness of breath with exertion or orthopnea. Patients with pulmonary embolism, option D, tend to have acute onset of shortness of breath, chest pain, and hemoptysis as likely symptoms. Sarcoidosis, option E, includes hilar and cervical adenopathy and hemoptysis, all of which this patient does not have. **Task:** A—History Taking and Performing Physical Examination

24. **Answer: B** This patient most likely aspirated a foreign body. The correct answer is bronchoscopy, option B, which is the procedure of choice when removing aspirated foreign bodies.
    Arterial blood gas analysis, option A, checks the oxygen and carbon dioxide levels in the blood and is not needed in this case. Contrast esophagography, option C, is a study that looks for abnormalities in the esophagus. The findings on chest x-ray study suggest a foreign body as the cause of this patient's symptoms; therefore, the esophagography is not helpful. Thoracotomy, option D, is performed if bronchoscopy fails, which only occurs in about 2% of cases. Upper gastrointestinal series, option E, evaluates the esophagus, stomach, and duodenum, which is not needed for this patient who has a suspected foreign body aspiration. **Task:** D2—Clinical Intervention

25. **Answer: C** The first sign of a rash, option C, is correct. The recommended treatment for HIV-related pneumocystis pneumonia, trimethoprim-sulfamethoxazole, is related to the severe and possibly fatal adverse effects of blood dyscrasia, Stevens-Johnson syndrome, toxic epidermal necrolysis, and hepatic necrosis. In each case, discontinuance of the medication is recommended if a rash appears.
    Esophageal reflux, option A, is not considered a serious adverse effect of this medication. New hyperglycemia, unresponsive hypokalemia, and worsening hypernatremia (options B, D, and E) are incorrect because use of this medication is associated with hypoglycemia, hyperkalemia, and hyponatremia. **Task:** D3—Pharmaceutical Therapeutics

26. **Answer: C** The findings on CT scan of this patient are indicative of idiopathic pulmonary fibrosis, option C. Compared with idiopathic interstitial pneumonias, the CT appearance of idiopathic pulmonary fibrosis is distinguished by the presence of fibrotic abnormalities, predominantly in the bases of the lower lobes, by subpleural reticulations, and by its hallmark honeycombing and traction bronchiectasis.
    Option A, acute interstitial pneumonia is marked by a CT scan that shows diffuse consolidation and ground-glass opacification, often with lobular sparing and late traction bronchiectasis. Cryptogenic pneumonia, option B, is marked by a CT scan that shows subpleural or peribronchial patchy consolidation or nodules. Neither sarcoidosis nor tuberculosis, options D and E, include honeycombing on CT scan of the lungs; therefore, these two options are incorrect. **Task:** C—Formulating Most Likely Diagnosis

27. **Answer: A** This patient has signs and symptoms of *Bordetella pertussis* infection, also known as whooping cough. She has passed the catarrhal stage of the disease, at which time she had anorexia, a night cough, and

malaise. She is now in the paroxysmal phase, where she has the high-pitched inspiration at the end of the coughing fit (whoop). She has never been vaccinated against pertussis during her childhood. Therefore, azithromycin, option A, is the correct answer because it is a macrolide antibiotic, which is the appropriate first-line antimicrobial of choice to treat pertussis.

None of the other types of antibiotics are macrolides. Therefore, they are inappropriate as first-line treatment for this patient. Clindamycin, option B, belongs to the lincosamide family of antibiotics. Neomycin and streptomycin, options C and D, belong to the class of antibiotics called aminoglycosides. Vancomycin, option E, is in a class of antibiotics called glycopeptide antibiotics. **Task:** D3—Pharmaceutical Therapeutics

28. **Answer: A** This patient has symptoms and physical examination findings that are consistent with bacterial pneumonia; however, his comorbid conditions and vital signs make his clinical presentation more severe. His pneumonia severity index score puts him at a risk class of IV, which warrants inpatient admission; however, laboratory studies are within normal limits, so he does not meet the criteria for admission to the ICU. Also, this patient has no risk factors for methicillin-resistant *Staphylococcus aureus* (MRSA) or pseudomonas infection. Therefore, treatment with ceftriaxone and azithromycin is most appropriate, option A.

As noted previously, this patient does not have any risk factors for MRSA or pseudomonas infection; therefore, he does not need to be admitted to the ICU, option B. While this patient's symptoms are consistent with bacterial pneumonia, his age, comorbid conditions, and vital signs warrant a higher level of care than outpatient antibiotic therapy, option C. This patient does not have any signs or symptoms of coccidioidomycosis, which is a fungal infection that includes dermatologic manifestations including erythema nodosum in a necklace distribution, symmetric arthralgia, fever, night sweats, and weight loss. Therefore, outpatient antifungal therapy with fluconazole is not appropriate treatment, option D. This patient has bacterial pneumonia as well as comorbid conditions; therefore, discharge to home with conservative management is not appropriate, option E. **Task:** D2—Clinical Intervention

29. **Answer: E** Hyaline membrane disease is a condition that results from a deficiency of surfactant production and inactivation, option E. The absence of surfactant results in poor lung compliance and atelectasis, which causes respiratory distress during the newborn period. G6PD deficiency and Rh incompatibility, options A and C, present with the development of hemolytic anemia and hyperbilirubinemia during the neonatal period. These options are less likely in this patient because he does not have pallor or jaundice on physical examination. Meconium aspiration, option B, is more common in term or post-term infants. Physical examination would show evidence of meconium staining of the skin, nails, and/or umbilical cord. Additional findings include respiratory distress with associated hypoxia, crackles, and rhonchi. Spontaneous pneumothorax, option D, results in diminished or absent breath sounds unilaterally. In this patient's case, rhonchi and crackles were heard bilaterally on physical examination. **Task:** E—Applying Basic Scientific Concepts

30. **Answer: A** This patient has sarcoidosis, as indicated by the shortness of breath and diffuse and symmetric hilar adenopathy noted on imaging studies. An elevated serum angiotensin-converting enzyme level, option A, is consistent with the diagnosis of sarcoidosis.

An elevated carcinoembryonic antigen level, option B, is consistent with a diagnosis of colon cancer. Elevations of D-dimer, option C, are indicative of conditions that include blood clots, such as deep venous thrombosis and pulmonary embolism, both of which this patient does not have. Elevated neutrophil and potassium levels, options D and E, are not diagnostic for this patient's condition. **Task:** B—Using Diagnostic and Laboratory Studies

31. **Answer: D** This patient is young, tall, and thin, and he had sudden onset of chest pain and shortness of breath. Also, unilateral diminished breath sounds are noted with hyperresonance to percussion over the affected side. These are all classic symptoms of pneumothorax, option D.

Costochondritis, option A, is inflammation of rib tissue generally secondary to an antecedent viral infection and is characterized by tenderness to palpation of the chest wall, which is absent in this patient. Options B and E, myocardial infarction and unstable angina, make up the acute coronary syndromes. These diagnoses are unlikely given the findings on pulmonary examination, the patient's age, and the absence of cardiovascular risk factors. Pneumonia, option C, is an infectious disease of the lung parenchyma. Patients with this condition have a history of fever and cough; this patient has had no recent illness. **Task:** C—Formulating Most Likely Diagnosis

32. **Answer: B** Ondansetron, option B, is correct because one of its primary indications is to treat and prevent chemotherapy-induced nausea and vomiting.

Chlorpromazine, promethazine, metoclopramide, and trimethobenzamide (options A, C, D, and E) are incorrect because they are not primarily indicated for chemotherapy-induced nausea and vomiting. Metoclopramide could be used, but ondansetron is more efficacious. Also, the risk of an adverse neurologic event is increased with the use of injectable metoclopramide. **Task:** D3—Pharmaceutical Therapeutics

33. **Answer: D** This patient has symptoms and findings on physical examination that are consistent with acute bronchitis, an infection most commonly caused by viruses. This typically causes a cough that lasts one to three weeks and may be associated with sputum production. It is appropriate to tell the patient that the condition is self-limited and expected to resolve within one to three weeks with conservative management, option D.

This patient does not have abnormal vital signs or signs of consolidation or crackles on examination that are consistent with a bacterial infection such as pneumonia. Therefore, antibiotic therapy, option A, is not appropriate. This patient has no history of asthma, and no wheezing, hypoxia, or tachypnea is noted on examination. Therefore, he does not have chronic asthma that will require corticosteroid therapy, option B. The patient does not have any signs of seasonal allergies, such as sneezing, itchy, watery eyes, rhinorrhea, or postnasal drip. Therefore, telling him that he needs to take daily antihistamines until winter, option C, is not appropriate education. The patient's symptoms and vital signs are reassuring, so there is no indication for him to go to the emergency department, option E. **Task:** D1—Health Maintenance, Patient Education, and Disease Prevention

34. **Answer: D** This question first asks the examinee to recognize the classic presentation of croup, or laryngotracheobronchitis, which is a common respiratory condition in young children between 6 months and 3 years of age. Croup is typically preceded by low fever and upper respiratory tract infection symptoms and results in a characteristic barking cough that is worse at night. After correctly identifying croup, the examinee then must recall the classic radiographic finding in this condition, which is the steeple sign, option D. This sign describes the appearance of subglottic tracheal stenosis on an x-ray study of the neck.

Egg-on-a-string sign, option A, is indicative of transposition of the great arteries. Option B, a football sign, is noted on x-ray study of a patient with massive pneumoperitoneum. A sail sign, option C, is noted on x-ray studies of patients with occult fractures of the elbow. A thumb sign, option E, on x-ray study is indicative of epiglottitis. **Task:** B—Using Diagnostic and Laboratory Studies

35. **Answer: E** Based on this patient's progressive shortness of breath over the preceding year and physical examination findings, it is apparent he has an emphysema-predominant chronic obstructive pulmonary disease (COPD). Unfortunately, the acceleration in the decline of lung function due to smoking is dose- and duration-dependent. At this late stage, the patient most likely has a significant loss of lung tissue elasticity and destruction of alveolar walls in the lung parenchyma. Patients with emphysema also frequently develop bullae on their lung surfaces that are prone to rupture with an ensuing pneumothorax. Thus, option E is the most likely pathophysiologic process resulting in the patient's acute respiratory distress.

The most common inherited cause of pulmonary embolism (PE) in Caucasians is the resistance of clotting factor V to activated protein C. Protein C is an important vitamin K–dependent glycoprotein that circulates in plasma. When protein C is activated, it, in turn, inactivates clotting factor V. A mutation in factor V, known as factor V Leiden (option A), interferes with normal binding with protein C resulting in a hypercoagulable state. Other than respiratory distress, this patient did not present with physical signs and symptoms consistent with a PE.

Bronchiectasis, option B, is a chronic process that results in abnormal and permanent dilation and destruction of bronchiolar walls. Cystic fibrosis accounts for half of the cases of bronchiectasis with tuberculosis, alpha$_1$-antitrypsin immunodeficiency, rheumatic diseases, and tumor accounting for the remaining pathophysiologies. Bronchiectasis should be distinguished from atelectasis, which is defined as a total or partial lung collapse. In this patient's case, he is experiencing atelectasis but not bronchiectasis. Mucus plugging, option C, is a pathophysiologic process in COPD and asthma and is most certainly contributing to this patient's longstanding shortness of breath. However, the question asks about the process involved in the patient's acute respiratory distress. The insidious nature of how mucus plugging contributes to emphysema makes this option an incorrect choice. The patient's profession as a long-haul truck driver and his history of smoking are significant risk factors for deep venous thrombosis and PE, option D. However, lung sounds in acute PE are typically clear or may exhibit basilar crackles or wheezes. Also, a sufficiently sized PE may result in signs of right-sided heart failure, such as jugular venous distension and peripheral edema. The absence of these findings makes option D incorrect. **Task:** E—Applying Basic Scientific Concepts

36. **Answer: C** Oseltamivir, option C, is an antiviral medication that is most appropriate for treatment of influenza A.

Options A and B, azithromycin and doxycycline, are antibiotics that are not indicated in the treatment of a viral condition. Also, chest x-ray study of this patient shows no consolidation, so there is no reason to cover for possible pneumonia with antibiotic therapy. Option D, remdesivir, is an antiviral medication used in the treatment of COVID-19. Option E, valacyclovir, is an antiviral medication used in the treatment of herpetic viral infections and not influenza. **Task:** D3—Pharmaceutical Therapeutics

Answer Key for this chapter begins on p. 181

37. **Answer: C** This patient presents with sudden onset of significant respiratory distress without a preexisting inciting event, such as chest trauma or obvious deep venous thrombosis. Two important factors to consider are that a similar event happened a few years earlier and that the patient has a genetic disorder, protein C deficiency, which induces a hypercoagulable state. With the patient being a professional driver with presumably long hours of sitting, she is at increased risk for thrombi formation, including pulmonary embolism (PE).

   If PE is suspected, numerous algorithms are available to determine its probability. One such algorithm is the Pulmonary Embolus Rule-out Criteria (PERC) that employs eight criteria. If all eight criteria are negative, the probability of PE is quite low. If one of the criteria is positive, a D-dimer assay (option C) should be obtained. An elevated D-dimer is an indication for further workup, typically with a CT scan. A D-dimer within normal limits does not warrant an imaging study.

   Brain natriuretic peptide (BNP), option A, is released from cardiac myocytes in response to stretching caused by increased ventricular blood volume. A BNP level is most useful as an indicator of congestive heart failure. C-reactive protein (CRP), option B, is an acute-phase reactant protein of hepatic origin that elevates in response to inflammatory processes.

   Determining a lactate (lactic acid) level, option D, is most commonly used in the evaluation of sepsis. Lactate also elevates during acidosis, strenuous activity, and heart failure. It is not a useful study in the evaluation of PE. Troponin T (TnT), option E, is a component of the troponin complex that includes proteins integral to the contractile mechanism in muscle cells. An elevated TnT level is indicative of cellular damage as a result of myocardial infarction. Note that right ventricular dysfunction as a result of PE may elevate CRP, BNP, and/or TnT, but none of these biomarkers are useful in the clinical decision-making process for pulmonary embolus. **Task:** B—Using Diagnostic and Laboratory Studies

38. **Answer: E** This patient has viral pneumonia, option E, based on the gradual onset of symptoms, the fact that she appears well, and the bilateral diffuse infiltrates noted on chest x-ray study.

   Acute bronchiolitis, option A, typically includes respiratory distress such as tachypnea and retractions with diffuse wheezing or crackles noted on auscultation of the lungs. Nonspecific changes would be noted in the chest x-ray study, including peribronchial thickening, patchy atelectasis, or hyperinflation. Children with bacterial pneumonia, option B, will typically have a more abrupt onset and a more ill/toxic appearance, respiratory distress, and focal findings on lung examination. Chest x-ray study findings in bacterial pneumonia may include alveolar infiltrates, segmental or lobar consolidation, or a "round" pneumonia. Croup, option C, is a viral laryngotracheitis that includes a barking cough and stridor and can progress to airway obstruction and respiratory distress. An upper respiratory tract infection, option D, is typically caused by a virus and includes cough, runny nose, and nasal congestion; a chest x-ray study will show no abnormalities. **Task:** C—Formulating Most Likely Diagnosis

39. **Answer: A** This patient has a pulmonary nodule that was noted incidentally on chest x-ray study. Therefore, additional imaging is needed to further evaluate the nodule and assess for the probability of malignancy. The preferred imaging modality is a CT scan of the chest, option A, without contrast, which will allow for a more precise characterization of the location, size, borders, and attenuation of the nodule.

   MRI and PET scans of the chest, options B and C, can also be used to further assess a pulmonary nodule, but these are not considered the best next step after a chest x-ray study. Repeat chest x-ray study, option D, will likely not give any additional information regarding the nodule. Ultrasonography of the chest, option E, does not have any role in the evaluation of a pulmonary nodule. **Task:** B—Using Diagnostic and Laboratory Studies

40. **Answer: B** Based on this patient's symptoms and vital signs, he has community-acquired pneumonia. This nonsevere case of pneumonia can be treated in the outpatient setting, and appropriate treatment includes a macrolide such as azithromycin, option B.

   Amoxicillin, option A, is a penicillin antibiotic and will not work to treat community-acquired pneumonia. Cefalexin, option C, is a cephalosporin and works best to treat other bacterial skin and urinary infections. Doxycycline, option D, is tetracycline and works best to treat infections other than community-acquired pneumonia. Metronidazole, option E, works best to treat fungal infections. **Task:** D3—Pharmaceutical Therapeutics

41. **Answer: C** This question tests the examinee's ability to recall the classification system for asthma severity from the National Heart, Lung, and Blood Institute. This classification system uses the frequency of symptoms, frequency of nighttime awakenings, frequency of short-acting beta agonist (SABA) use, and interference with normal activity to determine the severity of asthma. This patient has daily symptoms and daily SABA use, weekly nighttime awakenings, and some limitation in normal activity, which puts him in the moderate persistent category, option C.

   Intermittent severity, option A, refers to symptoms and SABA use less than two days a week, nighttime awakenings less than two days a month, and no interference with normal activity. Mild persistent asthma, option B, refers to symptoms and SABA use more than two days a week but not daily, nighttime awakenings two to four times per month, and minor interference with normal activity. Severe persistent,

option D, refers to symptoms and SABA use several times daily, nighttime awakenings greater than once a week and often nightly, and extreme limitation in normal activity. **Task:** A—History Taking and Performing Physical Examination

BIBLIOGRAPHY

Antman, E. M., & Loscalzo, J. (2018). Ischemic heart disease. In: J. Jameson, A. S. Fauci, D. L. Kasper, et al., (Eds.), *Harrison's principles of internal medicine* (20th ed.). McGraw-Hill.

Barson, W. J. (2020). Community-acquired pneumonia in children: Clinical features and diagnosis. In T. Post (Ed.), *UpToDate*. Waltham, MA: UpToDate.

Brink, D. S. (2012). Pathology of lung tumors. In A. J. Lechner, G. M. Matuschak, & D. S. Brink (Eds.), *Respiratory: An integrated approach to disease*. McGraw-Hill.

Chesnutt, A. N., Chesnutt, M. S., Prendergast, N. T., & Prendergast, T. J. (2021). Sarcoidosis. In M. A. Papadakis, S. J. McPhee, & M. W. Rabow (Eds.), *Current medical diagnosis & treatment 2021*. McGraw-Hill.

Chesnutt, A. N., Chesnutt, M. S., Prendergast, N. T., & Prendergast, T. J. (2021). Bronchial carcinoid tumors. In M. A. Papadakis, S. J. McPhee, & M. W. Rabow (Eds.), *Current medical diagnosis & treatment 2021*. McGraw-Hill.

Chesnutt, A. N., Chesnutt, M. S., Prendergast, N. T., & Prendergast, T. J. (2020). Chronic obstructive pulmonary disease. In M. A. Papadakis, S. J. McPhee, & M. W. Rabow (Eds.), *Current medical diagnosis & treatment 2020*. McGraw-Hill.

Chesnutt, A. N., Chesnutt, M. S., Prendergast, N. T., & Prendergast, T. J. (2021). Cystic fibrosis. In M. A. Papadakis, S. J. McPhee, & M. W. Rabow (Eds.), *Current medical diagnosis & treatment 2021*. McGraw-Hill.

Chesnutt, A. N., Chesnutt, M. S., Prendergast, N. T., & Prendergast, T. J. (2021). Pleural effusion. In M. A. Papadakis, S. J. McPhee, & M. W. Rabow (Eds.), *Current medical diagnosis & treatment 2021*. McGraw-Hill.

Chiles, C., & Gulla, S. M. (2010). Chapter 4. Radiology of the chest. In: M. M. Chen, T. L. Pope, & D. J. Ott (Eds.), *Basic radiology* (2nd ed.). McGraw-Hill.

Chow, A. W. (2015). Life-threatening infections of the head, neck, and upper respiratory tract.

Domino, F. J., Baldor, R. A., Golding, J., & Stephens, M. B. (2019). *The 5-minute clinical consult 2020*. Lippincott Williams & Wilkins.

Epocrates [online]. San Francisco, CA: Epocrates, Inc.; 2013. Updated continuously.

File, T. M. (2020). Acute bronchitis in adults. In T. Post (Ed.), *UpToDate*. Waltham, MA: UpToDate.

Force, A. D. T., Ranieri, V. M., Rubenfeld, G. D., Thompson, B., Ferguson, N., Caldwell, E., et al. (2012). Acute respiratory distress syndrome. *JAMA, 307*(23), 2526-2533.

Fort, G. (2021). Croup (Laryngotracheobronchitis). In F. Ferri (Ed.), *Ferri's clinical advisor 2021* (pp. 423.e3-423.e5). Philadelphia, PA: Elsevier, Inc.

Fox, D., & Takashima, M. (2020). Obstructive sleep apnea. In R. Kellerman & D. Rakel (Eds.), *Conn's current therapy 2020* (pp. 853-855). Philadelphia, PA: Elsevier, Inc.

Huffstetler, A. N., Muthusubramanian, A., & DeGeorge, K. C. (2019). *Bacterial pneumonia, Conn's current therapy 2020* (pp. 827-832). Elsevier.

Judson, M. (2021). *Sarcoidosis, Murray and Nadel's textbook of respiratory medicine* (pp. 1188-1206.e7). Saunders.

Kliegman, R. M., & Geme, J. (2020). *Nelson textbook of pediatrics* (7th ed., pp. 2266-2274).

Konkle, B. A. (2018). Bleeding and thrombosis. In: J. Jameson, A. S. Fauci, D. L. Kasper, et al., (Eds.), *Harrison's principles of internal medicine* (20th ed.). McGraw-Hill.

Linder, J. (2020). Influenza. In R. Kellerman & D. Rakel (Eds.), *Conn's current therapy 2020* (pp. 574-577). Philadelphia, PA: Elsevier, Inc.

Lung Cancer. Elsevier Point of Care. Updated June 4, 2020.

Macnee, W., Vestbo, J., Agusti, A. (2021). COPD: Pathogenesis and natural history. *Murray and Nadel's textbook of respiratory medicine*, 43, 751-766.e7. Saunders.

Mandell, D. (2020). *Bennett's principles and practice of infectious diseases*, 158, 2093-2103.e5. Elsevier.

Marcdante, K., & Kliegman, R. M. (2019). *Nelson essentials of pediatrics* (8th ed., pp. 519-526). Elsevier.

Marrie, T. J. (2015). Acute bronchitis and community-acquired pneumonia. In: M. A. Grippi, J. A. Elias, J. A. Fishman, et al., (Eds.), *Fishman's pulmonary diseases and disorders* (5th ed.). McGraw-Hill.

Nasir, M., Green, M., & Smith, M. A. (2019). Pulmonary embolism. In R. P. Usatine, M. A. Smith, & E. J. Mayeaux, Jr., et al. (Eds.), *The color atlas and synopsis of family medicine* (3rd ed.). McGraw-Hill.

Papadakis, M. A., McPhee, S. J., & Rabow, M. W. (2020). Chapter 32, Viral & rickettsial infections: *Current medical diagnosis & treatment 2020* (pp. 1437-1441). New York: McGraw-Hill Education.

Papadakis, M. A., McPhee, S. J., & Rabow, M. W. (2020). Chapter 33: Bacterial & chlamydial infections: *Current medical diagnosis & treatment 2020* (pp. 1486-1487). New York: McGraw-Hill Education.

Papadakis, M. A., McPhee, S. J., & Rabow, M. W. (2020). Chapter 9, Pulmonary disorders: *Current medical diagnosis & treatment 2020* (pp. 255-269). New York: McGraw-Hill Education.

Papadakis, M. A., McPhee, S. J., & Rabow, M. W. (2020). Chapter 9, Pulmonary disorders: *Current medical diagnosis & treatment 2020* (pp. 290-298). New York: McGraw-Hill Education.

Papadakis, M. A., & McPhee, S. J. (2021). *Current medical diagnosis & treatment 2020* (pp. 320-321).

Pertussis (whooping cough). The Centers for Disease Control. Published October 25, 2019.

Pneumocystis Pneumonia, Candidiasis, and Other Fungal Infections. In: J. Jameson, A. S. Fauci, D. L. Kasper, et al. (Eds.), (2020). *Harrison's manual of medicine* (20th ed.). McGraw-Hill.

Pollart, S., DeGeorge, K., & Kolb, A. (2020). Asthma in children. In R. Kellerman & D. Rakel (Eds.), *Conn's current therapy 2020* (pp. 1199-1206). Philadelphia, PA: Elsevier, Inc.

Powell, S., & Yates, P. D. (2020). Stridor in children. In A. K. Lalwani (Ed.), *Current diagnosis & treatment otolaryngology—head and neck surgery* (4th ed.). McGraw-Hill.

 Answer Key for this chapter begins on p. 181

Prevention Strategies for Seasonal Influenza in Healthcare Settings. The Centers for Disease Control. Published October 30, 2018.

Ramirez, J. A. (2020). Overview of community-acquired pneumonia in adults. In T. Post (Ed.), *UpToDate*. Waltham, MA: UpToDate.

Raghu, G., & Martinez, F. J. (2019). Interstitial lung disease. *Goldman-Cecil Medicine*, 86, 557-570.

Rubin, M. A., Ford, L. C., & Gonzales, R. (2018). Sore throat, earache, and upper respiratory symptoms. In: J. Jameson, A. S. Fauci, D. L. Kasper, et al. (Eds.), *Harrison's principles of internal medicine* (20th ed.). McGraw-Hill.

Sachdeva, A., & Matuschak, G. M. (2012). Pulmonary embolism. In A. J. Lechner, G. M. Matuschak, & D. S. Brink (Eds.), *Respiratory: An integrated approach to disease*. McGraw-Hill.

Semon, G., & McCarthy, M. *Chest wall, pneumothorax, and hemothorax, current surgical therapy* (pp. 1146-1150).

Sepah, Yasir Jamal, et al. Sarcoidosis. (2022). *Ryan's Retina*, 81, 1572-1585. Elsevier.

Sholl, L., & Mino-Kenudson, M. *Tumors of the lung and pleura. diagnostic histopathology of tumors* (pp. 225-272).

Smith, D. (2020). The newborn infant. In W. W. Hay Jr., M. J. Levin, M. J. Abzug, & M. Bunik (Eds.), *Current diagnosis & treatment: Pediatrics* (25th ed.). McGraw-Hill.

Targeted Tuberculosis Testing and Interpreting Tuberculin Skin Test Results. The Centers for Disease Control. Published August 31, 2016.

Tsukada, H. (2021). Pneumothorax, spontaneous. In F. Ferri (Ed.), *Ferri's clinical advisor 2021* (pp. 1120-1123.e1). Philadelphia, PA: Elsevier, Inc. 2021.

Walsh, E. E., & Janet, A. Englund. (2017). Respiratory syncytial virus.

Waxman, A. B., & Loscalzo, J. Pulmonary hypertension. In: J. Jameson, A. S. Fauci, D. L. Kasper, et al., (Eds.), *Harrison's principles of internal medicine* (20th ed.). McGraw-Hill.

Weinberger, S. E., Cockrill, B. A., & Mandel, J. (2018). *Principles of pulmonary medicine* (7th ed., pp. 194-205). Elsevier.

Weinberger, S. W., & McDermott, S. (2020). Diagnostic evaluation of the incidental pulmonary nodule. In T. Post (Ed.), *UpToDate*. Waltham, MA: UpToDate.

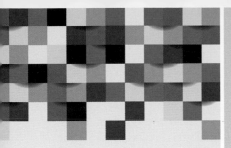

CHAPTER 13
Renal System

Questions

1. A 68-year-old woman with stage 4 chronic kidney disease comes to the primary care clinic for six-month follow-up. Her nephrologist recently told her that she would need to begin dialysis soon. The nephrologist also told her to adjust the amount of something in her diet, but she is unable to recall the specific dietary instruction. Which of the following dietary recommendations was most likely given to this patient by the nephrologist?
   A. Decrease intake of calcium by decreasing consumption of cheese, ice cream, and other dairy products
   B. Increase consumption of foods high in magnesium
   C. Increase protein intake as a percentage of total daily caloric intake
   D. Limit intake of foods high in potassium, such as avocados, nuts, legumes, and spinach
   E. Maintain consumption of sodium of at least 4g daily

2. A 4-year-old boy is brought to the office for routine well-child examination. Blood pressure is 146/96 mmHg. Physical examination shows a unilateral abdominal mass located in the right upper quadrant. Urinalysis shows gross hematuria. Which of the following is the most appropriate initial step in diagnosis?
   A. Abdominal ultrasonography
   B. CT scan of the kidneys, ureter, and bladder
   C. Cystoscopy
   D. Intravenous pyelography
   E. MRI of the kidneys, ureter, and bladder

3. A 54-year-old man comes to the primary care office for follow-up. Medical history includes type 2 diabetes mellitus that was diagnosed five years ago. Three months ago, the patient was told that his kidney function was abnormal, and he will require close monitoring for signs of progression. Lisinopril 5 mg daily was initiated at that time. Which of the following findings on history and physical examination is most likely to indicate progression toward chronic kidney disease in this patient?
   A. Bladder enlargement
   B. Decreased jugular venous pressure
   C. Decreased skin turgor
   D. Generalized pruritus
   E. Orthostatic hypotension

4. A 15-year-old girl is brought to the clinic because she has had worsening dysuria, hesitancy, and urgency for the past five days. She also has had fever with chills and back pain for the past day. Her most recent menstrual period was eight weeks ago, and she does not have any vaginal discharge. Medical history includes a urinary tract infection every year or so since menarche at 12 years of age. She has been otherwise healthy. Temperature is 39.7°C (103.4°F), pulse rate is 104/min, respirations are 12/min, and blood pressure is 130/88 mmHg. The patient appears acutely ill. Physical examination shows significant tenderness to palpation in the suprapubic region as well as the right costovertebral angle. Result of urine pregnancy test is positive. Urinalysis shows too-numerous-to-count white and red blood cells, is positive for nitrites, and shows many white blood cell casts on microscopic examination. The patient is admitted to the hospital pending results of urine culture and sensitivity. Empiric intravenous antibiotic therapy is planned. Which of the following antibiotic therapies is most appropriate for this patient?
   A. Azithromycin
   B. Doxycycline
   C. Gentamicin
   D. Piperacillin/tazobactam
   E. Trimethoprim-sulfamethoxazole

5. A 38-year-old woman comes to the emergency department because she has had nausea and vomiting as well as intermittent severe pain in the right back during the past two hours. She describes the pain as waxing and waning and rates the pain as a 9 on a 10-point scale. The patient appears to be in considerable discomfort. On physical examination, costovertebral tenderness is noted. The abdomen is soft with mild tenderness to palpation of the right lower quadrant. Results of urinalysis include the following:

Color	Yellow with >15–20 red blood cells/hpf
Appearance	Hazy with 0–3 white blood cells/hpf (N = 0–2/hpf)
Specific gravity	1.025 with few squamous epithelial cells (N = 1.005–1.030)
pH	6.0 with many monohydrate cells with a characteristic "dumbbell" appearance (N = 4.6–8.0)
Protein	Negative
Glucose	Negative
Ketones	Negative
Blood	Moderate
Nitrates	Negative
Leukocytes	Negative

Renal ultrasonography shows a large hypoechoic area in the center of the kidney extending into the parenchyma that is consistent with hydronephrosis. Which of the following is the most likely cause?
A. Acute cholecystitis
B. Appendicitis
C. Pelvic inflammatory disease
D. Pyelonephritis
E. Renal calculi

6. A 68-year-old man comes to the office because he has had decreased urine output for the past three days. Physical examination shows mild abdominal discomfort to deep palpation and a large, uniformly smooth prostate gland on digital rectal examination. Laboratory studies show serum creatinine level of 1.7 mg/dL (N = .75–1.27 mg/dL), which is increased from the previous baseline of 1.2 mg/dL at the patient's most recent annual physical examination four months ago. Urinalysis shows slight hematuria but is otherwise unremarkable. Ultrasonography of the abdomen shows bilateral hydroureters and hydronephrosis. Which of the following is the most appropriate initial management?
A. Admission to the hospital for observation
B. Alpha-adrenergic antagonist therapy
C. Bilateral nephrostomy tube placement
D. Bladder catheterization
E. Hemodialysis

7. A 34-year-old woman comes to the clinic for follow-up of stage 5 end-stage renal disease secondary to systemic lupus erythematosus. Current calculated glomerular filtration rate is 10 mL/min/1.73 m² (N = >90 mL/min/1.73 m²). The patient is on the renal transplant registry and currently undergoes dialysis three times per week. Which of the following hormone levels is most likely to be elevated as a secondary physiologic response to renal disease in this patient?
A. Erythropoietin
B. Gastrin
C. Insulin
D. Parathyroid hormone
E. Thyroid-stimulating hormone

8. A 73-year-old man with chronic obstructive pulmonary disease and type 2 diabetes mellitus is being evaluated in the hospital one day after undergoing total hip arthroplasty. Current medications include subcutaneous NPH insulin and regular insulin as well as intravenous fentanyl. On physical examination, the patient has worsening shortness of breath as well as confusion. Immediate arterial blood gas analysis shows pH of 7.12 (N = 7.35–7.45), pCO_2 of 88 mmHg (N = 35–45 mmHg), and HCO_3^- of 26 mEq/L (N = 22–26 mEq/L). Oxygen saturation is 84%. This patient most likely has which of the following acute conditions?
A. Metabolic acidosis
B. Metabolic alkalosis
C. Respiratory acidosis
D. Respiratory alkalosis

9. A 58-year-old man comes to the office for annual physical examination. Medical history includes hypertension that is well controlled with amlodipine 10 mg taken once daily. He smokes one pack of cigarettes every two days and has approximately two to six beers on the weekends. Physical examination shows no abnormalities. Results of laboratory studies are within normal limits. Urine dipstick test shows 2+ blood; one week later, repeat urine dipstick test shows similar results. Ultrasonography of the urinary system shows a 4.5-cm hypoechoic, solid mass in the inferior pole of the left kidney. Which of the following is the most likely diagnosis?
A. Amyloidosis
B. Perinephric abscess
C. Renal cell carcinoma
D. Simple renal cyst
E. Wilms tumor

10. An 18-month-old girl is brought to the clinic by her mother because she has had vomiting, diarrhea, and decreased oral intake during the past four days. The mother says that the patient has only had one wet diaper during the past 24 hours. Upon weighing the patient, a 10% decrease in total body weight is noted. Which of the following additional findings on history and physical examination is most likely?
   A. Bradycardia
   B. Capillary refill less than two seconds
   C. Increased thirst
   D. Slightly sunken fontanelle
   E. Tenting of the skin greater than two seconds

11. An 8-year-old boy is brought to the office by his father because he has had facial swelling and generalized malaise for the past two days. His urine has been dark and scant. Medical history includes streptococcal pharyngitis 10 days ago, but he has been otherwise healthy. Temperature is 37.2°C (99.0°F), pulse rate is 100/min (N = 59–123/min), and blood pressure is 118/78 mmHg (N = 95–110/60–73 mmHg). The patient appears fatigued. Physical examination shows periorbital edema. No other abnormalities are noted. Which of the following findings on examination of urine sediment is most specific for the suspected condition in this patient?
   A. Amorphous phosphate crystals
   B. Calcium oxalate crystals
   C. Neutrophils
   D. Red blood cell casts
   E. Transitional epithelial cells

12. A 59-year-old man with chronic kidney disease comes to the emergency department because he has had swelling of the lower extremities and shortness of breath for the past 24 hours. Pulse rate is 110/min, and blood pressure is 150/95 mmHg. Oxygen saturation is 94%. Physical examination shows bilateral basilar crackles and 3+ pitting edema of the lower extremities. The patient is admitted to the hospital and undergoes treatment for a few days before he is ready to be discharged to home. To decrease this patient's risk of future hospitalizations, it is most appropriate to encourage him to limit intake of which of the following substances?
   A. Calcium
   B. Glucose
   C. Phosphorus
   D. Potassium
   E. Sodium

13. A 29-year-old woman comes to the primary care office because she has had worsening flank pain over the past several weeks. Medical history includes no chronic disease conditions, and she takes no medications. Family medical history includes polycystic kidney disease in one of her parents. Physical examination shows bilateral tenderness to palpation at the costovertebral angles. Which of the following is the most appropriate initial diagnostic test?
   A. Genetic testing
   B. MRI of the kidneys
   C. Noncontrast CT scan of the abdomen and pelvis
   D. Renal biopsy
   E. Renal ultrasonography

14. A 66-year-old man with hypertension, type 2 diabetes mellitus, hyperlipidemia, and prominent atherosclerosis comes to the office for follow-up. Regarding the hypertension, he is currently taking the maximum dose of four medications, but home blood pressure monitoring shows it to consistently be around 160/100 mmHg. Current blood pressure is 170/105 mmHg; all other vital signs are within normal limits. On physical examination, bruits are present over the carotid, subclavian, renal, and iliac regions bilaterally. Arterial pulses in both feet are diminished. Which of the following additional findings is most likely to occur concomitantly with the extensive list of chronic diseases in this patient?
   A. Hemochromatosis
   B. Low QRS voltage
   C. Narrow pulse pressure
   D. Portal hypertension
   E. Prerenal azotemia

15. A 52-year-old man with cirrhosis is brought to the emergency department because he had a seizure three hours ago and has had a decrease in mental status since that time. Temperature is 36.7°C (98.1°F), pulse rate is 76/min, respirations are 18/min, and blood pressure is 110/75 mmHg. The patient is obtunded and not answering questions. On physical examination, the pupils are equal, round, and reactive to light. Cardiac auscultation shows regular rhythm, and the lungs are clear to auscultation. The abdomen is distended with palpable hepatomegaly and caput medusa. Chronic venous stasis changes and 1+ edema are noted in the extremities. Laboratory studies show serum sodium level of 100 mEq/L (N = 135–145 mEq/L). The most appropriate initial treatment is intravenous administration of which of the following?
   A. Calcium gluconate
   B. Diltiazem
   C. Furosemide
   D. Regular insulin
   E. 3% Saline

    Answer Key for this chapter begins on p. 196

16. A 66-year-old woman with end-stage renal disease comes to the emergency department because she has had generalized weakness since she missed her last two dialysis treatments. Physical examination shows diminished breath sounds at both lung bases. Peripheral 2+ edema is noted, bilaterally. Based on these findings, it is most appropriate to evaluate this patient for which of the following acute electrolyte abnormalities?
    A. Hyperkalemia
    B. Hypernatremia
    C. Hypocalcemia
    D. Hypomagnesemia
    E. Hypophosphatemia

17. A 52-year-old man comes to the clinic for follow-up of newly diagnosed nephrotic syndrome. Recent annual physical examination showed a blood pressure of 156/92 mmHg as well as 2+ pitting tibial edema. Current laboratory studies show serum albumin level of 2.5 g/dL (N = 3.4–5.4 g/dL) and total cholesterol level of 300 mg/dL (N = <200 mg/dL). Urinalysis shows protein of 80 mg/day (N = 0–60 mg/day) and trace hematuria. Initiation of which of the following medications is most appropriate at this time?
    A. Amlodipine
    B. Benazepril
    C. Clonidine
    D. Hydralazine
    E. Metoprolol

18. A 63-year-old woman is recovering in the hospital one day after undergoing resection of the bowel for treatment of a small-bowel obstruction. Aside from intravenous saline to address hypovolemia that was present at admission, the patient takes no medications and has no history of chronic disease conditions. Vital signs are within normal limits. Physical examination shows moist mucous membranes. No skin tenting or peripheral edema is noted. Findings on laboratory studies of serum include the following:

Creatinine	1.0 mg/dL (N = .75–1.27 mg/dL)
Sodium	130 mEq/L (N = 135–145 mEq/L)
Chloride	100 mEq/L (N = 97–108 mEq/L)
Potassium	4.9 mEq/L (N = 3.5–5.0 mEq/L)
Bicarbonate	22 mEq/L (N = 20–32 mEq/L)
Glucose	90 mg/dL (N = 65–99 mg/dL)

Which of the following is the most likely cause of the hyponatremia in this patient?
    A. Diuresis
    B. Heart failure
    C. Idiosyncratic drug reaction
    D. Mineralocorticoid deficiency
    E. Postoperative antidiuretic hormone release

19. A 7-year-old boy is brought to the pediatric clinic by his parents because he has had hematuria and mild swelling of the face for the past 24 hours. The parents say the patient had a sore throat a few weeks ago that resolved without intervention. Blood pressure is 135/88 mmHg; all other vital signs are within normal limits. Physical examination shows trace pretibial edema as well as mild edema of the periorbital tissues. Urinalysis shows hematuria and proteinuria. Damage to which of the following units of the kidney is most likely causing the symptoms in this patient?
    A. Collecting duct
    B. Distal tubule of the nephron
    C. Glomerulus
    D. Loop of Henle
    E. Proximal tubule of the nephron

20. A 53-year-old man with a six-year history of type 2 diabetes mellitus comes to the office for six-month follow-up. He has no acute symptoms, and vital signs are within normal limits. On physical examination, cardiac auscultation shows a regular rhythm without murmur. The lungs are clear to auscultation. The abdomen is soft and nontender to palpation. Examination of both legs shows 1+ pitting edema, and diminished sensation to monofilament is noted over the feet and toes, bilaterally. Laboratory studies show an estimated glomerular filtration rate of 24 mL/min (N = >60 mL/min), which has been stable for the past six months. Microalbumin-to-creatinine ratio is 45 mg/dL (N = <30 mg/dL). These findings are most consistent with which of the following stages of chronic kidney disease?
    A. Stage 1
    B. Stage 2
    C. Stage 3
    D. Stage 4
    E. Stage 5

21. An 82-year-old man is transferred by ambulance from a long-term residential treatment facility to the emergency department. Facility staff say that the patient has had vomiting and worsening lethargy and disorientation over the past six hours. Medical history includes Alzheimer disease, congestive heart failure, and myocardial infarction. Pulse rate is 88/min, respirations are 20/min, and blood pressure is 148/90 mmHg; he is afebrile. Oxygen saturation is 90% on room air. The patient appears drowsy and is not oriented to person, place, or time. On physical examination, mild tachypnea is noted. Auscultation of the chest shows bilateral basilar crackles, and 3+ pitting edema is noted up to the mid tibial area. Complete blood cell count shows no abnormalities. Results of complete metabolic panel show serum glucose and creatinine levels within normal limits but a serum sodium level of 122 mEq/L (N = 135–145 mEq/L). Measurement of serum osmolality is 262 mOsm/kg H_2O (N = 280–295 mOsm/kg H_2O). Urinalysis shows a sodium level of 8 mEq/L (N = spot urine >20 mEq/L). Chest x-ray study shows pulmonary congestion with blunting of both costovertebral angles. Which of the following is the most appropriate initial intravenous therapy?
    A. 5% Dextrose solution
    B. Furosemide 40 mg
    C. Mannitol 0.25 g/kg
    D. 0.9% Saline solution
    E. 10 U of regular insulin

22. A 32-year-old man comes to the clinic because he has had abdominal pain, hematuria, and morning headaches for the past week. Family medical history includes renal transplantation in his father. Blood pressure is 162/110 mmHg. Physical examination shows a bilateral mass in the abdomen that is not tender to palpation. Electrocardiography shows an S wave in V_1 and an R wave in V_6 ≥3.5 mV (35 mm).

Which of the following valvular abnormalities is most likely on echocardiography of this patient?
    A. Aortic regurgitation
    B. Aortic stenosis
    C. Mid systolic murmur
    D. Mitral valve prolapse
    E. Ventricular septal defect

23. Two days ago, a 32-year-old man was admitted to the surgical ICU after he sustained injuries when his lower extremities were crushed by a truck backing up to a loading dock platform. He sustained fractures in both lower extremities, compartment syndrome of the right calf area, and extensive damage to the muscles of the anterior and posterior compartments of both thighs. He underwent surgery to address the fractures and the compartment syndrome. Current laboratory studies show a serum creatinine level of 6.2 mg/dL (N = .84–1.21 mg/dL). Urinary output is approximately 40 mL/hr, and urine dipstick test shows 4+ blood; no blood is noted on microscopic examination of the sediment. Which of the following disorders related to renal pathophysiology is most likely?
    A. Acute tubular necrosis
    B. IgA nephropathy
    C. Interstitial nephritis
    D. Minimal change disease
    E. Pyelonephritis

24. A 65-year-old man is being treated in the hospital because he had an acute exacerbation of systolic congestive heart failure. He has been administered intravenous furosemide for the past two days. Which of the following is the most significant laboratory abnormality associated with this treatment?
    A. Hypercalcemia
    B. Hypermagnesemia
    C. Hyperphosphatemia
    D. Hypokalemia
    E. Metabolic acidosis

Answer Key for this chapter begins on p. 196

Answers

1. **Answer: D** Hyperkalemia and hypocalcemia are routinely observed in patients with stage 4 and 5 renal failure. While a balanced diet is the most appropriate advice for these patients, limiting the consumption of foods high in potassium, option D, is the most appropriate recommendation to this patient to avoid hyperkalemia.

   Hypocalcemia is a concern in patients with renal failure; therefore, decreasing calcium intake, option A, is the opposite of the desired outcome. The magnesium level in patients with predialysis chronic kidney disease for the most part remains within normal limits. Once dialysis is initiated in end-stage disease, the magnesium concentration in the dialysate is largely responsible for maintaining magnesium homeostasis. For these reasons, option B is incorrect. Increasing the percentage of protein in the diet, option C, will likely elevate blood urea nitrogen and is inconsistent with the recommendation of a balanced diet. A diet restricted to 4g of sodium daily, option E, is typically recommended to aid in the management of hypertension. According to the Dietary Guidelines for Americans published by the United States Department of Agriculture, individuals with not only hypertension but diabetes mellitus and chronic kidney disease should decrease their sodium intake to 1500 mg/day. **Task**: D1—Health Maintenance, Patient Education, and Disease Prevention

2. **Answer: A** This patient has signs and symptoms of a Wilms tumor, which is a nephroblastoma arising from the kidney that occurs in children. Wilms tumor accounts for 5% of all childhood malignancies and usually presents before 5 years of age. Most patients are asymptomatic with a rapidly growing abdominal mass. Thirty percent of patients have symptoms consistent with abdominal pain, malaise, gross hematuria, hypertension, and anemia. Abdominal ultrasonography, option A, is the most appropriate initial step in diagnosis because this study helps to localize the mass to the kidney.

   CT scan or MRI of the kidneys, ureter, and bladder, options B and E, are useful to identify additional information such as contralateral tumors, hemorrhage, abdominal lymph node enlargement, and renal vein thrombosis, but they are not the most appropriate initial step in diagnosis for this patient. Cystoscopy and intravenous pyelography, options C and D, are not useful in the diagnosis of Wilms tumor because these studies are used to examine the size and shape of the kidneys, ureters, and bladder and to assess their function. **Task**: B—Using Diagnostic and Laboratory Studies

3. **Answer: D** Generalized pruritis, option D, is the correct answer. Chronic kidney disease is defined as abnormalities of kidney function lasting greater than or equal to three months. As kidney disease progresses, pruritus is common due to an accumulation of toxic waste products in the body's circulation that are not excreted by the kidney.

   Bladder enlargement, option A, is seen in cases of acute renal failure caused by an obstruction within the urinary tract. Decreased jugular venous pressure, poor skin turgor, and orthostatic hypotension, options B, C, and E, are signs and symptoms that are manifestations of acute renal failure caused by hypovolemia. **Task**: A—History Taking and Performing Physical Examination

4. **Answer: D** This patient has signs and symptoms consistent with acute pyelonephritis. Her condition is further complicated by pregnancy and certainly warrants admission to the hospital. Piperacillin/tazobactam, option D, is the correct option, as its use is indicated as first-line therapy in complicated acute pyelonephritis. Azithromycin, option A, as well as other antibiotics in the macrolide class, is not indicated in the treatment of common urinary pathogens. Option B, doxycycline, similarly does not provide effective coverage of urinary pathogens. In addition, doxycycline is not advised in this patient due to pregnancy. While gentamicin, option C, provides excellent coverage for *Escherichia coli*, the most common causative organism for pyelonephritis, the drug is rated for pregnancy as category D and should be used only in life-threatening circumstances and when no other drug is available. Use of trimethoprim-sulfamethoxazole, option E, is certainly first-line treatment in nonresistant urinary tract infections and uncomplicated acute pyelonephritis. However, use of trimethoprim-sulfamethoxazole in the first and third trimesters of pregnancy is not advised. **Task**: D3—Pharmaceutical Therapeutics

5. **Answer: E** Hydronephrosis can be either unilateral or bilateral and occurs from ureteral or renal pelvic obstruction. Renal calculi, option E, is the most common cause of hydronephrosis. Other etiologies include, but are not limited to, pregnancy, benign prostatic hypertrophy, and malignancy. Eighty percent of calculi are calcium oxalate, which is consistent with findings on the microscopic urinalysis of this patient. Acute cholecystitis and appendicitis, options A and B, do not cause hydronephrosis. Acute cholecystitis presents with acute pain in the right upper quadrant with radiation to the right scapula. Patients may have fever and leukocytosis and display a positive Murphy sign. Appendicitis presents with symptoms of anorexia, nausea and vomiting, and localized abdominal pain.

Symptoms are usually vague with localization to the right lower quadrant (McBurney point) and increased with positive Rovsing and obturator sign. Pelvic inflammatory disease, option C, is typical in a sexually active young female with a history of fever, flank pain, and pyuria. Pyelonephritis, option D, can cause hydronephrosis, but patients with this disorder have fever, chills, flank pain, and pyuria. **Task**: C—Formulating Most Likely Diagnosis

6. **Answer: D** Option D, bladder catheterization, is the correct answer. This patient has the classic manifestations of postrenal acute kidney injury, which typically results from obstruction (e.g., by an enlarged prostate). Bladder catheterization bypasses the obstruction and allows the bladder and urinary system to decompress. Admitting the patient to the hospital for observation, option A, does not directly address the patient's problem. It may be necessary to observe the patient, but observation is not sufficient to address the acute kidney injury. Alpha-adrenergic antagonist therapy, option B, could address the symptoms of an enlarged prostate but not in a manner that would be timely enough to address the kidney injury present in this patient. Bilateral nephrostomy tube placement, option C, is incorrect because this will address the hydronephrosis and hydroureter, but it will not address the cause of the problem. Hemodialysis, option E, is incorrect. Because the acute kidney injury is expected to improve with decompression of the urinary system, hemodialysis is generally not needed. Furthermore, this degree of kidney injury is generally below the threshold for dialysis. **Task**: D2—Clinical Intervention

7. **Answer: D** There are several common findings in individuals with end-stage renal disease (ESRD). In addition to hypertension, acidosis, and uremic syndrome, laboratory studies consistently show anemia, hypocalcemia, hyperkalemia, and hyperphosphatemia. Each of these findings has a largely linear relationship with the declining glomerular filtration rate. When hypocalcemia and hyperphosphatemia occur, the body's natural physiologic response is to increase parathyroid hormone (PTH), option D. Indeed, PTH begins to rise as early as stage 3 renal disease, making it the correct option.
Erythropoietin, option A, is secreted primarily by the kidneys and serves a major role in stimulating erythropoiesis in the bone marrow. In stages 3 through 5 renal disease, a decreased erythropoietin level as a result of renal failure invariably leads to clinically significant anemia. Gastrin, option B, is a hormone secreted by the stomach and serves to promote the release of stomach digestive juices. An abnormally elevated gastrin level is found in patients with Zollinger–Ellison syndrome. There is no secondary relationship between gastrin and ESRD. The level of insulin,

option C, is not secondarily related to the renal disease in this patient. An elevated insulin level may be associated with insulin resistance or an insulinoma but not ESRD. An elevated thyroid-stimulating hormone level (TSH), option E, is observed in patients with hypothyroid states such as Hashimoto thyroiditis. There is no secondary relationship between TSH and ESRD. **Task**: E—Applying Basic Scientific Concepts

8. **Answer: C** This patient has acute respiratory acidosis, option C, marked by increased levels of pCO_2 and a decreased blood pH level. For the patient to have metabolic acidosis, option A, the level of HCO_3^- would need to be decreased and not high-normal. Both respiratory and metabolic alkalosis (options B and D) are incorrect since the patient's pH level is decreased and consistent with acidosis.
This scenario occurs frequently in patients with chronic obstructive pulmonary disease (COPD) who are hospitalized, especially if they are taking narcotics for pain management. Chronic respiratory acidosis is common in patients with COPD and is characterized by an elevation of pCO_2. Over time, this leads to compensatory elevations in HCO_3^- to maintain a relatively normal pH level. If the patient's breathing acutely decompensates due to narcotic respiratory depression, then the body is unable to properly ventilate and rid itself of excess carbon dioxide. This occurs more rapidly than the metabolic system can compensate, and thus the patient develops acidosis with decreased arterial pH. The HCO_3^- level in this patient is high-normal but not indicative of overt alkalosis and definitely not indicative of acidosis. **Task**: B—Using Diagnostic and Laboratory Studies

9. **Answer: C** This patient has several risk factors for renal cell carcinoma. The peak incidence of this disorder is in the sixth decade of life with a male-to-female ratio of 2:1. Cigarette smoking is the only environmental risk factor identified, and gross or microhematuria occurs in about 60% of cases. The results of ultrasonography showing a solitary, hypoechoic, and solid mass should be considered renal cell carcinoma, option C, until proven otherwise.
Amyloidosis, option A, is a systemic disease also affecting the kidneys whereby excess amyloid, an abnormally folded protein, is deposited within the glomeruli and renal parenchyma. Presenting signs of this disorder include proteinuria, a decreased glomerular filtration rate, and nephrotic syndrome. Although amyloid kidneys are frequently enlarged, the disorder does not present as a solitary mass. Perinephric abscess, option B, is characterized by a purulent, cystic structure typically located outside the renal parenchyma. A perinephric abscess consists of perirenal fat necrosis resulting from complications of pyelonephritis. Finally, the appearance of a perinephric abscess on

ultrasonography would not be solid in nature. Simple cysts, option D, account for approximately 70% of all renal masses. The solid nature of the mass observed on ultrasonography eliminates a fluid-filled structure such as a simple cyst or a renal abscess as the correct choice. Wilms tumor (option E), or nephroblastoma, occurs in children most commonly between 2 and 5 years of age. It is rare for the tumor to occur after 6 years of age. Hematuria and an intrarenal mass on ultrasonography in this age group should be considered a Wilms tumor until proven otherwise. **Task**: C—Formulating Most Likely Diagnosis

10. **Answer: E** This patient has signs and symptoms of severe hypovolemia, which is defined as volume depletion greater than or equal to 10%. Patients with severe hypovolemia typically have lethargy, confusion, decreased peripheral perfusion with a capillary refill greater than three seconds, cool and mottled extremities, absent tears, and tenting of the skin greater than two seconds, option E.
Bradycardia, capillary refill less than two seconds, increased thirst, and a slightly sunken fontanelle (options A through D) are symptoms consistent with mild to moderate dehydration. Also, by 18 months of age, the anterior fontanelles have typically closed. **Task**: A—History Taking and Performing Physical Examination

11. **Answer: D** This patient is suspected of having glomerulonephritis. Red blood cell casts, option D, in urine sediment is pathognomonic but not required for a diagnosis of glomerulonephritis.
Amorphous phosphate crystals, option A, are often seen in urinary sediment but usually are clinically insignificant. These crystals form when the pH is alkaline, and they are affected by diet. Calcium oxalate crystals, option B, can be found in normal urine or in patients with renal stones. Neutrophils, option C, are white blood cells and can be seen in glomerulonephritis but are more commonly associated with infections such as cystitis and pyelonephritis. Transitional epithelial cells, option E, is incorrect. It is common to find transitional epithelial cells in normal urine sediment. High numbers may indicate malignancy affecting the lining of the bladder. **Task**: B—Using Diagnostic and Laboratory Studies

12. **Answer: E** This patient has the classic manifestations of hypervolemia, likely due to his underlying kidney disease. Restriction of sodium intake, option E, will reduce the likelihood of recurrence.
Calcium, option A, does not contribute to volume status. Calcium derangements, with or without hyperparathyroidism, can be problematic in patients with advanced kidney disease, but they will not manifest with hypervolemia. Glucose, option B, does not factor

significantly into volume status. Phosphorus, option C, is related to the calcium derangements mentioned above and is incorrect for the same reasons. Potassium, option D, does not factor into volume status, though hyperkalemia is an important complication of chronic kidney disease. **Task**: D1—Health Maintenance, Patient Education, and Disease Prevention

13. **Answer: E** Option E, renal ultrasonography, is the correct answer. This patient has typical manifestations of polycystic kidney disease, along with a positive family history of this disorder, which is commonly an autosomal dominant condition. Renal ultrasonography is useful for screening and diagnosis of polycystic kidney disease due to its low cost and safety.
Genetic testing, option A, can be used as part of the diagnostic evaluation when imaging is equivocal or when a definitive diagnosis is needed, but it is not needed in straightforward cases such as with this patient. MRI of the kidneys, option B, is only rarely needed for evaluation of the kidneys. Noncontrast CT scan of the abdomen and pelvis, option C, is an appropriate second-line imaging study for polycystic kidney disease. CT scans are more expensive and expose the patient to radiation, without increasing the diagnostic reliability compared with ultrasonography. A CT scan is used if ultrasonography does not yield clear results. Renal biopsy, option D, does not generally have a role in diagnosing polycystic kidney disease. **Task**: B—Using Diagnostic and Laboratory Studies

14. **Answer: E** This patient has multiple chronic diseases, including extensive peripheral vascular disease. The presence of bilateral renal bruits is suggestive of a decrease in perfusion with resultant atherosclerotic ischemia of the kidney parenchyma. Renal artery stenosis occurs in approximately 5% of patients with hypertension, particularly those greater than 45 years of age. Serum creatinine and urea nitrogen (BUN) levels are typically elevated in these patients. Since the cause of the elevated BUN is due to decreased presentation to the glomerulus, the condition is considered prerenal azotemia, option E.
Hemochromatosis, option A, is a genetic disorder with a male-to-female preponderance of 5:1. This disorder results in an increase in iron absorption resulting in iron overload. Excess iron over time can result in diabetes mellitus, liver disease, and heart disease. There is no indication that this patient has hemochromatosis. A low QRS voltage, option B, is commonly seen in patients with obesity, emphysema, and cardiac tamponade. The description of this patient does not indicate he has any of these conditions. Pulse pressure is calculated by subtracting the diastolic from the systolic value. It is considered narrow if the sum is less than 40 mmHg. A narrow pulse pressure, option C, can indicate decreased cardiac

Answer Key for this chapter begins on p. 196

output and is a pathognomonic finding in cardiac tamponade. This patient shows no signs of tamponade. Portal hypertension, option D, secondary to cirrhosis is caused by obstruction of the normal flow of portal blood through the liver. The increased pressure in the portal vein typically results in ascites, esophageal varices, and gastrointestinal bleeding. Non-cirrhosis causes of portal hypertension include thrombosis of the portal or splenic veins, immunologic disorders, medications, or toxins. None of these conditions are present in this patient. **Task: E—Applying Basic Scientific Concepts**

15. **Answer: E** Hypertonic saline, or 3% saline (option E), is indicated for treatment of patients with hyponatremia who have neurologic deficit or mental status changes. Patients must have close monitoring of serum sodium due to the risk of osmotic demyelination syndrome with overrapid correction of serum sodium. Intravenous calcium gluconate, option A, is used to treat patients with hypocalcemia or hyperkalemia. Diltiazem, option B, is administered intravenously for treatment of tachycardia, arrhythmia, or hypertension. Intravenous furosemide, option C, is useful in treating patients with volume overload. Regular insulin, option D, is administered intravenously for treatment of hyperglycemia. **Task: D2—Clinical Intervention**

16. **Answer: A** Patients with chronic kidney disease (CKD) tend to develop hyperkalemia, option A. This results from decreased excretion of potassium from the nephron. Hyperkalemia is significant in this patient since she has missed two dialysis treatments and has generalized weakness, which is a common symptom of hyperkalemia. Failure to identify this life-threatening electrolyte abnormality may lead to cardiac arrhythmia and death. Hypernatremia, option B, is unlikely in this clinical scenario because the patient has edema and does not appear dehydrated. Hyponatremia is the more common abnormality due to fluid retention from the lack of dialysis. Hypocalcemia, hypomagnesemia, and hypophosphatemia (options C, D, and E) are unlikely to occur in patients with advanced CKD; elevation of electrolyte levels is much more likely in patients with these conditions. **Task: B—Using Diagnostic and Laboratory Studies**

17. **Answer: B** This patient has the classic signs and symptoms of nephrotic syndrome, such as hypertension, lower extremity edema, elevated cholesterol level, decreased albumin level, and significant proteinuria with minimal hematuria. Benazepril, option B, is a renin-angiotensin inhibitor that will lower both this patient's blood pressure and the nephrotoxic proteinuria. Diuretics and lipid-lowering medications are also indicated in this patient.

The other options (A, C, D, and E) are incorrect because they will lower blood pressure but will not treat the nephrotoxic proteinuria. Amlodipine, option A, is a calcium channel blocker. Clonidine, option C, is a central acting alpha-adrenergic agonist. Hydralazine, option D, is a direct vasodilator, and metoprolol, option E, is a beta-blocker. **Task: D3—Pharmaceutical Therapeutics**

18. **Answer: E** Option E, postoperative antidiuretic hormone release, is the correct answer. This patient has hyponatremia in the early postoperative period, and postoperative pain and nausea can lead to increased levels of antidiuretic hormone. This leads to water retention but sodium excretion, even when isotonic saline is administered, which results in hyponatremia. Diuresis, option A, is incorrect because the patient has no evidence of hypovolemia, which would be expected in the setting of hyponatremia due to that cause. Heart failure, option B, is incorrect because patients with hyponatremia due to heart failure are hypervolemic rather than euvolemic. Idiosyncratic drug reaction, option C, is incorrect because no other drugs are mentioned in this patient's history. Common drugs that cause such reactions include thiazide diuretics and angiotensin-converting enzyme inhibitors. A patient with mineralocorticoid deficiency, option D, would likely have hyperkalemia as well as hyponatremia. **Task: C—Formulating Most Likely Diagnosis**

19. **Answer: C** This patient has poststreptococcal glomerulonephritis. Damage to the basement membrane of the glomerulus, option C, results in spilling of blood and protein into the urine. In the case of poststreptococcal glomerulonephritis, this is caused by antibodies present from the body's response to the bacterial infection.

The other choices, options A, B, D, and E, are involved in a number of other functions of the nephron, but disruptions in function of these units of the kidney manifest with electrolyte abnormalities rather than hematuria and proteinuria. **Task: E—Applying Basic Scientific Concepts**

20. **Answer: D** Chronic kidney disease is diagnosed in patients who have markers of kidney damage and/or decreased renal filtration as demonstrated by a glomerular filtration rate (GFR) of less than 60 mL/min for three months or more. Microalbuminuria is significant, as it shows the glomeruli are filtering larger particles than normal and is often the first sign of kidney damage in a patient with diabetes mellitus. Also, some patients with inflammatory diseases of the kidney such as chronic glomerulonephritis may have chronic blood in the urine due to damaged and inflamed glomeruli. Blood in the urine requires investigation, as it can also

be a sign of a malignant process in the urinary tract. Both microalbuminuria and glomerular hematuria from chronic glomerulonephritis can occur in patients with a normal GFR but are signs that the kidneys are damaged. In the absence of known or demonstrated kidney damage, a GFR greater than 60 mL/min is considered normal and not at stage 1 or 2 of chronic kidney disease. The answer is stage 4 (option D), which includes a GFR of 15 to 29 mL/min with or without markers of kidney damage. These findings are consistent with this patient scenario.

Stage 1, option A, includes a normal GFR greater than 90 mL/min only if the patient has markers of kidney disease. Stage 2, option B, includes a GFR of 60 to 89 mL/min only if the patient has markers of kidney damage. Stage 3, option C, includes a GFR of 30 to 59 mL/min whether or not the patient has markers of kidney damage. Stage 5, option E, includes a GFR of less than 15 mL/min, which is the stage in which patients are often started on dialysis or renal replacement therapy. **Task:** B—Using Diagnostic and Laboratory Studies

21. **Answer: B** This patient has signs and symptoms consistent with congestive heart failure and hypervolemic hyponatremia. The decreased serum and urine sodium levels combined with a decreased serum osmolality are characteristic of a fluid overload state. Congestive heart failure, cirrhosis, nephrotic syndrome, and advanced renal failure are all contributors of hypervolemia. In the workup of hyponatremia, knowledge of the patient's volume status is crucial. Fluid restriction alone may correct many cases of hyponatremia. However, this patient has significant pulmonary and neurologic symptoms, presumably related to the electrolyte imbalance. A more aggressive treatment approach is warranted. Diuresis with furosemide, option B, will address the excess fluid and dilutional hyponatremia in this patient.

Option A, 5% dextrose solution, is indicated in the treatment of hypernatremia in patients with euvolemia or hypervolemia. Dextrose osmotically pulls intracellular water into the vascular space. The translocation of water thus lowers the serum sodium. Such a process is definitely not indicated in this patient. The same translocation of water process occurs with mannitol administration (option C). In fact, hyperglycemia, mannitol, sorbitol, glycerol, maltose, and radiocontrast agents all may induce osmotic hypertonic hyponatremia. Infusion with isotonic saline, option D, will only worsen this patient's pulmonary congestion and will not affect the serum sodium level. Normal saline is indicated in the treatment of hypernatremia with hypovolemia to restore euvolemia. Use of a 3% hypertonic saline solution is indicated but should be done with extreme caution and in an ICU setting. The administration of insulin along with glucose is an effective treatment for hyperkalemia. Insulin by itself, option E, will have no effect on volume status or sodium balance. **Task:** D2—Clinical Intervention

22. **Answer: D** This patient has autosomal dominant polycystic kidney disease, which is a genetic disease with multiple bilateral renal cysts that progresses to renal failure. It is rarely found in patients who are less than 30 years of age. However, patients may have abdominal/flank pain, lower back pain, hematuria, and symptoms of a urinary tract infection. Patients with larger kidneys tend to develop hypertension earlier in life, even before a decline in glomerular filtration rate. Complications include intracranial aneurysm, coronary artery aneurysm, and cardiovascular abnormalities. Echocardiography shows mitral valve prolapse, option D, and left ventricular hypertrophy.

Aortic regurgitation, option A, is a transient murmur that may be induced by the effects of volume overload. Aortic stenosis, option B, which is usually heard in elderly patients, is associated with increased age. Mid systolic murmur, option C, may occur in patients who are pregnant or who have thyrotoxicosis or anemia. Ventricular septal defect, option E, is associated with pulmonary hypertension. **Task:** B—Using Diagnostic and Laboratory Studies

23. **Answer: A** This patient has sustained significant tissue injury to his lower extremities, including injury to muscle. Damage to skeletal muscle cells, known as rhabdomyolysis, releases myoglobin into the circulation. The toxic effect of filtering excess myoglobin can result in acute tubular necrosis, option A, and renal failure. The elevated serum creatinine and oliguria are ominous signs of renal failure. The 4+ blood on urine dipstick test is actually myoglobin, not hemoglobin. Hence, no red blood cells are seen on microscopic examination.

IgA nephropathy (option B), or Berger disease, is characterized by deposition of IgA antibodies into the connective tissue of the glomerulus. The disorder can be primary in nature or secondary to disorders such as cirrhosis, celiac disease, or infectious agents including HIV and cytomegalovirus. Trauma is not an inciting event for IgA nephropathy. Interstitial nephritis, option C, accounts for about 10% of renal failure cases. It is an inflammatory disorder of the renal parenchyma resulting in edema, tubular damage, and proteinuria. The etiology of interstitial nephritis is not related to trauma but results from an inciting event such as an infectious disease, immunologic disorder, or drug reaction. To a lesser extent, interstitial nephritis may also be idiopathic. This disorder is characterized most often by fever, rash, and arthralgia. In addition to protein, the urine often contains white (95%) and red cell casts. Minimal change disease, option D, is the most common cause of proteinuria in children, accounting for approximately 80% of cases. The condition may be idiopathic but often follows a viral infection in children. In adults, the nephrotic syndrome associated with minimal change disease may be associated with neoplasia such as Hodgkin lymphoma, with use of drugs such as lithium and nonsteroidal anti-inflammatory drugs or hypersensitivity reactions to allergens (e.g., bee stings). Minimal change disease is self-limiting and is typically responsive to a course of corticosteroids for a few months. This condition is not associated with trauma. Pyelonephritis, option E, is an acute infectious inflammatory disease of the renal parenchyma and renal pelvis. The most common causative organisms include *Escherichia coli*, *Proteus*, *Klebsiella*, *Enterobacter*, and *Pseudomonas*. Along with fever, flank pain, shaking chills, and irritative voiding symptoms, urinalysis shows pyuria, heavy growth on culture, and the pathognomonic white blood cell casts. **Task:** B—Using Diagnostic and Laboratory Studies

24. **Answer: D** Furosemide is a loop diuretic that reversibly binds to and inhibits the Na^+-K^+-$2Cl^-$ cotransporter, which prevents salt transport in the thick ascending loop of Henle. This limits the resorption of calcium and magnesium, which leads to decreased serum levels and not hypercalcemia and hyperphosphatemia, making options A, B, and C incorrect. This also leads to a decrease in water resorption in the collecting duct and increased delivery of sodium to the distal nephron, which greatly enhances potassium excretion and causes hypokalemia, option D. Loop diuretics are known to cause contraction alkalosis with increased serum bicarbonate. Therefore, metabolic acidosis is unlikely in this clinical presentation as the patient tends to develop alkalosis, making option E incorrect. **Task:** D3—Pharmaceutical Therapeutics

BIBLIOGRAPHY

Adrogue, H. J., & Madias, N. E. Respiratory acidosis, respiratory alkalosis, and mixed disorders. *Comprehensive Clinical Nephrology*, 14, 170-183. E1.

Al-Awqati, Q. (2020). Disorders of sodium and water. In: *Goldman–cecil medicine* (26th ed). Philadelphia, PA: Elsevier; 2020. p. 712-723.

Arora, N., & Jefferson, J. Hyponatremia. In: M. A. Papadakis, S. J. McPhee & M. W. Rabow (Eds.), *Current medical diagnosis & treatment 2021*. McGraw-Hill.

Bargman, J. M., & Skorecki, K. L. (2018). Chronic kidney disease. In: J. Jameson, A. S. Fauci, D. L. Kasper, S. L. Hauser, D. L. Longo, & J. Loscalzo (Eds.), *Harrison's principles of internal medicine, 20e*. McGraw-Hill. https://accessmedicine-mhmedical-com.ezproxy. libraries.udmercy.edu/content.aspx?bookid=2129&section id=186950702.

Bashore, T. M., Granger, C. B., Jackson, K. P., & Patel, M. R. Pericardial effusion & tamponade. In: M. A. Papadakis, S. J. McPhee & M. W. Rabow (Eds.), *Current medical diagnosis & treatment 2021*. McGraw-Hill.

Curhan, G. C., Aronson, M. D., & Preminger, G. M. Kidney stones in adults: Diagnosis and acute management of suspected nephrolithiasis in adults. UpToDate. Reviewed through: Oct 2020. Updated: July 2, 2019.

Dirkx, T. C., & Woodell, T. B. Chronic kidney disease. In: M. A. Papadakis, S. J. McPhee & M.W. Rabow (Eds.), *Current medical diagnosis & treatment 2021*. McGraw-Hill.

Dirkx, T. C., & Woodell, T. B. Minimal change disease. In: M. A. Papadakis, S. J. McPhee & M. W. Rabow (Eds.), *Current medical diagnosis & treatment 2021*. McGraw-Hill.

Dirkx, T. C., & Woodell, T. B. Nephritic spectrum glomerular diseases. In: M. A. Papadakis, S. J. McPhee & M. W. Rabow (Eds.), *Current medical diagnosis & treatment 2021*. McGraw-Hill.

Dirkx, T. C., & Woodell, T. B. Renal artery stenosis. In: M. A. Papadakis, S. J. McPhee & M. W. Rabow (Eds.), *Current medical diagnosis & treatment 2021*. McGraw-Hill.

Dorsainvil, D., & Luciano, R. L. Chronic tubulointerstitial nephritis. In: E. V. Lerma, M. H. Rosner, & M. A. Perazella (Eds.), *Current diagnosis & treatment: Nephrology & hypertension* (2nd ed.). McGraw-Hill.

Friedman, L. S. Hemochromatosis. In: M. A. Papadakis, S. J. McPhee, M. W. Rabow (Eds.), *Current medical diagnosis & treatment 2021*. McGraw-Hill.

Friedman, L. S. Noncirrhotic portal hypertension. In: M. A. Papadakis, S. J. McPhee & M. W. Rabow (Eds.), *Current medical diagnosis & treatment 2021*. McGraw-Hill.

Dietary guidelines for Americans, 2020-2025. 2020.

Irazabal, M. V., & Torres, V. E. Cystic diseases of the kidney. In: E. V. Lerma, M. H. Rosner, & M. A. Perazella (Eds.), *Current diagnosis & treatment: Nephrology & hypertension* (2nd ed.). McGraw-Hill.

Kalantar-Zadeh, K., & Kopple, J. D. Chronic renal failure and the uremic syndrome: Nutritional issues. In: E. V. Lerma, M. H. Rosner & M. A. Perazella (Eds.), *Current diagnosis & treatment: Nephrology & hypertension* (2nd ed.). McGraw-Hill.

Keating, A. K., Knight-Perry, J., Maloney, K., Levy, J., Greffe, B. S., Franklin, A., et al. In: W. W. Jr. Hay, M. J. Levin, M. J. Abzug & M. Bunik (Eds.), *Current diagnosis & treatment: Pediatrics* (25th ed.). McGraw-Hill.

Lewis, J. B., & Neilson, E. G. Glomerular diseases. In: J. Jameson, A. S. Fauci, D. L. Kasper, S. L. Hauser, D. L. Longo & J. Loscalzo (Eds.), *Harrison's principles of internal medicine* (20th ed.). McGraw-Hill.

Mann, D. L. Management of heart failure patients with reduced ejection fraction. In: *Braunwald's heart disease* (4th ed., Chapter 25, pp. 490-522). Elsevier.

McDonald, K., Duffy, P., Chowdhury, T., & McHugh, K. (2013). Added value of abdominal cross-sectional imaging (CT or MRI) in staging of Wilms' tumours. Clinical Radiology. *The Royal College of Radiologists*, *68*(1), 16-20.

McQuaid, K. R. Zollinger–Ellison syndrome (gastrinoma). In: M. A. Papadakis, S. J. McPhee & M. W. Rabow (Eds.), *Current medical diagnosis & treatment 2021*. McGraw-Hill.

Mitchell, T., Deborah, L., Wendy, T., & Wilson Stephanie, R. (2014). *Diagnostic ultrasound* (Chapter 9, pp. 310-380). Elsevier.

Molitoris, B. A. (2020). Acute kidney injury. In: *Goldman–Cecil medicine* (26th ed.). Philadelphia, PA: Elsevier; 2020. p. 748-753.

Mount, D. B. Fluid and electrolyte disturbances. In: J. Jameson, A. S. Fauci, D. L. Kasper, S. L. Hauser, D. L. Longo & J. Loscalzo

(Eds.), *Harrison's principles of internal medicine* (20th ed.). McGraw-Hill.

Palmer, B. (2012). Individualizing the dialysate to address electrolyte disturbances in the dialysis patient. In: *Seldin and Giebisch's the kidney* (Chapter 93, pp. 3125-3150). Elsevier.

Papadakis, M. A., & McPhee, S. F. (2020). *Current medical diagnosis & treatment* (pp. 940-941). McGraw Hill.

Perrone, R. D., Neville, J., Chapman, A. B., Gitomer, B. Y., Miskulin, D. C., Torres, V. E., et al. (2015). Therapeutic area data standards for autosomal dominant polycystic kidney disease: A report from the Polycystic Kidney Disease Outcomes Consortium (PKDOC). *American Journal of Kidney Diseases*. 2015; *66*(4), 583-590. National Kidney Foundation. Accessed 11.11.2020.

Radhakrishnan, J., & Appel, G. B. (2020). Glomerular disorders and nephrotic syndromes. In: *Goldman–Cecil medicine* (26th ed.). Philadelphia, PA: Elsevier; 2020. p. 753-763.

Ritchey, M. L., Green, D. M., Breslow, N. B., & Guthrie, K. A. (1997). Comments on Wilms' tumor experience. *Pediatrics, 99*(3), 503.

Schade, G. R. Renal cell carcinoma. In: M. A. Papadakis, S. J. McPhee & M. W. Rabow (Eds), *Current medical diagnosis & treatment 2021*. McGraw-Hill.

Sorensen, M., Walsh, T. J., & Ostrowski, K. A. Genitourinary tract infections. In: M. A. Papadakis, S. J. McPhee & M. W. Rabow (Eds.), *Current medical diagnosis & treatment 2021*. McGraw-Hill.

Strasinger, S., & DiLorenzo, M. (2019). *Urinalysis and body fluids* (6th ed.), Textbook Solutions. 9780803639201ISBN-13: 0803639201ISBN. F A Davis.

Taal, M. (2019). Classification and management of chronic kidney disease. In: *Brenner and Rector's the kidney* 59, 1946-1976.e8. Elsevier.

Thomas, D. R., Cote, T. R., Lawhorne, L., Levenson, S. A., Rubenstein, L. Z., Smith, D. A., et al. (2008). Understanding clinical dehydration and its treatment. *Journal of the American Medical Directors Association*, *9*(5), 292-301. American Medical Directors Association.

Torres, V. E., Bennett, W. M., & Perrone, R. D. Autosomal dominant polycystic kidney disease (ADPKD) in adults: Epidemiology, clinical presentation, and diagnosis. UpToDate. Literature review current through: Oct 2020. This topic last updated: September 23, 2020.

Torres, V. E., & Harris, P. C. (2020). Cystic diseases of the kidney . In: *Brenner and Rector's the kidney* (11th ed.). Philadelphia, PA: Elsevier; 2020. 1490-1534.

Waikar S. S., & Bonventre J. V. (2018). Acute kidney injury. In: Jameson, J., Fauci A. S., Kasper D. L., Hauser S. L., Longo D. L., & Loscalzo J (Eds.), *Harrison's principles of internal medicine* (20th ed.). McGraw-Hill.

Yancy, C. W., Januzzi, J. L., Jr., Allen, L. A., Butler, J., Davis, L. L., Fonarow, G. C., et al. (2018). 2017 ACC expert consensus decision pathway for optimization of heart failure treatment: Answers to 10 pivotal issues about heart failure with reduced ejection fraction: A report of the American College of Cardiology Task Force on expert consensus decision pathways. *Journal of the American College of Cardiology*, *71*(2), 201-230.

Answer Key for this chapter begins on p. 196

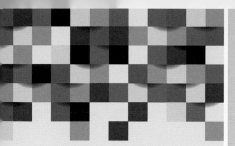

CHAPTER 14
Reproductive System

Questions

1. A 32-year-old woman, gravida 2, para 1, comes to the office because she has had abnormal uterine bleeding and pelvic pain for the past three months. Medical history includes spontaneous abortion at 10 weeks' gestation four years ago. Physical examination shows no abnormalities. Result of pregnancy test is negative. Ultrasonography of the pelvis shows multiple large leiomyomas. Preservation of fertility is discussed, and myomectomy is scheduled. Removal of the tumors from which of the following areas is most likely?
   A. Body of the uterus
   B. Detrusor muscle
   C. Fallopian tube
   D. Paraovarian area
   E. Pouch of Douglas

2. Physical examination of a 2-day-old male neonate shows pallor of the nail beds. After delivery, the infant had rapid development of jaundice within the first 24 hours of life. The patient's mother is a 28-year-old White woman, gravida 2, para 2, and she did not receive routine prenatal care. The patient's current vital signs are within normal limits. Laboratory studies show elevated serum bilirubin level, and peripheral blood smear shows a predominant number of nucleated red blood cells with few spherocytes. Which of the following is the most likely diagnosis?
   A. G6PD deficiency
   B. Hereditary spherocytosis
   C. Rh incompatibility
   D. Sepsis
   E. Thalassemia

3. A 22-year-old woman with recently diagnosed infectious cervicitis calls the clinic because she has questions about the diagnosis. She says she was evaluated at the free clinic, given some antibiotics, and told not to have sex for a week. The patient also says that she was told to have her partner treated as well. She wants to know which sexually transmitted infection caused the cervicitis. It is most appropriate to tell this patient that which of the following pathogens is the most likely cause?
   A. Candidiasis
   B. Chlamydia
   C. Herpes simplex virus
   D. *Staphylococcus aureus*
   E. Trichomoniasis

4. A 70-year-old woman, gravida 4, para 4, comes to the primary care office because she has had a vaginal mass for the past three months. She says she feels as if something is obstructing her vaginal canal. The patient has not had dysuria, back pain, flank pain, or difficulty with bowel movements. Medical history includes hysterectomy. Pelvic examination shows mild-to-moderate vaginal prolapse. The patient says that she does not want to undergo surgical intervention at this time. Which of the following is the most appropriate management to recommend?
   A. Oral estrogen therapy
   B. Oral progesterone therapy
   C. Referral for physical therapy for pelvic floor retraining
   D. Testosterone injection
   E. Use of a pessary

5. A 38-year-old woman comes to the office because she has had intermittent breast pain during the past four months. She is concerned because her cousin was recently diagnosed with breast cancer. She says that just before her menstrual cycle begins, she experiences bilateral breast fullness and tenderness that improves a few days after her menstrual cycle begins. The patient has not had weight loss, appetite changes, fever, chills, fatigue, or generalized weakness. Physical examination shows mild-to-moderate bilateral breast tenderness to palpation along with palpable areas of thickening and nodularity noted throughout the breasts. No axillary lymphadenopathy, retraction, dimpling, or nipple discharge is noted. Based on these findings, which of the following is the most likely diagnosis?
   A. Breast abscess
   B. Breast cancer
   C. Fibroadenoma
   D. Fibrocystic changes
   E. Lipoma

6. A 34-year-old woman, gravida 2, para 1, comes to the emergency department because she has had light, painless vaginal bleeding for the past two hours. She has not received any prenatal care but thinks she is at 30 weeks' gestation. She says her other child was delivered vaginally five years ago. Pulse rate is 72/min, and blood pressure is 115/84 mmHg. Fetal heart rate is stable at 150/min. Ultrasonography shows a low-lying placenta that is partially covering the internal os. Membranes have not ruptured. Which of the following is the most likely diagnosis?
   A. Abruptio placentae
   B. Placenta accreta
   C. Placenta percreta
   D. Placenta previa
   E. Vasa previa

7. A 26-year-old woman, gravida 1, para 0, who is at 36 weeks' gestation comes to the emergency department because she had recent onset of headache, blurred vision, shortness of breath, and right upper quadrant pain. Pulse rate is 96/min, respirations are 20/min, and blood pressure is 175/115 mmHg; she is afebrile. Oxygen saturation is 94% on room air. On physical examination, Doppler ultrasonography shows fetal heart tones at 160/min, and measurement of fundal height is consistent with gestational age. Auscultation of the chest show bilateral basilar crackles, and 2+ pitting edema is noted in the pretibial areas bilaterally. Laboratory studies show a mild elevation of serum hepatic transaminases. Urine dipstick test shows 3+ proteinuria and 2+ glucose. Which of the following medications is most appropriate to initiate in the emergency department while preparations are being made to deliver the fetus?
   A. Aliskiren (Tekturna)
   B. Enalapril
   C. Hydralazine
   D. Lisinopril
   E. Losartan

8. A 35-year-old woman comes to the office because she has had menstrual irregularity during the past six months. She also has had increased vaginal dryness, hot flashes, night sweats, and irritability during this time. Medical history includes cancer in the left breast treated with mastectomy, chemotherapy, and radiation. She says that she has not resumed her menstrual cycle since she completed radiation six months ago. The patient has not had any recent changes in weight, medication, or activity level. Physical examination shows vaginal atrophy. Laboratory studies show that serum thyroid-stimulating hormone, prolactin, and free testosterone levels are within normal limits. Follicle-stimulating hormone and luteinizing hormone levels are elevated, and estradiol level is decreased. Beta-human chorionic gonadotropin test is negative. Which of the following is the most likely cause of the amenorrhea in this patient?
   A. Anorexia nervosa
   B. Increased emotional stress
   C. Intrauterine pregnancy
   D. Polycystic ovary syndrome
   E. Premature menopause

9. A 38-year-old woman, gravida 4, para 3, who is at 35 weeks' gestation comes to the emergency department because she has had fluid flowing from her vagina down her leg for the past six hours. She has no pelvic or abdominal pain. Vital signs are within normal limits. Fetal heart tones are 160/min. Physical examination shows fluid in the vaginal area. Results of nitrazine and fern tests are positive. Which of the following next steps is contraindicated in the management of this patient?
   A. Cervical cultures
   B. Digital cervical examination
   C. Facilitation of delivery
   D. Pelvic ultrasonography
   E. Sterile speculum examination

10. A 24-year-old primigravida woman comes to the clinic 11 days postpartum because she has had worsening left breast pain over the past 24 hours. She says that breastfeeding had been going well until today when feeding from the left breast became too painful. Temperature is 37.7°C (99.8°F); all other vital signs are within normal limits. Physical examination shows diffuse edema and erythema of the upper-outer quadrant of the left breast. The overlying skin is warm to touch. Tender left axillary lymphadenopathy is noted, and a small amount of purulent discharge is easily expressed from the nipple. Infection with which of the following organisms is most likely?
A. *Clostridium difficile*
B. *Lactobacillus casei*
C. *Moraxella catarrhalis*
D. *Staphylococcus aureus*
E. *Streptococcus mutans*

11. A 29-year-old woman comes to the OB/GYN office for examination because she wants to become pregnant within the next six months. Medical history includes a recent diagnosis of celiac disease. Her only medication was an oral contraceptive which she stopped taking three months ago. Which of the following topics is most appropriate to discuss with this patient to promote a healthy pregnancy prior to conception?
A. Initiating an exercise regimen
B. Maintaining adequate hydration
C. Monitoring basal body temperatures
D. Practicing proper sleep hygiene
E. Taking a multivitamin with folic acid

12. A 54-year-old woman comes to the urgent care clinic because she has abdominal pain 15 minutes after she was involved in a motor vehicle collision in which she was the restrained driver traveling at 45 miles/hr. She has had three children via uncomplicated vaginal birth. The patient's most recent menstrual period was six years ago. Screening abdominal ultrasonography shows a 3-cm unilocular ovarian cyst on the right. Which of the following is the most appropriate next step?
A. CT scan of the pelvis
B. Refer to general surgery
C. Refer to an OB/GYN
D. Repeat ultrasonography in three months
E. Repeat ultrasonography in six months

13. A 24-year-old woman, gravida 0, para 0, comes to the primary care office because she has an eight-month history of cyclical bloating, breast tenderness, and severe cramping that usually occur approximately five days prior to menses. The patient does not have depression or mood fluctuations associated with these symptoms, and the symptoms do not interfere with her ability to work or interact with friends and family. She has regular menstrual cycles that occur every 28 to 30 days. Which of the following is the most likely diagnosis?
A. Borderline personality disorder
B. Generalized anxiety disorder
C. Polycystic ovary syndrome
D. Premenstrual dysphoric disorder
E. Premenstrual syndrome

14. A 22-year-old woman comes to the emergency department because she has had sharp, constant, nonradiating pain in the right lower quadrant of her abdomen for the past six hours. She rates the pain as a 6 on a 10-point scale. She has not had any gastrointestinal or urinary symptoms. The patient's most recent menstrual period was three months ago. She has not had any vaginal discharge or dyspareunia. Medical history includes no chronic disease conditions, and she has no history of surgery. Vital signs are within normal limits. On physical examination, the abdomen is flat and soft. Light palpation of the abdomen elicits tenderness in the right lower quadrant. No rebound, guarding, or masses are noted. Pelvic examination exacerbates the pain. The cervical vault is clear, and no inflammation or discharge is noted at the cervical os. Laboratory studies show a positive result on beta-human chorionic gonadotropin testing, and transvaginal ultrasonography shows an inhomogeneous adnexal mass. Which of the following laboratory studies is the most appropriate next step?
A. Complete blood cell count
B. Measurement of serum follicle-stimulating hormone level
C. Measurement of serum luteinizing hormone level
D. Measurement of serum progesterone level
E. Rh factor blood test

15. A 25-year-old woman comes to the office because she has had mild vulvovaginal erythema and thin, grayish-white vaginal discharge for the past two weeks. Medical history includes human papillomavirus with normal cytology. She is sexually active with one partner. Vital signs are within normal limits. Bacterial vaginosis is suspected. Which of the following findings on analysis of vaginal secretions is most likely to confirm this diagnosis?
A. Clue cells greater than 20% on microscopy
B. Increased polymorphonuclear cells on normal saline preparation
C. Motile trichomonads on normal saline preparation
D. Positive whiff test
E. Pseudohyphae on microscopy

    Answer Key for this chapter begins on p. 209

16. A 20-year-old woman comes to the primary care clinic to request postcoital contraception. She says she had unprotected sexual intercourse 48 hours ago. She has no history of pregnancy, and her most recent menstrual period was five days ago. Medical history is unremarkable. The patient takes no medications and has no allergies. Physical examination shows no abnormalities. Therapy with ulipristal acetate is planned. Which of the following best explains the mechanism of action of this drug?
    A. Delays ovulation
    B. Inflames the uterine wall
    C. Modulates estrogen
    D. Prevents sperm–egg adhesion

17. A 33-year-old woman who is six weeks postpartum and breastfeeding comes to the office because she has new onset of fever and body aches. Two weeks ago she completed a course of antibiotics for treatment of mastitis of the left breast. Current temperature is 38.1°C (100.6°F). Physical examination shows a localized area of fluctuant erythema with tenderness to palpation just lateral to the nipple of the left breast. Which of the following is the most appropriate next step?
    A. Perform incision and drainage of the abscess and initiate antibiotic therapy
    B. Perform ultrasound-guided needle aspiration of the abscess and initiate antibiotic therapy
    C. Recommend she apply warm compresses to the breast and take analgesic medication as needed
    D. Recommend she continue nursing on the affected side to ensure drainage of the breast
    E. Refer the patient for surgical drainage of the abscess

18. A 32-year-old woman, gravida 3, para 2, who is at 28 weeks' gestation is referred to the clinic for consultation three weeks after gestational diabetes was diagnosed. She has received nutritional counseling and has been modifying her diet as instructed. The patient also has been walking 30 minutes daily. Family medical history includes type 2 diabetes mellitus. Blood pressure is 142/84 mmHg. Fasting serum glucose level is 118 mg/dL (N = <95 mg/dL), and one-hour postprandial serum glucose level is 152 mg/dL (N = <140 mg/dL). Which of the following is the most appropriate recommendation to give this patient?
    A. Initiate testing for urine ketones
    B. Initiate therapy with lisinopril for treatment of hypertension
    C. Initiate therapy with sitagliptin for control of serum glucose level

    D. Keep the fasting serum glucose level less than 95 mg/dL
    E. Test serum glucose level when fasting and preprandial

19. A 22-year-old woman, gravida 0, para 0, comes to the urgent care clinic because she has had pelvic pain and foul-smelling vaginal discharge for the past two weeks. She says she recently had sexual intercourse with three male partners, and she did not use condoms. Medical history includes placement of an intrauterine device two years ago and infection with chlamydia one year ago. Physical examination shows cervical motion tenderness, cloudy white discharge from the cervical os, and erythematous mucosa of the vaginal wall. Results of cultures and urinalysis are pending. Which of the following is the most likely diagnosis?
    A. Herpes simplex virus type 2
    B. Human papillomavirus
    C. Pelvic inflammatory disease
    D. Syphilis
    E. Urinary tract infection

20. An 18-year-old woman, gravida 1, para 0, who is at 30 weeks' gestation comes to the emergency department because she was slapped in the face and punched in her belly by her boyfriend yesterday and wants to make sure her baby is okay. She does not have pelvic pain, vaginal bleeding, or vaginal discharge. Vital signs are within normal limits. Physical examination shows no abnormalities. Fetal heart rate is 140/min. Based on these findings, this patient is at increased risk for which of the following?
    A. Eclampsia
    B. Gestational diabetes
    C. Postterm delivery
    D. Preeclampsia
    E. Preterm delivery

21. A 27-year-old woman comes to the clinic because she has had severe pelvic pain with menstruation and dyspareunia during the past three years. She says she has been trying to get pregnant for the past 15 months but has been unsuccessful. Pelvic examination elicits significant pain, and enlarged, immobile ovaries are noted. Which of the following is the most likely diagnosis?
    A. Adenomyosis
    B. Endometriosis
    C. Pelvic inflammatory disease
    D. Primary dysmenorrhea
    E. Uterine fibroids

22. A 28-year-old woman, gravida 1, para 1, comes to the OB/GYN clinic for routine six-week postpartum follow-up. The patient says that she has feelings of sadness and anxiety any time she looks at her newborn, which are not feelings that she expected to have. She says she has limited interest in breastfeeding, although she has continued to attempt to successfully do so. She has not had suicidal thoughts or feelings of wanting to abandon her child. Which of the following is the most appropriate initial treatment?
A. Antipsychotics
B. Benzodiazepines
C. Lithium salts
D. Selective serotonin reuptake inhibitors
E. Tricyclic antidepressants

23. A 31-year-old woman comes to the office with her husband for counseling regarding infertility. The couple has been trying to conceive for more than a year without success. The patient has a history of regular periods up until about eight months ago when they became sporadic. Her most recent menstrual period was about four months ago. She has no history of chronic disease conditions, and she has not had hot flashes or vaginal dryness. Vital signs are within normal limits, and physical examination shows no abnormalities. Result of a pregnancy test is negative. On laboratory studies of serum, prolactin level is within normal limits, follicle-stimulating and luteinizing hormone levels are significantly elevated, estrogen level is decreased, and anti-Müllerian hormone level is less than 1.0 ng/mL (N = 1.0-4.0 ng/mL). Karyotyping shows the normal chromosomal complement. Pelvic ultrasonography shows small ovaries without evidence of growing follicles. Which of the following is the most likely diagnosis?
A. Anovulatory cycles
B. Menopause
C. Polycystic ovary syndrome
D. Primary ovarian insufficiency
E. Streak gonads

24. A 28-year-old woman comes to the emergency department because she has had painful vaginal bleeding for the past five days. Her most recent normal menstrual period was two weeks ago. Medical history includes no chronic disease conditions. Vital signs are within normal limits. Pelvic examination shows blood in the vaginal vault. Complete blood cell count is within normal limits. Result of urine pregnancy test is negative. Which of the following is the most appropriate initial step in diagnosis?
A. Dilation and curettage
B. Endometrial biopsy

C. Hysteroscopy
D. MRI of the pelvis
E. Pelvic ultrasonography

25. Results of a Pap smear obtained from a 33-year-old woman show atypical glandular cells of undetermined significance. Results of testing for the presence of human papillomavirus are negative. Which of the following is the most appropriate next step in management?
A. Carbon dioxide laser treatment
B. Cryotherapy
C. Endocervical biopsy
D. Loop electrosurgical excision procedure
E. Repeat Pap testing every six months for one year

26. A 38-year-old woman, gravida 4, para 3, who is at 37 weeks' gestation is brought to the emergency department by ambulance on a backboard and wearing a cervical collar. She has had very painful vaginal bleeding and abdominal pain since she was involved in a high-speed motor vehicle collision just prior to arrival. After clearing the patient off the board and removing the collar, dark-colored blood is noted on the patient's underwear. Fetal heart rate is 90/min. Based on these findings, which of the following is the most likely diagnosis?
A. Abruptio placentae
B. Placenta previa
C. Premature rupture of membranes
D. Threatened miscarriage
E. Vaginal laceration

27. A 15-year-old girl is brought to the clinic by her mother because she has irregular periods, facial acne, and noticeable thinning of her hair that have been worsening over the past year. Medical history includes no acute or chronic diseases, and she takes no medications. Body mass index is 34 kg/m² (N = 18.5-24.9 kg/m²). Vital signs are within normal limits. Physical examination shows numerous closed and open comedones on the mandibular area, cheeks, chin, and upper neck. There is prominent darkened hair above the superior lip. Blood glucose measured by finger stick shows 180 mg/dL (N = 70-99 mg/dL). Initiation of which of the following therapies is most appropriate to decrease the excess androgen production in this patient?
A. Metformin
B. Rosiglitazone
C. Simvastatin
D. Spironolactone
E. Tamoxifen

28. A 22-year-old woman comes to the office for follow-up four days after she had a spontaneous abortion at eight weeks' gestation. The patient is distraught and would like to know the cause of the miscarriage. The practitioner explains to the patient that there are several possible causes, such as infection and chromosomal abnormalities. If an infection is suspected, which of the following infections is most likely to have caused the spontaneous abortion in this patient?
    A. Bacterial vaginosis
    B. Chlamydia trachomatis
    C. Herpes simplex virus
    D. HIV
    E. Human papillomavirus

29. A 36-year-old woman comes to the office for follow-up six weeks after she delivered her first baby. Since the delivery, she says she has had difficulty bonding with her baby and feels down and sad most days. The patient has no appetite and finds it difficult to concentrate. She has not had thoughts of harming herself or the baby. Which of the following findings on history taking most significantly increases this patient's risk of developing postpartum depression?
    A. History of miscarriage
    B. Lack of social support
    C. Not breastfeeding the infant
    D. Personal history of depression
    E. Symptoms of a thyroid disorder

30. A 22-year-old woman is being treated in the delivery room immediately after undergoing a live birth that was assisted by forceps due to fetal distress. Successful delivery of the placenta occurred five minutes ago. Physical examination shows ongoing postpartum hemorrhage of bright red blood; estimated blood loss is 800 mL. The uterus is firm and well contracted. Examination of the episiotomy site shows slight ooze but no hematoma. Which of the following is the most appropriate next step?
    A. Infuse oxytocin 20 to 40 U/L in crystalloid
    B. Insert vaginal packing and reevaluate in 15 minutes
    C. Locate and stop the bleeding
    D. Perform vigorous uterine massage
    E. Place an inflatable abdominal binder

Answers

1. **Answer: A** Body of the uterus, option A, is correct because leiomyomas are benign tumors of smooth muscle origin located within the myometrium.
Option B, detrusor muscle, is the contractile muscle of the urinary bladder and has no anatomic relationship to the myometrium. Options C and D, fallopian tube and paraovarian area, describe areas of the female reproductive tract unrelated to the myometrium. Option E, pouch of Douglas, is the name given to the recess located between the rectum and uterus. This area, anatomically known as the rectouterine pouch, while of clinical importance, is not directly related to the myometrium. **Task:** E— Applying Basic Scientific Concepts

2. **Answer: C** Rh incompatibility, option C, is correct because this disorder usually occurs in a second-born Rh positive baby to a mother who is Rh negative. It is one of the leading causes of hemolytic disease in the newborn. Newborns may present with varying degrees of anemia and hyperbilirubinemia. Women who undergo routine prenatal screening found to be Rh negative receive prophylactic treatment to prevent Rh-mediated hemolytic disease.
G6PD deficiency, option A, most commonly occurs in babies of African or Mediterranean descent. Bite or blister cells are noted on peripheral blood smear. Hereditary spherocytosis, option B, is incorrect because peripheral blood smear is characterized by uniform spherocytes. Sepsis, option D, is incorrect because temperature instability, physical examination findings, and a septic workup of blood, urine, and cerebrospinal fluid cultures would differentiate the diagnosis. Thalassemia, option E, most commonly presents in infants of Southeast Asian, Indian, or Middle Eastern descent. Peripheral blood smear would show hypochromic, microcytic anemia. **Task:** C—Formulating Most Likely Diagnosis

3. **Answer: B** Chlamydia trachomatis, option B, is the most common cause of cervicitis and is responsible for up to 50% of cases. The majority of women with endocervical chlamydial infection are asymptomatic.
Candidiasis or yeast infections, option A, are caused by a fungus and are not considered sexually transmitted infections. Genital herpes simplex virus, option C, is marked by genital pain and lesions. It can lead to cervicitis but is not the most common cause. *Staphylococcus aureus*, option D, is not a culprit in sexually transmitted diseases and does not lead to cervicitis. Trichomoniasis, option E, is caused by a parasite and may lead to cervicitis but is not the most common cause. **Task:** E—Applying Basic Scientific Concepts

4. **Answer: E** Vaginal prolapse is common in parous women and is often described as having fullness or something protruding from the vagina. Pelvic organ or vaginal prolapse is often associated with urinary incontinence. Diagnosis is made based on history and physical examination findings. Treatment options usually involve referral to a surgeon or more conservative treatment with a pessary device, option E. A pessary is a medical-grade device that comes in various shapes and sizes. This device can be appropriately fitted and placed into the vagina to support the prolapsing vaginal walls or to help with continence. Up to 90% of women can be adequately fitted for a pessary device if indicated. Pessaries are inexpensive and provide immediate relief of symptoms, while surgical interventions come with a multitude of risks associated. As a result, pessary devices have become the first-line treatment for vaginal prolapse.
There is no role for oral or injected hormone therapy, options A, B, and D, in a postmenopausal woman with vaginal prolapse. Pelvic floor retraining, option C, is appropriate treatment for urinary incontinence. However, this therapy will not resolve the anatomic change that has caused vaginal prolapse in this patient. **Task:** D2—Clinical Intervention

5. **Answer: D** This patient has fibrocystic changes (option D) due to fibrocystic breast disease, which is a benign condition associated with bilateral breast pain, tenderness, and nodularity that fluctuates in size with the menstrual cycle.
Although a breast abscess, option A, is painful, this condition typically occurs unilaterally, and symptoms do not fluctuate with the menstrual cycle. Although this patient is concerned about breast cancer, option B, her history and physical examination findings make this option less likely. Breast cancer is associated with a painless, hard, fixed mass or nodule that does not fluctuate in size with the menstrual cycle. Fibroadenoma, option C, is the most common benign breast tumor in premenopausal women. This condition typically presents unilaterally with the presence of a painless, well-circumscribed nodule that does not fluctuate with the menstrual cycle. A lipoma, option E, is usually painless and occurs unilaterally, whereas fibrocystic changes are painful and occur bilaterally. **Task:** A—History Taking and Performing Physical Examination

6. **Answer: D** This patient comes to the emergency department with vaginal bleeding, presumably in her second or third trimester. Signs and symptoms that must be considered are that the bleeding is light, the mother and baby appear hemodynamically

stable, membranes have not ruptured, and the internal cervical os is partially covered by placental tissue and not by vasculature alone. From these findings, the correct answer is placenta previa (option D). Multiparity and advanced maternal age are risk factors for placenta previa. Other risk factors include prior uterine surgery for any reason, history of prior cesarean delivery, and multiple gestations.

Abruptio placenta, option A, includes a premature separation of the placenta from the uterine wall after 20 weeks' gestation and prior to delivery. The triad for abruptio placenta includes fetal distress or death, uterine contractions, and uterine bleeding that may be external (vaginal) or concealed between the placenta and uterine wall. Abruptio placenta may be diagnosed with ultrasonography by the presence of hemorrhage or hematoma positioned in a retroplacental location. Differences in characteristics on ultrasonography will distinguish abruptio placenta from placenta previa.

Patients with placenta previa are at increased risk for developing placenta accreta or percreta. Placenta accreta, option B, includes a placenta that has grown or developed too deeply into the uterus such that there is no functional decidua basalis. The result of this formation is that the placenta does not separate normally from the uterus after delivery. Placenta accreta poses a risk of severe vaginal bleeding at the time of eventual placental separation. This disorder is also the most common indication for emergency peripartum hysterectomy. Placenta percreta, option C, includes placental tissue with transmural extensions across the myometrium with a serosal breach. Invasion into surrounding viscera is possible. This pattern of abnormal placental growth is typically detected by ultrasonography. The condition is rare but constitutes the most severe form of placental adherence. Complications of placenta percreta include uterine rupture and catastrophic peripartum vaginal hemorrhage.

Vaginal bleeding can occur with vasa previa, option E. The condition occurs when placental vessels cross the internal os but are not within nor supported by the cotyledons. Evidence of this ectopic vascularity is observed on ultrasonography. As the vessels are unsupported by the placenta, normal rupture of the fetal membranes can lacerate the placental-derived vessels, resulting in significant hemorrhage, fetal exsanguination, and death. Rates of neonatal survival are as high as 97% with antenatal diagnosis. However, in pregnancies complicated by vasa previa, the fetal mortality rate exceeds 50%. **Task:** C—Formulating Most Likely Diagnosis

7. **Answer: C** This patient is exhibiting signs and symptoms consistent with severe preeclampsia. At 36 weeks' gestation, prompt delivery of the fetus is indicated to avoid serious risk to the mother and fetus. Early management of the patient's significant hypertension is

indicated, and hydralazine (option C), labetalol, and nifedipine are considered safe throughout pregnancy. All drug classes that have an inhibitory effect at some point in the renin-angiotensin system should generally be avoided in pregnant patients. While they are not specifically contraindicated, none would be selected over hydralazine. Aliskiren (Tekturna), option A, is a direct renin inhibitor that interferes with conversion of angiotensinogen to angiotensin I. As with angiotensin-converting enzyme (ACE) inhibitors and angiotensin II receptor blockers, aliskiren should be avoided in pregnancy. Enalapril and lisinopril, options B and D, are both ACE inhibitors and should be avoided in pregnancy, particularly in the second and third trimesters. Intrauterine growth restriction, oligohydramnios, renal failure, and death have all been observed with ACE inhibitor use in pregnancy. Losartan, option E, selectively antagonizes or blocks angiotensin II receptors in the blood vessels, kidneys, and adrenal cortices. Like ACE inhibitors, losartan should be avoided in the second and third trimesters. **Task:** D3—Pharmaceutical Therapeutics

8. **Answer: E** This patient is experiencing premature ovarian failure and subsequent premature menopause (option E), which is most likely caused by the chemotherapy and radiation received to treat her breast cancer. Premature menopause occurs when ovarian failure occurs before the age of 40.

Anorexia nervosa, option A, is incorrect because the patient has not had any recent weight changes. Anorexia nervosa is a risk factor for development of functional or hypothalamic amenorrhea. Functional or hypothalamic amenorrhea occurs when there are decreased gonadotropin-releasing hormone pulsations released from the hypothalamus in the absence of a pathologic process. Causes include strict dieting, vigorous exercise, organic illness, and anorexia nervosa. Laboratory results will show luteinizing hormone (LH) or follicle-stimulating hormone (FSH) levels that are decreased or within normal limits rather than increased. Increased emotional stress, option B, is incorrect. Although being diagnosed with breast cancer can cause emotional stress, based on this patient's laboratory results, signs, and symptoms, this is not likely the cause. Similar to anorexia, emotional stress can cause functional or hypothalamic amenorrhea. Laboratory results will show LH or FSH levels that are decreased or within normal limits rather than increased. Intrauterine pregnancy, option C, is incorrect because the patient's beta-human chorionic gonadotropin test is negative. Polycystic ovary syndrome, option D, is associated with an elevated free serum testosterone level and LH/FSH ratio. In this case, the patient's testosterone level is within normal limits, making polycystic ovary syndrome an unlikely cause. **Task:** B—Using Diagnostic and Laboratory Studies

abdominal pain with associated abnormal vaginal discharge, dyspareunia, vaginal itching or discomfort, and intermittent vaginal bleeding. Classic physical examination findings for pelvic inflammatory disease are cervical motion tenderness, mucopurulent cervical discharge, adnexal tenderness, and cervical friability. Herpes simplex virus type 2, human papillomavirus, and syphilis, options A, B and D, can be considered in this patient, but they are less likely because there is no rash or known exposure. Urinary tract infection, option E, can be considered and ruled out in this patient without urinalysis because she does not have dysuria, increased urgency or frequency of urination, back pain, or flank pain. **Task:** A—History Taking and Performing Physical Examination

20. **Answer: E** Women who have had physical abuse during pregnancy have an increased risk of preterm delivery, option E, independently from a large set of sociodemographic and behavioral characteristics usually recognized as determinants of preterm birth. Eclampsia, option A, is marked by signs and symptoms of preeclampsia with the addition of seizures. Gestational diabetes, option B, is marked by abnormal blood glucose levels in pregnancy and is not associated with physical abuse. Postterm delivery, option C, is delivery of the fetus after 42 weeks' gestation, and physical abuse is not a known risk factor. Preeclampsia, option D, is marked by high blood pressure, edema of the hands and feet, and protein in the urine during pregnancy. It is not associated with physical abuse in pregnancy. **Task:** D1—Health Maintenance, Patient Education, and Disease Prevention

21. **Answer: B** Endometriosis, option B, is the most common form of secondary dysmenorrhea, occurring most commonly in women from 25 to 29 years of age. Women typically experience cyclic menstrual pain, with pain out of proportion to physical findings during pelvic examination. Women may also experience infertility and may have enlarged, immobile ovaries due to adhesions. Adenomyosis, option A, usually manifests in the fourth or fifth decade of life, is associated with menorrhagia, and includes a large, tender uterus noted on pelvic examination. Pelvic inflammatory disease, option C, usually presents with cervical or vaginal mucopurulent discharge and cervical motion tenderness. Primary dysmenorrhea, option D, typically presents shortly after menarche, and physical examination findings are usually unremarkable. Uterine fibroids, option E, typically present with menorrhagia and an enlarged, nontender uterus on pelvic examination. **Task:** A—History Taking and Performing Physical Examination

22. **Answer: D** This patient is showing signs and symptoms of postpartum depression, which is defined as

a major depressive episode with an onset of mood symptoms that occurs most commonly within two key time frames after childbirth: 2 to 4 weeks and/ or 10 to 14 weeks postpartum. Symptoms associated with postpartum depression include depressed mood, insomnia, anxiety, irritability, fatigue, anhedonia, change in appetite, feeling overwhelmed or inadequate as a parent, and thoughts of self-harm or harming the infant. Postpartum depression can go unrecognized because some of the above symptoms, including changes in sleep and appetite, may be attributed to normal pregnancy and postpartum adjustments. The diagnosis is made based on history taking with specific focus placed on screening questions during each postpartum visit. The most appropriate therapy for postpartum depression is selective serotonin reuptake inhibitors (SSRIs), option D, which are the mainstay of pharmacologic treatment because of the low levels at which these medications are excreted into breastmilk. Antipsychotics, option A, are not the standard of care for major depressive disorder or postpartum depression. Benzodiazepines, option B, are medications reserved for the treatment of anxiety disorders. Lithium salts, option C, are used for treatment of bipolar disorder and are a pregnancy category D drug, which are not recommended for breastfeeding women. Tricyclic antidepressants, option E, have been historically used during pregnancy and postpartum, but this medication type has an increased risk for anticholinergic side effects. As a result, SSRIs are still preferred over tricyclic antidepressants. **Task:** D3—Pharmaceutical Therapeutics

23. **Answer: D** This patient has primary ovarian insufficiency, option D. Formally called primary ovarian failure, this condition occurs prior to 40 years of age and is accompanied by ovaries that fail to respond to signaling from higher elements of the hypothalamus-pituitary axis. All of this patient's laboratory and imaging results are consistent with primary ovarian insufficiency. An anovulatory cycle, option A, occurs when a menstrual cycle fails to ovulate an egg. Without ovulation, a corpus luteum fails to sustain the uterine lining and menses soon follows. Anovulatory cycles may be sporadic in their occurrence. However, ultrasonography shows follicular development, and the anti-Müllerian hormone level is within normal limits. Menopause, option B, is signaled by 12 months since a patient's most recent menstruation, typically occurs after the age of 40, and is accompanied by hot flashes, vaginal dryness, and sleep disturbances. Although this patient's laboratory studies are consistent with menopause, her physical symptoms are not consistent with this condition. Characteristics of polycystic ovary syndrome, option C, include numerous cysts on ultrasonography

of the ovaries, diabetes mellitus, obesity, hirsutism, and acne. Results of this patient's ultrasonography alone exclude option C as the correct answer. Streak gonads, option E, is also known as gonadal dysgenesis. This congenital disorder is characterized by normal reproductive tissues being replaced by functionless, fibrous tissue. This patient had a normal menstrual history until recently, which makes this option incorrect. **Task:** C—Formulating Most Likely Diagnosis

24. **Answer: E** Transvaginal pelvic ultrasonography, option E, should be the first-line imaging modality for abnormal uterine bleeding in the emergency setting because it is quick, is noninvasive, and will potentially rule out any emergent causes of the vaginal bleeding in this patient.

Dilatation and curettage, option A, is no longer the standard of care for the initial assessment of the endometrium. It is a blind procedure, with sampling errors and risks of complications similar to hysteroscopy. Endometrial biopsy, option B, is not performed as an initial assessment in the emergency department setting. Hysteroscopy, option C, is an invasive surgical procedure and is not an appropriate initial assessment, especially in the emergency department. MRI of the pelvis, option D, is rarely used to assess the endometrium in patients who have menorrhagia. It may be helpful to map the exact location of fibroids in planning surgery and prior to therapeutic embolization for fibroids. It may also be useful in assessing the endometrium when transvaginal ultrasonography or instrumentation of the uterus cannot be performed. **Task:** B—Using Diagnostic and Laboratory Studies

25. **Answer: C** Women with atypical glandular cells of undetermined significance (AGUS) have an approximately 50% chance of having significant underlying pathology ranging from cervical intraepithelial neoplasia (CIN II/III) to invasive cancer. All patients with AGUS should immediately undergo colposcopy with directed biopsies and endocervical sampling, option C. The human papillomavirus status is not relevant to the management of this patient.

Use of a carbon dioxide laser, cryotherapy, and loop electrosurgical excision procedure (options A, B, and D) are all therapies used to treat CIN II and III. All three techniques result in destruction of the tissues, making them unavailable for pathologic evaluation. Thus, with AGUS on a Pap cytology report, a biopsy must first be performed to determine the invasiveness of the lesion prior to excision. Repeat Pap testing every six months for one year, option E, is one of the options suggested for managing low-grade dysplasia, such as atypical squamous cells of undetermined significance

(ASCUS). Repeat testing for monitoring purposes is never indicated if glandular cells are observed on the cytology report. **Task:** D2—Clinical Intervention

26. **Answer: A** This patient has signs suggestive of abruptio placentae, option A. Placental separation can be associated with blunt trauma to the abdomen. In such cases, the cause appears to be shearing of a nonelastic placenta from the easily distorted elastic uterine wall at the time of traumatic impact. Vaginal bleeding occurs in 70% of patients with abruptio placentae, and blood is characteristically dark.

Placenta previa, option B, usually presents with painless, bright red vaginal bleeding. This is not likely in this patient because of the presence of trauma, which causes the separation of the placenta from the uterine wall. Premature rupture of membranes, option C, usually includes a clear watery discharge and not dark-colored discharge. Threatened miscarriage, option D, may be the sequelae of the abruptio placentae but does not explain the symptoms in this patient. Vaginal laceration, option E, may cause bleeding but is not likely in the setting of a motor vehicle collision. **Task:** A—History Taking and Performing Physical Examination

27. **Answer: D** This patient has many of the physical and physiologic characteristics of polycystic ovary syndrome (PCOS). Three of the most prominent pathophysiologic mechanisms in PCOS are insulin resistance, ovulatory function, and androgen excess. Thus, therapy is targeted toward managing blood sugar, normalizing hormone levels, and decreasing the androgen load. In addition to its aldosterone-blocking effect as a potassium-sparing diuretic, spironolactone (option D) acts as an androgen antagonist. Acne, hirsutism, and alopecia associated with PCOS are all addressed with the addition of low-dose spironolactone to the therapy regimen.

Metformin or rosiglitazone, options A and B, are indicated to address the insulin resistance. Of course, prior to initiating either medication, adolescents who are obese with a diagnosis of PCOS should undergo a formal oral glucose tolerance test to confirm the diagnosis of diabetes mellitus. Simvastatin, option C, is an HMG-CoA reductase inhibitor used to lower cholesterol. Hypercholesterolemia is a comorbidity in up to 70% of women with PCOS. However, while simvastatin may address the dyslipidemia, it has no antiandrogen effect in symptom management. Tamoxifen, option E, selectively binds to estrogen receptors, resulting in antiestrogen effect on receptor-positive breast cancer cells and an agonist effect on estrogen receptors in the hypothalamus. Tamoxifen does not have the mechanism of action needed to treat PCOS. **Task:** D3—Pharmaceutical Therapeutics

28. Answer: B Chlamydia trachomatis, option B, is correct because this infection is most likely to cause first-trimester spontaneous abortions. Bacterial vaginosis, herpes simplex virus, HIV, and human papillomavirus (options A, C, D, and E) are infections that can occur during pregnancy but are not common causes of spontaneous abortions in the first trimester. **Task:** E—Applying Basic Scientific Concepts

29. Answer: D Having a personal history of depression, option D, significantly increases this patient's risk of developing postpartum depression. Postpartum depression occurs in 5% to 9% of women. Clinical diagnostic criteria include feeling depressed or hopeless most of the day for at least two consecutive weeks. History of miscarriage, lack of social support, and not breastfeeding the infant (options A, B, and C) are all risk factors for postpartum depression, but the most significant risk factor for postpartum depression is having a personal history of depression. Symptoms of a thyroid disorder, option E, is incorrect because this condition does not increase the patient's risk of postpartum depression. However, before a patient can be diagnosed with postpartum depression, they should be screened for thyroid disorders that may mask as depression. **Task:** D1—Health Maintenance, Patient Education, and Disease Prevention

30. Answer: C Locate and stop the bleeding, option C, is correct because ongoing bleeding when the uterus is firm and well contracted suggests a laceration. Infuse oxytocin 20 to 40 U/L in crystalloid, option A, and perform vigorous uterine massage, option D, are not indicated when the uterus is firm and well-contracted. These treatments may be beneficial in a patient with an atonic uterus. Insert vaginal packing and reevaluate in 15 minutes, option B, is not appropriate. When needed, uterine packing, and not vaginal packing, is used to control uterine hemorrhage. Place an inflatable abdominal binder, option E, is not indicated in a patient with postpartum hemorrhage. **Task:** D2—Clinical Intervention

REFERENCES

Ambrose, G., & Berlin, D. (2019). *Roberts and Hedges' clinical procedures in emergency medicine and acute care* (7th ed., Chapter 37, pp. 738-773). Elsevier.

American College of Obstetricians and Gynecologists. (2014). *Guidelines for women's health care: A resource manual* (4th ed.). Washington, DC: American College of Obstetricians and Gynecologists.

Barter, C. M., Dunne, L., & Jardim, C. (2020). Abdominal complaints. In J. E. South-Paul, S. C. Matheny, & E. L. Lewis (Eds.), *CURRENT diagnosis & treatment: Family medicine* (5th ed.). McGraw-Hill.

CDC. (2015, June 4). *Pelvic inflammatory disease: 2015 sexually transmitted diseases treatment guidelines*. CDC website.

Clinical Overview. (2019, August 14). *Hemolytic disease of the newborn*. Elsevier point of care.

Clinical Overview. (2019, May 31). *Gestational diabetes*. Elsevier point of care.

Clinical Overview. (2020, January 6). *Dysmenorrhea*. Elsevier Point of Care.

Committee on Practice Bulletins-Gynecology, American College of Obstetricians and Gynecologists. (2007). ACOG practice bulletin no. 79: Pelvic organ prolapse. *Obstetrics and Gynecology*, *109*(2 Pt 1), 461-473.

de Jong, A., Dondorp, W., Frints, S. G., de Die-Smulders, C. E., & de Wert, G. M. (2011). Advances in prenatal screening: The ethical dimension. *Nature Reviews. Genetics*, *12*, 657-663.

Domino, F. J., Baldor, R. A., Golding, J., & Stephens, M. B. (2019). *The 5-minute Clinical Consult 2020*. Lippincott: Williams & Wilkins.

Dukhovny, S., & Wilkins-Haug, L. (2022, August 24). *Open neural tube defects: Risk factors, prenatal screening and diagnosis, and pregnancy management*. UpToDate [online serial]. Waltham, MA: UpToDate. Updated August 24, 2020.

Epocrates [online]. San Francisco, CA: Epocrates, Inc.; 2013. http://www.epocrates.com . Updated continuously.

Fibrocystic condition, breast. (2019). In M. A. Papadakis, S. J. McPhee, & J. Bernstein (Eds.), *Quick medical diagnosis & treatment 2020*. McGraw-Hill.

Fitzgerald, P. A. (2021). Secondary amenorrhea & menopause. In M. A. Papadakis, S. J. McPhee, & M. W. Rabow (Eds.), *Current medical diagnosis & treatment 2021*. McGraw-Hill.

Friedman, S. (2015). Irritable Bowel syndrome. In N. J. Greenberger, R. S. Blumberg, & R. Burakoff (Eds.), *CURRENT diagnosis & treatment: Gastroenterology, hepatology, & endoscopy* (3th ed.). McGraw-Hill.

Garcia, L. M., & Holschneider, C. H. (2019). Premalignant & Malignant Disorders of the Uterine Cervix. In A. H. DeCherney, L. Nathan, N. Laufer, & A. S. Roman (Eds.), *CURRENT diagnosis & treatment: Obstetrics & gynecology* (12th ed.). McGraw-Hill.

Geisler, W. M. *Diseases caused by chlamydiae* (Chapter 302, pp. 1977-1983.e2). Goldman-Cecil Medicine.

Greenberger, N. J., Blumberg, R. S., & Burakoff, R. (2016). First-trimester abortion. In B. L. Hoffman, J. O. Schorge, L. M. Halvorson, C. A. Hamid, M. M. Corton, & J. I. Schaffer (Eds.), *Williams gynecology* (4th ed.). McGraw-Hill.

Hall, J. E. (2018). Menstrual disorders and pelvic pain. In J. Jameson, A. S. Fauci, D. L. Kasper, S. L. Hauser, D. L. Longo, & J. Loscalzo (Eds.), *Harrison's principles of internal medicine* (20th ed.). McGraw-Hill.

Heniff, M., & Fleming, H. B. (2020). Abdominal and pelvic pain in the nonpregnant female. In J. E. Tintinalli, O. Ma, D. M. Yealy, G. D. Meckler, J. Stapczynski, D. M. Cline, & S. H. Thomas (Eds.), *Tintinalli's emergency medicine: A comprehensive study guide* (9th ed.). McGraw-Hill.

Hoffman, B. L., & Moreno, W. (2020). Ectopic pregnancy. In B. L. Hoffman, J. O. Schorge, L. M. Halvorson, C. A. Hamid, M. M. Corton, & J. I. Schaffer (Eds.), *Williams gynecology* (4th ed.). McGraw-Hill.

with pulmonary embolism, option D. Pyelonephritis, option E, is incorrect and does not directly cause any ECG changes. **Task**: C—Formulating Most Likely Diagnosis

18. **Answer: A** Current research suggests that the national standard goal is for patients with ST-segment elevation myocardial infarction (STEMI) to receive percutaneous coronary intervention (PCI) within 90 minutes of presentation to the emergency department (ED), option A.
Options B, C, and D have time frames that are longer than the national standard for patients with STEMI to receive PCI. Finally, option E is incorrect; an electrocardiogram (ECG) and subsequent serial ECGs should be obtained early and often in a patient with

chest pain. When a STEMI is identified, nothing should delay transfer to PCI. Treatments certainly may be initiated in the ED as the patient is prepped without delaying care. **Task**: D2—Clinical Intervention

19. **Answer: B** In order to ensure safe and effective patient transfer of care, it is always best to speak directly to the receiving provider, option B. If possible, transmit the 12-lead electrocardiogram that reflects the ST-segment elevation myocardial infarction, as this will expedite care and minimize costly delays. The other options are possible; however, they will not have the same impact on patient safety. **Task**: F—Entry-Level Professional Practice—Physician/PA Relationship

BIBLIOGRAPHY

Akbar, H., Foth, C., Kahloon, R. A., Mountfort, S. (2022). Acute ST elevation myocardial infarction: *StatPearls [Internet]*. Treasure Island, FL: StatPearls Publishing.

Chow, C. K., Pell, A. C., Walker, A., O'Dowd, C., Dominiczak, A. F., & Pell, J. P. (2007). Families of patients with premature coronary heart disease: an obvious but neglected target for primary prevention. *British Medical Association*, 335(7618), 481-485

Foreman, K. J., Marquez, N., Dolgert, A., Fukutaki, K., Fullman, N., McGaughey, M., et al. (2018). Forecasting life expectancy, years of life lost, and all-cause and cause-specific mortality for 250 causes of death: reference and alternative scenarios for 2016–2040 for 195 countries and territories. *Lancet*, 392(10159), 2052-2090.

Ismail, T. F. (2020). Acute pericarditis: Update on diagnosis and management. *Clinical Medicine (London, England)*, 20(1), 48-51.

LaRosa, J. C. (2000). Statins and risk of coronary heart disease. *Journal of the American Medical Association*, 283(22), 2935-2936.

Mechanic, O. J., Gavin, M., & Grossman, S. A. (2022). Acute myocardial infarction: *StatPearls [Internet]*. Treasure Island, FL: StatPearls Publishing.

Messerli, F. H., Bangalore, S., Bavishi, C., & Rimoldi, S. F. (2018). Angiotensin-Converting Enzyme Inhibitors in Hypertension: To Use or Not to Use? *Journal of the American College of Cardiology*, 71(13), 1474-1482.

Rochlani, Y., Pothineni, N. V., Kovelamudi, S., & Mehta, J. L. (2017). Metabolic syndrome: pathophysiology, management, and modulation by natural compounds. *Therapeutic Advances in Cardiovascular Disease*, 11(8), 215-225.

Sequist, T. D., Marshall, R., Lampert, S., Buechler, E. J., & Lee, T. H. (2006). Missed opportunities in the primary care management of early acute ischemic heart disease. *Archives of Internal Medicine*, 166(20), 2237-2243.

Shrestha, S. K. (2017). Acute STEMI management—Mnemonic based approach [Internet]. *Epomedicine*.

Srinutta, T., Chewcharat, A., Takkavatakarn, K., Praditpornsilpa, K., Eiam-Ong, S., Jaber, B. L., et al. (2019). Proton pump inhibitors and hypomagnesemia: A meta-analysis of observational studies. *Medicine*, 98(44), e17788.

Stark, M., Kerndt, C. C., & Sharma, S. (2022). Troponin: *StatPearls [Internet]*. Treasure Island, FL: StatPearls Publishing.

Switaj, T. L., Christensen, S. R., & Brewer, D. M. (2017). Acute coronary syndrome: Current treatment. *American Family Physician*, 95(4), 232-240.

Szary, N. M., Sarwal, A., Boshard, B. J., & Hall, L. W. (2010). Transfer of care communication: improving communication during interfacility patient transfer. *Missouri Medicine*, 107(2), 127-130.

Vahdatpour, C., Collins, D., & Goldberg, S. (2019). Cardiogenic Shock. *Journal of the American Heart Association*, 8(8), e011991.

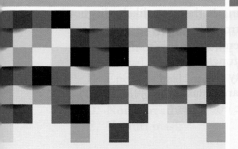

CASE STUDY 2
Cardiovascular System

Questions

Case Section I: Chief Complaint and History of Present Illness

A 40-year-old woman comes to the emergency department because she has had shortness of breath for the past four weeks. She says that she initially experienced shortness of breath on exertion when walking to her mailbox, but she recently has been experiencing it at rest. The patient also says that she occasionally wakes up at night due to shortness of breath, which improves if she sits on the edge of the bed. She has not had chest pain, cough, fever, syncope/near-syncope, or recent changes in weight; she has no history of similar episodes, nor has she been evaluated in the past for cardiopulmonary disorders. She is four weeks postpartum with a cesarean delivery (gravida 4, para 4), and her previous three pregnancies were uncomplicated. Medical history includes no chronic disease conditions, and she takes no medications. Family medical history includes heart disease in her father, who had a myocardial infarction at 51 years of age. The patient has a history of smoking one pack of cigarettes per day for 10 years but quit smoking five years ago. She does not drink alcoholic beverages or use illicit drugs.

1. Based on this patient's presentation, which of the following is the most likely differential diagnosis that could potentially be life-threatening?
   A. Cardiac deconditioning
   B. Chronic obstructive pulmonary disease
   C. Heart failure
   D. Pneumonia
   E. Sleep apnea

2. During the interview, the patient says that she experienced significant fatigue prior to the development of dyspnea. Which of the following is the most likely cause of this patient's fatigue?
   A. Arrythmia
   B. Congestion

   C. Hypoperfusion
   D. Hypovolemia
   E. Ischemia

3. Which of the following clinical findings in this patient is most likely to be associated with right heart failure?
   A. Altered mental status
   B. Ascites
   C. Fatigue
   D. Pleural effusion
   E. Pulmonary edema

Case Section II: Objective Findings, Assessment, and Plan

Weight is 216 lb. Temperature is 37.0°C (98.6°F), pulse rate is 96/min, respirations are 20/min, and blood pressure is 162/90 mmHg. Oxygen saturation is 90% on room air. The patient appears well developed and well nourished. She is in mild distress due to dyspnea. On physical examination, jugular venous distention is noted. Cardiac auscultation shows a regular rate and rhythm; an S_3 gallop is noted. Auscultation of the lungs shows fine crackles in both bases. The abdomen is soft and nontender to palpation; bowel sounds are active. Moderate abdominal ascites is noted, which the patient says is abnormal. A cesarean scar is noted in the pelvic region and is healing with no erythema, edema, or discharge. The extremities are dry and warm, and pulses are brisk and symmetric in both upper and lower extremities; 2+ pretibial edema is noted in the lower extremities.

4. Which of the following findings on physical examination is most specific for this patient's condition?
   A. Ascites
   B. Bilateral basilar fine crackles
   C. Hypoxia
   D. Jugular venous distention
   E. Pretibial edema

6. Which of the following additional findings of the lesion on physical examination is most likely to indicate malignant melanoma as a possible diagnosis?
   A. Diameter of 4 mm
   B. Symmetrical shape
   C. Ulceration
   D. Uniform color
   E. Well-defined borders

Due to the location of the lesion and the potential for it being malignant, the decision is made to refer the patient to a local dermatologist. The dermatologist elects to initially evaluate the lesion by dermoscopic examination.

7. Which of the following is the most likely benefit of this procedure?
   A. Decreases the number of unnecessary biopsies
   B. Does not require training to provide an advantage over the naked eye
   C. Increases the specificity of melanoma detection but has no effect on the sensitivity
   D. Is routinely performed in the primary care setting
   E. Mostly used to diagnosis nonpigmented lesions

Dermoscopic evaluation of the lesion shows an atypical pigment network with irregular streaks. Based on these findings, a biopsy is scheduled.

8. Which of the following types of biopsy is most appropriate?
   A. Curettage
   B. Excisional
   C. Fine-needle aspiration
   D. Punch
   E. Shave

Biopsy of the lesion confirms malignant melanoma with extension of the cancerous cells into the dermis.

9. Based on the location of the lesion and the patient's demographics, which of the following types of melanoma is most likely?
   A. Acral lentiginous melanoma
   B. Lentigo maligna melanoma
   C. Melanoma in situ
   D. Nodular melanoma
   E. Superficial spreading melanoma

Case Section III: Comorbidity
Further evaluation of the biopsy along with additional studies, including a PET scan, confirms stage IV disease with the following designation: T2aN3cM1. The meaning of designations within the TNM classification system can vary depending on the tissue.

10. Regarding the patient's TNM result, which of the following best describes a characteristic that can also apply to most solid tumor masses?
    A. Bilateral involvement
    B. Central necrosis
    C. Metastasis to distant viscera
    D. Presence of satellite lesions
    E. Presence on both sides of the diaphragm

Case Section IV: Professional Practice
The patient and his wife are told that he has malignant melanoma, and they are devastated and disappointed that they did not address this sooner.

11. Which of the following may be the most reasonable cultural-related explanation as to why this patient delayed seeking medical attention for the lesion?
    A. Concerns about relying on others for transportation
    B. Expense of seeking medical attention
    C. Mistrust of health care providers
    D. Pressure from his wife
    E. Too busy to deal with the lesion

At the conclusion of the primary care office visit with the patient, a copy of the dermatologist's biopsy report is provided to the patient.

12. Which of the following is most important for ensuring continuity of care for this patient?
    A. Advise the patient to contact the office for his future primary care needs after conclusion of cancer treatment
    B. Have the patient sign a release of information form that will ensure that the office continues to receive reports related to his future cancer care
    C. Instruct the patient to contact his insurance company for a referral for cancer treatment
    D. Remind the patient about his next follow-up appointment with the dermatologist prior to him leaving the office
    E. Tell the patient that someone from the office will call him regarding next steps

13. Which of the following is the best way to assess a patient's health literacy?
    A. Administer a published survey on health literacy
    B. Ask the patient to read a prepared statement
    C. Have the patient verify that he understands the instructions
    D. Make sure the patient's spouse is included in all discussions
    E. Obtain and document a complete review of systems

14. If this patient underwent excisional biopsy via a physician assistant (PA) in the clinical setting, which of the following is the primary determinant of the PA's ability to actually perform such a surgical procedure?
    A. Geographic proximity to the PA's practice site
    B. The Accreditation Review Commission on Education for the Physician Assistant, Inc.
    C. The National Commission on Certification of Physician Assistants
    D. The supervising physician
    E. Years of experience

Answer Key for this chapter begins on p. 234

The other options (A, B, D, and E) are frequently encountered issues in the decision to seek medical attention. However, they apply to all persons and are not specifically related to race or ethnicity. **Task:** F—Entry-Level Professional Practice—Patient Care and Communication

12. **Answer: D** Because of the extent of this patient's illness, he will be requiring extensive care from specialists over the ensuing months, starting with the dermatologist who performed the biopsy. To avoid a breakdown in communication and to ensure continuity of care, it is most appropriate for the office to contact the dermatologist for an appointment date and time and to remind the patient of this appointment prior to him leaving the office, option D.

    Option A is incorrect since it would be more appropriate to schedule the primary care appointments rather than wait for a more urgent care issue to arise. Since the office referred the patient to the dermatologist, a medical information release (option B) is unnecessary as both offices are entitled to the patient's medical records. Referrals are typically made between providers, not insurance companies. Thus, option C is incorrect. Although a common practice, having the office contact the patient at a later time to arrange for future care, option E, frequently leads to a breakdown in the communication link. **Task:** F—Entry-Level Professional Practice—Patient Care and Communication

13. **Answer: A** Possessing health literacy means having the capacity to obtain, integrate, and comprehend basic health information in written and/or oral forms in order to make appropriate decisions related to one's health care. Numerous published health literacy surveys are available and provide an accurate assessment of this important aspect of health care delivery. Thus, option A is correct.

    Health literacy involves much more than simply the ability to read; therefore, option B in incorrect. Options C, D, and E rely on the assumption that medical information is understood. This all-too-often misperception of what practitioners tell patients and what patients internalize provides the rationale for the need to assess health literacy. **Task:** F—Entry-Level Professional Practice—Patient Care and Communication

14. **Answer: D** In most states, the scope of practice of the physician assistant (PA) in the outpatient setting is determined by the supervising (or collaborating) physician, option D. While state law often defines how a PA is utilized, it is typically up to the supervising physician to determine the extent of health care delivery. State statutes dictating how far a supervising physician can be from where the PA is practicing have largely been removed from practice acts over the past few decades. While option A would have been correct in the early years of the profession, such statutory language is now largely antiquated. The Accreditation Review Commission on Education for the Physician Assistant Inc., option B, is the organization that accredits PA programs. It has no authority over scope of practice. The National Commission on Certification of Physician Assistants (NCCPA), option C, is the organization that develops and administers the national certifying examination for PAs. The NCCPA has no authority over regulating scope of practice. While years of experience, option E, may contribute to the level of health care a PA brings to a practice, it is not a primary factor in determining a PA's scope of practice. **Task:** F—Entry-Level Professional Practice—Physician/PA relationship

BIBLIOGRAPHY

Armstrong, K., Ravenell, K. L., McMurphy, S., & Putt, M. (2007). Racial/ethnic differences in physician distrust in the United States. *American Journal of Public Health, 97*(7), 1283-1289. https://doi.org/10.2105/AJPH.2005.080762.

Diagnostic errors. (2017). In: R. M. Wachter & K. Gupta (Eds.), *Understanding patient safety* (3rd ed.). McGraw Hill.

Fiessinger, L. A. (2022). Nevi and melanoma. In C. Soutor & M. K. Hordinsky (Eds.), *Clinical dermatology: diagnosis and management of common disorders* (2nd ed.). McGraw Hill.

Grumbach, K., Braveman, P., Adler, N., & Bindman, A. B. (2016). Vulnerable populations, health disparities, and health equity: an overview. In T. E. King & M. B. Wheeler (Eds.), *Medical management of vulnerable and underserved patients: principles, practice, and populations* (2nd ed.). McGraw Hill.

Hassel, J. C., & Enk, A. H. (2019). Melanoma. In S. Kang, M. Amagai, A. L. Bruckner, A. H. Enk, D. J. Margolis, A. J. McMichael, & J. S. Orringer (Eds.), *Fitzpatrick's dermatology* (9th ed.). McGraw Hill.

Healthcare: people, roles, and third-party partners. In: S. P. Murphy (Ed.), *Healthcare information security and privacy, 2018.* McGraw Hill.

How communication fails. In: R. L. Kravitz, & R. L. Street Jr. (Eds.), *Understanding clinical negotiation, 2021.* McGraw Hill.

https://scopeofpracticepolicy.org/practitioners/physician-assistants/

https://www.staffcare.com/locum-tenens-blog/news/the-future-of-physician-assistant-practice-authority-sop/

López, L., & Betancourt, J. R. (2022). Racial and ethnic disparities in health care. In J. Loscalzo, A. Fauci, D. Kasper, S. Hauser, D. Longo, & J. Jameson (Eds.), *Harrison's principles of internal medicine* (21st ed.). McGraw Hill.

Rudd, R. E., Groene, O. R., Navarro, D., & Reid, S. (2022). Health literacy: an update. In M. L. Boulton & R. B. Wallace (Eds.), *Maxcy-Rosenau-Last public health & preventive medicine* (16th ed.). McGraw Hill.

Sabath, D. E. (2019). Diseases of white blood cells, lymph nodes, and spleen. In M. Laposata (Ed.), *Laposata's laboratory medicine: diagnosis of disease in the clinical laboratory* (3rd ed.). McGraw Hill.

Schiff, G. (2022). Diagnosis: reducing errors and improving quality. In J. Loscalzo, A. Fauci, D. Kasper, S. Hauser, D. Longo, & J. Jameson (Eds.), *Harrison's principles of internal Medicine* (21st ed.). McGraw Hill.

Swanson, D. L. (2017). Nevi and melanoma. In C. Soutor & M. K. Hordinsky (Eds.), *Clinical dermatology*. McGraw Hill.

Vail, B. (2020). Diabetes mellitus. In J. E. South-Paul, S. C. Matheny, & E. L. Lewis (Eds.), *CURRENT diagnosis & treatment: family medicine* (5th ed.). McGraw Hill.

Vestergaard, M. E., Macaskill, P., Holt, P. E., & Menzies, S. W. (2008). Dermoscopy compared with naked eye examination for the diagnosis of primary melanoma: a meta-analysis of studies performed in a clinical setting. *The British Journal of Dermatology*, *159*(3), 669.

Washington, C. V., Mishra, V., & Soon, S. L. (2016). Melanomas. In A. Kelly, S. C. Taylor, H. W. Lim, & A. Serrano (Eds.), *Taylor and Kelly's dermatology for skin of color* (2nd ed.). McGraw Hill.

Answer Key for this chapter begins on p. 234

14. Which of the following findings on funduscopic examination is most likely to suggest glaucoma in this patient?
    A. Arteriovenous nicking
    B. Cotton wool spots and optic disc swelling
    C. Cup-to-disc ratio of 1/6
    D. Engorgement of the retinal veins
    E. Generalized atrophic appearance

15. Besides the time to onset of symptoms, acute angle-closure glaucoma and open angle-closure glaucoma differ in which of the following ways?
    A. Changes in intraocular pressure
    B. Effect of trabecular meshwork and its ability to drain aqueous fluid
    C. Potential irreversible loss of vision
    D. Preservation of foveal acuity until end-of-stage progression
    E. Treatment options, including surgery

16. Which of the following is a known risk factor for the development of open angle-closure glaucoma?
    A. Celiac disease
    B. Herpes simplex virus
    C. Irritable bowel syndrome
    D. Myopia
    E. Osteoarthritis

17. After further testing, the patient receives a diagnosis of open angle-closure glaucoma. Which of the following is the most efficacious initial treatment for this condition?
    A. Alpha-adrenergic agonists
    B. Beta-blockers
    C. Carbonic anhydrase inhibitors
    D. Cholinergics
    E. Prostaglandin analogues

18. It is most appropriate to tell this patient that despite receiving full and adequate treatment for primary open angle-closure glaucoma, what percentage of patients usually progress to blindness?
    A. 1%
    B. 7%
    C. 14%
    D. 45%
    E. 95%

19. According to the American Academy of Ophthalmology, in order to have prevented this condition, this patient should have undergone screening with an eye examination and tonometry at which of the following ages and intervals?
    A. Less than 40 years of age; follow-up every two to four years
    B. At 50 years of age; follow-up every two to four years
    C. At 55 years of age; follow-up every five years
    D. Between 55 and 64 years of age; follow-up every one to three years
    E. At 65 years of age; follow-up every one to two years

Case Section IV: Professional Practice

The patient initiates treatment for glaucoma and returns to the office for follow-up several months later. At today's appointment, the patient is wearing a headscarf. She is of Middle Eastern descent and is also of the Muslim faith.

20. Which of the following factors is most significant when making shared decisions with this patient in consideration of her faith?
    A. Cost-effective medication options
    B. Health Insurance Portability and Accountability Act compliance
    C. Health insurance status
    D. Level of education
    E. Touch during examinations

During the interview, the patient begins to have difficulty explaining that she has lost complete vision in her left eye. The patient is then transported via ambulance to the closest emergency department, where she receives a diagnosis of acute stroke and is admitted to the hospital. During the patient's hospital course, she is administered a thrombolytic agent.

21. Which of the following is most likely to result in an error of commission during this patient's hospital stay?
    A. Failure to administer a correct dosage of the thrombolytic agent because of using an inaccurate weight for calculation
    B. Failure to order incentive spirometry postoperatively if surgery was indicated for this patient
    C. Failure to raise the bedside rails after accompanying the patient back to the bed from toileting
    D. Failure to remove a Foley catheter postoperatively if surgery was indicated for this patient
    E. Failure to wear precautionary garments and use a disposable stethoscope when examining the patient in the hospital room

Answers

1. **Answer: B** It is most appropriate to ask this patient about the presence or absence of neurologic symptoms, including change in vision, option B, as this will help determine the likelihood of a transient ischemic attack (TIA). TIA can present with dizziness in addition to other common symptoms, including vision change, upper and lower extremity weakness, headache, numbness, gait disturbance, and difficulty with facial movement, speech, and swallowing.

   Option A is an essential question to include since it will aid in ruling out TIA, but it more closely aligns with the diagnosis of benign paroxysmal positional vertigo (BPPV). Asking if this patient has nausea and vomiting, option C, does not exclude the likelihood of TIA as nausea and vomiting are common symptoms of multiple differential diagnoses that can include TIA, BPPV, and Meniere disease. Asking about tinnitus, option D, is not correct as it is not specific enough to aid in ruling out TIA. Weight loss is commonly associated with an etiology of malignancy, and while an important question to ask, option E is also not specific. **Task:** A—History Taking and Performing Physical Examination

2. **Answer: B** Orthostatic hypotension caused by antihypertensive medications can cause symptoms including dizziness; therefore, asking if this patient checks her blood pressure at home (option B) is appropriate.

   Asking about using medications for psoriasis, occupation, other adverse effects she experiences from sulfa drugs, and when she had her most recent DEXA scan (options A, C, D, and E) are unlikely to help determine the cause of this patient's symptoms. **Task:** A—History Taking and Performing Physical Examination

3. **Answer: E** Provocation of dizziness with head movement, option E, is specific, and it supports a differential diagnosis of benign paroxysmal positional vertigo. A patient may use terms to describe dizziness, such as "light-headedness," "vertigo," "woozy sensation," or "unsteady on my feet" among others. These terms and phrases are quite subjective; therefore, options A and B are of little value in determining a differential diagnosis. The presence or absence of symptoms such as fatigue or nausea in options C and D also add little value to determining the differential diagnosis as the symptoms are rather generic and may or may not be associated with each patient. **Task:** C—Formulating Most Likely Diagnosis

4. **Answer: A** Acoustic neuroma, option A, is a benign tumor involving the vestibular branch of cranial nerve VIII with common symptoms including unilateral hearing loss, tinnitus, facial pain, dysphagia, dizziness, and headache. Audiometry is one diagnostic study used to evaluate hearing loss as a result of acoustic neuroma. Neuroimaging with MRI of the brain can aid in the diagnosis of both central paroxysmal positional vertigo and transient ischemic attack; therefore, options B and C are incorrect. Audiometry is not used to test for trigeminal neuralgia, option D, as hearing loss is not present in this disorder. Presenting symptoms are rather unilateral paroxysmal pain in the distribution of cranial nerve V. Electronystagmography is used in the diagnosis of vestibular neuritis, option E, which does not present with hearing loss. **Task:** B—Using Diagnostic and Laboratory Studies

5. **Answer: A** The presence of flulike symptoms in option A is found in a viral prodrome. Vestibular neuritis is caused by inflammation of the vestibular nerve caused by a viral infection with a viral prodrome as a common presentation.

   Asking this patient if she takes chronic opioid medications, option B, is an important question as the adverse effects of opioids can cause dizziness and worsen her symptoms. However, this question is not pertinent in determining an inflammatory etiology. Asking if she has ever taken medications for similar episodes in the past or if she's ever lost consciousness (options C and D) are questions to include in the interview. However, they are also not pertinent to this etiology. Asking about previous surgeries, option E, is not contributory to determining if this patient's symptoms are of an inflammatory etiology. **Task:** A—History Taking and Performing Physical Examination

6. **Answer: D** A positive Dix-Hallpike maneuver, option D, is considered the gold standard for diagnosis of BPPV.

   Absence of dizziness with head position or motion, option A, is indicative of Meniere disease. Diminished unilateral hearing loss, option B, is not a finding in BPPV. Facial pain, option C, is found on examination in patients with trigeminal neuralgia and acoustic neuroma. Spontaneous nystagmus, option E, is suggestive of Meniere disease, as nystagmus in BPPV is more commonly provoked on physical examination, especially when the patient is lying on their side. **Task:** A—History Taking and Performing Physical Examination

7. **Answer: D** The best explanation of the pathology of the cause of BPPV is free-floating calcium carbonate crystals within the semicircular canals, option D.

BIBLIOGRAPHY

Aboul-Enein, B. H., & Aboul-Enein, F. H. (2010). The cultural gap delivering health care services to Arab American populations in the United States. *Journal of Cultural Diversity, 17*(1), 20-23.

American Academy of Ophthalmology. *Policy statement: Frequency of ocular examinations—2015*. AAO website. Revised March 2015.

American Academy of Ophthalmology. *Preferred practice pattern: Primary open-angle glaucoma—2020*.

Baloh, R. W. (2003). Clinical practice. Vestibular neuritis. *The New England Journal of Medicine, 348*(11), 1027-1032.

Bendtsen, L., Zakrzewska, J. M., Abbott, J., Braschinsky, M., Di Stefano, G., Donnet, A., et al. (2019). European Academy of Neurology guideline on trigeminal neuralgia. *European Journal of Neurology, 26*(6), 831-849.

Bhattacharyya, N., Gubbels, S. P., Schwartz, S. R., Edlow, J. A., El-Kashlan, H., Fife, T., et al. (2017). Clinical practice guideline: Benign paroxysmal positional vertigo (update). *Otolaryngology—Head and Neck Surgery, 156*(3_suppl), S1-47.

Bhattacharyya, N., Gubbels, S. P., Schwartz, S. R., Edlow, J. A., El-Kashlan, H., Fife, T., et al. (2017). Clinical practice guideline: Benign paroxysmal positional vertigo (update) executive summary. *Otolaryngology—Head and Neck Surgery, 156*(3), 403-416.

Casani, A. P., Nacci, A., Dallan, I., Panicucci, E., Gufoni, M., & Sellari-Franceschini, S. (2011). Horizontal semicircular canal benign paroxysmal positional vertigo: Effectiveness of two different methods of treatment. *Audiology & Neuro-Otology, 16*, 175.

Coscas, G., Loewenstein, A., Augustin, A., Bandello, F., Battaglia Parodi, M., Lanzetta, P., et al. (2011). Management of retinal vein occlusion—consensus document. *Ophthalmologica, 226*(1), 4-28.

Easton, J. D., Saver, J. L., Albers, G. W., Alberts, M. J., Chaturvedi, S., Feldmann, E., et al. (2009). Definition and evaluation of transient ischemic attack: A scientific statement for healthcare professionals from the American Heart Association/American Stroke Association Stroke Council; Council on Cardiovascular Surgery and Anesthesia; Council on Cardiovascular Radiology and Intervention; Council on Cardiovascular Nursing; and the Interdisciplinary Council on Peripheral Vascular Disease. The American Academy of Neurology affirms the value of this statement as an educational tool for neurologists. *Stroke, 40*(6), 2276-2293.

Edlow, J. A., & Newman-Toker, D. (2016). Using the physical examination to diagnose patients with acute dizziness and vertigo. *The Journal of Emergency Medicine, 50*(4), 617-628.

Fife, T. D., & von Brevern, M. (2015). Benign paroxysmal positional vertigo in the acute care setting. *Neurologic Clinics, 33*(3), 601-ix.

Fife, T. D., et al. (2017). Meniere disease. In J. Stein (Ed.), *Reference module in neuroscience and biobehavioral psychology* (pp. 33746). Elsevier.

Fife, T. D., Iverson, D. J., Lempert, T., Furman, J. M., Baloh, R. W., Tusa, R. J., et al. (2008). Practice parameter: Therapies for benign paroxysmal positional vertigo (an evidence-based review): Report of the Quality Standards Subcommittee of the American Academy of Neurology. *Neurology, 70*, 2067.

Glaucoma Research Foundation. *How often should I have my eyes tested?* GRF website. Reviewed October 17, 2019.

Goldman, B., & Johns, P. (2020). Vertigo. In J. E. Tintinalli, O. Ma, D. M. Yealy, G. D. Meckler, J. Stapczynski, D. M. Cline, & S. H. Thomas (Eds.), *Tintinalli's emergency medicine: A comprehensive study guide* (9th ed.). McGraw Hill.

Grober, E. D., & Bohnen, J. M. A. (2005). Defining medical error. *Canadian Journal of Surgery, 48*(1), 39-44.

Gupta, D., & Chen, P. P. (2016). Glaucoma. *American Family Physician, 93*(8), 668-674.

Ha, A., Kim, C. Y., Shim, S. R., Chang, I. B., & Kim, Y. K. (2022). Degree of myopia and glaucoma risk: A dose-response meta-analysis. *American Journal of Ophthalmology, 236*, 107-119.

Helminski, J. O., Janssen, I., & Hain, T. C. (2008). Daily exercise does not prevent recurrence of benign paroxysmal positional vertigo. *Otology & Neurotology, 29*, 976.

Herdman, S. J., & Tusa, R. J. (1996). Complications of the canalith repositioning procedure. *Archives of Otolaryngology—Head & Neck Surgery, 122*, 281.

Horton, J. C. (2018). Disorders of the eye. In J. Jameson, A. S. Fauci, D. L. Kasper, S. L. Hauser, D. L. Longo, & J. Loscalzo (Eds.), *Harrison's principles of internal medicine* (20th ed.). McGraw Hill.

Juraschek, S. P., Daya, N., Rawlings, A. M., Appel, L. J., Miller, E. R., 3rd, Windham, B. G., et al. (2017). Association of history of dizziness and long-term adverse outcomes with early vs later orthostatic hypotension assessment times in middle-aged adults. *JAMA Internal Medicine, 177*(9), 1316-1323.

Kapaki, V., & Souliotis, K. (2018). Defining adverse events and determinants of medical errors in healthcare. In S. StawickiM. (2018). Firstenberg (Eds.), *Vignettes in patient safety* (Vol. 3). IntechOpen.

Kim, J. -S., & Zee, D. S. (2014). Clinical practice. Benign paroxysmal positional vertigo. *The New England Journal of Medicine, 370*(12), 1138-1147.

Mandalà, M., Pepponi, E., Santoro, G. P., Cambi, J., Casani, A., Faralli, M., et al. (2013). Double-blind randomized trial on the efficacy of the Gufoni maneuver for treatment of lateral canal BPPV. *The Laryngoscope, 123*, 1782-1786.

Mantravadi, A. V. (2015). Glaucoma. *Primary Care, 42*(3), 437-449.

Mitchell, P., Liew, G., Gopinath, B., & Wong, T. Y. (2018). Age-related macular degeneration. *Lancet, 392*, 1147-1159.

Parnes, L. S., Agrawal, S. K., & Atlas, J. (2003). Diagnosis and management of benign paroxysmal positional vertigo (BPPV). *Canadian Medical Association Journal, 169*(7), 681-693.

Johns, P., & Quinn, J. (2020). Clinical diagnosis of benign paroxysmal positional vertigo and vestibular neuritis. *Canadian Medical Association Journal, 192*(8), E182-E186.

Rodziewicz, T. L., Houseman, B., & Hipskind, J. E. (2022). Medical error reduction and prevention. In *StatPearls*. StatPearls Publishing.

Savitz, S. I., & Caplan, L. R. (2005). Vertebrobasilar disease. *The New England Journal of Medicine, 352*(25), 2618-2626.

Soto-Varela, A., Rossi-Izquierdo, M., Sánchez-Sellero, I., & Santos-Pérez, S. (2013). Revised criteria for suspicion of non-benign positional vertigo. *The Quarterly Journal of Medicine, 106*(4), 317-321.

Stern, S. C. (2020). Benign paroxysmal positional vertigo (BPPV). In S. C. Stern, A. S. Cifu, & D. Altkorn (Eds.), *Symptom to diagnosis: An evidence-based guide* (4th ed.). McGraw Hill.

Tanimoto, H., Doi, K., Katata, K., & Nibu, K. I. (2005). Self-treatment for benign paroxysmal positional vertigo of the posterior semicircular canal. *Neurology, 65*, 1299.

van de Beek, D., Cabellos, C., Dzupova, O., Esposito, S., Klein, M., Kloek, A. T., et al. (2016). ESCMID guideline: Diagnosis and treatment of acute bacterial meningitis. *Clinical Microbiology and Infection, 22*(suppl 3), S37-62.

van den Broek, E. M., van der Zaag-Loonen, H. J., & Bruintjes, T. D. (2014). Systematic review: Efficacy of Gufoni maneuver for treatment of lateral canal benign paroxysmal positional vertigo with geotropic nystagmus. *Otolaryngology—Head and Neck Surgery, 150,* 933.

Vannucchi, P., Giannoni, B., & Pagnini, P. (1997). Treatment of horizontal semicircular canal benign paroxysmal positional vertigo. *Journal of Vestibular Research, 7,* 1-6.

Vishwanath, S., Mukhopadhyay, C., Prakash, R., Pillai, S., Pujary, K., & Pujary, P. (2012). Chronic suppurative otitis media: Optimizing initial antibiotic therapy in a tertiary care setup. *Indian Journal of Otolaryngology and Head and Neck Surgery, 64*(3), 285-289.

Walker, M. F., & Daroff, R. B. (2018). Dizziness and vertigo. In J. Jameson, A. S. Fauci, D. L. Kasper, S. L. Hauser, D. L. Longo, & J. Loscalzo (Eds.), *Harrison's principles of internal medicine* (20th ed.). McGraw Hill.

Weinreb, R. N., & Khaw, P. T. (2004). Primary open-angle glaucoma. *Lancet, 363*(9422), 1711-1720.

Wong, T. Y., & Mitchell, P. (2004). Hypertensive retinopathy. *The New England Journal of Medicine, 351,* 2310.

Wormald, M. R. P., & Jones, M. E. (2015). Glaucoma: Acute and chronic primary angle-closure. *BMJ Clinical Evidence, 2015,* 0703.

Answer Key for this chapter begins on p. 247

Medications that decrease flatulence, smooth muscle relaxants, and bulk laxatives are helpful in decreasing symptoms of IBS, thus making options A, B, and E incorrect. Compounds known as FODMAPs are poorly absorbed in the intestines and are fermented in the colon to produce gas and osmotically active carbohydrates. A diet low in FODMAPs typically improves the pain, bloating, and constipation of IBS. Thus, option C is incorrect. **Task:** D3—Pharmaceutical Therapeutics

7. **Answer: D** Without knowledge of the results of antibody studies at this point, IBS (option D) is the most likely diagnosis. An absence of specific physical findings, along with the patient's gender and long history of unchanging symptoms, makes IBS the correct choice at this time.
Crohn disease and ulcerative colitis, options A and E, are considered inflammatory in nature. As a consequence, blood in the stool is a common finding. While a single negative occult blood test is not equivocal, it suggests inflammation is not the most likely etiology. Dumping syndrome, option B, describes a process whereby stomach contents are propelled into the duodenum before appropriate intragastric digestion has taken place. Symptoms include nausea, abdominal cramping, and possibly postprandial reactive hypoglycemia. Constipation and pain are not predominant symptoms of dumping syndrome, which makes option B incorrect. Functional constipation, option C, is similar to constipation-dominant IBS in terms of frequency of stools and bloating. Where the two conditions differ significantly is that abdominal pain is associated with IBS and is not typically associated with functional constipation. **Task:** C—Formulating Most Likely Diagnosis

8. **Answer: A** Due to the chronic nature of the disorder, patients with IBS frequently experience depression and anxiety, which makes option A correct.
Diverticulosis (option B), while a condition of the colon, is typically found in men and in patients over the age of 40. Diverticulosis is rare under the age of 30. Iron deficiency anemia, option C, is common in women who menstruate or those who suffer from indolent gastrointestinal blood loss from disease (i.e., inflammatory bowel disease). However, this type of anemia is not associated with IBS. Mesenteric adenitis, option D, is an acute inflammatory condition of abdominal lymph nodes, usually lasting a few days, which follows a viral gastroenteritis. While the abdominal discomfort of mesenteric adenitis may mimic that of IBS, the two conditions are of different etiologies and are not associated with one another. Polycystic ovarian syndrome, option E, essentially

shares none of the symptomatology or pathophysiology of IBS. **Task:** D1—Health Maintenance, Patient Education, and Disease Prevention

9. **Answer: D** All of these disorders include symptoms that are present in this patient. However, chronic constipation symptoms along with intermittent bouts of diarrhea are most suggestive of IBS. Thus, symptomatology alone makes option D correct.
The negative results of the antibody studies effectively rule out celiac disease and inflammatory bowel diseases. Therefore, options A and C are incorrect. Symptoms related to gluten insensitivity, option B, are more acute following ingestion of gluten-containing foods. Furthermore, constipation is not typically a predominant symptom of gluten insensitivity, but it is the predominant symptom in this patient. Lactose intolerance, option E, includes symptoms such as abdominal pain and bloating, which is similar in IBS. However, constipation is not the predominant symptom related to lactose intolerance. If lactose intolerance needed to be ruled out in this patient, a hydrogen breath test is the optimal laboratory study for this disorder. **Task:** C—Formulating Most Likely Diagnosis

10. **Answer: D** Hematochezia, option D, refers to blood in the stool. This symptom, if present, should direct the clinician to a potentially more destructive process such as ulcerative colitis, Crohn disease, or colon cancer.
Typical symptoms associated with IBS include abdominal pain, bloating, flatulence, and constipation and/or diarrhea. Therefore, options A, B, and E support a diagnosis of IBS. IBS occurs most commonly in young females. Thus, option C is consistent with the disease and an incorrect choice. **Task:** A—History Taking and Performing Physical Examination

11. **Answer: A** The gastric balloon procedure, option A, involves placing a saline-filled balloon in the stomach via endoscopy and removing it by the same route six months later. This is appropriate to recommend to this patient because it is a nonsurgical, temporary, and reversible treatment for weight loss.
The gastric band procedure, option B, involves placing an inflatable band around the stomach via laparoscopy. While it is reversible, it is not intended to be a temporary weight loss measure. The gastric sleeve procedure, option C, involves removing a portion of the stomach to create a smaller pouch. It is not reversible. Roux-en-Y and vertical banded gastroplasty, options D and E, describe similar surgical procedures. Neither surgical modifications are designed to be temporary nor reversible, thus making these options incorrect. **Task:** D2—Clinical Intervention

12. **Answer: C** Lubiprostone, option C, is designed to increase fluid secretion into the small bowel to ease the passage of stool. It is approved for the treatment of IBS with constipation in women with severe symptoms who have not responded to other treatments.

Eluxadoline and rifaximin, options B and D, are indicated in IBS in which diarrhea is the predominant symptom. Adalimumab and ustekinumab, options A and E, are biologic preparations used in the treatment of ulcerative colitis and/or Crohn disease. Neither drug is indicated for the treatment of IBS. **Task:** D3—Pharmaceutical Therapeutics

13. **Answer: C** Linaclotide, option C, is the correct choice. While lubiprostone has a similar pharmacotherapeutic effect, it is indicated only in women, while linaclotide has no gender-related limitation.

Alendronate, option A, is a bisphosphonate used in the treatment of osteoporosis; it is not indicated to treat IBS. Aripiprazole, option B, is used for the treatment of schizophrenia, bipolar disorder, and depression. While individuals with IBS frequently receive concomitant treatment for depression, option B has no action directly related to IBS. Sulfasalazine, option D, is a relatively old drug used in the treatment of ulcerative colitis and Crohn disease. Vedolizumab, option E, is a biologic agent used in the treatment of moderately severe inflammatory bowel disease. It is not indicated for the treatment of constipation-predominant IBS. **Task:** D3—Pharmaceutical Therapeutics

14. **Answer: D** Unfortunately, because IBS can be difficult to diagnose, patients frequently undergo unnecessary surgical procedures, including exploratory laparoscopy, cholecystectomy, and others. Therefore, option D is correct.

An estrogen antagonist like leuprolide, option A, is not indicated in the treatment of IBS. Reluctance to seek health care, option B, is incorrect because this is the opposite of what actually occurs in patients with IBS. Unfortunately, IBS is a disease mostly of exclusion; therefore, multiple providers are usually consulted before a correct diagnosis is made. Repetitive ordering of antibody titers, option C, is incorrect because once a negative titer is obtained, it is not likely to be repeated. **Task:** D1—Health Maintenance, Patient Education, and Disease Prevention

15. **Answer: A** An electronic health record, option A, is an interorganizational collection of patient health information designed to allow the primary care office and the gastroenterologist office, being within the same provider network, to share digital information.

A health maintenance organization, option B, is a type of insurance program that links patients with a group of member providers. A patient portal, option C, provides access for patients to view their electronic health record. It is not the format one provider would use to examine the medical record from another provider. TRICARE, option D, is the name of the health insurance program for uniformed service members and their families. **Task:** F—Entry-Level Professional Practice—Medical informatics

16. **Answer: B** Heightened security risk, option B, is a well-recognized drawback to use of an electronic medical record (EMR). Despite advances in encryption and strict policies on removing medical information-containing hardware from practice sites, breeches in EMR are reported regularly. Therefore, option B is correct.

EMRs have been around for more than 50 years. Many benefits are associated with their use as well as some notable drawbacks. Of the benefits, coordination of patient care (option A) and creation of a patient-centered mechanism for individuals to view their own medical information (option E) are significant advances. The efficiency of EMR resides in the elimination of stacks of paper, reducing the duplication of testing (option C), and decreasing the frequency of medical errors (option D). Thus, options C and D are incorrect. **Task:** F—Entry-Level Professional Practice—Medical informatics

17. **Answer: B** Empathy, option B, is a patient-centered quality of understanding and relating to this patient's experience and emotion with her disease.

Eliciting this patient's agenda, option A, is a way of asking questions to bring focus to a patient's purpose of the visit. Phrasing questions like, "How may I help you today?" is an example yet clearly does not equate to understanding disease from this patient's perspective. Shared decision-making, option C, is a mechanism that invites the patient into the medical or surgical plan. As it is not related to understanding illness from the patient's perspective, option D is an incorrect choice. Sympathy, option D, is by definition much different than empathy. Sympathy refers to an awareness of a patient's disease from the provider's perspective. In essence, sympathy relates more to your own feelings, whereas empathy is being more aware of your patient's feelings. **Task:** F—Entry-Level Professional Practice—Patient Care and Communication

BIBLIOGRAPHY

Cosgrove, T. (2018). Care should be monitored and recorded for auality. In *The cleveland clinic way: Lessons in excellence from one of the world's leading healthcare organizations*. McGraw Hill.

Friedman, S. (2016). Irritable bowel syndrome. In N. J. Greenberger, R. S. Blumberg, & R. Burakoff (Eds.), *CURRENT diagnosis & treatment: Gastroenterology, hepatology, & endoscopy* (3th ed.). McGraw Hill.

Hettema, J. E., Neumann, C., Samuel, B., Lessler, D. S., & Dunn, C. (2016). Promoting behavior change. In T. E. King & M. B. Wheeler (Eds.), *Medical management of vulnerable and underserved patients: Principles, practice, and populations* (2th ed.). McGraw Hill.

Levine, J. S., & Burakoff, R. (2016). Inflammatory bowel disease: Medical considerations. In N. J. Greenberger, R. S. Blumberg, & R. Burakoff (Eds.), *CURRENT diagnosis & treatment: Gastroenterology, hepatology, & endoscopy* (3th ed.). McGraw Hill.

Luo, J. N., & Tavakkoli, A. (2020). Surgical Weight Management. In G. M. Doherty (Ed.), *Current diagnosis & treatment: Surgery* (15th ed.). McGraw Hill.

Murphy, S. P. (Eds.). (2018). Impact of information privacy and security on health IT. In: *Healthcare information security and privacy*. McGraw Hill.

Nicoll, D., Lu, C. M., & McPhee, S. J. (2017). *Guide to diagnostic tests* (7th ed.). Lange.

Owyang, C. (2018). Irritable bowel syndrome. In J. Jameson, A. S. Fauci, D. L. Kasper, S. L. Hauser, D. L. Longo, & J. Loscalzo (Eds.), *Harrison's principles of internal medicine* (20th ed.). McGraw Hill.

Sharkey, K. A., & MacNaughton, W. K. (2017). Gastrointestinal motility and water flux, emesis, and biliary and pancreatic disease. In L. L. Brunton, R. Hilal-Dandan, & B. C. Knollmann (Eds.), *Goodman & Gilman's: The pharmacological basis of therapeutics* (13th ed.). McGraw Hill.

Answer Key for this chapter begins on p. 255

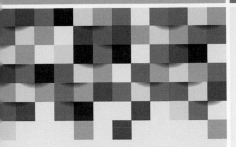

Genitourinary/Reproductive System—Male

Questions

Case Section I: Chief Complaint and History of Present Illness

A 79-year-old man is brought to the clinic by a neighbor because he has had frequent urination for the past three months. He says that he has been unable to get a good night's sleep because he has to get up multiple times to urinate. The patient has no history of trauma, fever, chills, body aches, dysuria, or hematuria. He says he also has had lower back pain for years, but he attributes it to part of getting older. Medical history includes hypertension, for which he takes hydrochlorothiazide 25 mg daily. He has no known drug allergies.

1. Which of the following is the most pertinent question to ask this patient to help rule out a communicable infectious etiology?
   A. Do you engage in sexual intercourse?
   B. Do you have abdominal pain?
   C. Do you have a skin rash?
   D. Have you been around any sick contacts?
   E. How much alcohol do you drink per week?

2. Which of the following differential diagnoses is an emergency and needs to be ruled out when evaluating this patient's back pain?
   A. Cauda equina syndrome
   B. Diabetes insipidus
   C. Kidney stone
   D. Overactive bladder
   E. Reactive arthritis

3. Which of the following is an important follow-up question to ask this patient regarding his symptoms when considering an obstructive etiology?
   A. Does your urine have a foul odor?
   B. Do you experience burning pain with urination?
   C. Do you have difficulty making it to the bathroom in time to urinate?
   D. Do you have a slow or decreased force of urinary stream?
   E. Is your urine cloudy?

4. Which of the following findings thus far in this patient's case is most likely to impact continuity of care?
   A. Advanced age
   B. Chronic lower back pain
   C. Dependence on the neighbor to bring him to the clinic
   D. Frequent urination
   E. Insomnia

Case Section II: Objective Findings, Assessment, and Plan

Temperature is 36.6°C (97.8°F), pulse rate is 70/min, respirations are 17/min, and blood pressure is 140/90 mmHg. Oxygen saturation is 98% on room air. Physical examination of the abdomen shows no abnormalities.

5. Which of the following findings on physical examination of the prostate gland is most likely to indicate cancer in this patient?
   A. Bogginess
   B. No abnormalities
   C. Palpable nodules
   D. Secretions on massage
   E. Tenderness to palpation

6. If this patient had sudden onset of fever, chills, malaise, defecation pain, and a tender, enlarged prostate gland on physical examination, which of the following acute conditions would be the most likely diagnosis?
   A. Bacterial prostatitis
   B. Cystitis
   C. Epididymitis
   D. Orchitis
   E. Proctitis

7. If prostate cancer is diagnosed in this patient and active surveillance is planned, which of the following best describes this treatment approach?
   A. Active monitoring of complications arising from undergoing a radical prostatectomy
   B. Adjuvant therapy to manage patients with more extensive disease
   C. A method that monitors cancer progression for palliative care of symptoms without plans for definitive treatment
   D. Postponement of definitive treatment to eradicate cancer until a higher risk of metastasis is determined, at which time treatment would be undertaken
   E. A way to monitor for cancer recurrence after curative treatment has been implemented

8. If this patient's initial symptoms included stress urinary incontinence, which of the following would be the most common cause?
   A. Bladder infection
   B. Mental illness
   C. Overactive bladder
   D. Prostatectomy
   E. Urethral stricture

9. If this patient is diagnosed with prostate cancer, which of the following lymph nodes is most likely to be affected?
   A. Abdominal visceral
   B. Axillary parasternal
   C. Common iliac
   D. Supraclavicular
   E. Thoracic parietal

10. If this patient has acute prostatitis, which of the following is the most likely etiology of this type of infection?
    A. *Candida albicans*
    B. *Escherichia coli*
    C. Human papillomavirus
    D. Tinea cruris
    E. Toxoplasmosis

11. If this patient has benign prostatic hyperplasia without erectile dysfunction, which of the following classes of medications is an appropriate first-line treatment to relax bladder neck muscles and muscle fibers?
    A. Alpha-blockers
    B. 5-Alpha-reductase inhibitors
    C. Anticholinergic agents
    D. Phosphodiesterase-5 inhibitors

12. If this patient has prostate cancer, which of the following drugs is most likely to cause prostate-specific antigen levels to decrease despite his having prostate cancer?

A. Fluoxetine
B. Hydrochlorothiazide
C. Lisinopril
D. Metformin
E. Testosterone

13. If this patient were suspected of having acute bacterial prostatitis, which of the following secondary differential diagnoses is most appropriate to consider?
    A. Cystitis
    B. Meningitis
    C. Myocarditis
    D. Pleuritis
    E. Uveitis

14. Which of the following is a major risk factor for the development of prostate cancer in this patient?
    A. Advanced age
    B. Chronic lower back pain
    C. Hypertension
    D. Interrupted sleep patterns
    E. Polyuria

15. After physical examination and testing, benign prostatic hyperplasia is diagnosed. Which of the following is the most appropriate initial step?
    A. Alpha-blocker therapy
    B. Beta-3 agonist therapy
    C. Lifestyle modifications
    D. Phosphodiesterase-5 inhibitor therapy

16. Which of the following medications is most likely to suppress this patient's serum prostate-specific antigen level by approximately 50%?
    A. 5-Alpha-reductase inhibitors
    B. Angiotensin-converting enzyme inhibitors
    C. Biguanides
    D. Corticosteroids
    E. Nonsteroidal anti-inflammatory drugs

Case Section III: Comorbidity

During the interview, the patient says he has not had sexual intercourse since his wife died four years ago. He says he has tried to have an intimate relationship with his current girlfriend, but he often thinks of his wife, feels guilty and sad, and then has difficulty getting and maintaining an erection.

17. Based on the findings in this patient, which of the following is the most likely cause of erectile dysfunction?
    A. Cardiovascular factors
    B. Endocrine disorder
    C. Medication
    D. Neurologic factors
    E. Psychosocial factors

18. If this patient was also taking nitrates for treatment of heart disease, which of the following medications for benign prostatic hyperplasia would be contraindicated?
    A. Alpha-blockers
    B. 5-Alpha-reductase inhibitors
    C. Phosphodiesterase-5 inhibitors
    D. Saw palmetto

19. Which of the following types of drugs is most appropriate to prescribe to this patient to treat erectile dysfunction and benign prostatic hyperplasia?
    A. Alpha-blockers
    B. 5-Alpha-reductase inhibitors
    C. Calcium channel blockers
    D. Phosphodiesterase-5 inhibitors
    E. Thiazide diuretics

20. The erectile dysfunction in this patient can be considered an early warning sign for which of the following types of disease?
    A. Autoimmune
    B. Cardiovascular
    C. Hepatic
    D. Pulmonary
    E. Renal

Case Section IV: Professional Practice
This patient is a Native American/Indigenous person who strongly identifies with his culture and tribe. He lives alone on a Native American reservation that is geographically isolated. His income level is below the poverty line, and he is unable to get to the clinic on his own. He also has had difficulty filling his prescriptions in a timely manner due to lack of transportation.

21. Which of the following factors determines if this patient is eligible to receive health care services under the Indian Health Service?
    A. DNA test proving Native American heritage
    B. Socioeconomic status
    C. Home address as long as it is on a Native American reservation
    D. Maternal lineage to determine Native American blood quantum
    E. Native American status as determined by the federal government

22. The most appropriate initial step in cultural competency is to understand how this patient's health and well-being are influenced by which of the following?
    A. Care from a medicine man or woman
    B. Economic status
    C. Herbal remedies
    D. Historical and generational trauma
    E. Worldview

23. On what basis does the Federal government provide Indian Health Services to Native Americans, such as this patient?
    A. Affiliated tribal sovereignty
    B. Economic status
    C. Ethnicity
    D. Race

Answer Key for this chapter begins on p. 262

Answers

1. **Answer: A** This patient has frequent urination, which could be a sign of a urinary tract infection. The most important question to ask to rule out communicable disease is whether or not he is sexually active, option A.

   The other options are incorrect because abdominal pain and a skin rash, options B and C, are not specific enough manifestations to rule out the communicable disease of the genitourinary (GU) system. Asking if he has been around any sick contacts, option D, is incorrect because this patient does not have fever, chills, or body aches. Option E is incorrect because alcohol intake has no direct bearing on the infectious etiology of the GU system. **Task:** A—History Taking and Performing Physical Examination

2. **Answer: A** This patient's symptom of long-standing back pain requires some attention to rule out cauda equina syndrome, option A. Cauda equina syndrome is a serious nerve compression condition that includes lower back pain, altered bladder function, and saddle (i.e., groin, anus, genitals, buttocks) numbness or altered sensations. Decompression of the nerve is an urgent matter to decrease the risk of permanent damage and morbidity.

   Option B is incorrect because diabetes insipidus is an uncommon condition relating to dysfunction of antidiuretic hormone (ADH) production or decreased sensitivity of ADH receptors that is unrelated to back pain. Kidney stone, option C, is a possibility but is not as serious because most kidney stones are able to pass through the urinary system without causing permanent damage. Kidney stones that are severely obstructing can be removed with function fully restored. Overactive bladder, option D, is incorrect because, while interfering with the quality of life, the condition does not necessitate urgent intervention to preserve life or function. Finally, reactive arthritis, option E, is incorrect because while the infection causes joint pain and discomfort of the urethra, it is not a life-threatening or permanently debilitating condition if the infection is not immediately treated. **Task:** C—Formulating Most Likely Diagnosis

3. **Answer: D** A slow or decreased urinary stream, option D, clues the clinician into an obstructive etiology for urinary system symptoms. Obstruction causes the flow of urine to become impeded in some physical way.

   Options A, B, C, and E are good general questions to ask a patient with urinary symptoms, but they do not address issues specific to an obstructed flow. **Task:** A—History Taking and Performing Physical Examination

4. **Answer: C** Being dependent on another individual to access care is critical to the continuity of receiving care. Therefore, option C is correct. It is unclear if this patient must always rely on his neighbor or someone else to bring him into the clinic; therefore, follow-up questions are in order.

   Advanced age, option A, is incorrect because there is nothing to signify in the history that this patient is frail due to advanced age. Chronic lower back pain, frequent urination, and insomnia, options B, D, and E, are symptoms the patient is experiencing that, once treated, should not impact continuity of care. **Task:** D1—Health Maintenance, Patient Education, and Disease Prevention

5. **Answer: C** Adenocarcinoma of the prostate gland, or glandular prostate cancer, typically presents as nodules on the prostate gland, option C. It is the most common type of cancer found in the prostate gland. Other prostate cancer findings often include an enlarged prostate gland; therefore, option B is incorrect. A boggy prostate, option A, and a tender prostate, option E, are more indicative of prostatitis. Secretions on massage of the prostate gland, option D, is a nonspecific finding. **Task:** A—History Taking and Performing Physical Examination

6. **Answer: A** If this patient had sudden onset of fever, chills, malaise, pain on defecation, and a tender, enlarged prostate gland on physical examination, the most likely diagnosis would be acute bacterial prostatitis, option A. This condition includes the acute onset of symptoms relating to infection.

   Cystitis, option B, is incorrect because this is a bladder infection that does not typically involve a tender, enlarged prostate. Epididymitis and orchitis, options C and D, are incorrect because this patient does not have pain in the testicles. Also, both conditions do not involve a tender and enlarged prostate. Proctitis, option E, is incorrect as the symptoms in this condition are limited to the rectum and do not involve the prostate gland. **Task:** A—History Taking and Performing Physical Examination

7. **Answer: D** For patients with low-risk, low-grade prostate cancer, active surveillance is a treatment choice. Active surveillance is a method of treatment that postpones other treatment options to avoid risks

and adverse effects. It involves monitoring the localized stage of prostate cancer until further treatment is needed to halt or cure the disease, option D.

Options A, B, C, and E are definitions of other viable courses to take in the management of prostate cancer, but they are not describing active surveillance. **Task: D2—Clinical Intervention**

8. **Answer: D** In men, surgery to remove the prostate gland to treat prostate cancer is the most common cause of stress incontinence. Therefore, option D is correct.

Bladder infection and overactive bladder, options A and C, are more likely to cause urge incontinence. While mental illness, option B, and stress incontinence may coincide, the degree to which mental illness such as depression causes incontinence is unknown. Urethral stricture, option E, is more likely to cause overflow incontinence. **Task: A—History Taking and Performing Physical Examination**

9. **Answer: C** The lymph nodes responsible for draining the prostate are the common iliac nodes, option C.

The other lymph nodes, options A, B, D, and E, are not involved in collecting lymph from the prostate gland. **Task: E—Applying Basic Scientific Concepts**

10. **Answer: B** The majority of cases of acute bacterial prostatitis are caused by an ascending urethral infection or intraprostatic reflux. The most common pathogens are gram-negative bacteria such as *Escherichia coli*, option B.

Candida albicans, option A, usually only causes prostatitis in immunocompromised patients. Human papillomavirus, option C, is a common infection transmitted through direct sexual contact with an infected individual. The infection can cause warts on the genitals and sometimes leads to the development of cancer. Tinea cruris, option D, is a dermatophyte affecting the skin and nails primarily. Toxoplasmosis, option E, may cause inflammation of the prostate, but it is not the most common cause of prostatitis in an immunocompetent patient. **Task: E—Applying Basic Scientific Concepts**

11. **Answer: A** Alpha-blockers, option A, relax the prostate muscles and provide symptomatic relief of the most common symptoms of benign prostatic hyperplasia (BPH). However, they do not shrink the prostate gland or address underlining causes.

5-Alpha-reductase inhibitors, option B, block the production of dihydrotestosterone production which results in decreasing the size of the prostate gland. Anticholinergic agents, option C, are typically used for overactive bladder; however, they may occasionally and cautiously be used to treat similar symptoms experienced with BPH. Phosphodiesterase-5 inhibitors, option D, relax smooth muscles, but they are currently used primarily for the treatment of erectile dysfunction. This medication is primarily used when treating both BPH and erectile dysfunction. **Task: D3—Pharmaceutical Therapeutics**

12. **Answer: B** This patient has hypertension and is taking hydrochlorothiazide for treatment, which is a thiazide diuretic, option B. This medication can also lower prostate-specific antigen (PSA) levels and can possibly mask the disease processes of the prostate gland.

Fluoxetine, lisinopril, metformin, and testosterone (options A, C, D, and E) have not been shown to decrease PSA levels. **Task: D3—Pharmaceutical Therapeutics**

13. **Answer: A** Bladder pathologies such as cystitis, option A, should be ruled out in patients with suspected infections of the lower urinary tract. Symptomology for infection of the prostate gland and bladder can be similar and simultaneous.

Meningitis and pleuritis, options B and D, are unlikely to occur due to bacterial infection of the prostate gland. Option C, myocarditis, is a possible but rare complication caused by bacterial infection of the prostate gland and thus is low on the differential diagnosis list. Uveitis, option E, may be present due to reactive arthritis or Reiter syndrome in this patient; however, this has a lower priority on the differential diagnosis list. **Task: C—Formulating Most Likely Diagnosis**

14. **Answer: A** The risk of developing prostate cancer is most directly associated with age; chances for developing prostate cancer increase significantly, on average, after the age of 50 years, and this patient is 79 years of age. Therefore, option A is correct.

Options B through E are factors that are either less clear or are not implicated in the risk of developing prostate cancer. **Task: D1—Health Maintenance, Patient Education, and Disease Prevention**

15. **Answer: C** The most appropriate initial step for benign prostatic hyperplasia is to begin with lifestyle modifications and behavioral interventions, option C. These modifications include avoiding drinking fluids before going to bed, avoiding caffeinated drinks that have a diuretic effect, eating more fiber to prevent constipation which can worsen symptoms, and emptying the bladder as much as possible with each urination, also referred to as double voiding.

Once lifestyle modifications have been employed, the use of prescriptive medications may be useful to gain further symptomatic relief if necessary. These medications include alpha-blockers, beta-3 agonists, or phosphodiesterase-5 inhibitors, options A, B, and D. **Task: D2—Clinical Intervention**

16. **Answer: A** Caution is advised when interpreting prostate-specific antigen (PSA) levels in men who take 5-alpha-reductase inhibitors, option A. Studies have shown that this type of medication decreases the production of PSA by up to 50%.
Options B through E can also affect PSA production but not to the same extent as 5-alpha-reductase inhibitors. **Task:** D3—Pharmaceutical Therapeutics

17. **Answer: E** Based on the findings in this case, psychological factors (option E) are the most likely contributing cause of this patient's erectile dysfunction. Psychological erectile dysfunction causes and/or worsens problems of getting and/or maintaining an erection. Options A through D are possible causes of erectile dysfunction; however, these causes require further workup and evaluation of the patient to ascertain. **Task:** A—History Taking and Performing Physical Examination

18. **Answer: C** If this patient were taking nitrates, the concomitant use of phosphodiesterase-5 (PDE5) inhibitors would be most contraindicated. Simultaneous use of nitrates and PDE5 inhibitors can cause a substantial increase in cGMP accumulation, thereby significantly decreasing blood pressure.
Alpha-blockers, 5-alpha-reductase inhibitors, and saw palmetto are not contraindicated for use with PDE5 inhibitors. **Task:** D3—Pharmaceutical Therapeutics

19. **Answer: D** Tadalafil, a phosphodiesterase-5 inhibitor (option D), is the most commonly prescribed agent to treat patients with both erectile dysfunction (ED) and benign prostatic hyperplasia (BPH).
Alpha-blockers, option A, will treat symptoms of BPH, but they will not be as effective in treating symptoms of ED. Over time, 5-alpha-reductase inhibitors, option B, will decrease the size of the prostate, thereby relieving BPH symptoms. However, they will not have an effect on the ED. Calcium channel blockers and thiazide diuretics, options C and E, do not have an effect on treating either symptoms of BPH or ED. **Task:** D3—Pharmaceutical Therapeutics

20. **Answer: B** Erectile dysfunction may be an early warning sign of cardiovascular disease in this patient, option B. This is thought to be due to the pathology related to the endothelium of the blood vessels and inadequate blood flow to smooth muscle cells. This process contributes to atherosclerosis.
Autoimmune, hepatic, pulmonary, and renal disease (options A, C, D, and E) are unlikely to be heralded by erectile dysfunction. **Task:** D1—Health Maintenance, Patient Education, and Disease Prevention

21. **Answer: E** Indian Health Service is a health care system for federally recognized Native American and Alaskan Natives in the United States. It is not a health care provider, so care can only be given through federal hospitals and clinics, which makes accessibility of services challenging for a lot of the population it serves.
Options A through D are often misconceptions about eligibility. **Task:** F—Entry-Level Professional Practice—Patient Care and Communication

22. **Answer: E** The most appropriate initial step in the approach to cultural competency, after a practitioner has explored their own worldview of health and well-being, is to seek to understand the worldview of the individual patient regarding health and well-being, option E. These influences will help guide the practitioner in uncovering specific and individual influences that need to be incorporated into the health care plan.
Options A through D are considerations that can influence health and well-being; however, without first exploring the worldview perspective of the patient, it can be falsely assumed that he believes that care from a medicine man or woman, economic status, herbal remedies, and historical and generational trauma have an effect on his health and well-being. **Task:** F—Entry-Level Professional Practice—Legal/Medical Ethics

23. **Answer: A** The United States Constitution allows for tribal nations to act as sovereign entities that engage with the United States Government. Providing health care services to Native Americans is a result of political engagement and signed treaties between the United States Government and the tribal nation. Therefore, option A is the answer.
Options B, C, and D are myths and misconceptions about the political relationship that exists between the federal government and the Native Americans. **Task:** F—Entry-Level Professional Practice—Legal/Medical Ethics

BIBLIOGRAPHY

American Cancer Society. (2016). *Prostate cancer risk factors*. Cancer.org; American Cancer Society.

American Cancer Society. (2018). Prostate Cancer. Retrieved from Cancer.org website.

Beasley, C., Jones-Locklear, J., & Jacobs, M. A. (2021). Cultural competence with American Indian clients: workforce and personal development. *North Carolina medical journal*, *82*(6), 423-426.

Centers for Disease Control and Prevention. (2019). STD Facts – Gonorrhea. Retrieved from CDC website.

Coker, T. J., & Dierfeldt, D. M. (2016). Acute Bacterial Prostatitis: Diagnosis and Management. *American Family Physician, 93*(2), 114-120.

CultureCard A Guide to Build Cultural Awareness American Indian and Alaska Native. (n.d.). Retrieved from https://store.samhsa.gov/sites/default/files/d7/priv/sma08-4354.pdf

Erectile dysfunction: Find out how it's linked to heart disease. (n.d.). Retrieved from Mayo Clinic website.

Huang, S. A., & Lie, J. D. (2013). Phosphodiesterase-5 (PDE5) inhibitors in the management of erectile dysfunction. *Pharmacy and therapeutics, 38*(7), 407.

Indian Health Service, The Federal Health Program for American Indians and Alaskan Natives. Department of Health and Human Services, https://www.ihs.gov/

Jarow, J. (n.d.). *Interpretation of Serum PSA in Men Taking 5α-Reductase Inhibitors.* Retrieved from CDC website.

Mayo Clinic. (2018). Benign prostatic hyperplasia (BPH) – Diagnosis and treatment – Mayo Clinic. Retrieved from Mayo Clinic website.

Mayo Clinic. (2018). Erectile dysfunction - Symptoms and causes. Retrieved from Mayo Clinic website.

McVary, K. Medical treatment of benign prostatic hyperplasia. *UpToDate* [online serial]. Waltham, MA: UpToDate.

Nash, C. (n.d.). External iliac lymph nodes | Radiology Reference Article | Radiopaedia.org. Retrieved from Radiopaedia website.

National Institute of Diabetes and Digestive and Kidney Diseases. (2019). Prostate Enlargement (Benign Prostatic Hyperplasia). Retrieved from National Institute of Diabetes and Digestive and Kidney Diseases website.

Preminger, G. (2019). Urinary Tract Obstruction. Retrieved from Merck Manuals Consumer Version website.

Prostate Cancer Prevention and Early Detection. (n.d.). Retrieved from: https://www.cancer.org/content/dam/CRC/PDF/Public/6673.00.pdf

Sharp, V. J., Takacs, E. B., & Powell, C. R. (2010). Prostatitis: Diagnosis and Treatment. American Family Physician, 82(4), 397-406.

Stress incontinence - Symptoms and causes. (2017). Retrieved from Mayo Clinic website.

Wiseman, D. (2019). Cauda Equina Syndrome – Symptoms, Causes, Diagnosis and Treatments. Retrieved from Aans.org website.

Answer Key for this chapter begins on p. 262

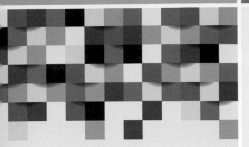

CASE STUDY 8

Genitourinary/Reproductive System—Female

Questions

Case Section I: Chief Complaint and History of Present Illness

A 19-year-old woman comes to the clinic because she has had fever, dyspareunia, malaise, and joint pain in her right knee and ankle for the past 48 hours. She also has had pain in the lower abdomen, urinary frequency, and vaginal discharge for the past five days. The patient says she has a constant urge to urinate. She does not have rash, dysuria, hematuria, or back pain.

1. Based on the patient's acute symptoms of dyspareunia and vaginal discharge, which of the following is the most appropriate question to ask this patient?
   A. Do you have a history of sexual abuse?
   B. Do you have a history of sexually transmitted infections?
   C. How heavy have your menstrual cycles been?
   D. How many urinary tract infections have you had in your lifetime?
   E. What form of birth control do you use?

2. If this patient had associated symptoms of back pain and hematuria and fever and the other presenting symptoms, which of the following would be the most likely diagnosis?
   A. Chronic cystitis
   B. Interstitial cystitis
   C. Poststreptococcal glomerulonephritis
   D. Pyelonephritis
   E. Acute uncomplicated cystitis

3. Which of following symptoms is most likely indicative of an acute viral illness as the source of the findings in this patient?
   A. Dyspareunia
   B. Fever and malaise
   C. Pain in the lower abdomen
   D. Urinary urgency
   E. Vaginal discharge

4. If pelvic inflammatory disease is the differential diagnosis, which of the following are the two most common causal agents of this infection?
   A. *Chlamydia trachomatis* and *Neisseria gonorrhoeae*
   B. Herpes simplex virus and condyloma acuminata
   C. *Mycoplasma genitalium* and nongonococcal urethritis
   D. Syphilis and trichomoniasis
   E. Tuberculosis and *Escherichia coli*

Case Section II: Objective Findings, Assessment, and Plan

The patient has one child who is three years of age. Currently, she says she has an intrauterine device (IUD) in place and has infrequent, irregular light menses. She is sexually active with multiple partners and uses protection most of the time. Medical history includes a gonococcal sexually transmitted infection one year ago that she says was treated appropriately. She has chronic migraines and takes a prescription medication daily for migraine prevention, but she is unsure of the name of the drug. The patient smokes marijuana socially, drinks three to four beers each week, and does not use illicit drugs. She has no known drug allergies.

5. Which of the following additional findings on history taking is most likely to increase this patient's risk of pelvic inflammatory disease?
   A. Early menarche
   B. Frequent urinary tract infections
   C. History of vaginal childbirth
   D. IUD placed less than three weeks ago
   E. Previous use of oral contraceptives

6. Which of the following is a nonmodifiable risk factor that increases the risk of a sexually transmitted infection?
   A. Age less than 25 years
   B. Early menarche
   C. Illicit drug use
   D. Inconsistent condom use
   E. Tobacco use

7. Which of the following medications for the treatment of migraine is most likely to increase this patient's risk of calculi formation and potentially lead to an acute renal obstruction?
   A. Hydrocodone
   B. Metoclopramide
   C. Propranolol
   D. Sumatriptan
   E. Topiramate

Temperature is 38.0°C (100.4°F), pulse rate is 124/min, and blood pressure is 117/60 mmHg. Oxygen saturation is 98% on room air. The patient is not in acute distress and appears to be well developed and well nourished. On physical examination, the lungs are clear to auscultation, bilaterally. Cardiac auscultation shows tachycardia with a regular rhythm and no murmurs. Palpation of the abdomen shows no rebound tenderness, but adnexal tenderness is noted on the left. No costovertebral angle tenderness is noted. The right knee is warm, erythematous, and edematous.

8. Which of the following is the most appropriate next step in evaluation?
   A. Contrast-enhanced CT scan of the abdomen and pelvis
   B. Knee arthrocentesis
   C. Pelvic examination
   D. Transfer to the emergency department
   E. Urine culture

9. If Grey Turner or Cullen signs were present on physical examination of this patient, which of the following urologic disorders would most likely be on the list of differential diagnoses?
   A. Colovesical fistula
   B. Nephrolithiasis
   C. Pyelonephritis
   D. Retroperitoneal hematoma
   E. Vesicoureteral reflux

10. According to the CDC guidelines, which of the following findings must be present on pelvic examination of this patient in order to make a presumptive diagnosis of pelvic inflammatory disease?
    A. Lesions in the vaginal introitus
    B. Pain in the lower abdomen
    C. Purulent cervical drainage
    D. Uterine tenderness
    E. Vaginal discharge

11. On further abdominal examination, the patient has exquisite tenderness in the right upper quadrant.

Which of the following disease processes most likely explains this finding?
    A. Diverticulitis
    B. Dressler syndrome
    C. Fitz-Hugh-Curtis syndrome
    D. Hiatal hernia
    E. Tertiary syphilis

12. Which of the following best depicts the triad of signs and symptoms that is most likely to increase the specificity of a diagnosis of pelvic inflammatory disease in this patient?
    A. Abdominal pain, urinary frequency, and vaginal discharge
    B. Cervical friability, elevated erythrocyte sedimentation rate, and white blood cells on potassium hydroxide preparation of vaginal fluid
    C. Elevated C-reactive protein level, lower back pain, and abdominal tenderness
    D. Elevated white blood cell count, abdominal pain, and tachycardia
    E. Fever, malaise, and joint pain

13. Which of the following dermatologic findings on a physical examination of this patient is most likely to indicate the need for an antibody titer for a spirochete *Borrelia burgdorferi* infection?
    A. Bull's eye rash on the lower extremity
    B. Clusters of fluid-filled vesicles on an erythematous base
    C. Generalized diffuse annular macules with central clearing
    D. Multiple small dark spots on the palms and soles
    E. Red patches on extensor surfaces with silver scaling

14. Which of the following findings is most likely to contraindicate the use of arthrocentesis on this patient's knee in the clinic?
    A. Fever
    B. Pain
    C. Pregnancy
    D. Septic joint
    E. Surgical knee prosthesis

15. If a disseminated sexually transmitted infection is the source of the arthralgia in this patient, which of the following is the most likely finding on analysis of synovial fluid from the right knee?
    A. Branching hyphae with budding yeast
    B. Calcium pyrophosphate crystals
    C. Gram-negative diplococci
    D. Gram-negative rods
    E. Presence of Lewy bodies

Answer Key for this chapter begins on p. 270

16. Pelvic examination is performed and shows a friable cervix and cervical motion tenderness, which are concerning for pelvic inflammatory disease. Which of the following is the most appropriate next step in diagnosis?
    A. Colposcopy
    B. Contrast-enhanced CT scan of the abdomen and pelvis
    C. Exploratory laparoscopy
    D. MRI of the abdomen
    E. Transvaginal ultrasonography

17. On physical examination, the patient has a positive chandelier sign. Which of the following is meant by this finding?
    A. Adnexal tenderness
    B. Cervical motion tenderness
    C. Costovertebral angle tenderness
    D. Pneumaturia
    E. Rebound tenderness

18. Which of the following values on a urine dipstick test is most specific for a urinary tract infection in this patient?
    A. Nitrites
    B. Protein
    C. Red blood cells
    D. Specific gravity
    E. Urine creatinine

Case Section III: Comorbidity

19. Based on age and gender, which of the following is the most common causative organism if pyelonephritis is diagnosed in this patient?
    A. *Clostridium difficile*
    B. *Enterococcus*
    C. *Escherichia coli*
    D. *Proteus mirabilis*
    E. *Pseudomonas*

20. A CT scan of the abdomen and pelvis with and without contrast is ordered. Which type of stone composition would be expected if this patient had a history of frequent urinary tract infections, an elevated urine pH, and a large staghorn calculus noted on CT scan?
    A. Calcium oxalate
    B. Cystine
    C. Struvite
    D. Triamterene
    E. Uric acid

21. If this patient has a calcium-based calculus, which of the following hormones is most appropriate to measure to rule out an endocrine disorder?
    A. Aldosterone
    B. Cortisol
    C. Parathyroid hormone
    D. Renin
    E. Thyroid-stimulating hormone

22. This patient has a history of high-risk sexual behavior and previous sexually transmitted infection (STI). If she receives a diagnosis of chlamydia as the cause of her current symptoms, which of the following other STIs is most appropriate to test for at this time?
    A. Condylomata acuminata
    B. Herpes simplex virus
    C. HIV
    D. Human papillomavirus
    E. Trichomoniasis

23. Because this patient has tenderness in the left adnexal region, which of the following tests is most appropriate to rule out an emergent condition?
    A. Nucleic acid amplification probe of the cervix
    B. Rapid plasma reagin test
    C. Rapid serum HIV
    D. Urine culture
    E. Urine pregnancy

24. If a disseminated gonococcal infection is diagnosed in this patient, which of the following is the most appropriate initial pharmacologic treatment?
    A. Intramedullary penicillin G
    B. Intravenous ceftriaxone
    C. Intravenous gentamycin
    D. Oral doxycycline and metronidazole
    E. Topical erythromycin

Case Section IV: Professional Practice
The patient is a single mother with good social support from her parents and extended family and friends. She is very motivated to decrease her risk for future STIs.

25. To avoid reinfection, which of the following is the most appropriate immediate instruction to give the patient regarding her sexual partners?
    A. Tell her that all sexual partners need to be notified and treated if symptoms develop
    B. Tell her that all sexual partners need to undergo STI testing in three months
    C. Tell her that all sexual partners should avoid intercourse for one week to monitor for symptoms
    D. Tell her that expedited partner therapy needs to be started for all sexual partners within the past 60 days regardless of symptoms
    E. Tell her to give all of her sexual partner's educational material about signs and symptoms of STIs

The patient comes to the clinic three days after beginning treatment and says that she continues to have persistent abdominal pain, fever, and malaise despite taking the antibiotics as prescribed. Ultrasonography is ordered and shows a tubo-ovarian abscess.

26. According to the CDC, which of the following is the most appropriate next step?
    A. Admit the patient to the hospital for parenteral antimicrobial therapy and further evaluation
    B. Discharge the patient to home with the current treatment and provide reassurance
    C. Recommend the patient schedule follow-up with her OB/GYN
    D. Refer the patient for surgical consultation regarding possible oophorectomy
    E. Stop the current antibiotic regimen and switch to a second-line antimicrobial agent

27. The patient asks how likely it is that her STI could lead to pelvic inflammatory disease (PID). Which of the following best represents the percentage of women with endocervical *Neisseria gonorrhoeae* infections who will eventually develop PID?
    A. 0%; *Neisseria gonorrhoeae* is not a cause of PID
    B. 10% to 15%
    C. 50%
    D. 70% to 75%
    E. 90%

28. It is important to initiate treatment if PID is suspected in this patient because of the risk of potential complications. Which of the following potential complications is most likely to develop if treatment is delayed?
    A. Cervical cancer
    B. Depression
    C. Ectopic pregnancy
    D. Recurrent STIs
    E. Secondary fungal infection

29. The patient says that she would like to have more children in the future. The practitioner tells her that PID and recurrent PID further increases risk of infertility due to the infection damaging or disrupting which of the following structures?
    A. Cervix
    B. Fallopian tubes
    C. Hypothalamic-pituitary-ovarian axis
    D. Ovaries
    E. Uterine lining

30. During routine follow-up, the patient says that she has heard that STIs can cause cancer. It is most appropriate to discuss vaccination with the patient to prevent which of the following types of gynecologic malignancy?
    A. Breast
    B. Cervical
    C. Endometrial
    D. Fallopian tube
    E. Ovarian

Answer Key for this chapter begins on p. 270

Answers

1. **Answer: B** Based on the patient's symptoms, the differential diagnoses include sexually transmitted infection (STI) and pelvic inflammatory disease (PID). Although no single historical physical examination or laboratory finding is both sensitive and specific for PID, a history of STIs increases the risk of recurrent STIs, new STIs, and complications of PID. Therefore, option B is correct.

   Asking if the patient has a history of sexual abuse, choice A, is a valid question but is not the most appropriate specific inquiry to determine a diagnosis of this acute illness. Asking this patient about the heaviness of her menstrual cycles or about her method of birth control, options C and E, does not directly correlate to the differential diagnosis but to her reproductive history. Finally, asking the patient about her lifetime number of urinary tract infections, option D, is unlikely to provide information that is useful in the diagnosis of STI/PID. **Task:** A—History Taking and Performing Physical Examination

2. **Answer: D** The classic triad of presentation for pyelonephritis, option D, is fever, back pain, and hematuria. Chronic cystitis, option A, is chronic inflammation and irritation of the bladder. It typically causes only localized symptoms and is not abrupt in onset as in this patient's presentation. Interstitial cystitis, option B, is a chronic bladder/pelvic pain syndrome but can be associated with hematuria. Poststreptococcal glomerulonephritis, option C, is a sequelae of untreated streptococcus infection and is an insidious progression to renal failure. It is not typically painful or acute. Acute uncomplicated cystitis, option E, is an infection of the lower urinary bladder and can be associated with hematuria. However, once fever and back pain develop, an upper urinary tract infection would be the more likely diagnosis. **Task:** C—Formulating Most Likely Diagnosis

3. **Answer: B** The symptoms of fever and malaise, option B, is most likely to indicate that a viral illness is the cause of the findings in this patient.

   Dyspareunia, pain in the lower abdomen, and urinary urgency, options A, C, and D, are nonspecific for STIs and could often be related to any number of genitourinary or gynecologic infections or abnormalities. Evaluation of vaginal discharge, option E, is a very sensitive test for STIs but not very specific for a disseminated illness causing other symptoms like fever and malaise. **Task:** A—History Taking and Performing Physical Examination

4. **Answer: A** *Chlamydia trachomatis* and *Neisseria gonorrhoeae*, option A, are the two most common causal agents of PID.

   Options B through E are all potential infecting organisms that are rare or not specific for PID. Herpes simplex virus and condyloma acuminata, option B, are incorrect. Herpes simplex virus is a viral infection often spread via sexual contact, but it is not associated with PID. Condyloma acuminata is a viral infection that causes genital warts but not PID. *Mycoplasma genitalium* and nongonococcal urethritis, option C, are organisms that cause STIs and potentially PID, but they are classically associated with localized urethritis and not a common cause of PID. For option D, syphilis is an STI that is not associated with PID but instead can progress to a late-stage neurologic disorder if untreated, and trichomoniasis is a common protozoal parasite that causes an STI but is not associated with PID. Tuberculosis and *Escherichia coli*, option E, are incorrect. Tuberculosis is a rare cause of PID and is more commonly seen in patients who have HIV or who are immunocompromised. *E. coli* is not a cause of PID. **Task:** E—Applying Basic Scientific Concepts

5. **Answer: D** Placement of an intrauterine device within the past three weeks, option D, is most likely to increase this patient's risk of PID.

   A history of early menarche, frequent urinary tract infections, vaginal childbirth, and use of oral contraceptives (options A, B, C, and E) are not known to increase a patient's risk of PID. **Task:** D1—Health Maintenance, Patient Education, and Disease Prevention

6. **Answer: A** Age less than 25 years, option A, is the only nonmodifiable risk factor listed that increases the risk of an STI.

   Early menarche, option B, is a nonmodifiable risk factor that does not increase the risk of STIs. Illicit drug use, inconsistent condom use, and tobacco use, choices C, D, and E, are all modifiable risk factors. However, illicit drug use and inconsistent condom use increase risk of STIs. **Task:** D1—Health Maintenance, Patient Education, and Disease Prevention

7. **Answer: E** Treatment with topiramate, option E, causes systemic metabolic acidosis, markedly lower urinary citrate excretion, and increased urinary pH. These changes increase the propensity to form calcium phosphate calculi.

None of the other options increases the risk of calculi formation. Hydrocodone, option A, is a narcotic analgesic used to decrease severe migraine symptoms and should not be used as migraine prevention. It is not known to increase the risk of calculi. Metoclopramide, option B, is an antiemetic commonly used for migraine with aura and associated nausea, but it is not used as a maintenance drug. Propranolol, option C, is a beta-blocker that can be used as migraine prevention but is not related to renal calculi. Sumatriptan, option D, is a migraine treatment that blocks pain pathways in the brain but is not related to formation of calculi. **Task:** D3—Pharmaceutical Therapeutics

8. **Answer: C** Because this patient has dyspareunia, vaginal discharge, and adnexal tenderness, the most appropriate next step in evaluation is pelvic examination, option C.
CT scan, knee arthrocentesis, transfer to the emergency department, and urine culture (choices A, B, D, and E) are not the most appropriate next step. At some point, and as the clinician gains more information about this patient, these options may be appropriate. **Task:** D2—Clinical Intervention

9. **Answer: D** Positive Grey Turner and Cullen signs are most likely associated with retroperitoneal hematoma, option D. Traumatic abdominal injuries and pancreatitis are associated with these clinical signs.
Colovesical fistula, nephrolithiasis, pyelonephritis, and vesicoureteral reflux (options A, B, C, and E) are all urologic conditions, but they are not associated with the specific clinical signs of Cullen and Grey Turner. **Task:** C—Formulating Most Likely Diagnosis

10. **Answer: D** According to CDC guidelines, patients are at increased risk of PID if they have cervical motion, uterine, or adnexal tenderness on pelvic examination. Therefore, option D is correct.
Lesions in the vaginal introitus, pain in the lower abdomen, purulent cervical drainage, and vaginal discharge (options A, B, C, and E) are nonspecific findings that may be present on examination if a patient has an STI. According to the CDC, these findings are not included in the minimum criteria for a diagnosis of PID. **Task:** B—Using Diagnostic and Laboratory Studies

11. **Answer: C** Exquisite tenderness in the right upper quadrant is a symptom of perihepatitis. Fitz-Hugh-Curtis syndrome, option C, is a rare complication from an STI that can lead to perihepatitis.
Diverticulitis, option A, typically presents with pain in the left lower quadrant. This patient has no other gastrointestinal symptoms that would be related to diverticulitis. Dressler syndrome, option B, is a complication from pericarditis and typically includes fever and chest pain. Hiatal hernia, option D, does not cause pain in the right upper quadrant of the abdomen. Tertiary syphilis, option E, is a progressive neurologic disease resulting from untreated syphilis. **Task:** A—History Taking and Performing Physical Examination

12. **Answer: B** A diagnosis of PID without positive findings on imaging studies will rely heavily on the history and physical examination of this patient. Most of the symptoms of PID can be very nonspecific. However, cervical friability, white blood cells on potassium hydroxide preparation of vaginal fluid, an elevated erythrocyte sedimentation rate (ESR) and C-reactive protein (CRP) level, as well as a temperature above 38.6°C (101.4°F) are the most specific. Therefore, option B is correct.
The other options are nonspecific and can be associated with a large number of genitourinary and gynecologic infections. Elevated ESR and CRP level are markers of inflammation and infection that are nonspecific in the absence of other more specific symptoms of PID. **Task:** B—Using Diagnostic and Laboratory Studies

13. **Answer: A** The spirochete *Borrelia burgdorferi* is the bacteria known to cause Lyme disease. The bull's eye rash, option A, is commonly found with this infection. Clusters of fluid-filled vesicles on an erythematous base, option B, indicates a herpetic infection such as herpes zoster or varicella-zoster virus infection. Generalized diffuse annular macules with central clearing, option C, is indicative of a tinea or pityriasis rash. Multiple small dark spots on the palms and soles, option D, is descriptive of a secondary syphilis rash. Red patches on extensor surfaces with silver scaling, option E, is descriptive for psoriatic rash. **Task:** B—Using Diagnostic and Laboratory Studies

14. **Answer: E** If a patient has a prosthetic joint, option E, arthrocentesis performed by a nonspecialist in the outpatient setting is contraindicated. Bacteremia (not fever) and an overlying skin infection are also contraindications.
Fever, pain, and a septic joint (options A, B, and D) are often indications for arthrocentesis. Pregnancy, option C, is not a contraindication for arthrocentesis. **Task:** D2—Clinical Intervention

15. **Answer: C** Gram-negative diplococci, option C, is consistent with *Neisseria gonorrhoeae* infection which is an STI that can cause disseminated disease.
Branching hyphae with budding yeast, option A, is indicative of a fungal infection. Calcium pyrophosphate crystals, option B, indicates gouty arthritis. Gram-negative rods, option D, is a typical finding for *Escherichia coli* but not a disseminated STI. Presence of Lewy bodies, option E, is not related to synovial

fluid but is found in the brain and is associated with dementia. **Task: B**—Using Diagnostic and Laboratory Studies

16. **Answer: E** Transvaginal ultrasonography, option E, is the most appropriate initial imaging study to obtain to confirm a diagnosis of PID. This study is not invasive and does not expose the patient to unnecessary radiation.

    CT scan or MRI of the abdomen, options B and D, are indicated for some of this patient's symptoms especially if the history and physical examination findings indicated intra-abdominal pathology. However, if PID is the concern, these studies are not the most appropriate initial steps if ultrasonography is available. Colposcopy and exploratory laparoscopy, options A and C, are not imaging studies but rather invasive scopes that can be diagnostic and therapeutic. Colposcopy is not indicated in the diagnosis or treatment of PID. Exploratory laparoscopy may be needed later in this patient's course if an etiology is still undetermined. **Task: B**—Using Diagnostic and Laboratory Studies

17. **Answer: B** "Chandelier sign" is a colloquial term used to indicate the presence of cervical motion tenderness, option B, on pelvic examination.

    Adnexal tenderness, costovertebral angle tenderness, and rebound tenderness, options A, C, and E, are all possible findings on physical examination, but they are not referred to as a chandelier sign. Pneumaturia, option D, occurs when a patient voids air bubbles in the urine. Usually this is associated with a colovesicular fistula. **Task: A**—History Taking and Performing Physical Examination

18. **Answer: A** Nitrites, option A, are highly specific for a urinary tract infection (UTI) with a urea splitting bacteria such as *Escherichia coli* or *Proteus mirabilis*.

    Protein, option B, can be detected with UTIs if a patient also has red blood cells in the urine; however, this value is not the most specific for UTI since it can indicate intrinsic renal insufficiency as well. Red blood cells, option C, are often detected with UTIs but also with other urologic etiologies such as kidney calculi and bladder cancer. Specific gravity, option D, is a measurement of the concentration of the urine. Urine creatinine, option E, is not evaluated on urine dipstick testing. **Task: B**—Using Diagnostic and Laboratory Studies

19. **Answer: C** *Escherichia coli*, option C, is still the most common bacterial pathogen in upper and lower UTIs. This organism is most prevalent even in adolescent female patients.

    Clostridium difficile, option A, is the cause of colitis and is not a common cause of genitourinary infections.

Enterococcus, option B, is a common bacterial pathogen in elderly patients. *Proteus mirabilis*, option D, is a fairly common bacterial cause of UTIs, but it is more prevalent in hospitalized patients. *Pseudomonas*, option E, is incorrect because this is not the most common cause of pyelonephritis and is typically associated with catheter-acquired UTIs. **Task: E**—Applying Basic Scientific Concepts

20. **Answer: C** Struvite calculi, option C, are known as "infection stones" and are composed of magnesium, ammonium phosphate (struvite), and calcium carbonate-apatite. The ammonia increases the urinary pH.

    Options A, B, D, and E are all different types of renal stones, but they are associated with elevated oxalate, uric acid, calcium, or cysteine levels as well as triamterene use. **Task: B**—Using Diagnostic and Laboratory Studies

21. **Answer: C** If this patient has a calcium-base calculus, then parathyroid hormone, option C, should be measured. Hyperparathyroidism causes hypercalcemia leading to "stones, abdominal groans, and psychiatric overtones." Calcium phosphate is the most common type of stone associated with hyperparathyroidism.

    Aldosterone and thyroid-stimulating hormone, choices A and E, are hormones that are not related to the formation of renal calculi. Cortisol, option B, is a hormone secreted by the adrenal gland that is not associated with stone formation. Renin, option D, is a hormone produced by the kidney, but it is not associated with stone formation. **Task: B**—Using Diagnostic and Laboratory Studies

22. **Answer: C** The CDC recommends testing for HIV for any patient diagnosed with an STI. Therefore, option C is correct.

    Routine testing for condylomata acuminata, herpes simplex virus, human papillomavirus (HPV), and trichomoniasis (options A, B, D, and E) is not necessary unless this patient has a specific symptom or has been exposed to a partner who tested positive for these STIs. In a female, HPV is routinely tested for every three to five years and is not indicated for this patient in the acute setting. **Task: B**—Using Diagnostic and Laboratory Studies

23. **Answer: E** With tenderness in the left adnexal region, ectopic pregnancy is possible. Therefore, a urine pregnancy test, option E, must be done in order to rule out an ectopic pregnancy in this patient.

    Nucleic acid amplification probe of the cervix, option A, is an appropriate test for a suspected STI, but results of this test will not come back rapidly, which is necessary in an emergent situation. Rapid plasma reagin test, option B, is a test for syphilis that is not typically a cause of abdominal pain. Also, it is not an appropriate initial test to rule out an emergent condition since it is not a rapid test. Rapid serum HIV test, option C, should be included if an STI is diagnosed in this patient, but it is not necessary in this emergent situation. Urine culture, option D, is appropriate if a UTI is suspected in this patient. However, results of a urine culture take at least 72 hours to return, which is not helpful in an emergency. **Task:** B—Using Diagnostic and Laboratory Studies

24. **Answer: B** Intravenous ceftriaxone, option B, is the most appropriate initial treatment for a patient with a disseminated gonococcal infection.
Intramedullary penicillin G, option A, is appropriate treatment for syphilis but not gonorrhea. Intravenous gentamycin, option C, is not an appropriate treatment for gonorrhea. Oral doxycycline and metronidazole, option D, is an appropriate secondary treatment option for gonorrhea/chlamydia/trichomoniasis infections, but it is inappropriate as an initial treatment choice. Topical erythromycin, option E, is not appropriate for a disseminated infection. **Task:** D3—Pharmaceutical Therapeutics

25. **Answer: D** Even if sexual partners are asymptomatic, the CDC recommends that all sexual contacts begin treatment, option D.
The other options (A, B, C, and E) are incorrect because treatment should be initiated immediately, and all sexual partners need to avoid sexual contact for seven to 10 days while undergoing treatment. The CDC does recommend following up in three months to repeat tests to make sure there is no recurrent infection. **Task:** F—Entry-Level Professional Practice—Public Health

26. **Answer: A** If the patient has a tubo-ovarian abscess or persistent symptoms 72 hours after beginning treatment, the CDC guidelines are to admit the patient to the hospital for parenteral treatment, option A.
Discharging the patient to home or stopping the current antibiotic regimen, options B and E, are not appropriate when managing a suspected tubo-ovarian abscess. Scheduling follow-up with an OB/GYN, option C, is not appropriate as a first-line option without first implementing hospitalization and parenteral treatment. Oophorectomy, option D, may be warranted later if the patient does not respond to parenteral treatment. **Task:** F—Entry-Level Professional Practice—Professional Development

27. **Answer: B** According to national statistics, infection with *Neisseria gonorrhoeae* progressing to PID occurs in approximately 10% to 15% of infections (option B). However, PID is relatively uncommon with a lifetime prevalence of 4.5%. Options A, C, D, and E are incorrect. **Task:** E—Applying Basic Scientific Concepts

28. **Answer: C** Delay in treatment of PID can cause chronic pain, infertility, and ectopic pregnancy, option C. Cervical cancer, depression, recurrent STIs, and secondary fungal infection (options A, B, D, and E) are not potential complications if treatment for PID is delayed. **Task:** D2—Clinical Intervention

29. **Answer: B** PID increases the risk of infertility due to severe damage and occlusion of the fallopian tubes, option B.
The cervix, ovaries, and uterine lining (options A, D, and E) are not likely to be damaged from PID infection, and the hypothalamic-pituitary-ovarian axis, option C, is not affected by PID directly. **Task:** D1—Health Maintenance, Patient Education, and Disease Prevention

30. **Answer: B** Human papillomavirus (HPV) is a common STI that can cause cervical cancer, option B. The HPV vaccine is recommended for ages 9 to 45 to prevent certain strains of HPV and the resulting cervical cancer that is caused by certain strains of HPV.
Currently, there are no vaccinations that decrease the risk of developing cancers in the breast, endometrium, fallopian tubes, and ovaries (options A, C, D, and E). **Task:** D1—Health Maintenance, Patient Education, and Disease Prevention

BIBLIOGRAPHY

Atlanta, G. A., & Centers for Disease Control and Prevention, (2011). *Sexually transmitted disease surveillance 2010*. U.S. Department of Health and Human Services.

Atri, M., Leduc, C., Gillett, P., Bret, P. M., Reinhold, C., Kintzen, G., et al. (1996). Role of endovaginal sonography in the diagnosis and management of ectopic pregnancy. *Radiographics, 16*, 755.

Bethel, J. (2012). Acute pyelonephritis: risk factors, diagnosis and treatment. *Nursing Standard, 27*(5), 51-56. quiz 58.

Branda, J. A., & Steere, A. C. (2021). Laboratory diagnosis of Lyme borreliosis. *Clinical Microbiology Reviews, 34*(2), e00018-e00019.

Capriotti, T. (2018). HIV/AIDS: an update for home healthcare clinicians. *Home Healthc Now, 36*(6), 348-355.

Carnevale-Maffé, G., & Modesti, P. A. (2015). Out of the blue: the Grey-Turner's sign. *Internal and Emergency Medicine, 10*(3), 387-388.

Chou, R., Selph, S., Dana, T., Bougatsos, C., Zakher, B., Blazina, I., et al. (2012). Screening for HIV: systematic review to update the 2005 U.S. Preventive Services Task Force recommendation. *Annals of Internal Medicine, 157*(10), 706.

Cortes, E. G., & Adamski, J. J. (2021). Chandelier Sign. StatPearls [Internet].

Cox, J. T., & Palefsky, J. M. *Human papillomavirus vaccination.* UpToDate. Waltham, MA. Accessed 15.09.2018.

de Carvalho, N. S., Botelho, A. B., Mauro, D. P., Ferreira, K. A., Amaro, L. C., Mendes, P. C., et al. (2016). Sexually transmitted infections, pelvic inflammatory disease, and the role from intrauterine devices: myth or fact? *Journal of Biomedical Science, 6,* 1.

Di Tucci, C., Di Mascio, D., Schiavi, M. C., Perniola, G., Muzii, L., & Benedetti Panici P. (2018). Pelvic inflammatory disease: possible catches and correct management in young women. *Case Reports in Obstetrics and Gynecology, 2018,* 5831029.

Doxanakis, A., Hayes, R. D., Chen, M. Y., Gurrin, L. C., Hocking, J., Bradshaw, C. S., et al. (2008). Missing pelvic inflammatory disease? Substantial differences in the rate at which doctors diagnose PID. *Sexually Transmitted Infections, 84*(7), 518-523.

Flannigan, R., Choy, W. H., Chew, B., & Lange, D. (2014). Renal struvite stones—pathogenesis, microbiology, and management strategies. *Nature Reviews Urology, 11*(6), 333. Epub 2014 May 13.

Fouks, Y., Cohen, Y., Tulandi, T., Meiri, A., Levin, I., Almog, B., et al. (2019 Jann). Complicated clinical course and poor reproductive outcomes of women with tubo-ovarian abscess after fertility treatments. *Journal of Minimally Invasive Gynecology, 26*(1), 162-168.

Gaitán, H., Angel, E., Diaz, R., Parada, A., Sanchez, L., & Vargas, C. (2002). Accuracy of five different diagnostic techniques in mild-to-moderate pelvic inflammatory disease. *Infectious Diseases in Obstetrics and Gynecology, 10*(4), 171-180.

Ganesan, C., Weia, B., Thomas, I. C., Song, S., Velaer, K., Seib, C. D., et al. (2020). Analysis of primary hyperparathyroidism screening among US veterans with kidney stones. *JAMA Surgery, 155,* 861.

Garza, I., & Schwedt, T. J. (2015). Chronic migraine. UpToDate [Internet]. Waltham, Mass. UpToDate.

Golden, M. R., Whittington, W. L., Handsfield, H. H., Hughes, J. P., Stamm, W. E., Hogben, M., et al. (2005). Effect of expedited treatment of sex partners on recurrent or persistent gonorrhea or chlamydial infection. *The New England Journal of Medicine, 352,* 676-685.

Goldfarb, D. S., Ferraro, P. M., Sas, D. J., & Baum, M. A. Cystinuria and cystine stones. Section Editors: Stanley Goldfarb, Glenn M Preminger. Deputy Editor: Albert Q Lam, UpToDate.

Grandison, M. (2012). Pelvic inflammatory disease. *American Family Physician, 85*(8), 791-796.

Haggerty, C. L., & Ness, R. B. (2006). Epidemiology, pathogenesis and treatment of pelvic inflammatory disease. *Expert Review of Anti-infective Therapy, 4,* 235-247.

Hook, E. W., III, & Holmes, K. K. (1985). Gonococcal infections. *Annals of Internal Medicine, 102*(2), 229.

Hook, E. W., III, & Handsfield, H. H. (2008). Gonococcal infections in the adult. In K. K. Holmes, P. F. Sparling, & W. E. Stamm, P. Piot, J. Wasserheit, L. Corey, & M. Cohen, *Sexually Transmitted Diseases* (4th ed). New York, NY: McGraw-Hill.

Hu, L. T. (2016 May 3). Lyme disease. *Annals of Internal Medicine, 164*(9), ITC65-ITC80.

Huether, S. (2019). Alterations of renal and urinary tract function. In K. McCance & S. Huether (Eds.), *Pathophysiology: The biologic basis for disease in adults and children* (8th ed, pp. 1246-1277). St. Louis: MO: Elsevier.

Jaiyeoba, O., & Soper, D. E. (2011). A practical approach to the diagnosis of pelvic inflammatory disease. *Infectious Diseases in Obstetrics and Gynecology, 2011,* 753037.

Jarvis, W. R., & Martone, W. J. (1992). Predominant pathogens in hospital infections. *The Journal of Antimicrobial Chemotherapy, 29,* 19-24.

Khine, H., Wren, S. B., Rotenberg, O., & Goldman, D. L. (2019). Fitz-Hugh-Curtis syndrome in adolescent females: a diagnostic dilemma. *Pediatric Emergency Medicine Practice, 35*(7), e121-e123.

Klausner, J. D. (2019). Disseminated gonococcal infection. UpToDate, T. W. Post (Ed.), UpToDate, Waltham, MA.

Kreisel, K., Torrone, E., Bernstein, K., Hong, J., & Gorwitz, R. (2017). Prevalence of pelvic inflammatory disease in sexually experienced women of reproductive age—United States, 2013-2014. *MMWR. Morbidity and Mortality Weekly Report, 66.3,* 80.

Lamb, E. J., Stevens, P. E., & Nashef, L. (2004). Topiramate increases biochemical risk of nephrolithiasis. *Annals of Clinical Biochemistry, 41*(Pt 2), 166-169.

Mandell, S. P., Bulger, E. M., Collins, K. A. (Eds.) Overview of the diagnosis and initial management of traumatic retroperitoneal injury. *UpToDate* [online serial]. Waltham, MA: UpToDate.

Markowitz, L. E., Dunne, E. F., Saraiya, M., Chesson, H. W., Curtis, C. R., Gee, J., et al. (2014). Human papillomavirus vaccination: recommendations of the Advisory Committee on Immunization Practices (ACIP). *MMWR Recommendations and Reports, 63,* 1.

Ness, R. B., Randall, H., Richter, H. E., Peipert, J. F., Montagno, A., Soper, D. E., et al. (2004). Condom use and the risk of recurrent pelvic inflammatory disease, chronic pelvic pain, or infertility following an episode of pelvic inflammatory disease. *American Journal of Public Health, 94*(8), 1327-1329.

Owen, D. S., Weiss, J. J., & Wilke, W. S. (1990). When to aspirate and inject joints. *Patient Care, 24,* 128-145.

Park, S. T., Lee, S. W., Kim, M. J., Kang, Y. M., Moon, H. M., & Rhim, C. C. (2017). Clinical characteristics of genital chlamydia infection in pelvic inflammatory disease. *BMC Women's Health, 17*(1), 5.

Pathela, P., Braunstein, S. L., Blank, S., & Schillinger, J. A. (2013). HIV incidence among men with and those without sexually transmitted rectal infections: estimates from matching against an HIV case registry. *Clinical Infectious Diseases, 57,* 1203-1209.

Plumptre, I., Mulki, O., Granados, A., Gayle, C., Ahmed, S., Low-Beer, N., et al. (2017). Standardizing bimanual vaginal examination using cognitive task analysis. *International Journal of Gynaecology and Obstetrics, 139*(1), 114-119.

Preminger, G. M., Curhan, G. C., & O'Leary, M. P. (2021). Kidney stones in adults: Struvite (infection) stones. UpToDate. A. Q. Lam (Ed.), Wolters Kluwer, Philadelphia, PA. [UpToDate]

Raszka, W. V., Jr., MD, & Khan, O., MD. (2005). MedlinePlus medical encyclopedia on pyelonephritis. *Pediatrics in Review, 26*(10).

Revzin, M. V., Mathur, M., Dave, H. B., Macer, M. L., & Spektor, M. (2016). Pelvic inflammatory disease: Multimodality imaging approach with clinical-pathologic correlation. *Radiographics., 36*(5), 1579-1596.

Risser, W. L., Risser, J. M., & Risser, A. L. (2017). Current perspectives in the USA on the diagnosis and treatment of pelvic inflammatory disease in adolescents. *Adolescent Health, Medicine and Therapeutics, 8,* 87-94.

Rosen, C. J. (2019). Parathyroid hormone/parathyroid hormone-related protein analogs for osteoporosis. *UpToDate* [online serial]. Waltham, MA: UpToDate.

Schillinger, J. A., Kissinger, P., Calvet, H., Whittington, W. L., Ransom, R. L., Sternberg, M. R., et al. (2003). Patient-delivered partner treatment with azithromycin to prevent repeated Chlamydia trachomatis infection among women: A randomized, controlled trial. *Sexually Transmitted Diseases, 30*(1), 49-56.

Seeras, K., Qasawa, R. N., Akbar, H., & Lopez, P. P. Colovesicular Fistula. [Updated 2022 Jul 25]. In: StatPearls [Internet]. Treasure Island (FL): StatPearls Publishing; 2022.

Sellors, J., Mahony, J., Goldsmith, C., Rath, D., Mander, R., Hunter B., et al. (1991). The accuracy of clinical findings and laparoscopy in pelvic inflammatory disease. *American Journal of Obstetrics and Gynecology*, *164*(1 Pt 1), 113-120.

Shikino, K., & Ikusaka, M. (2019). Fitz-Hugh-Curtis syndrome. *BMJ Case Reports*, *12*(2). [PMC free article] [PubMed].

Sholter, D., Russell, A., & Calderwood, S. B. "Synovial fluid analysis." UpToDate, Waltham Accessed 16 (2017).

Singh, R. H., Erbelding, E. J., Zenilman, J. M., & Ghanem., K. G. (2007). The role of speculum and bimanual examinations when evaluating attendees at a sexually transmitted diseases clinic. *Sexually Transmitted Infections*, *83*(3), 206-210. Published online 2006 Nov 15.

Soper, D. E. (2010). Pelvic inflammatory disease. *Obstetrics and Gynecology*, *116*(2 pt 1), 419-428.

St John, A., Boyd, J. C., Lowes, A. J., & Price, C. P. (2006). The use of urinary dipstick tests to exclude urinary tract infection: A systematic review of the literature. *American Journal of Clinical Pathology*, *126*(3), 428-436.

Tulandi, T., Barbieri, R. L., & Falk, S. J. Ectopic pregnancy: Clinical manifestations and diagnosis. *UpToDate* [online serial]. Waltham, MA: UpToDate.

US Preventive Services Task Force. (2005). Screening for gonorrhea: recommendation statement. *Annals of Family Medicine*, *3*(3), 263-267.

Wald, R. Urinalysis in the diagnosis of kidney disease. *UpToDate* [online serial]. Waltham, MA: UpToDate.

Welch, B. J., Graybeal, D., Moe, O. W. & Maalouf, N. M. Biochemical and stone-risk profiles with topiramate treatment. *Khashayar Sakhaee*. PMID: 16997051.

Weintrob, A. C., & Sexton, D. J. "Emphysematous urinary tract infections." UpToDate. Accessed 18th July (2010).

Wiesenfeld, H. C., Hillier, S. L., Meyn, L. A., Amortegui, A. J., & Sweet, R. L. (2012). Subclinical pelvic inflammatory disease and infertility. *Obstetrics and Gynecology*, *120*, 37-43.

Workowski, K. A., Bolan, G. A., & Centers for Disease Control and Prevention. (2015). Sexually transmitted diseases treatment guidelines, 2015. *MMWR Recommendations and Reports*, *64*(RR-03), 1.

Workowski, K. A., Berman, S., & Centers for Disease Control and Prevention (CDC). (2010). Sexually transmitted diseases treatment guidelines, 2010. *MMWR Recommendations and Reports*, *59*(RR-12), 1-110.

Zetola, N. M., Bernstein, K. T., Wong, E., Louie, B., & Klausner, J. D. (2009). Exploring the relationship between sexually transmitted diseases and HIV acquisition by using different study designs. *Journal of Acquired Immune Deficiency Syndromes*, *50*, 546-551.

Zuber, T. J. (2002). Knee joint aspiration and injection. *American Family Physician*, *66*(8), 1497-1501.

 Answer Key for this chapter begins on p. 270

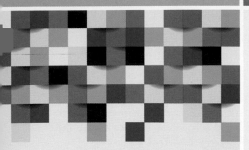

CASE STUDY 9

Hematologic System

Questions

Case Section I: Chief Complaint and History of Present Illness

A 34-year-old woman, gravida 0, para 0, comes to the office for routine gynecologic examination, including a Pap smear. During the interview, she says that her menses, which are regular, have become heavier over the past year. Menses lasts four to five days, and she has to change her pad every four hours. She has no history of abdominal pain, change in stools, or rectal bleeding. The patient has not had fatigue or shortness of breath. She has been sexually active with one partner for the past six months, and they consistently use condoms for contraception. Medical history includes mild anemia that has never specifically been evaluated, diagnosed, or treated. She takes no medications.

1. Based on this history, which of the following gynecologic conditions is most appropriate to include in the differential diagnosis as the cause of increased menstrual bleeding and anemia in this patient?
   A. Condyloma acuminata
   B. Cystocele
   C. Endometriosis
   D. Ovarian tumor
   E. Uterine leiomyoma

2. Because of her history of mild anemia, which of the following questions is most appropriate to ask this patient?
   A. Do you smoke cigarettes?
   B. Have you ever had bacterial vaginosis?
   C. Have you ever taken birth control pills?
   D. How much exercise do you get each week?
   E. What type of foods do you eat?

3. The presence of which of the following physical examination findings is the most sensitive and specific indication that this patient has moderate to severe anemia?
   A. Bradycardia
   B. Conjunctival pallor
   C. Enlarged, tender lymph nodes
   D. Facial flushing
   E. Strong, sturdy fingernails

Case Section II: Objective Findings, Assessment, and Plan

The patient does not smoke cigarettes, she gets a moderate amount of weekly exercise, she has never taken birth control pills, and she has never had bacterial vaginosis. Her diet consists of yogurt and fruit for breakfast, sandwich and chips or fast food burger and fries for lunch, and chicken and rice or a salad for dinner; she usually has one glass of wine with dinner. The patient says that she usually snacks on something sweet, like cookies, between lunch and dinner. Vital signs are within normal limits. Body mass index is 23 kg/m² (N=18.5–24.9 kg/m²). Physical examination, including pelvic and rectal examinations, shows no abnormalities. Results of a complete blood cell count (CBC) include the following:

Red blood cell count	6.21 million/mm³ (N = 4.2–5.4 million/mm³)
Red cell distribution width	14.1% (N = 11.5–14.5%)
Hematocrit	34.8% (N = 34–47%)
Hemoglobin	10.7 g/dL (N = 12–16 g/dL)
White blood cell count	4900/mm³ (N = 4800–10,800/mm³)
Mean corpuscular hemoglobin	17.2 pg/cell (N = 27–31 pg/cell)
Mean corpuscular hemoglobin concentration	30.6 g/dL (N = 33–37 g/dL)
Mean corpuscular volume	56 μm³ (N = 80–99 μm³)
Comments: Moderate number of target cells seen; marked microcytosis; moderate to marked hypochromasia	

4. Which of the following measurements on CBC indicates the size of the erythrocytes in this patient?
   A. Hematocrit
   B. Hemoglobin
   C. Mean corpuscular volume
   D. Red blood cell count
   E. Red cell distribution width

5. The red cell distribution width on CBC is most likely to be elevated if this patient has which of the following types of anemias?
   A. Anemia of chronic disease
   B. Aplastic anemia
   C. Hereditary spherocytosis
   D. Iron deficiency anemia
   E. Thalassemia trait

6. To confirm the technologist's comment on the presence of hypochromasia in this patient, it is most appropriate for the practitioner to review which of the following measurements on CBC?
   A. Hemoglobin
   B. Mean corpuscular hemoglobin concentration
   C. Mean corpuscular volume
   D. Red blood cell count
   E. Red cell distribution width

Based on this patient's history and results on CBC, further laboratory studies are obtained and show serum iron level of 84 μg/dL (N = 50–175 μg/dL), total iron-binding capacity of 326 μg/dL (N = 250–460 μg/dL), and ferritin level of 20 μg/dL (N = 11–22 μg/dL).

7. The serum ferritin level indicates that which of the following is normal?
   A. Body iron stores
   B. Erythropoiesis
   C. Iron absorption by intestines
   D. Iron concentration bound to transferrin
   E. Removal of senescent red blood cells

8. Based on the findings in this patient thus far, which of the following is the most likely diagnosis?
   A. Anemia of chronic disease
   B. Folate deficiency
   C. Iron deficiency anemia
   D. Lead poisoning
   E. Thalassemia minor

9. Which of the following questions on history taking is most appropriate to ask this patient next?
   A. Do you have a family history of anemia?
   B. Do you have a personal history of sexually transmitted infections?
   C. Have you experienced easy skin bruising?
   D. Have you noticed any blood in your urine?
   E. Have you taken folic acid supplementation in the past?

Hemoglobin electrophoresis is ordered for laboratory confirmation of the suspected diagnosis and shows hemoglobin-binding protein A of 89.5% (N = 95.8–98.5%), fetal hemoglobin of 2.8% (N = 0.0–2.0%), and hemoglobin A2 of 7.7% (N = 1.8–4.2%).

10. Which of the following questions, if not already asked, is most important to ask now?
    A. Are you experiencing recurring epistaxis?
    B. Have you been a frequent blood donor?
    C. Have you had any known toxic exposures?
    D. Is there a family history of sickle cell trait?
    E. What is your race and ethnicity?

On further questioning, the patient says that she has not had recurring epistaxis, is not a frequent blood donor, has not been exposed to any toxins, and has no information on family medical history. She also says that she is 75% Filipino and 25% White.

11. Based on these findings, which of the following is the most likely diagnosis?
    A. Alpha-thalassemia minor
    B. Beta-thalassemia minor
    C. Hereditary spherocytosis
    D. Sickle cell disease
    E. Sickle cell trait

12. Which of the following best describes the underlying pathophysiology of this patient's anemia?
    A. Continuous bleeding
    B. Defects in synthesis of hemoglobin chains
    C. Hypoproliferative bone marrow
    D. Nutritional deficiency
    E. Underlying chronic illness

Four weeks later, the patient returns to the office to discuss the results of testing and the cause of the anemia.

13. Which of the following is the most appropriate intervention to recommend at this time?
    A. Administration of erythropoietin
    B. Administration of intramuscular vitamin B_{12}
    C. Iron chelation therapy
    D. Referral for genetic counseling
    E. Referral for splenectomy

14. Which of the following is most appropriate to tell this patient regarding treatment of this type of anemia?
    A. As the condition worsens, frequent blood transfusions will be necessary
    B. Bone marrow transplantation is necessary for treatment
    C. Folic acid supplementation is necessary to help prevent severe anemia
    D. No pharmacologic therapy is necessary to treat this disease
    E. Therapy with hydroxyurea is necessary to prevent progression of disease

Case Section III: Comorbidity

The patient returns to the office for follow-up in one year. She says that her menses remain the same, but she feels this is normal for her. During the interview, she says that she recently found out that a distant Filipino cousin's 18-month-old son was diagnosed with a "bad" anemia and had to have blood transfusions.

15. Based on hereditary patterns of anemia, this cousin's son most likely has which of the following conditions?
    A. Acute leukemia
    B. Beta-thalassemia major
    C. Congenital pernicious anemia
    D. Congenital sideroblastic anemia
    E. Sickle cell trait

16. Currently, the only curative treatment for the anemia in the 18-month-old child is which of the following?
    A. Chimeric antigen receptor T-cell immunotherapy
    B. Iron chelation
    C. Life-long red blood cell transfusions
    D. Splenectomy
    E. Stem cell transplantation

17. If the 18-month-old child is treated with long-term red blood cell transfusion, which of the following is the most common complication?
    A. Disseminated intravascular coagulation
    B. Gastrointestinal bleeding
    C. Henoch-Schönlein purpura
    D. Hypokalemia
    E. Iron overload

18. If the original 34-year-old female patient has beta-thalassemia minor and conceives a child with a partner who also has beta-thalassemia minor, which of the following best indicates the approximate chance she will have a child with beta-thalassemia major?
    A. 10%
    B. 25%
    C. 50%
    D. 75%
    E. 100%

As noted earlier, the patient is 75% Filipino and 25% White. The practitioner tells her that both alpha- and beta-thalassemia are inherited conditions that occur often in persons of Southeast Asian and African descent.

19. Additionally, beta-thalassemia occurs commonly in which of the following populations?
    A. Ashkenazi Jewish persons
    B. Hispanics
    C. North Germanic ethnic groups
    D. Pacific Islanders
    E. People of Mediterranean descent

Case Section IV: Professional Practice
20. If this patient's 18-month-old distant cousin has a serious genetic condition, the most appropriate initial step is for the practitioner responsible for the child's care to do which of the following?
    A. Advise the child's parents that they have the duty to warn family members of the condition
    B. Contact and inform the patient's distant family members of the disease, with or without the parents' consent
    C. Contact the patient's insurance company so they can review family member's health records
    D. Tell the parents that the clinical laboratory will notify family members of this genetic disorder

Answers

1. **Answer: E** Uterine leiomyomas (option E), or fibroids, are benign tumors of the uterus. Uterine fibroids may put pressure against the uterine lining, causing more bleeding than usual.
Condyloma acuminata, option A, refers to warty growth on the vulva, perianal area, vaginal walls, or cervix. The most common symptom is itching or discomfort. A cystocele, option B, is a bulge of the bladder into the vagina that can cause pelvic pressure. Endometriosis, option C, includes aberrant growth of endometrium outside of the uterus; the most common symptoms are dysmenorrhea and dyspareunia. Ovarian tumors, option D, cause vague gastrointestinal discomfort or pelvic pain. **Task:** A—History Taking and Performing Physical Examination

2. **Answer: E** Nutritional anemias due to iron, folate, or vitamin B_{12} deficiencies are common and are evaluated by diet history and appropriate laboratory testing. Therefore, option E is correct.
Smoking cigarettes, option A, does not cause anemia. Bacterial vaginosis, option B, is a nonsexually transmitted polymicrobial overgrowth of bacteria in the vagina and not related to anemia. Birth control pills, option C, cause less menstrual bleeding and less iron deficient anemia in women. Only extreme, excessive exercise, option D, could cause anemia by depleting iron stores. **Task:** A—History Taking and Performing Physical Examination

3. **Answer: B** Studies show that conjunctival pallor, option B, is useful to detect moderate to severe anemia but is insensitive to detect mild anemia. Observed conjunctival pallor correlates with a decreased hemoglobin level.
Severe anemias cause a compensatory tachycardia (increased heart rate) and not bradycardia (decreased heart rate); therefore, option A is incorrect. Enlarged, tender lymph nodes, option C, are most often due to infections. Skin paleness rather than flushing, option D, is associated with anemia. Fingernails, option E, in iron deficiency anemia can be brittle and spoon-shaped rather than strong and sturdy. **Task:** A—History Taking and Performing Physical Examination

4. **Answer: C** Mean corpuscular volume (MCV), option C, is a laboratory value that measures the average size and volume of red blood cells. Based on the MCV, red blood cells are classified as microcytic, normocytic, or macrocytic.
Hematocrit, option A, is the packed red cell volume. Hemoglobin, option B, is the measurement of protein molecule in red blood cells that carry oxygen. The red blood cell count, option D, is the number of red blood cells per microliter. Red cell distribution width, option E, measures the variation in red blood cell width. **Task:** B—Using Diagnostic and Laboratory Studies

5. **Answer: D** Red cell distribution width (RDW) is most often elevated in nutritional anemias, such as iron deficiency anemia (option D), because there is a wide variation in the size of the red blood cells. RDW is also elevated in anemias due to deficiency in vitamin B_{12} or folic acid.
Patients with anemia of chronic disease, aplastic anemia (anemia resulting from an inability of the bone marrow to produce red blood cells), and hereditary spherocytosis (options A, B, and C) have a normal RDW. In thalassemia trait, option E, the RDW is usually normal; however, there are exceptions in which it is elevated. **Task:** B—Using Diagnostic and Laboratory Studies

6. **Answer: B** Hypochromasia means that red blood cells lack their red coloring, and they are pale in color. It is most appropriate for the practitioner to review the mean corpuscular hemoglobin concentration (MCHC), option B, to confirm hypochromasia, because this is a measure of the average concentration of hemoglobin inside a single red blood cell. The MCHC gives an absolute average of the hemoglobin in a red blood cell expressed in picograms; it does not take into account the size of the cell. One would expect large cells to have more hemoglobin and small cells less. The MCHC is expressed as a percentage, thereby eliminating the issue of the size of the cells.
The hemoglobin measurement, option A, measures the hemoglobin in whole blood, not the concentration inside a red blood cell. Mean corpuscular volume and red cell distribution width, options C and E, are incorrect because they have nothing to do with the amount of hemoglobin in the cell. Option D, red blood cell count, is the number of red corpuscles in a given volume of blood and does not measure hemoglobin in the cells. **Task:** B—Using Diagnostic and Laboratory Studies

7. **Answer: A** Ferritin is a blood protein that contains iron and is a marker for body iron stores, option A. If serum ferritin is decreased, this indicates that the body's iron stores are low and the patient may have iron deficiency.
Option B is incorrect because erythropoiesis is the production of red blood cells in the bone marrow. Intestinal absorption of iron, option C, can be affected by diseases such as celiac sprue and by surgery affecting

the intestines, but the ferritin level does not measure absorption. The amount of iron bound to transferrin, option D, is measured by a serum iron level not the ferritin level. Option E is incorrect, because red blood cells are removed from circulation at approximately 120 days, and they are not measured by a ferritin level. **Task:** B—Using Diagnostic and Laboratory Studies

8. **Answer: E** Thalassemia minor, option E, is most likely in this patient. Her anemia is mild, marked microcytosis is present, the red cell distribution width is normal, and a mild relative erythrocytosis is present, which are all consistent with thalassemia minor.

   In anemia of chronic disease, option A, the serum iron level is usually decreased, ferritin level is either within normal limits or increased, and total iron-binding capacity (TIBC) is decreased or within normal limits; all three of these results are in the normal reference range for this patient. Anemia associated with folate deficiency, option B, is a macrocytic anemia. This patient's serum iron and ferritin levels are within normal limits, which makes iron deficiency anemia unlikely (option C). Also, in iron deficiency, the TIBC is usually elevated. In anemia associated with lead poisoning, option D, the technologist will often note basophilic stippling in red blood cells; iron deficiency often coexists with lead poisoning. **Task:** C—Formulating Most Likely Diagnosis

9. **Answer: A** Thalassemias are inherited blood disorders characterized by decreased hemoglobin production (hemoglobinopathies). Because they are genetic, knowing family history is helpful, option A.

   Sexually transmitted infections, option B, does not cause anemia, so asking about this is not appropriate. Easy skin bruising, option C, is associated with a decreased platelet count. Blood in the urine, option D, is associated with urinary tract infections and cancer of the urinary tract. Anemias due to blood loss are iron deficient. Folic acid deficiency, option E, causes a macrocytic anemia. **Task:** A—History Taking and Performing Physical Examination

10. **Answer: E** Asking this patient about her race and ethnicity, option E, is the appropriate question to ask at this time. Clinicians cannot assume race or ethnicity by looking at a patient; direct inquiry is necessary. Since thalassemia is an inherited condition, it is not surprising that the frequency of thalassemia varies widely depending on the ethnic population.

    Patients who experience recurring epistaxis or who are frequent blood donors, options A and B, are at increased risk for iron deficiency anemia. Lead and copper toxicities, option C, can cause microcytic anemias, but this is uncommon. The evaluation process for microcytic anemia tests for the common causes

such as iron deficiency anemia, thalassemia, and anemia of chronic disease. If evaluation for these three causes is inconclusive, then the clinician pursues less common causes of microcytic anemia. Based on the results of the hemoglobin electrophoresis, sickle cell trait, option D, is not a consideration in this patient. **Task:** A—History Taking and Performing Physical Examination

11. **Answer: B** The correct answer is beta-thalassemia minor, option B. Hemoglobin electrophoresis identifies abnormal hemoglobin variants. An increase in hemoglobin A2 to about 4 to 8% indicates beta-thalassemia minor when present in the correct clinical context. This patient has findings on complete blood cell count that are consistent with thalassemia minor. Persons from Southeast Asia, including the Philippines, are at increased risk for beta-thalassemia. In patients with alpha-thalassemia minor and hereditary spherocytosis, options A and C, hemoglobin electrophoresis shows no abnormalities. With sickle cell disease, option D, electrophoresis shows only hemoglobin S and hemoglobin F (fetal hemoglobin). In sickle cell trait, option E, patients have a mixture of both the normal hemoglobin A and hemoglobin S. **Task:** A—History Taking and Performing Physical Examination

12. **Answer: B** Beta-thalassemia is caused by decreased (minor) or absent (major) synthesis of beta-globin chains, option B. Alpha-thalassemia is caused by decreased (minor) or absent (major) synthesis of alpha-globin chains.

    Continuous bleeding, option A, is a cause of iron deficiency anemia. An example of anemia caused by hypoproliferative bone marrow, option C, is aplastic anemia. Anemias caused by nutritional deficiencies, option D, include iron deficiency, vitamin B_{12} (cobalamin) deficiency, and folic acid deficiency. Anemia of chronic disease is a multifactorial anemia generated by activation of the immune system due to a chronic illness, option E. **Task:** E—Applying Basic Scientific Concepts

13. **Answer: D** Genetic counseling, option D, is integral and necessary for persons with thalassemia minor. People inherit the genes for beta-thalassemia from their parents. If this patient conceives a child with a partner who also has beta-thalassemia minor, there is a chance of that child having beta-thalassemia major (also called Cooley anemia). Beta-thalassemia major is a severe and life-threatening anemia.

    Erythropoietin, option A, is most often administered for anemia due to chronic kidney disease, which this patient does not have. Administration of vitamin B_{12}, option B, is used for anemia due to cobalamin deficiency and is not useful for treatment of thalassemia. Iron chelation therapy, option C, is often required when a patient receives ongoing blood transfusions. Splenectomy, option E, is performed in some patients with beta-thalassemia major, for hereditary spherocytosis, and for autoimmune hemolytic anemias. However, there is no reason to perform it for this patient with beta-thalassemia minor. **Task:** D2—Clinical Intervention

14. **Answer: D** Persons with uncomplicated alpha- or beta-thalassemia minor can have mild anemia but do not have symptoms nor do they have progression of disease; therefore, they require no pharmacologic treatment (option D).
Typically, there is no progression of the disease over time, and patients have a normal life span. Therefore, options A, B, C, and E are incorrect. No pharmacologic treatment or long-term monitoring is needed. Also, iron should not be prescribed unless there is coexisting iron deficiency. Long-term use of iron supplements when there is no deficiency can lead to iron overload. The body cannot excrete excess iron, so it stores excess iron in certain organs, notably the liver, heart, and pancreas, which can lead to organ damage. **Task:** D1—Health Maintenance, Patient Education, and Disease Prevention

15. **Answer: B** A risk factor for developing thalassemia major, option B, is a family history of thalassemia. This patient has thalassemia trait, so we know there are thalassemia genes in the family tree.
Acute leukemia, option A, in children is usually acute lymphoblastic leukemia. There are a few known risk factors for childhood leukemia, and genetic risk factors have not been identified. There is no known history of pernicious or sideroblastic anemia or sickle cell trait in this patient's family (options C, D, and E). **Task:** A—History Taking and Performing Physical Examination

16. **Answer: E** The only definitive treatment at present is allogeneic hematopoietic stem cell transplantation, option E, in transfusion-dependent patients with greater than 90% success rate if it takes place before the damage related to iron overload occurs.
Chimeric antigen receptor T-cell immunotherapy, option A, is used to treat childhood leukemia and not anemia. Iron chelation, red blood cell transfusions, and splenectomy, options B, C, and D, are all treatments used for beta-thalassemia major, but none of them are curative. **Task:** D2—Clinical Intervention

17. **Answer: E** With multiple blood transfusions and continued absorption of intestinal iron, iron overload develops (option E). Iron is deposited in visceral organs (mainly the heart, liver, and endocrine glands), and most patient deaths are caused by cardiac complications.
Infections can occur with blood cell transfusions, and disseminated intravascular coagulation (option A) can be the result of infections, but this is a rare complication. Gastrointestinal bleeding, option B, is an indication for red blood cell transfusion and not a complication of this treatment. Henoch-Schönlein purpura, option C, is an autoimmune disorder and not related to transfusions. The use of stored blood for transfusions is followed by an elevation of serum potassium levels, not a decrease, or hypokalemia, option D. **Task:** D2—Clinical Intervention

18. **Answer: B** Thalassemia major (Cooley disease) is inherited when two carrier parents who have thalassemia minor pass it on to their child. Each child of two carrier parents has a 25% of having beta-thalassemia major. Therefore, option B is the correct answer. Thalassemia minor is inherited when two carrier parents pass it on to their child. Each child of two carrier parents has a 50% chance of having beta-thalassemia minor. In general, thalassemia is inherited in an autosomal recessive manner. **Task:** E—Applying Basic Scientific Concepts

19. **Answer: E** People of Mediterranean descent, option E, are at risk for beta-thalassemia. The frequency of beta-thalassemia varies widely, depending on the ethnic population. The disease is reported most commonly in Mediterranean (Greek and Italian), Southeast Asian, and African populations. Alpha-thalassemia mutations are very common in people of Asian descent; the Mediterranean and Middle Eastern regions also have a high frequency of this genetic disorder. Ashkenazi Jewish people, Hispanic people, North Germanic ethnic groups, and Pacific Islanders (options A through D) are not at risk for this condition. **Task:** E—Applying Basic Scientific Concepts

20. **Answer: A** Genetic information is unique because of its familial nature and ability to predict future health. The legal duty to warn family members is first imposed on the patient, or in this case, the patient's parents. Therefore, option A is correct.
Contacting the patient's relatives with or without consent, option B, is incorrect because practitioners must preserve patient confidentiality as a default. Under some circumstances, the clinician would be obligated to warn family members at risk, but this is not an initial action. Options C and D are incorrect because neither insurance companies nor clinical laboratories contact family members about genetic disorders. **Task:** F—Entry-Level Professional Practice: Legal/medical ethics

BIBLIOGRAPHY

AMA Journal of Ethics: Illuminating the Art of Medicine. journalof-ethics.ama-assn.org/article/genetic-diseases-and-duty-disclose/2012-08

Galanello, R., & Origa, R. (2010). Beta-thalassemia. *Orphanet Journal of Rare Diseases*, 5-11. https://doi.org/10.1186/1750-1172-5-11.

Lee, M. *Basic skills in interpreting laboratory data* (4th ed., pp. 340-343, 350). American Society of Health-System Pharmacists.

Papadakis, M. A., & McPhee, S. J. (2020a). *Current medical diagnosis & treatment* (pp. 515, 519-521, 791-792). McGraw Hill.

Sheth, T. N., Choudhry, N. K., Bowes, M., & Detsky, A. S. (1997). The relation of conjunctival pallor to the presence of anemia. *Journal of General Internal Medicine*, *12*(2), 102-106. McGraw Hill.

Sheth, T. N., Choudhry, N. K., Bowes, M., & Detsky, A. S. (1997). The relation of conjunctival pallor to the presence of anemia. *Journal of general internal medicine*, 12(2), 102-106.

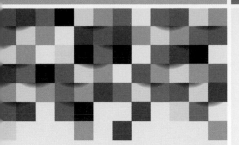

CASE STUDY 10
Infectious Diseases

Questions

Case Section I: Chief Complaint and History of Present Illness

A 7-year-old girl is brought to the office by her parents because she has had a raised, red rash for the past 24 hours. The parents say that the rash initially started on the patient's face but now has spread down her trunk including both upper arms and thighs. Four days ago, the patient had development of a low-grade fever to 37.9°C (100.2°F) as well as fatigue, dry cough, runny nose, and red teary eyes. The fever improved with acetaminophen, and the other symptoms are somewhat better today. Medical history includes perennial allergic rhinitis, for which she has been taking loratadine 5 mg daily for over a year; the patient is allergic to penicillin, which results in development of hives.

1. Which of the following is the most likely differential diagnosis?
   A. Drug allergy
   B. Erythema infectiosum
   C. Measles
   D. Roseola infantum

2. Which of the following parts of this patient's history is key to confirming the likely diagnosis?
   A. Family history
   B. Immunization status
   C. Medical history
   D. Neonatal history
   E. Recent medication use

3. If roseola infantum is the primary differential diagnosis for this patient, which of the following symptoms, besides the rash, is most likely to indicate this diagnosis?
   A. Conjunctivitis
   B. Coryza
   C. Cough
   D. Fatigue
   E. Fever

4. If measles is the primary differential diagnosis for this patient, which of the following rash distributions and evolutions is most likely?
   A. On the bilateral cheeks only with no spread
   B. On the trunk only with no spreading
   C. Starting at the head and spreading down to the trunk
   D. Starting on the face and spreading down the whole body
   E. Starting on the trunk and spreading outward to the limbs and head

5. If erythema infectiosum is the primary differential diagnosis, this patient's rash is most likely to be concentrated over which of the following areas of the body?
   A. Face
   B. Neck
   C. Trunk
   D. Extremities
   E. Palms and soles

Case Section II: Objective Findings, Assessment, and Plan

Temperature is 38.0°C (100.4°F), pulse rate is 95/min, respirations are 17/min, and blood pressure is 98/68 mmHg. Oxygen saturation is 99% on room air. The patient is crying and appears to be in mild distress. Physical examination shows bilateral conjunctival injection with clear lacrimation and clear rhinorrhea. The buccal mucosa and soft palate have scattered 2-mm lesions that are grayish and elevated with erythematous bases, as shown in image A. Many of the lesions appear to be sloughing off. The pharynx appears erythematous, but no exudates are noted on the tonsils. Cervical lymphadenopathy is noted. The lungs are clear to auscultation bilaterally with no wheezes, rhonchi, or crackles. A generalized erythematous maculopapular rash is noted over the entire body with a few lesions on the palms and soles, as shown in image b. The rash blanches on palpation.

6.

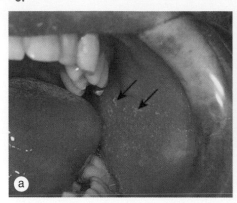 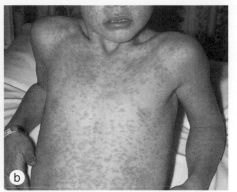

Based on these physical examination findings, which of the following is the most likely diagnosis?
A. Erythema infectiosum
B. Hand, foot, and mouth disease
C. Measles
D. Roseola infantum

7. Based on this clinical presentation, which of the following is the most likely etiology of this patient's disease?
A. Adverse effect of a drug
B. Autoimmune disorder
C. Genetic syndrome
D. Hypersensitivity reaction
E. Infectious disease

8. Which of the following physical examination findings in this patient is pathognomonic for one specific disease process?
A. Constellation of conjunctivitis and rash
B. Constellation of conjunctivitis, rhinorrhea, and lymphadenopathy
C. Constellation of generalized maculopapular rash and fever
D. Lesions found on buccal mucosa
E. Presence of rash on the palms and soles

9. Which of the following tests is most likely to confirm the diagnosis?
A. Allergy testing with radioallergosorbent testing
B. Bacterial culture
C. Complete blood cell count with differential
D. CT scan of the head and neck with contrast
E. Serology

10. Which of the following additional physical examination findings is most likely to indicate a potentially fatal complication of this patient's disease?
A. Adventitious breath sounds
B. Injected tympanic membranes
C. Maxillary sinus tenderness
D. New heart murmur
E. Tenderness to palpation in the abdomen

Case Section III: Comorbidity

During the interview, the patient's parents say that she did not complete all of her recommended childhood vaccinations, including measles, mumps, and rubella (MMR) and varicella. The mother says that they missed that well-child check and forgot to reschedule but would like to get caught up. The patient attends daycare twice a week, and one of the other children at school had a fever and was not feeling well recently and was subsequently sent home. The parents are fully immunized. They do not know if all the children at the daycare are immunized because it is run by a family friend.

11. Based on these new findings, this patient most likely has which of the following diseases?
A. Chickenpox
B. Measles
C. Mumps
D. Roseola infantum

12. This patient's disease was most likely acquired via which of the following pathways?
A. Bloodborne
B. Fecal-oral route
C. Inhalation
D. Inoculation via infected fomites

13. If this patient has measles, how long does the rash associated with this disease typically last?
A. One day
B. Two days
C. Four days
D. Seven days
E. Two weeks

14. Which of the following is the most common complication of this disease?
A. Appendicitis
B. Corneal ulceration
C. Diarrhea
D. Myocarditis
E. Pneumonia

15. Measles is most often acquired during which of the following times of the year?
    A. Fall
    B. Spring
    C. Summer
    D. Winter
    E. No specific time of year

16. Which of the following is the most appropriate first-line treatment of this disease?
    A. Antihistamines
    B. Antiviral therapy
    C. Broad-spectrum antibiotics
    D. Monoclonal antibodies
    E. Supportive treatment

17. Which of the following body systems is most likely to develop complications after recovery from measles?
    A. Endocrine
    B. Integumentary
    C. Neurologic
    D. Renal
    E. Reproductive

Case Section IV: Professional Practice
The parents say that they are considering moving the patient to a different daycare facility.

18. It is most appropriate to recommend the parents ensure that the new daycare does which of the following to prevent the spread of this disease in the future?
    A. Has cafeteria staff using gloves and hairnets while preparing food
    B. Has hand sanitizer readily available
    C. Follows the three feet of social distancing rule
    D. Requires cloth masks except while actively eating or drinking
    E. Requires full childhood vaccination series

19. In addition to notifying this disease to the state Centers for Disease Control and Prevention and the daycare, which of the following is the most appropriate next step with regard to the patient and isolation?
    A. Allow the patient to return to daycare tomorrow
    B. Allow the patient to return to normal activities immediately
    C. Discharge to home with directions to isolate for three days
    D. Discharge to home with directions to isolate for five days
    E. Discharge to home with directions to isolate for seven days

20. Which of the following represents the percentage that herd immunity needs to reach in order for this patient's disease to not be able to spread to immunocompromised individuals who cannot be vaccinated?
    A. 50%
    B. 60%
    C. 70%
    D. 80%
    E. 90%

21. The vaccine for measles is live attenuated, which means that it is contraindicated in patients with a history of which of the following?
    A. Chronic kidney disease
    B. Lymphoma who are being treated with chemotherapy
    C. Previous bout of the disease
    D. Sickle cell anemia
    E. Type 2 diabetes mellitus

22. Which of the following childhood diseases would this patient have been protected from if she received a full childhood vaccination series?
    A. Erythema infectiosum
    B. Hand, foot, and mouth disease
    C. Herpangina
    D. Roseola infantum
    E. Rubella

At 14 years of age, the patient is brought to the pediatric office because she has had uncontrollable jerking movements for the past week. Her mother says that she has not been able to concentrate in school, has been exhibiting uncharacteristic behavior, and has been feeling lethargic over the past year.

23. Which of the following rare but fatal complications of measles is this patient most likely experiencing?
    A. Essential myoclonus
    B. Juvenile myoclonic epilepsy
    C. Lennox-Gastaut syndrome
    D. Periodic limb movement disorder
    E. Subacute sclerosing panencephalitis

24. If this patient had not experienced this complication and had recovered fully from this disease, which of the following would have been the best next step in management at 7 years of age?
    A. Catch up on vaccinations
    B. Obtain baseline bloodwork
    C. Obtain chest x-ray studies
    D. Schedule routine annual physical examinations
    E. Switch to a different antihistamine

Answer Key for this chapter begins on p. 286

Answers

1. **Answer: C** Measles, option C, is the most likely differential diagnosis at this point, based on the patient's cough, conjunctivitis, and coryza, as well as the rash distribution.

   Option A, drug allergy, is incorrect because the rash associated with this condition is pruritic and typically starts on the trunk then spreads to the rest of the body. Also, a drug allergy is associated with a new medication and is not necessarily associated with the cough, coryza, or conjunctivitis. Option B, erythema infectiosum, is incorrect because the rash with this disease is concentrated on the cheeks of the face first. Also, the symptoms of this disease do not include cough or conjunctivitis. Option D, roseola infantum, is incorrect because patients with this disease usually have a high fever, and the rash starts on the neck and trunk and then spreads to the face and extremities. **Task: C—Formulating Most Likely Diagnosis**

2. **Answer: B** Immunization status, option B, is correct because a diagnosis of measles is more likely if the patient is not fully immunized to measles, mumps, and rubella. Risk factors include not being immunized, partial immunization, those immunized with poor response to the vaccine, and those who travel to endemic areas.

   With measles being an infectious disease that is highly contagious (90% who contact it develop disease), options A, C, and D are incorrect. Family, medical, and neonatal history do not prevent nor protect the patient from acquiring measles. Option E, recent medication use, is not correct because medications do not cause measles; however, this would be important if the differential diagnosis were a drug exanthem. **Task: A—History Taking and Performing Physical Examination**

3. **Answer: E** Option E, fever, is correct because roseola infantum is mainly suspected if the patient has a very high fever (40.0°C [104.0°F]) for a few days then develops a rash. Conjunctivitis, coryza, cough, and fatigue (options A through D) can occur but are not as specific for this disease. A low-grade fever, as seen in this patient, therefore makes roseola infantum less likely. **Task: A—History Taking and Performing Physical Examination**

4. **Answer: C** Starting at the head and spreading down to the trunk, option C, is the correct rash distribution and evolution that corresponds with measles, which is the primary differential diagnosis for this patient's case. On the bilateral cheeks only and starting on the face and spreading down the whole body, options

A and D, are incorrect as they are representative of erythema infectiosum. On the trunk only with no spreading, option B, is indicative of a drug exanthem. Starting on the trunk and spreading outward to the limbs and head, option E, is representative of roseola infantum. **Task: A—History Taking and Performing Physical Examination**

5. **Answer: A** Face, option A, is correct because erythema infectiosum is characterized by a concentrated vasculitis-type rash on the cheeks of the face. It can occur all over the body as well, but the cheeks are the key to diagnosis. Options B through E are incorrect because the rash is not concentrated on those areas in erythema infectiosum. **Task: A—History Taking and Performing Physical Examination**

6. **Answer: C** Based on the findings on physical examination, this patient has measles, option C. Examination shows the characteristic measles rash, Koplik spots in the mouth, as well as rhinorrhea and conjunctivitis. Erythema infectiosum, option A, is not correct because this patient does not have a slapped-cheek rash, nor does she have a lacelike rash on the trunk and extremities. Also, Koplik spots are not indicative of erythema infectiosum. Hand, foot, and mouth disease, option B, is not correct because this patient's rash is not concentrated on the hands, feet, arms, upper thighs, and buttocks, nor is it vesicular, which is indicative of hand, foot, and mouth disease. The oral lesions are most commonly found on the buccal mucosa and tongue and are erythematous macules that evolve into ulcers with a grayish/yellow base and erythematous margins. Roseola infantum, option D, is incorrect because this patient's fever is not high enough to be roseola infantum. Also, the oral lesions that are indicative of roseola, called Nagayama spots, are on the uvulo-palatoglossal junction and are macular or frank ulcerations, not papules like Koplik spots. **Task: A—History Taking and Performing Physical Examination**

7. **Answer: E** This patient has measles, which is an infectious disease, option E. Fever, lymphadenopathy, conjunctivitis, rhinorrhea, cough, and exanthem point toward an infectious etiology and not to one caused by an adverse effect of a drug, autoimmune disorder, genetic syndrome, or hypersensitivity reaction (options A through D). **Task: E—Applying Basic Scientific Concepts**

8. **Answer: D** Lesions found on the buccal mucosa, option D, are Koplik spots which are pathognomonic for one specific disease—measles.

Conjunctivitis and rash, option A, can be found in other diseases such as roseola infantum and rubella. Conjunctivitis, rhinorrhea, and lymphadenopathy, option B, are symptoms that can be found in viral conjunctivitis caused by an upper respiratory tract virus such as adenovirus. Generalized maculopapular rash and fever, option C, are found in many viral exanthems. Rash on the palms and soles, option E, is incorrect because there are several diseases that can cause rashes on the palms and soles such as Rocky Mountain spotted fever and syphilis. **Task: E—Applying Basic Scientific Concepts**

9. **Answer: E** Serology, option E, is the most common diagnostic test for this disease. IgM titers of measles antibodies are the test of choice, but another option to diagnose measles is viral RNA RT-PCR. Allergy testing with radioallergosorbent testing, option A, is incorrect since measles is not caused by a reaction to an allergen. Bacterial culture, option B, is incorrect because measles is a virus and not a bacterium. Complete blood cell count with differential, option C, will not show a measles-specific pattern. CT scan of the head and neck with contrast, option D, will not show the infectious etiology of measles, but it can detect the complications of the disease. **Task: B—Using Diagnostic and Laboratory Studies**

10. **Answer: A** Adventitious breath sounds, option A, indicate pneumonia which is the most common fatal complication of measles.
Injected tympanic membranes, option B, indicate otitis media which is not a potentially fatal complication of measles. Maxillary sinus tenderness, option C, is incorrect because it is not a common finding of measles and not specifically that of a fatal complication of this disease. A new heart murmur, option D, could indicate myocarditis or pericarditis which can be a complication of measles, but they are not usually fatal. Tenderness to palpation of the abdomen, option E, is incorrect because while it could indicate hepatitis, appendicitis, or gastroenteritis, which are complications of measles, they are not usually fatal. **Task: A—History Taking and Performing Physical Examination**

11. **Answer: B** Measles, option B, is the most likely diagnosis based on the characteristic rash, presence of Koplik spots, and now the known partially immunized status of the patient. Risk factors for being infected with measles include those who have not received a second dose of MMR, like this patient. She was likely infected by the other sick contact at daycare.
The rash associated with chickenpox, option A, is pustular and vesicular with pruritis. Varicella also does not cause cough, coryza, conjunctivitis, or Koplik spots. This patient is at risk for this without completing the varicella series. Mumps, option C, does not present with a rash, but the patient is more at risk for this without having both doses of MMR. Roseola infantum, option D, is incorrect because this patient does not have a high fever, and the rash did not start on the neck and trunk and then spread to the face and extremities. **Task: A—History Taking and Performing Physical Examination**

12. **Answer: C** This patient has measles, which is acquired via inhalation of infected respiratory secretions (option C).
Option A is incorrect because measles is not a blood-borne pathogen. Measles is not spread via the fecal-oral route, option B, like gastrointestinal microbes. Inoculation via infected fomites, option D, is incorrect because measles is not thought to be spread via fomites. **Task: E—Applying Basic Scientific Concepts**

13. **Answer: D** Option D is correct as the measles rash usually lasts six to seven days. Options A, B, and C are incorrect as the measles rash does not resolve that quickly. Option E is incorrect as the measles rash does not last that long. **Task: E—Applying Basic Scientific Concepts**

14. **Answer: C** Diarrhea, option C, is the most common complication of measles. Appendicitis, corneal ulceration, myocarditis, and pneumonia (options A, B, D, and E) are possible complications of measles; however, they occur less often than diarrhea. **Task: C—Formulating Most Likely Diagnosis**

15. **Answer: E** Option E is correct because measles can be acquired any time of the year. While there may be peak incidence in late winter or early spring in temperate regions, many regions have no temporal pattern. Options A through D are therefore incorrect. **Task: E—Applying Basic Scientific Concepts**

16. **Answer: E** Measles is treated with supportive treatment only, option E.
Measles is not a hypersensitivity reaction; therefore, antihistamines (option A) is incorrect. There are no antiviral medications or monoclonal antibodies available for the treatment of measles, therefore options B and D are incorrect. Measles is not caused by bacteria; it is caused by a virus. Therefore, broad-spectrum antibiotic therapy, option C, is not appropriate treatment. **Task: D2—Clinical Intervention**

17. **Answer: C** Option C, neurologic, is correct due to the risk for encephalitis, acute disseminated encephalomyelitis, and subacute sclerosing panencephalitis in patients who are recovering from, or have recovered from, measles. Pulmonary, gastrointestinal, ocular, and cardiovascular complications can also happen.

The endocrine, integumentary, renal, and reproductive systems (options A, B, D, and E) are not affected after recovery from measles. **Task:** C—Formulating Most Likely Diagnosis

18. **Answer: E** It is most appropriate that the new daycare requires full childhood vaccination series, option E, to prevent the spread of this disease in the future because measles is so contagious and airborne, vaccination is the best prevention strategy. If vaccination cannot be done, airborne precautions would be necessary with respirators.

    Having cafeteria staff use gloves and hairnets, option A, is incorrect because measles is not spread via the fecal-oral route where food safety precautions could prevent spread. Having hand sanitizer readily available, option B, is incorrect because measles is not primarily spread by fomite contact or fecal-oral route which would be prevented by handwashing. Following the three feet of social distancing rule, option C, will not be effective because measles can remain airborne for up to two hours, thereby making social distancing ineffective. Cloth masks, option D, will not filter out measles virus; only N95 respirators would be able to do this. **Task:** F—Entry-Level Professional Practice—Public Health

19. **Answer: C** Isolate for three days, option C, is correct because the recommended isolation period for measles is four days after rash onset. Since this patient's rash began one day ago, three more days of isolation are needed.

    Options A and B are incorrect because they will lead to spread of measles at the daycare and wherever this patient is participating in normal activities. Options D and E are incorrect because the time of isolation, five and seven days, is too long. **Task:** F—Entry-Level Professional Practice—Public Health

20. **Answer: E** Option E is correct as it takes between 85% and 95% for herd immunity to be reached for measles. Options A through D would not be sufficient and would leave those unimmunized patients unprotected from measles. **Task:** F—Entry-Level Professional Practice—Public Health

21. **Answer: B** Patients with lymphoma who are being treated with chemotherapy, option B, cannot receive live attenuated vaccines such as MMR.

    Options A, D, and E are incorrect because a history of these conditions does not cause a patient to be severely immunocompromised; therefore, patients with these diseases can receive live attenuated vaccines. A patient with a previous bout of the measles, option C, can receive the vaccine, although it is usually not needed because they are considered immune. **Task:** F—Entry-Level Professional Practice—Public Health

22. **Answer: E** Rubella, option E, is correct since rubella is part of the MMR vaccine.

    Options A through D do not have any vaccines on the market currently. Candidate vaccines were tried with parvovirus B19, which causes erythema infectiosum, but efforts were abandoned. **Task:** D1—Health Maintenance, Patient Education, and Disease Prevention

23. **Answer: E** Subacute sclerosing panencephalitis, option E, usually begins 7 to 10 years after diagnosis with measles and starts with lethargy, behavioral and personality changes, and difficulty in school. It progresses to myoclonus, motor and sensory neuron disease, and dementia. It finally progresses to autonomic dysfunction, flaccid paralysis, or decorticate rigidity which then devolves into a vegetative state and eventual death.

    Essential myoclonus, option A, is incorrect because patients are also cognitively normal, they only have the myoclonus. Juvenile myoclonic epilepsy, option B, is incorrect because patients with this condition have normal cognitive function and may show other types of seizures. Lennox-Gastaut syndrome, option C, is incorrect because there are no seizures present which predominate in Lennox-Gastaut syndrome along with the myoclonus, intellectual disability, and psychotic symptoms. Periodic limb movement disorder, option D, does not present with cognitive changes or behavioral changes and is characterized by myoclonus during sleep only. **Task:** C—Formulating Most Likely Diagnosis

24. **Answer: A** Catching up on vaccinations, option A, is correct since this patient did not receive the recommended vaccinations at well-child visits prior to her initial presentation in this case. She needs the second dose of MMR and varicella since she is in daycare with other children who do not have known vaccination statuses and are at risk for other communicable diseases. Obtaining baseline bloodwork, option B, is not necessary at this time in a child who is 7 years of age and otherwise healthy. Chest x-ray studies, option C, are not needed at this time if the patient did not have symptoms suspicious for pneumonia. Scheduling routine annual physical examinations, option D, is important but is not as pressing as getting caught up on vaccinations. Switching to a different antihistamine, option E, is not appropriate since the patient has not complained of worsening seasonal allergies and is currently doing well with loratadine. **Task:** D1—Health Maintenance, Patient Education, and Disease Prevention

BIBLIOGRAPHY

Albrecht, M. A. (2021). Clinical features of varicella-zoster virus infection: Chickenpox. In J. Mitty (Ed.), *UpToDate* [online serial]. Waltham, MA: UpToDate.

Albrecht, M. A. (2021). Mumps. In E. L. Baron (Ed.), *UpToDate* [online serial]. Waltham, MA: UpToDate.

Bircher, A. J. (2021). Exanthematous (maculopapular) drug eruption. In R. Corona (Ed.), *UpToDate* [online serial]. Waltham, MA: UpToDate.

Caviness, J. N. (2021). Classification and evaluation of myoclonus. In A. F. Eichler (Ed.), *UpToDate* [online serial]. Waltham, MA: UpToDate.

Drutz, J. E. (2021). Measles, mumps, and rubella immunization in infants, children, and adolescents. In M. M. Torchia, MM (Ed.), *UpToDate* [online serial]. Waltham, MA: UpToDate.

Edwards, M. S. (2021). Rubella. In M. Bogorodskaya (Ed.), *UpToDate* [online serial]. Waltham, MA: UpToDate.

Gans, H., & Maldonado, Y. A. (2021). Measles: Clinical manifestations, diagnosis, treatment, and prevention. In E. L. Baron (Ed.), *UpToDate* [online serial]. Waltham, MA: UpToDate.

Gans, H., & Maldonado, Y. A. (2021). Measles: Epidemiology and transmission. In E. L. Baron (Ed.), *UpToDate* [online serial]. Waltham, MA: UpToDate.

Hibberd, P. L. (2021). Measles, mumps, and rubella immunization in adults. In E. L. Baron (Ed.), *UpToDate* [online serial]. Waltham, MA: UpToDate.

Hicks, C. B., & Clement, M. (2021). Syphilis: Epidemiology, pathophysiology, and clinical manifestations in patients without HIV. In J. Mitty (Ed.), *UpToDate* [online serial]. Waltham, MA: UpToDate.

Jacobs, D. S. (2021). Conjunctivitis. In J. Givens (Ed.), *UpToDate* [online serial]. Waltham, MA: UpToDate.

Jordan, J. A. (2021). Clinical manifestations and diagnosis of parvovirus B19 infection. In M. Bogorodskaya (Ed.), *UpToDate* [online serial]. Waltham, MA: UpToDate.

Jordan, J. A. (2021). Treatment and prevention of parvovirus B19 infection. In M. Bogorodskaya (Ed.), *UpToDate* [online serial]. Waltham, MA: UpToDate.

Korff, C. M. (2021). Juvenile myoclonic epilepsy. In J. F. Dashe (Ed.), *UpToDate* [online serial]. Waltham, MA: UpToDate.

Lopez, F. A., & Sanders, C. V. (2021). Fever and rash in an immunocompetent patient. In *UpToDate* [online serial]. Waltham, MA: UpToDate.

Romero, J. R. (2021). Hand, foot, and mouth disease and herpangina. In M. M. Torchia (Ed.), *UpToDate* [online serial]. Waltham, MA: UpToDate.

Sexton, D. J., & McClain, M. T. (2021). Clinical manifestations and diagnosis of Rocky Mountain spotted fever. In J. Mitty (Ed.), *UpToDate* [online serial]. Waltham, MA: UpToDate.

Tremblay, C., & Brady, M. T. (2021). Roseola infantum (exanthem subitum). In M. M. Torchia (Ed.), *UpToDate* [online serial]. Waltham, MA: UpToDate.

Wilfong, A. (2021). Epilepsy syndromes in childhood. In J. F. Dashe (Ed.), *UpToDate* [online serial]. Waltham, MA: UpToDate.

   Answer Key for this chapter begins on p. 286

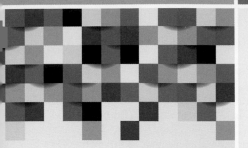

CASE STUDY 11
Musculoskeletal System

Questions

Case Section I: Chief Complaint and History of Present Illness

A 36-year-old transgender woman comes to the clinic because she has had pain in her lower back for the past six weeks. She says the pain has been persistent during this time and began shortly after she did weighted squats at the gym. Physical examination shows difficulty with flexion of the lumbar spine.

1. Based on the limited information thus far, which of the following is at the top of the differential diagnosis list?
   A. Ankylosing spondylitis
   B. Cauda equina syndrome
   C. Lumbar strain
   D. Psoriatic arthritis
   E. Spondylolisthesis

2. Which of the following questions is most important to ask this patient at this time?
   A. Do you have a history of back pain?
   B. Do you take multivitamins?
   C. Have you ever had surgery?
   D. Have you lost sensation around the rectum?
   E. Have you taken any medications for the pain?

3. Which of the following studies is considered the gold standard to determine if this patient has a herniated disk?
   A. Electromyelography
   B. Lumbar puncture
   C. MRI
   D. Plain-film x-ray studies
   E. Ultrasonography

4. Which of the following findings, if noted on further inquiry into this patient's history, is most likely to cause concern for neoplasm of the spine?
   A. Abrupt nature of onset of back pain
   B. Persistence of pain
   C. Previous back surgery
   D. Radiculopathy
   E. Weight loss

5. Testing of which of the following parameters is most likely to help determine if this patient has an impingement of the L5 nerve root?
   A. Dorsiflexion of the fifth toe
   B. Extension of the spine
   C. Patellar reflex
   D. Sensation to pinprick of the great toe
   E. Straight-leg raise

6. Which of the following studies is the most appropriate initial diagnostic study to order at this time?
   A. CT scan of the lumbar spine
   B. Electromyelography
   C. MRI of the lumbar spine
   D. Nerve conduction studies
   E. Plain-film x-ray studies of the lumbar spine

Imaging studies of the spine show no abnormalities. After a period of rest, the patient's symptoms remain unchanged. She returns for follow-up two weeks later to discuss treatment options.

7. Which of the following is the most appropriate next step?
   A. Continue the current exercise routine in the gym
   B. Refer for physical therapy
   C. Refer to a neurosurgeon
   D. Refer to an orthopedic surgeon
   E. Refer to a pain management clinic

8. If herniated nucleus pulposus is diagnosed in this patient, which of the following disk spaces is most commonly injured in patients with this same diagnosis?
   A. L2–L3
   B. L3–L4
   C. L4–L5
   D. L5–S1

9. If cauda equina syndrome is diagnosed in this patient, which of the following is the most appropriate management?
   A. Bed rest
   B. Immediate referral to a neurosurgical specialist
   C. Intramuscular injection of corticosteroids
   D. Nonsteroidal anti-inflammatory drugs and follow-up in one week
   E. Physical therapy

10. If ankylosing spondylitis is suspected in this patient, which of the following laboratory studies is most likely to confirm this diagnosis?
    A. Anti-cyclic citrullinated peptide antibody test
    B. HLA-B27 test
    C. Measurement of C-reactive protein level
    D. Measurement of erythrocyte sedimentation rate
    E. Rheumatoid factor assay

Case Section II: Objective Findings, Assessment, and Plan

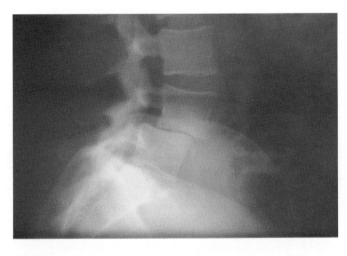

Two years later, the patient comes to the clinic for follow-up and says that she continues to have lower back pain. Close monitoring and conservative treatment during the past two years have not provided relief. Physical examination shows a positive straight-leg raising test. Plain-film x-ray study of the lower lumbar spine is shown.

11. Which of the following best describes the findings on the x-ray study?
    A. Compression fracture of the L4 vertebral body
    B. Herniated disk at L3–L4
    C. Loss of disk height between L3–L4
    D. Spondylolisthesis of L4–L5
    E. Normal findings

12. Which of the following diagnoses is most appropriate to consider in this patient if she has headache and sudden onset of fever in addition to lower back pain?
    A. Meningitis
    B. Migraine
    C. Osteoarthritis
    D. Spina bifida occulta
    E. Tension headache

Case Section III: Comorbidity

The patient is treated appropriately and her pain is managed. Eight years later, she comes to the clinic because she has had bilateral shoulder and hip pain that has progressively worsened over the past three months. More recently, she says that it has become difficult to dress herself because of the pain. She is otherwise healthy and has no history of recent illness. Physical examination shows no tenderness over the muscular areas, but stiffness is noted with active range of motion of the hips and shoulders. No edema or redness of the joints and no skin rashes are noted.

13. Based on these findings, which of the following is the most likely diagnosis?
    A. Gouty arthropathy
    B. Polymyalgia rheumatica
    C. Polymyositis
    D. Rheumatoid arthritis

14. Which of the following laboratory studies is most likely to help evaluate the course of this disease?
    A. Analysis of synovial fluid
    B. Antinuclear antibody test
    C. Epstein-Barr nuclear antigen test
    D. Measurement of complete blood cell count
    E. Measurement of erythrocyte sedimentation rate

15. Which of the following is the most effective treatment for this patient's condition?
    A. Bisphosphonate
    B. Conservative management
    C. Corticosteroids
    D. Disease-modifying antirheumatic drugs
    E. Pain management with opiates

16. If polymyositis is diagnosed in this patient, a history of which of the following is most consistent with this diagnosis?
    A. Alcohol use
    B. Injury to the muscle
    C. Joint pain
    D. Migraine headaches
    E. Progressive muscle weakness

    Answer Key for this chapter begins on p. 293

17. Which of the following studies is most likely to confirm polymyositis as the definitive diagnosis in this patient?
    A. Complete blood cell count
    B. Electromyography
    C. Erythrocyte sedimentation rate
    D. MRI of the spine
    E. Muscle biopsy

Case Section IV: Professional Practice

Nine years later, the patient who is now 55 years of age comes to the office for routine physical examination. She is up-to-date on all routine health maintenance including colonoscopy and vaccinations. She says that she has had daily pain and stiffness in her lower back during the past several months. The pain seems to improve with rest and worsens with movement. The patient has no history of fever, night sweats, or weight loss. Plain-film x-ray studies show multiple osteophytes on the lumbosacral spine.

18. Which of the following is the most likely diagnosis?
    A. Ankylosing spondylitis
    B. Degenerative joint disease
    C. Reactive arthritis
    D. Rheumatoid arthritis
    E. Psoriatic arthritis

19. If rheumatoid arthritis is suspected in this patient, which of the following is the most sensitive and specific study to confirm this diagnosis?
    A. Anti-cyclic citrullinated peptide antibody test
    B. Antinuclear antibody test
    C. Plain-film x-ray studies of the hands
    D. Rheumatoid factor assay
    E. Uric acid level

20. Which of the following findings on history taking and physical examination is most likely to increase this patient's risk of osteoarthritis?
    A. Anorexia
    B. Obesity

C. Regular weight-bearing exercise
D. Use of nonsteroidal anti-inflammatory drug
E. Use of vitamin supplements

21. If the patient has osteoarthritis, which of the following treatment options is most appropriate?
    A. Acetaminophen
    B. Disease-modifying antirheumatic drugs
    C. Nonsteroidal anti-inflammatory drugs
    D. Opiates
    E. Oral glucocorticoids

22. Long-term therapy for osteoarthritis is planned. Which of the following laboratory values is most appropriate to monitor while she is taking this medication?
    A. Complete blood cell count
    B. Erythrocyte sedimentation rate
    C. Serum glucose level
    D. Serum urea nitrogen/creatinine ratio
    E. Serum uric acid level

The billing office contacts the practitioner regarding the most recent office visit for this patient with osteoarthritis. The practitioner performed a detailed history and only examined the patient's joints, but the practitioner coded the visit at a higher level than needed.

23. Which of the following is the most appropriate next step?
    A. Falsify the documentation to meet the billing standard
    B. Have the patient return to the office for a more thorough history
    C. Have the patient return to the office for a more thorough physical examination
    D. Revise the coding and bill at a lower level
    E. Do nothing and keep the same coding level

Answers

1. **Answer: C** Lumbar strain, option C, is the most likely differential diagnosis because of the length of the mechanism of injury and the absence of any red flag symptoms or neuropathic complaints.
Ankylosing spondylitis and spondylolisthesis, options A and E, include neuropathic symptoms, of which this patient does not have. Patients have saddle anesthesia and loss of bowel and bladder function with cauda equina syndrome, option B. Finally, psoriatic arthritis, option D, is unlikely to present in the spine. **Task:** A—History Taking and Performing Physical Examination

2. **Answer: D** The most appropriate question to ask this patient is to determine if she has saddle anesthesia (option D), which is a red flag and could mean that she has cauda equina syndrome, a surgical emergency. Options A, B, C, and E are appropriate questions to ask this patient, but they are not the most important or critical question to ask at this time. **Task:** A—History Taking and Performing Physical Examination

3. **Answer: C** Because herniated disks are soft-tissue structures, the gold standard for determining if a disk is herniated is MRI, option C.
Electromyelography and lumbar puncture, options A and B, do not allow for visualization of disk spaces in the spine. Plain-film x-ray studies, option D, are appropriate when determining if a patient has a bone abnormality in the spine. Although ultrasonography, option E, will visualize a disk, it is not the most sensitive study to visualize a herniated disk. **Task:** B—Using Diagnostic and Laboratory Studies

4. **Answer: E** A history of back pain with weight loss, option E, could possibly indicate that a patient has a neoplasm of the spine.
Abrupt nature of onset of back pain, option A, is not concerning for neoplasm since the back pain associated with neoplasm typically occurs more gradually. A history of persistent pain or back surgery, options B and C, are not specific enough to diagnose cancer. Radicular symptoms, option D, can be common in multiple back pain complaints. **Task:** A—History Taking and Performing Physical Examination

5. **Answer: E** The straight-leg raising test, option E, is the most sensitive tool in an outpatient setting to determine if a patient has impingement of the L5

nerve root. The test result is positive if the patient experiences pain in the lower limb in the same distribution of L5.
Testing dorsiflexion of the fifth toe, option A, is not appropriate, because the fifth metatarsals are not in the same nerve root distribution as L5; however, impingement of the L5 nerve root would impact dorsiflexion of the great toe. Extension of the spine, option B, can exacerbate many forms of back pain and not just impingement of the L5 nerve root. Testing the patellar reflex, option C, will determine if there are abnormalities in the L2–L4 nerve roots. Sensation to pinprick of the great toe, option D, is also under the influence of L4 and would not be of diagnostic value in this case. **Task:** A—History Taking and Performing Physical Examination

6. **Answer: E** Plain-film x-ray studies of the lumbar spine, option E, are the least expensive and least invasive initial diagnostic tool for this patient, especially since she does not have any red flag symptoms. CT scan, electromyography, MRI, and nerve conduction studies, options A through D, are appropriate next steps if abnormalities are noted on plain-film x-ray studies of this patient's lumbar spine. **Task:** B—Using Diagnostic and Laboratory Studies

7. **Answer: B** Referring this patient for physical therapy, option B, is the most appropriate next step since the majority of cases of lower back pain are functional. Currently, the patient has no red flag symptoms and appears to otherwise be in good health. A trial of physical therapy along with nonsteroidal anti-inflammatory drugs (NSAIDs) are the most appropriate next steps in management.
If this patient continues her current regimen in the gym, option A, she will further exacerbate her pain. Referral to a neurosurgeon or an orthopedic surgeon, options C and D, is not warranted at this time since the patient has not yet tried conservative management. Referring the patient to a pain management clinic, option E, is not appropriate since she has yet to see if her pain subsides with conservative management with physical therapy and NSAIDs. **Task:** D2—Clinical Intervention

8. **Answer: D** L5–S1, option D, is the most commonly injured disk space found in 90% of patients with a herniated lumbar disk. Options A, B, and C can also

Answer Key for this chapter begins on p. 293

be damaged in lower back injuries, but they are not the most commonly injured area. **Task:** E—Applying Basic Scientific Concepts

9. **Answer: B** The most appropriate next step is immediate referral to a neurosurgical specialist, option B, as this patient could have long-lasting detrimental functional and neurologic deficits if not treated immediately.

   Bed rest, injection of corticosteroids, nonsteroidal anti-inflammatory drugs, or physical therapy, options A, C, D, and E, are inappropriate because choosing these treatment options will delay treatment of the underlying problem (cauda equina), which could harm the patient and lead to lasting deficits. **Task:** D2—Clinical Intervention

10. **Answer: B** HLA-B27 antigen, option B, is found in the majority of patients with ankylosing spondylitis (AS).

    Anti-cyclic citrullinated peptide antibody test and rheumatoid factor assay, options A and E, are negative serologic factors in patients with ankylosing spondylitis. While C-reactive protein level and erythrocyte sedimentation rate, options C and D, can be elevated in patients with AS, they are not specific enough for the diagnosis. **Task:** B—Using Diagnostic and Laboratory Studies

11. **Answer: D** The plain-film x-ray study of the patient's lower lumbar spine shows significant slippage of the L4 vertebra consistent with degenerative spondylolisthesis. Thus, option D is correct.

    Compression fracture of the L4 vertebral body, option A, is incorrect because the body appears completely intact with no evidence of collapse of height indicative of a compression fracture. Herniated disk at L3–L4, option B, is incorrect because this condition would not likely be diagnosed via plain-film x-ray study and would require imaging by MRI for confirmation. Loss of disk height between L3–L4, option C, is incorrect because the disk spacing is consistent with the spacing observed between L2–L3 (barely in image) and L5–S1. However, loss of disk height between L4–L5 is clearly evident. Normal findings, option E, is incorrect because the lumbar x-ray is not normal and shows significant evidence of degenerative spondylolisthesis.
    Task: B—Using Diagnostic and Laboratory Studies

12. **Answer: A** In patients with headache, stiffness and pain in the spine or neck, and fever, meningitis (option A) should be quickly ruled out with a lumbar puncture, and empiric therapies should be initiated as quickly as possible.

    Migraine, osteoarthritis, and tension headache, options B, C, and E, do not include sudden onset of fever. Spina bifida occulta, option D, is typically diagnosed serendipitously and not associated with meningeal signs. **Task:** C—Formulating Most Likely Diagnosis

13. **Answer: B** The correct answer is B, polymyalgia rheumatica. This diagnosis usually follows a pattern of pain affecting the bilateral shoulders, hips, and pelvic girdle. The pain progresses over time until muscle weakness generally develops. Unlike some of the other systemic rheumatologic disorders such as rheumatoid arthritis (option D), constitutional symptoms such as fever are usually rare.

    Gouty arthropathy, option A, is commonly monoarticular. Polymyositis, option C, is a disease that affects the muscular tissue and presents with myalgia rather than joint pain. **Task:** A—History Taking and Performing Physical Examination

14. **Answer: E** Due to the inflammatory process in polymyalgia rheumatica, the most common marker for disease progression or regression is an erythrocyte sedimentation rate, option E, or a C-reactive protein level.

    Analysis of synovial fluid, antinuclear antibody test, or Epstein-Barr nuclear antigen test (options A, B, and C) will rule out other infectious or gouty processes but will not help to monitor the disease over time. Complete blood cell count, option D, is not useful, as this is not an infectious process. **Task:** B—Using Diagnostic and Laboratory Studies

15. **Answer: C** Due to the inflammatory process associated with polymyalgia rheumatica, the mainstay treatment usually begins with corticosteroids, option C. These medications block inflammatory markers that contribute to both pain and stiffness in the joints. Other treatments after corticosteroid use consist of calcium and vitamin D supplementation and methotrexate.

    Bisphosphonates, option A, are not appropriate since the patient does not have any changes in bone density. Conservative management, option B, will allow polymyalgia rheumatica to progress and can lead to long-term consequences. Disease-modifying antirheumatic drugs, option D, is an appropriate option but in patients who have failed initial management or who have refractory disease. Opioid therapy, option E, may help with pain but will not address the underlying condition. **Task:** D3—Pharmaceutical Therapeutics

16. **Answer: E** Polymyositis can also lead to progressive muscle weakness, option E, as with polymyalgia rheumatica. Generally, the weakness of polymyositis

begins proximally and spreads distally over time. This bilateral muscle weakness worsens and can eventually lead to difficulty with swallowing and breathing.

Injury to the muscle, option B, is not an inciting factor for polymyositis. Alcohol use, joint pain, and migraine headaches (options A, C, and D) are not directly correlated with this disease. **Task:** A—History Taking and Performing Physical Examination

17. **Answer: E** Muscle biopsy, option E, is required for a definitive diagnosis of polymyositis. A biopsy of the muscle tissue typically shows mononuclear infiltrates of the endomysium and changes in the muscle fibers themselves.

    Complete blood cell count and MRI, options A and D, are not specific enough to diagnose polymyositis. Electromyography and erythrocyte sedimentation rate, options B and C, can assist with determining the degree of muscle weakness and the progression of disease, but they also are not specific enough to confirm the polymyositis. **Task:** B—Using Diagnostic and Laboratory Studies

18. **Answer: B** The most likely diagnosis based on this patient's age and presenting symptoms is degenerative joint disease or osteoarthritis (OA), option B. Most patients with OA have pain that worsens throughout the day and stiffness in the affected joints.

    Ankylosing spondylitis, option A, is diagnosed more commonly in young White men, and patients usually have spinal pain from the cervical region through the lumbar region. Reactive arthritis, option C, typically includes more systemic symptoms and is secondary to recent infection. Rheumatoid arthritis, option D, typically affects smaller joints and is associated with more systemic symptoms. Psoriatic arthritis, option E, is more commonly monoarticular and less commonly affects the spine. **Task:** C—Formulating Most Likely Diagnosis

19. **Answer: A** Anti-cyclic citrullinated peptide (anti-CCP) antibody test, option A, is the most sensitive and specific test to confirm a diagnosis of rheumatoid arthritis (RA).

    Option B, antinuclear antibody test, is a screening tool for autoimmune disease and is particularly useful for the diagnosis of systemic lupus erythematosus. It can be elevated in some patients with RA but not all. Plain-film x-ray studies of the hands, option C, may provide diagnostic features, but these features may overlap with other rheumatic disorders. While rheumatoid factor assay, option D, can be used as a diagnostic tool to diagnose RA, it is not as sensitive or specific as the anti-CCP antibody test. Uric acid level, option E, provides a diagnostic reference for gouty arthropathy and not RA. **Task:** B—Using Diagnostic and Laboratory Studies

20. **Answer: B** Obesity, option B, is most likely to increase this patient's risk of osteoarthritis (OA) because increased weight puts a mechanical burden on the joints.

    Anorexia, option A, is characterized by a loss of appetite for food, which usually results in weight loss. Weight loss is not a risk factor for OA. Regular weight-bearing exercise and use of vitamin supplements, options C and E, are protective factors of OA and not risk factors. Use of nonsteroidal anti-inflammatory drugs, option D, does not increase the risk of OA but can be used as part of the treatment regimen. **Task:** D1—Health Maintenance, Patient Education, and Disease Prevention

21. **Answer: C** Nonsteroidal anti-inflammatory drugs (NSAIDs), option C, are the most appropriate treatment of this patient's condition, which is osteoarthritis (OA). Although acetaminophen, option A, is used more commonly in patients with OA, NSAIDs actually provide the most amount of relief even in the setting of this noninflammatory condition. Disease modifying antirheumatic drugs, option B, are not necessary since this patient does not have an inflammatory condition. Opiates, option D, are never an appropriate option for patients with OA due to their addictive properties. Option E, glucocorticoids are not routinely used in patients with OA due to the progression of the condition and risk for long-term use. **Task:** D3—Pharmaceutical Therapeutics

22. **Answer: D** This patient has osteoarthritis and is taking long-term nonsteroidal anti-inflammatory drugs (NSAIDs) for treatment. Therefore, it is most appropriate to monitor serum urea nitrogen/creatinine ratio, option D. In patients chronically taking NSAIDs, there can be long-lasting damage to the renal system. Complete blood cell count, erythrocyte sedimentation rate, serum glucose level, and serum uric acid level (options A, B, C, and E) are not necessary to monitor as they do not provide information on the renal function of a patient. **Task:** D1—Health Maintenance, Patient Education, and Disease Prevention

23. **Answer: D** It is most appropriate for the practitioner to only bill for the level of services provided. Therefore, the practitioner needs to revise the coding and bill at a lower level, option D.

    Falsifying medical documentation is fraudulent, therefore, option A is incorrect. Having the patient return to the office for more thorough history and physical examination, options B and C, are not appropriate methods of handling this billing issue. Doing nothing, option E, is incorrect because it would be fraudulent to perform billing at a level in which sufficient documentation has not been provided to meet the standard for that level of billing. **Task:** F—Entry-Level Professional Practice—Medical Informatics

Answer Key for this chapter begins on p. 293

BIBLIOGRAPHY

Mantegazza R, Bernasconi P. Inflammatory Myopathies: Dermatomyositis, Polymyositis and Inclusion Body Myositis. In: Madame Curie Bioscience Database [Internet]. Austin (TX): Landes Bioscience; 2000-2013.

Hellmann, D. B., & Imboden, J. B. (2020). Rheumatologic, immunologic and allergic disorders. Current medical diagnosis and treatment. 59th ed. United States of America: Mc Graw Hill Education.

Luke, A., & Ma, C. B. (2020). Sports Medicine and Outpatient Orthopedics (2020). Current medical diagnosis and treatment. 59th ed. United States of America: Mc Graw Hill Education.

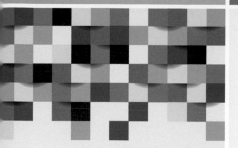

CASE STUDY 12
Neurologic System

Questions

Case Section I: Chief Complaint and History of Present Illness

A 15-year-old boy is transported via ambulance from home to the emergency department after he suddenly fell to the floor and had jerking movements of all four limbs for about a minute. The patient's parents say that as he was standing at the kitchen sink, he cried out something unintelligible, and then collapsed and started jerking. After he stopped jerking, the patient lied on the floor and did not respond to his parents who were trying to arouse him. By the time the ambulance arrived 20 minutes later, the parents were able to arouse the patient, but he remained disoriented and extremely groggy. Medical history includes glaucoma that was diagnosed at 6 years of age; he has been otherwise healthy and has no history of a motor disorder. Currently, the patient is lying comfortably in the bed and is asleep. Physical examination shows a sizable birthmark on the right side of the face.

1. Which of the following best describes the type of seizure that he experienced?
   A. Absence
   B. Atonic
   C. Focal seizure with retained awareness
   D. Gelastic
   E. Tonic-clonic

2. Which of the following disorders is the most likely cause of the new onset seizure experienced by this patient?
   A. Batten disease
   B. Cerebral palsy
   C. Dravet syndrome
   D. Sturge-Weber syndrome
   E. Tay-Sachs disease

3. Which of the following seizure types or conditions typically occurs without a postictal state and thus can be excluded from the differential diagnosis?
   A. Focal seizures with retained awareness
   B. Generalized tonic-clonic seizure

   C. Lennox-Gastaut syndrome
   D. Progressive myoclonic epilepsy
   E. Tonic seizure

4. Which of the following seizure types or conditions is typically devoid of convulsive jerking or repetitive motor activity and thus can be excluded from the differential diagnosis?
   A. Absence
   B. Clonic
   C. Febrile
   D. Focal seizure with impaired awareness
   E. Lennox-Gastaut syndrome

5. Which of the following is a common trigger for seizure activity in epilepsy, particularly among adolescents such as this patient?
   A. Excessive exercise
   B. Foods with a high tryptophan content
   C. Lack of sleep
   D. Tanning bed use
   E. Use of prescription tretinoin

Case Section II: Objective Findings, Assessment, and Plan

After a brief period in the emergency department, the patient awakens and becomes communicative. Vital signs are within normal limits. Physical examination shows no abnormalities of the heart or lungs, and neurologic examination shows no focal deficits. Near the end of the examination, the patient suddenly becomes rigid and does not respond to commands. The left arm then begins to jerk followed a few seconds later by the same abnormal movements appearing in the right arm and bilateral lower extremities. The jerking movements continue for approximately six minutes.

6. Which of the following intravenous medications is the most appropriate immediate first-line therapy?
   A. Midazolam
   B. Naloxone
   C. Oxycodone
   D. Succinylcholine
   E. Thorazine

7. Which of the following initial laboratory studies is most appropriate to obtain to investigate a possible metabolic cause of the seizures in this patient?
   A. Plasma cyclic citrullinated antibody level
   B. Serum ferritin level
   C. Serum fructosamine level
   D. Serum glucose level
   E. Urine vanillylmandelic acid level

The ectopic motor activity experienced by the patient in the emergency department is quickly suppressed by pharmaceutical means. After eight hours of observation, the patient regains normal mentation and does not experience further seizure activity. A follow-up appointment with his primary care provider is scheduled, and the patient is discharged to home in the care of his parents.

8. Which of the following discharge instructions is most appropriate to tell this patient's parents if he experiences another seizure at home?
   A. Attempt to restrain the patient's limbs to prevent injury
   B. Call 911 if the seizure lasts more than five minutes
   C. Move the patient to a flat, hard surface (e.g., tile floor)
   D. Place a wooden spoon or similar object in the patient's mouth to prevent him from biting or severing his tongue
   E. Position furniture such as a couch or chairs adjacent to the patient to decrease the chance of injury

Case Section III: Comorbidity

Two weeks later, the patient is brought back to the emergency department by his parents after he had another seizure at home. His parents say that the jerking activity during this seizure lasted at least 10 minutes. Vital signs are within normal limits. Physical examination, including neurologic examination, shows no abnormalities. The patient is admitted to the hospital for further workup and observation.

9. Which of the following imaging modalities or procedures related to the central nervous system is the most appropriate initial study?
   A. CT angiography of the head
   B. Electroencephalography
   C. MRI of the brain
   D. Noncontrast CT scan of the head
   E. Overnight polysomnography

10. Because this patient's most recent seizure was excessive in length, a prescription for which of the following rescue medications is most appropriate to provide on discharge?
    A. Albuterol hydrofluoroalkane inhaler
    B. Epinephrin autoinjector
    C. Intranasal naloxone
    D. Oral leucovorin
    E. Rectal diazepam gel

Case Section IV: Professional Practice

An imaging study of the head shows no anatomic defect. After a brief and uneventful hospital stay, the patient is discharged to home with a diagnosis of epilepsy. Prescriptions for seizure-suppressive medications are provided.

11. Which of the following patient care instructions is most important to communicate to the patient and his parents at the time of discharge?
    A. Any missed doses of antiseizure medication should be doubled up the following day
    B. Avoid getting a learner's permit to drive
    C. Avoid participating in contact sports in high school
    D. Do not seek afterschool employment in a restaurant setting
    E. He can swim unattended while on antiseizure medication

12. Which of the following anticipatory recommendations regarding this patient's life with epilepsy is most appropriate to communicate to the patient and his parents?
    A. As an adult with epilepsy, the patient will experience unemployment and underemployment similar to the general population
    B. The parents need to work with the patient to consider the psychosocial aspects of living with epilepsy
    C. The patient must abstain completely from alcohol during his collegiate years
    D. The patient must maintain regular hours of sleep, particularly as he enters his high school years, or breakthrough seizures can occur
    E. The patient will never be able to live alone

The patient is eventually prescribed an antiseizure medication, but the drug is expensive and is not produced in a generic form. The patient's parents are advised by the local pharmacist that they should apply to the pharmaceutical company to obtain the drug through a prescription assistance program (PAP).

13. The patient and his family must meet which of the following requirements in order to be accepted into a PAP program?

A. Completed at least a 90-day trial of the tradename drug

B. Failed at least one generic drug available to treat the condition

C. Have documentation that they have been denied drug coverage through the state's Medicaid program

D. Have an income below a defined level

E. Prove that they are citizens of the United States

Answer Key for this chapter begins on p. 300

Answers

1. **Answer: E** This patient has had a tonic-clonic seizure. These seizures are characterized by a tonic phase where muscles stiffen, causing the patient to fall to the floor. A clonic phase ensues, resulting in the limbs jerking rapidly and rhythmically for a few minutes. Once the convulsion concludes, a postictal state resulting in a slow return of consciousness and awareness begins. Urinary incontinence is also a possible feature of tonic-clonic seizures. While incontinence is not mentioned in the vignette, the other features of the seizure exhibited by the patient make tonic-clonic seizures, option E, correct.

   Absence-type seizures (option A), also known as petit mal, are characterized by lapses in awareness lasting a few seconds. Jerking movements and postictal confusion are not characteristics of absence seizures. An atonic seizure (option B), also known as a drop seizure, is characterized by the body becoming limp. If the patient is standing, they immediately drop to the floor, hence the name. Jerking movements are not typical of atonic seizures. Focal seizures with retained awareness, option C, are the most common type of seizure and are characterized by brief focal neurologic symptoms (i.e., jerking of a limb, flashing lights, speech difficulties) during which the patient retains awareness and awakeness. Gelastic seizures, option D, are characterized by bouts of uncontrolled laughter or giggling and often begin as early as 10 months of age. The symptom usually occurs when falling asleep and lasts for 10 to 20 seconds. None of these characteristics describe this patient, thus making this option incorrect. **Task**: A—History Taking and Performing Physical Examination

2. **Answer: D** Sturge-Weber syndrome (SWS), option D, results from a noninherited mutation of the *GNAQ* gene. Over 80% of infants born with SWS have a characteristic port-wine stain in the scalp or facial area, as in this patient. Upwards of 99% of individuals with SWS develop seizures in adolescence.

   Batten disease, option A, is a rare, inherited disease included in the class of lysosomal storage diseases. Tragically, symptoms of most forms of Batten disease begin in early childhood and are typically fatal in the teenage years. The motor-related symptoms of cerebral palsy, option B, typically manifest by 18 to 24 months of age. There is no indication that this patient has impaired motor function. Dravet syndrome, option C, is also known as severe myoclonic epilepsy of infancy. This option is incorrect due to the early age of onset of seizure activity. Option E, Tay-Sachs disease, was historically concentrated in people of Ashkenazi Jewish descent. More recently, the disease has been observed in individuals with other ethnic backgrounds. Nonetheless, the neurologic symptoms of Tay-Sachs disease typically begin around the age of 3 to 6 months with death occurring between 3 and 5 years of age. **Task**: A—History Taking and Performing Physical Examination

3. **Answer: A** Focal seizure with retained awareness, option A, is characterized by brief focal neurologic symptoms (i.e., jerking of a limb, flashing lights, speech difficulties) during which the patient retains awareness and awakeness. There is no classic postictal phase in this type of seizure; therefore, option A is correct.

   A postictal phase is characterized by a gradual return to consciousness and is a consistent feature of generalized tonic-clonic seizures, option B. Lennox-Gastaut syndrome, progressive myoclonic epilepsy, and tonic seizures, options C, D, and E, all have a postictal phase as a possible or a consistent feature. **Task**: C—Formulating Most Likely Diagnosis

4. **Answer: A** Absence seizures, option A, are characterized as a lapse in awareness as if in a daydreaming state. Convulsions or jerking of extremities are not associated with absence-type seizures; therefore, option A is correct.

   The seizure types listed in options B through E all have convulsions (febrile, Lennox-Gastaut), jerking (clonic), or motor automatisms (focal seizure with impaired awareness) as characteristic ectopic motor activities. **Task**: C—Formulating Most Likely Diagnosis

5. **Answer: C** Lack of sleep, option C, is a common trigger for seizure activity, particularly in the adolescent population. Other common triggers include flashing/bright lights, stress, and overstimulation (like playing video games excessively, which also is related to a lack of sleep).

   Excessive exercise and tanning bed use, options A and D, are not identified as triggers for seizure activity. Foods with a high tryptophan content, option B, include chicken, turkey, red meat, pork, tofu, fish, beans, milk, nuts, seeds, oatmeal, and eggs. None of these have been identified as a trigger for seizures. While tretinoin, option E, has a plethora of adverse effects, seizure activity is not one of them. **Task**: A—History Taking and Performing Physical Examination

6. **Answer: A** The seizure activity described in the vignette is characteristic of a tonic-clonic seizure. This seizure type presents as an initial tonic phase

(the patient becoming rigid) followed by a clonic phase (the jerking movements). By definition, a seizure lasting five minutes or more constitutes status epilepticus and should be aggressively suppressed with intravenous administration of medication. Drugs of the benzodiazepine class, such as midazolam, lorazepam, and diazepam, are first-line agents for treating status epilepticus. Therefore, midazolam, option A, is correct. Naloxone, option B, is an opioid antagonist that reverses typical opioid effects by binding to opioid receptors in the central nervous system. It has no effect on seizure activity. Because of its powerful opioid effect, oxycodone (option C), will likely suppress motor activity. However, opioids are not first-line agents when treating status epilepticus and should generally be avoided altogether due to their long duration and suppressive effects on respiration. Paralyzing agents such as succinylcholine, option D, should only be used briefly during status epilepticus for the purpose of intubation. They are not indicated as first-line agents for treating the seizure itself. Thorazine, option E, is among the first-generation phenothiazines used as antipsychotics and anxiolytics. Phenothiazines are avoided when treating seizures. **Task**: D3—Pharmaceutical Therapeutics

7. **Answer: D** There are numerous causes for a first-time seizure. In addition to the multitude of intracranial conditions that can result in an increase in ectopic neural activity, external factors include high fever, increased or decreased blood glucose level, and alcohol or drug withdrawal. Thus, obtaining a serum glucose level, option D, is the most appropriate initial laboratory study.

Cyclic citrullinated antibodies (anti-CCP), option A, are observed in rheumatoid arthritis (RA). The presence of anti-CCP antibodies along with a positive rheumatoid factor provides strong support for a diagnosis of RA. There is no reported correlation between anti-CCP antibodies and seizure disorders in the adolescent population. Ferritin, option B, is a protein that functions as the storage form of iron. Ferritin levels are decreased in iron deficiency anemia but are unaffected by seizure disorders. Fructosamine, option C, is a glycated serum protein that provides a quantitative assessment of average serum glucose levels over the preceding two to three weeks. There are several clinical reasons for obtaining a fructosamine level over a hemoglobin A_{1c} level, including hemoglobinopathies (e.g., sickle cell disease), hemolytic anemia, and when a more rapid measure of glucose control is needed. However, the fructosamine level is not affected by seizures. A urine vanillylmandelic acid (VMA) level, option E, is obtained in the workup for pheochromocytoma. An elevated VMA level signifies excess degradation of catecholamines but is not related to seizure activity. **Task**: B—Using Diagnostic and Laboratory Studies

8. **Answer: B** The list of instructions for caregivers of a patient who has had a first-time seizure is lengthy. The most important instruction is to tell the parents that they must call 911 if the patient has another seizure lasting longer than five minutes, option B. Such a lengthy seizure is considered status epilepticus and a medical emergency.

Options A, C, D, and E describe actions that a caregiver should not do in the event of another seizure. No attempt should be made to restrain the limbs of a seizing patient, and the patient should be placed on a flat, carpeted (soft, not hard) surface. Nothing should be placed in the patient's mouth because of the high risk of damage to oral structures. Also, the area where the patient is seizing should be cleared of furniture and other objects to decrease the risk of injury. **Task**: D1—Health Maintenance, Patient Education, and Disease Prevention

9. **Answer: C** MRI of the brain, option C, is the most appropriate initial study in the workup of seizure. An MRI provides exceptional detail of the central nervous system parenchyma and is optimal at resolving an anatomic reason for seizure.

CT angiography, option A, is indicated in the investigation of a potential intracranial vascular-related issue. While angiography may identify a vascular etiology for seizure (e.g., aneurysm, arteriovenous malformation), it is not the most appropriate initial study. Electroencephalography, option B, may be essential in the workup of seizure but not as an initial study. A noncontrast CT scan of the head, option D, is the study of choice in the workup of stroke to rule out an intra- or extracerebral hemorrhage. Unfortunately, a CT scan does not provide the detail needed to resolve neuroanatomical reasons for a seizure workup. Overnight polysomnography (option E), also known as a sleep study, is not indicated in the initial workup of seizure. While polysomnography is used in investigations of epilepsy, the procedure is not used in the initial workup. **Task**: B—Using Diagnostic and Laboratory Studies

10. **Answer: E** All of these medications are considered rescue agents for a particular condition. Rectal diazepam gel, option E, is the only agent indicated to interrupt seizure activity. In addition to treating acute seizures, the benzodiazepine class of drugs is also indicated in the emergent treatment of status epilepticus, which by definition is a seizure lasting more than five minutes or multiple seizures within a five-minute time frame.

                     Answer Key for this chapter begins on p. 300

Albuterol inhalers, option A, are indicated as rescue medications for asthma. An epinephrine autoinjector, option B, is indicated for emergent treatment of anaphylaxis. Intranasal naloxone, option C, is indicated for acute toxicity from opioid overdose. Leucovorin, option D, which is a folic acid analogue, is typically given to patients to counteract the effects of methotrexate therapy or overdose. It is not used in the treatment of seizures. **Task**: D3—Pharmaceutical Therapeutics

11. **Answer: B** While this patient is at the age of beginning to drive, any person with incompletely controlled epilepsy should not be allowed to do so. Since the patient is only now starting antiseizure medication, it is inaccurate to describe his disease as controlled. Therefore, option B is correct.

   Doubling a missed dose of an antiseizure medication, option A, is not prudent, as it increases the chance of an unwanted adverse effect. There is no reason to prohibit the patient from participating in contact sports, option C. While no general restriction regarding after school employment in a restaurant is described (option D), activities such as climbing ladders, operating unguarded machinery, and working from heights is expressly discouraged. It is never acceptable for a person with epilepsy, even if taking antiseizure medication, to swim unattended. Therefore, option E is incorrect. **Task**: F—Entry-Level Professional Practice—Patient care and communication

12. **Answer: B** It is well recognized that individuals with epilepsy are often stigmatized and bullied in American culture. To prevent feelings of inferiority, particularly among school-aged patients, the parents need to work diligently with the patient to consider the psychosocial aspects of living with epilepsy, option B.

Unemployment and underemployment, option A, occurs in approximately half of all individuals with epilepsy. While alcohol is often a trigger for seizure, moderating alcohol consumption and not completely abstaining (option C), particularly during the college years, is the current recommendation. While lack of sleep is a common trigger for seizure, option D, failure to take antiseizure medication as prescribed is by far the number one reason breakthrough seizures occur. There is no formal recommendation against living alone as a patient with epilepsy, option E. In fact, upwards of 20% of people with epilepsy do indeed live alone. **Task**: F—Entry-Level Professional Practice—Patient care and communication

13. **Answer: D** Eligibility requirements for acceptance into a prescription (or patient) assistance program (PAP) vary among pharmaceutical manufacturers. Ubiquitous among PAP programs is the need to demonstrate a financial reason for the discounted or free medication. This is usually accomplished by confirming that the family is at or below a given income level or below a certain percentage of the federal poverty level, option D.

   PAPs do not typically inquire as to whether the patient has taken the requested drug prior to submitting the PAP, option A. Also, they do not typically inquire as to what other medication the patient has taken or what prior medication has failed, option B. Option C is incorrect because there is no direct connection between a PAP and a state's Medicaid program. While some charitable entities require proof of US citizenship, option E, PAPs typically are available to everyone who qualifies through financial hardship. **Task**: F—Entry-Level Professional Practice—Patient care and communication

BIBLIOGRAPHY

Diagnostic testing in neurologic disease. Ropper A. H., & Samuels M. A., & Klein J. P., & Prasad S. (Eds.), (2019). *Adams and Victor's Principles of Neurology, 11e*. McGraw Hill.

Epilepsy and other seizure disorders. Ropper A. H., & Samuels M. A., & Klein J. P., & Prasad S. (Eds.), (2019). *Adams and Victor's Principles of Neurology, 11e*. McGraw Hill.

Fitzgerald, P. A. (2017). Adrenal medulla and paraganglia. In D. G. Gardner & D. Shoback (Eds.), *Greenspan's basic & clinical endocrinology* (10th ed.). McGraw Hill.

Kobau, R., Cui, W., Kadima, N., Zack, M. M., Sajatovic, M., Kaiboriboon, K. et al. Tracking psychosocial health in adults with epilepsy—estimates from the 2010 National Health Interview Survey. *Epilepsy & Behavior, 41*, 66-73.

Kobau, R. (2015). Nearly one in five adults with active epilepsy lives alone based on findings from the 2010 and 2013 US National Health Interview Surveys. US Centers for Disease Control and Prevention, Epilepsy Program. *Epilepsy & Behavior, 51*, 259-260.

Messer, R., Schreiner, T. L., Walleigh, D., Yang, M. L., Martin, J. A., & Demarest, S. (2020). Neurologic & muscular disorders. In W. E. Hay Jr., M. J. Levin, M. J. Abzug, & M. Bunik (Eds.), *Current diagnosis & treatment: pediatrics* (25th ed.). McGraw Hill.

Middleton, D. B. (2020). Seizures. In J. E. South-Paul, S. C. Matheny, & E. L. Lewis (Eds.), *Current diagnosis & treatment: family medicine* (5th ed.). McGraw Hill.

Shah, S., Hagopian, T., Klinglesmith, R., & Bonfante, E. (2014). Diagnostic neuroradiology. In K. M. Elsayes & S. A. Oldham (Eds.), *Introduction to diagnostic radiology*. McGraw Hill.

Shih, T. (2019). Epilepsy & seizures. In J. M. Brust (Ed.), *Current diagnosis & treatment: neurology* (3rd ed.). McGraw Hill.

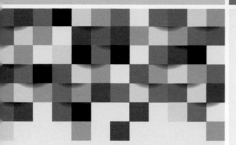

CASE STUDY 13
Psychiatry/Behavioral Science

Questions

Case Section I: Chief Complaint and History of Present Illness

A 33-year-old man is brought to the office by his new girlfriend because he has had "bizarre" behavior over the past eight days that has caused significant functional impairment. She says he is only sleeping a few hours per night, but he does not feel tired when he wakes up. His speech is rapid and pressured, and he is easily distracted. The girlfriend says that he has made several expensive credit card purchases during the past few days, and he exaggerates his accomplishments when speaking to others. Medical history does not include any recent injuries, and she does not know if he is taking any medications. The patient says that he has been sober from alcohol and other substances for the past six months.

The patient's girlfriend says that she called his ex-wife who noted that he has had similar episodes with accompanying hallucinations about once per year since high school. He also has had periods of depressed dark moods, fatigue, weight loss, diminished libido, and a preoccupation about death that lasted for months. The patient's mother has a history of similar episodes.

1. Which of the following is the most likely diagnosis?
   A. Bipolar I disorder
   B. Borderline personality disorder
   C. Cyclothymia
   D. Schizoaffective disorder
   E. Schizophrenia

2. If this patient has bipolar I disorder, which of the following is of most concern once the patient leaves the office?
   A. Becoming a victim of domestic violence
   B. Distancing himself from family and friends
   C. Homicidal ideation of nonfamily members
   D. Kleptomania
   E. Suicidality

3. Which of the following screening tests is most likely to help determine the diagnosis?
   A. Alcohol Use Disorders Identification Test
   B. Generalized Anxiety Disorder-7
   C. Mood Disorder Questionnaire
   D. Opioid Use Disorder Screening Tool
   E. Patient Health Questionnaire-9

4. If schizophrenia and bipolar I disorder are on the differential diagnosis list, which of the following findings in this patient is more consistent with the diagnosis of schizophrenia?
   A. Age at onset of symptoms
   B. Genetic predisposition
   C. History of substance abuse
   D. Male gender
   E. White race

5. Which of the following criteria is required to make a diagnosis of bipolar I disorder?
   A. At least one hypomanic and one major depressive episode occurring one after the other
   B. At least one hypomanic and one psychotic episode in a lifetime
   C. At least one manic and one major depressive episode occurring one after the other
   D. At least one manic and one substance-induced hypomanic episode
   E. At least one manic episode in a lifetime lasting at least one week

6. If this patient has bipolar II disorder, which of the following diagnostic features is most specific to this disorder?
   A. Depressive episodes
   B. Hallucinations
   C. Hypomania
   D. Inflated self-esteem
   E. Psychotic features

7. Which of the following symptoms, if displayed by this patient, would favor schizophrenia over bipolar I disorder as the most likely diagnosis?
   A. Catatonic behavior
   B. Grandiosity
   C. Hallucinations
   D. Paranoia
   E. Pressured speech

Case Section II: Objective Findings, Assessment, and Plan

Temperature is 36.6°C (97.9°F), pulse rate is 99/min, respirations are 16/min, and blood pressure is 130/82 mmHg. The patient has a torn shirt that is buttoned inappropriately. His hair is unkempt, and he is unshaven. He is pacing in the examination room and opening drawers. When asked to sit in the chair by his girlfriend, he is unable to be still and begins to pace again. The patient's mood is euphoric, but he also exhibits irritability when asked certain questions. His speech is rapid and pressured, and he switches topics repeatedly. He is alert to person, place, and time. Laboratory studies show no abnormalities in serum electrolyte levels, thyroid function, glucose level, liver enzymes, or renal function. Results of serum alcohol measurement and urine drug screen are negative.

8. Which of the following imaging studies is the most appropriate next step to support a psychiatric cause for the patient's presenting symptoms?
   A. Carotid Doppler ultrasonography
   B. CT angiography of the head
   C. MRI of the brain
   D. PET scan of the brain
   E. SPECT scan of the brain

9. Which of the following medications is the most appropriate initial management for this patient's acute symptoms?
   A. Duloxetine
   B. Fluoxetine
   C. Lamotrigine
   D. Lorazepam
   E. Quetiapine

10. When considering pharmaceutical management for this patient, which of the following medications is considered an atypical or second-generation antipsychotic but has extrapyramidal symptoms as a frequent adverse effect?
    A. Alprazolam
    B. Fluoxetine
    C. Lithium
    D. Phenelzine
    E. Risperidone

11. If lithium is prescribed to this patient, which of the following clinical scenarios is most likely to increase his risk of lithium toxicity?
    A. Cirrhosis of the liver
    B. Excessive water intake
    C. High-protein diet
    D. High-sodium diet
    E. Vomiting and diarrhea

12. Therapy with olanzapine is prescribed for this patient. Which of the following conditions is most likely to be associated with the chronic administration of this drug?
    A. Acute tubular necrosis
    B. Amaurosis fugax
    C. Metabolic syndrome
    D. Serotonin syndrome
    E. Torsades de pointes

The patient's ex-wife tells his girlfriend that he was prescribed a medication for a similar episode several years ago that caused polyuria and intense thirst. A review of medical records indicates that urine osmolality was decreased at that time, and after a water-deprivation challenge, the urine osmolality failed to increase.

13. Which of the following is the most likely medication that caused the drug-induced thirst and renal symptoms?
    A. Aripiprazole
    B. Lamotrigine
    C. Lithium
    D. Olanzapine
    E. Risperidone

14. Which of the following types of drugs is most likely to unmask the underlying mania in this patient?
    A. Antiepileptics
    B. Antipsychotics
    C. Benzodiazepines
    D. Dopamine antagonists
    E. Selective serotonin reuptake inhibitors

15. After a period of stabilization, lamotrigine is initiated in this patient for maintenance therapy. Which of the following is a serious adverse effect of this drug?
    A. Adrenal insufficiency
    B. Diabetes insipidus
    C. Hyperosmolar hyperglycemia
    D. Hypertensive crisis
    E. Stevens-Johnson syndrome

Case Section III: Comorbidity

A review of the patient's medical record shows that he was hospitalized two years ago for a similar episode involving significant psychosis, and it became clear that he had been using methamphetamines daily for two weeks. He had also been struggling with an addiction to opioid pain killers at that time.

16. Which of the following best describes the mechanism of action of amphetamine-induced psychosis, such as what occurred in this patient?
    A. Act as cholinesterase inhibitors
    B. Function as a dopamine receptor antagonist
    C. Function as a muscarinic receptor antagonist
    D. Increase monoamine levels in the neuronal synapse
    E. Inhibit the release of glutamate

The girlfriend says that the patient's primary care provider encouraged him to enroll in a medication-assisted treatment (MAT) program last year to help with his opioid addiction.

17. Which of the following medications is a partial μ-opioid receptor agonist most commonly used in MAT programs?
    A. Buprenorphine
    B. Chlordiazepoxide
    C. Disulfiram
    D. Naloxone
    E. Varenicline

18. When considering nonpharmacologic treatment options for this patient with a comorbid substance use disorder, which of the following is the most appropriate first-line therapy?
    A. Aversion therapy
    B. Electroconvulsive therapy
    C. Eye movement desensitization and reprocessing therapy
    D. Integrated group therapy
    E. Narrative exposure therapy

Case Section IV: Professional Practice

During the interview, the patient says that he was laid off from his job two months ago and currently has no income or health insurance. He could not afford refills of his mental health medications after he lost his insurance. He says that he called his former primary care provider to ask for less expensive medications but was informed an office visit was required. He could not afford the visit and subsequently ran out of medications several weeks ago.

19. When considering whether to hospitalize this patient, which of the following best describes the practice of an inpatient civil commitment of a person with mental illness?

    A. The federal government becomes the guardian for a citizen who is admitted involuntarily to a psychiatric facility
    B. Federal law mandates that a mentally ill individual must have committed a crime in order to meet criteria for involuntary commitment
    C. Mentally ill individuals with bipolar disorder who have been off their medications typically exhibit violent behaviors necessitating inpatient commitment to the hospital
    D. The physician in charge makes the ultimate decision on whether to uphold the commitment
    E. When civilly committing an individual to a psychiatric facility, they lose the right of autonomy regarding their own health care decisions

The practitioner decides to refer the patient to the local community mental health center to help him with counseling, integration of care, and medications.

20. Which of the following best describes the primary objective of the Community Mental Health Act of 1963 that helped to establish community mental health centers such as this?
    A. Decrease the incidence of suicide in patients with mental illness
    B. Decrease the number of individuals with mental illness involved in the corrections system
    C. Deinstitutionalize state mental hospitals
    D. Improve rights for individuals in long-term institutional care
    E. Provide funding for inpatient mental health treatment in rural communities

The patient's girlfriend says she has heard about Assertive Community Treatment (ACT) programs and wants to know more information.

21. Which of the following best describes how an ACT program works to assist those with mental illness?
    A. It is an intensive inpatient psychiatric program focused on pharmacologic stabilization
    B. It is an outpatient program for patients with symptoms of mild mental illness that is designed to prevent progression of the disorder
    C. It provides electronic ankle monitoring for criminal offenders with mental illness under house arrest to avoid incarceration
    D. It provides a team-based approach designed to stabilize community living for those with severe mental illness
    E. It is a residential program for pregnant women suffering from mental illness

Answers

1. **Answer: A** Bipolar I disorder, option A, is associated with at least one lifetime episode of mania, present for at least one week (or less than one week if hospitalization is required), and it must cause significant functional impairment. Individuals may experience major depressive and hypomanic episodes, but they are not required for the diagnosis. Psychosis may occur, but only when mania or major depression is present. All of these symptoms are displayed by the patient, which makes bipolar I disorder the answer.
Borderline personality disorder, option B, is associated with intense mood swings that may manifests as viewing things in extremes, intense and unstable relationships, distorted sense of self, and loss of anger control. Self-harming behavior, such as cutting, is also characteristic of borderline personality disorder. This disorder is characterized by shorter periods of aberrant behavior. Cyclothymia, option C, involves numerous periods of depression and elevated mood for at least two years, with periods of stable moods lasting only two months at most. Patients suspected of this disorder must not meet criteria for major depression or mania during this time. Schizoaffective disorder, option D, involves manic and major depressive episodes, but psychosis occurs for at least two weeks, in the absence of any mood symptoms. Schizophrenia, option E, involves chronic or recurrent psychosis with impairment in social and occupational functioning. Symptoms include delusions, hallucinations, disorganized speech, grossly disorganized or catatonic behavior, and flat affect or apathy. Cognitive and motor impairment are present, and mood and anxiety symptoms are common. **Task:** A—History Taking and Performing Physical Examination

2. **Answer: E** Assessing for suicidal ideation is crucial, as 10% to 15% of patients with bipolar I disorder die by suicide, option E. A lifetime risk of suicide in individuals with bipolar disorder is at least 15 times that of the general population.
Being the perpetrator rather than the victim of domestic violence, option A, is associated with untreated bipolar disorder. While individuals with bipolar disorder often experience abrupt involvement or cessation with relationships, distancing himself from family and friends, option B, is not characteristic of the disorder. The potential for homicide, option C, in bipolar disease has been studied and was found to be increased during the depressive phase and most frequently involved family members. Kleptomania, option D, is defined as an irresistible urge to steal and is not associated with bipolar disorder. **Task:** D1—Health Maintenance, Patient Education, and Disease Prevention

3. **Answer: C** Those who screen positive on the Mood Disorder Questionnaire, option C, should be interviewed further to establish a diagnosis of bipolar disorder.
The Alcohol Use Disorders Identification Test, option A, is used to screen for unhealthy alcohol use. The Generalized Anxiety Disorder-7 test, option B, is used to screen for generalized anxiety disorder. Opioid Use Disorder Screening Tool, option D, is a screening tool that is also called OWLS (Overuse, Worried, Lose interest, Sedated) and checks for opioid use disorder. The Patient Health Questionnare-9, option E, is used to assess depression symptoms. **Task:** B—Using Diagnostic and Laboratory Studies

4. **Answer: D** Schizophrenia is observed more frequently in males, while there is an equal gender frequency in bipolar I disorder. Thus, option D is correct.
Options A, B, C, and E are all incorrect in that they are observed in equal frequency in both disorders. Note that the age of onset of schizophrenia in females is typically in the late 20s and early 30s. Had this patient been female, this would also have been a correct option. **Task:** A—History Taking and Performing Physical Examination

5. **Answer: E** Criteria for at least one lifetime manic episode lasting at least one week, option E, must be met in order to diagnose bipolar I disorder.
Although hypomania and major depression are common in bipolar I disorder, they are not required for the diagnosis, making options A and C incorrect. Although hypomania and psychosis occur in bipolar I disorder, they are not required for the diagnosis, making option B incorrect. Option D is incorrect, as the manic episode must not be attributable to the direct physiological effects of a substance, medication, or other medical condition. **Task:** A—History Taking and Performing Physical Examination

6. **Answer: C** The primary distinction between the two types of bipolar disorder is that bipolar I is characterized by manic episodes while bipolar II is characterized by the less disruptive hypomanic episodes. Thus, option C is correct.
Depressive episodes and inflated self-esteem, options A and D, are observed in both types of bipolar disease and not just bipolar II disorder. By definition, hallucinations (option B) are a dominant component of psychosis. Psychotic features, option E, are only observed in patients with bipolar I disorder. **Task:** A—History Taking and Performing Physical Examination

7. **Answer: A** Catatonic behavior, option A, is a distinguishing feature of schizophrenia; catatonia does not occur in patients with bipolar disorder.

   Grandiosity, hallucinations, and paranoia (options B, C, and D) are all present in patients with bipolar disorder and will not specifically direct a practitioner to a diagnosis of schizophrenia. Pressured speech, option E, is common during mania of bipolar I disorder while disorganized or incoherent speech is frequently observed in schizophrenia. **Task: A**—History Taking and Performing Physical Examination

8. **Answer: C** Supporting a psychiatric cause for the patient's symptoms means that an organic or neuroanatomic cause must be ruled out. The normal results from the laboratory studies help to rule out an organic cause. The next step would be to examine the brain. MRI of the brain, option C, provides a very detailed view of white and gray matter structures within the central nervous system and is the correct answer.

   A carotid Doppler ultrasound, option A, will only provide information on the patency of the carotid circulation. CT angiography of the head, option B, is an appropriate choice. However, this test focuses on vascular structures and will generally not provide sufficient detail on cortical and subcortical structures. PET and SPECT scans of the brain, options D and E, are used primarily to note the presence of cancerous cells and cardiac stress, respectively. They are not appropriate imaging studies to examine the neuroanatomical integrity of the brain. **Task: B**—Using Diagnostic and Laboratory Studies

9. **Answer: E** Use of an atypical antipsychotic agent, such as quetiapine (option E) is an effective first-line agent in the treatment of bipolar disorder. Lithium, while effective and widely used, has a narrow therapeutic window and requires expensive laboratory monitoring. Thus, it may not be an appropriate choice for many patients.

   Selective serotonin and norepinephrine reuptake inhibitor antidepressants should be avoided as first-line agents as they may trigger mania. Thus, options A and B are incorrect. A mood stabilizer like lamotrigine, option C, is an effective medication for maintenance treatment but is not indicated in the initiation of treatment. Benzodiazepines, option D, and other drugs with addictive potential should be avoided. **Task: D3**—Pharmaceutical Therapeutics

10. **Answer: E** Risperidone, option E, is an atypical antipsychotic medication with extrapyramidal symptoms as an adverse effect. As a general rule, all atypical antipsychotics may induce extrapyramidal symptoms. Benzodiazepines, selective serotonin reuptake inhibitors, lithium, and monoamine oxidase inhibitors (options A through D) typically do not have extrapyramidal symptoms as a possible adverse effect. **Task: D3**—Pharmaceutical Therapeutics

11. **Answer: E** Although lithium is prescribed less often for bipolar disorder now than in past decades, its use is still frequently encountered. Unfortunately, lithium has a rather narrow therapeutic window with a blood level between 0.6 and 1.2 mEq/L considered safe. Dehydration due to vomiting and/or diarrhea, option E, results in a hemoconcentration of the drug. Severe toxicity, which may be life-threatening, happens at blood levels at and above 2.0 mEq/L. Blood levels of 3.0 mEq/L and higher are considered a medical emergency.

    Cirrhosis of the liver, excessive water intake, high-protein diet, or high-sodium diet (options A through D) have no demonstrable effect on lithium levels and are thus incorrect choices. **Task: D3**—Pharmaceutical Therapeutics

12. **Answer: C** Olanzapine is an excellent medication for treating bipolar disorder. However, of the many serious potential reactions associated with the drug, hyperglycemia, diabetes mellitus, and diabetic ketoacidosis occur most often. Thus, metabolic syndrome, option C, is correct.

    The remaining options (A, B, D, and E) are not associated with olanzapine use or with the entire atypical antipsychotic class of drugs. **Task: D3**—Pharmaceutical Therapeutics

13. **Answer: C** Lithium, option C, is widely recognized to cause drug-induced nephrogenic diabetes insipidus. Options A, B, D, and E have their own wide range of potential serious adverse effects, but none have an antidiuretic hormone-blocking effect on the collecting ducts as is observed with the use of lithium. **Task: D3**—Pharmaceutical Therapeutics

14. **Answer: E** Antidepressants should generally be avoided in the treatment of bipolar type I disorder because of their potential to elevate the risk of provoking a switch from depression to mania. If depression persists, an antidepressant may be used in bipolar type II, but the risk of inciting hypomania does exist. Thus, selective serotonin reuptake inhibitors, option E, is correct.

    Seizure disorder and bipolar disorder frequently coexist. However, medications to control seizure activity, option A, are not known to trigger mania. Since most first- and second-generation antipsychotic medications are dopamine antagonists, both options B and D are incorrect. Benzodiazepines, option C, do not trigger mania but, in fact, may be used to sedate a patient having an acute, serious manic episode. **Task: D3**—Pharmaceutic Therapeutics

Answer Key for this chapter begins on p. 306

15. **Answer: E** Severe and life-threatening hypersensitivity reactions such as Stevens-Johnson syndrome and toxic epidermal necrolysis are associated with lamotrigine, option E. Options A through D, while serious by themselves, are not listed as serious or common adverse reactions to this drug. **Task:** D3—Pharmaceutical Therapeutics

16. **Answer: D** Monoamines include serotonin, norepinephrine, and dopamine. Amphetamines, such as methamphetamine, increase the concentration of monoamines in the synaptic cleft by both increasing their release and inhibiting their reuptake, option D. Amphetamines do not function as noted in options A, B, C, or E. Cholinesterase inhibitors, option A, are used to treat myasthenia gravis and dementia. Dopamine receptor antagonists, option B, include antiemetic drugs. Atropine is the prototypical muscarine receptor antagonist, option C. Drugs that inhibit glutamate release, option E, are used to treat Alzheimer disease and amyotrophic lateral sclerosis. **Task:** E—Applying Basic Scientific Concepts

17. **Answer: A** Buprenorphine (option A), used alone or combined with naloxone as a single tablet, is used widely in medication-assisted treatment programs for opioid addiction. Buprenorphine acts as a partial μ-opioid receptor agonist while naloxone, option D, is an opioid antagonist.
Chlordiazepoxide, option B, is a long-acting benzodiazepine receptor agonist used in the treatment of acute alcohol withdrawal. Disulfiram, option C, is used as deterrent therapy in individuals with alcohol addiction and exerts its effect by inhibiting aldehyde dehydrogenase. Varenicline, option E, is a nicotinic receptor antagonist used in the treatment of nicotine addiction. **Task:** D3—Pharmaceutical Therapeutics

18. **Answer: D** Patients with comorbid mental health disorders and substance use disorder have worse clinical outcomes. Integrated group therapy, option D, addresses both bipolar disorder and substance use disorder simultaneously, using cognitive behavioral therapeutic principles. Therefore, this is the most appropriate first-line therapy option.
Aversion therapy, option A, exposes the patient to noxious or unpleasant experiences in order to eliminate undesirable behavior or symptoms; it is not commonly used today. Electroconvulsive therapy, option B, has been found to be effective and safe for the treatment of severe and drug-resistant bipolar disorder, but it would not be a first-line option. Eye movement desensitization and reprocessing therapy, option C, is a form of psychotherapy that has been used in the treatment of post-traumatic stress disorder (PTSD). The patient recalls distressing experiences while moving their eyes side to side or while tapping either side

of the body. Opinions are mixed on the effectiveness of the technique, but it has been suggested that it might be a form of exposure therapy. Narrative exposure therapy, option E, is conditionally recommended by the American Psychological Association for the treatment of PTSD. **Task:** D2—Clinical Intervention

19. **Answer: E** An inpatient civil commitment, emergency order of detention, or other name used by the different states, is a commitment of an individual, usually up to 72 hours, whose behavior is such that they are considered high risk of imminent and immediate harm to themselves or others. As they may be committed against their will, they are essentially stripped of all personal liberties guaranteed by the Constitution, including the right of autonomy. Thus, option E is correct.
Involuntary commitment falls under the jurisdiction of the state and not the federal government, option A. Criminal activity, option B, is not needed for commitment. Involuntary commitment is a legal process. There is an extensive body of literature that concludes that individuals with mental illness who are appropriately medicated are at no greater risk of committing violence than the general population. However, the risk of violent behavior is increased versus the general population in those with serious mental illness who are not under active medical treatment. This observation does not apply to everyone with mental illness and by itself is not a reason for involuntary commitment. Thus, option C is incorrect. While many health care professionals including physician assistants (PAs) may admit a patient into commitment, a judge (not a physician or PA) must agree and sign the order for the commitment to remain in force. Thus, option D is incorrect. **Task:** F—Entry-Level Professional Practice—Legal/Medical Ethics

20. **Answer: C** The Community Mental Health Act of 1963 was designed to shift the care of individuals with mental illness from long-term stays in state institutions to the community setting, and many individuals with severe mental illness were released from state mental hospitals (deinstitutionalized). Therefore, option C is correct. Although funding is consistently limited, much progress has been made over the years to develop high-quality community mental health centers that integrate physical and mental health care. This patient would likely benefit from the services offered in this type of system.
The act was not specifically intended to decrease the incidence of suicide in those with mental illness, option A. As a result of the act, many mentally ill individuals ended up incarcerated given the inability for the system to adequately care for them in the community, option B. While the act was developed in response to concerns about inhumane conditions in the state

mental hospitals, improving rights for institutionalized individuals was not the intended goal, option D. The act offered support to construct community mental health centers, but the provision of funding for inpatient mental health care was not the primary focus, option E. **Task:** F—Entry-Level Professional Practice—Patient Care and Communication

21. **Answer: D** An Assertive Community Treatment (ACT) program is a team-based approach designed to stabilize community living for persons with severe mental illness, option D. Even though the individual may be living independently or semi-independently, they are at high risk for psychiatric rehospitalization, incarceration, or homelessness. Most services are provided in the community rather than at a mental health center. ACT team members work closely together to address the various needs of the individual, which may involve regular home visits in order to coordinate services.

Option A is incorrect, as the purpose of ACT is to assist individuals in the community setting. Option B is incorrect as the program is not designed for those with mild mental illness. Option C is incorrect since the program is not designed as a monitoring program for criminal offenders. Finally, option E is incorrect because ACT is not a residential program, **Task:** F—Entry-Level Professional Practice—Patient Care and Communication

BIBLIOGRAPHY

Depression and related disorders. In: R. C. Smith, G. G. Osborn, F. C. Dwamena, D. D'Mello, L. Freilich, & H. S. Laird-Fick (Eds), *Essentials of psychiatry in primary care: Behavioral health in the medical setting, 2019*. McGraw Hill.

Dieterich, M., Irving, C. B., Park, B., & Marshall, M. (2010). Intensive case management for severe mental illness. *Cochrane Database of Systematic Reviews, 2010*. https://doi.org/10.1002/14651858.CD007906.pub2.

Drake, R. E., & Latimer, E. (2012). Lessons learned in developing community mental health care in North America. *World Psychiatry, 11*(1), 47-51.

Erden, A., Karagöz, H., Basak, M., Karahan, S., Cetinkaya, A., Avci, D., et al. (2013). Lithium intoxication and nephrogenic diabetes insipidus: A case report and review of literature. *International Journal of General Medicine, 6*, 535-539.

Harris, E. C., & Barraclough, B. (1997). Suicide as an outcome for mental disorders. A meta-analysis. *British Journal of Psychiatry, 170*, 205.

Hirschfeld, R. M., Williams, J. B., Spitzer, R. L., Calabrese, J. R., Flynn, L., Keck, P. E., et al. (2000). Development and validation of a screening instrument for bipolar spectrum disorder: the Mood Disorder Questionnaire. *American Journal of Psychiatry, 157*, 1873.

Knott, S., Forty, L., Craddock, N., & Thomas, R. H. (2015). Epilepsy and bipolar disorder. *Epilepsy & Behavior, 52*, 267-274.

Major depression and related disorders. In: R. C. Smith, G. G. Osborn, F. C. Dwamena, D. D'Mello, L. Freilich, & H. S. Laird-Fick (Eds.), *Essentials of psychiatry in primary care: Behavioral health in the medical setting, 2019*. McGraw Hill.

Meyer, J. M. (2017). Pharmacotherapy of psychosis and mania. In L. L. Brunton, R. Hilal-Dandan, & B. C. Knollmann (Eds.), *Goodman & Gilman's: The pharmacological basis of therapeutics* (13th ed.). McGraw Hill.

Neuropharmacology. (2017). In L. L. Brunton, R. Hilal-Dandan, & B. C. Knollmann (Eds.), *Goodman & Gilman's: The pharmacological basis of therapeutics* (13th ed.). McGraw Hill.

Psychotic disorders. (2019). In R. C. Smith, G. G. Osborn, F. C. Dwamena, D. D'Mello, L. Freilich, & H. S. Laird-Fick (Eds.), *Essentials of psychiatry in primary care: Behavioral health in the medical setting*. McGraw Hill.

Raj, K. S., Williams, N., & DeBattista, C. (2022). Mood disorders (depression & mania). In M. A. Papadakis, S. J. McPhee, M. W. Raboew, & K. R. McQuaid (Eds.), *Current medical diagnosis & treatment 2022*. McGraw Hill.

Rueve, M. E., & Welton, R. S. (2008). Violence and mental illness. *Psychiatry (Edgemont), 8*, 34-48.

Shah, S., Hagopian, T., Klinglesmith, R., & Bonfante, E. (2014). Diagnostic neuroradiology. In K. M. Elsayes & S. A. Oldham (Eds.), *Introduction to diagnostic radiology*. McGraw Hill.

Testa, M., & West, S. G. (2010). Civil commitment in the United States. *Psychiatry (Edgemont), 10*, 30-40.

www.nimh.nih.gov/health/statistics/bipolar-disorder

www.nimh.nih.gov/health/statistics/schizophrenia

Yoon, J.-H., Kim, J. H., Choi, S. S., Lyu, M. K., Kwon, J. H., Jang, Y. I., et al. (2012). Homicide and bipolar I disorder: a 22-year study. *Forensic Science International, 10*, 113-118.

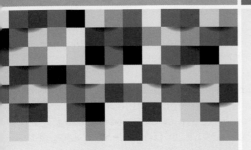

CASE STUDY 14
Pulmonary System

Questions

Case Section I: Chief Complaint and History of Present Illness

A 72-year-old man is brought to the clinic by his wife who says that the patient has had worsening fatigue and weight gain over the past few months and increasing confusion over the past week. She says that his symptoms have progressed to the point of him no longer having the energy or inclination to tend to his garden. Medical history includes a mild stroke three years ago, hypertension for which he takes losartan 50 mg daily, and hyperlipidemia that is well-controlled with simvastatin 20 mg daily. He also takes one 81-mg aspirin daily. His wife says that he drinks about six beers on the weekends and has smoked one pack of cigarettes per day since he was a teenager. The patient says he has had a smoker's cough in the morning for the past 10 years; however, the cough seems to be worsening and he has noticed occasional flecks of blood in his handkerchief over the past month or so. The patient retired eight years ago following a 40-year career working in glass manufacturing. He has no known drug allergies.

1. Which of the following is high on the differential diagnosis list and must be investigated during this patient's visit?
   A. Babesiosis
   B. Carcinoma of the lung
   C. Cor pulmonale
   D. Left-sided heart failure
   E. Tuberculosis

2. Which of the following screening tests administered to the patient is most likely to help clarify what his wife describes as "increasing confusion"?
   A. AD8 Dementia Screening Interview
   B. Brief Psychiatric Rating Scale
   C. Informant Questionnaire on Cognitive Decline in the Elderly
   D. Mini Mental Status Examination
   E. Positive and Negative Syndrome Scale

3. Which of the following is the most likely etiology of the patient's increasing confusion?
   A. Alzheimer disease
   B. Delirium
   C. Lewy body dementia
   D. Normal pressure hydrocephalus
   E. Vascular dementia

4. Which of the following disorders is this patient at increased risk of having based on his long career in the glass manufacturing industry?
   A. Brucellosis
   B. Byssinosis
   C. Hypersensitivity pneumonitis
   D. Mesothelioma
   E. Pneumoconiosis

5. Based on this patient's symptoms and overall history, which of the following laboratory studies is most likely to link these diverse elements and help determine the most likely diagnosis?
   A. Ceruloplasmin level
   B. Complete blood cell count
   C. D-Dimer assay
   D. Electrolyte study
   E. Thyroid-stimulating hormone level

Case Section II: Objective Findings, Assessment, and Plan

Temperature is 36.6°C (97.9°F), pulse rate is 92/min, respirations are 24/min, and blood pressure is 145/98 mmHg. Oxygen saturation is 88% on room air. Physical examination shows signs of anasarca, labored breathing with bilateral crackles, and 2+ pitting pedal edema. No jugular venous distension is noted, and the hepatojugular reflux is absent. Laboratory studies show a serum glucose level of 92 mg/dL (N = 60–100 mg/dL), potassium level of 5.2 mEq/L (N = 3.5–5.0 mEq/L), sodium level of 111 mEq/L (N = 135–145 mEq/L), and creatinine level of 1.2 mg/dL (N = 0.5-1.5 mg/dL). Chest x-ray study shows a widened mediastinum, increased vascular markings in the lower lung fields, and blunting of the bilateral costodiaphragmatic recesses.

6. Which of the following is the most likely cause of the anasarca in this patient?
   A. Bronchogenic carcinoma
   B. Carcinoid syndrome
   C. Congestive heart failure
   D. Emphysema
   E. Superior vena cava syndrome

7. Overproduction of which of the following is most likely responsible for the anasarca?
   A. Albumin
   B. Brain natriuretic peptide
   C. Parathyroid hormone-related peptide
   D. Thyroxine
   E. Vasopressin

8. Which of the following is most likely to result from progression of this patient's disease state?
   A. Grey-Turner sign
   B. Painless jaundice
   C. Pancoast syndrome
   D. Sister Mary Joseph nodule
   E. Tic douloureux

9. If the hyponatremia in this patient is related to a diagnosis of pulmonary cancer, which of the following is the most likely histologic or serologic type?
   A. Human epidermal growth factor 2 (HER2) positive
   B. Mesothelioma
   C. Reed-Sternberg cells
   D. Small-cell carcinoma
   E. Transitional cell carcinoma

10. If this patient's signs and symptoms are the result of syndrome of inappropriate antidiuretic hormone secretion (SIADH), which of the following laboratory findings is most likely?
    A. Decreased serum osmolality
    B. Decreased urine osmolality
    C. Decreased urine sodium level
    D. Decreased urine specific gravity
    E. Increased daily urine output

11. Cytology of the pleural effusion shows malignant cells. Referral to which of the following services is most appropriate?
    A. Brachytherapy
    B. Memory care center
    C. Palliative care
    D. Proton therapy
    E. Respite services

Case Section III: Comorbidity

During the interview, the patient mentions that he was hospitalized about 10 years ago because his sodium level was very low during a bout of pneumonia. Although the details are absent, he recalls symptoms of confusion and considerable cough and is concerned that he has the same illness as he had in the past.

12. Infection with which of the following organisms is most consistent with community-acquired pneumonia with concomitant hyponatremia?
    A. *Haemophilus influenzae*
    B. *Klebsiella pneumoniae*
    C. *Legionella pneumophila*
    D. *Staphylococcus aureus*
    E. *Streptococcus pneumoniae*

13. The pathophysiology of the patient's past hyponatremic episode with pneumonia and the current hyponatremia are most consistent with which of the following endocrinopathies?
    A. Hyperaldosteronism
    B. Hypercortisolism
    C. Hyperparathyroidism
    D. Multiple endocrine neoplasia type 1
    E. Posterior pituitary dysfunction

14. Which of the following structures has a significant role in regulating serum sodium balance and will be significantly suppressed in this patient?
    A. Adrenal medulla
    B. Alpha and beta cells of the pancreatic islets
    C. Hypothalamus
    D. Liver
    E. Parathyroid glands

15. If the patient is found to have a paraneoplastic tumor of the lung, ectopic secretion of which of the following hormones is most likely to result in a dilutional hyponatremia?
    A. Adrenocorticotropic hormone
    B. Aldosterone
    C. Angiotensin II
    D. Cortisol
    E. Vasopressin

Case Section IV: Professional Practice

Despite aggressive chemotherapy, the patient's condition progressively declines over the next eight months. At a current follow-up visit, the patient says that he wants to stop further efforts at treating his terminal disease and has decided he would like to begin care with hospice.

Answer Key for this chapter begins on p. 313

16. Which of the following is the most appropriate next step in arranging for hospice care for this patient?
    A. Ensuring that the patient continues to receive all other Medicare-covered benefits and treatments while in hospice
    B. Making sure the patient has Medicare Part D benefits
    C. Making the patient aware that hospice care is only for six months
    D. Obtaining certification by a hospice nurse
    E. Obtaining written certification that the patient is foregoing curative care

17. Which of the following provides direction to the health care team on the patient's wishes for end-of-life care?
    A. Durable attorney for health care
    B. Health care proxy
    C. Living will
    D. Referral for palliative care
    E. Successor trustee

Answers

1. **Answer: B** Carcinoma of the lung, option B, is correct because any patient with a long history of smoking and worsening cough and hemoptysis requires workup for this condition.

   Babesiosis, option A, is a tick-borne illness that can present with flulike symptoms. Since the patient does not have body aches, fever, chills, or headache, this is incorrect. Cor pulmonale and left-sided heart failure (options C and D) are incorrect because this patient does not have the universal symptom of these conditions, which is jugular venous distension. While hemoptysis is consistent with tuberculosis (option E), the patient does not describe other constitutional symptoms such as unintentional weight loss, night sweats, or fever and chills. **Task:** C—Formulating Most Likely Diagnosis

2. **Answer: D** The Mini Mental Status Examination, option D, is correct because this test can provide a quantitative measure of the severity of cognitive impairment at a given point in time.

   Being able to quantify the symptom of "increasing confusion" is helpful. With confusion, it is important to distinguish between an insidious or acute onset. An insidious progression of confusion is consistent with dementia. However, in this patient's case the onset is rather acute, thus screening tests for dementia, options A and C, are incorrect. The Brief Psychiatric Rating Scale (BPRS), option B, has been in use since the early 1960s and focuses on identifying conditions such as depression, anxiety, and psychoses. Since the BPRS is not used to quantify a state of confusion, this is incorrect. Option E, the Positive and Negative Syndrome Scale, is the most widely used measure of symptom severity in schizophrenia. The acute nature of this patient's symptoms is more consistent with delirium, making option E an incorrect choice. **Task:** B—Using Diagnostic and Laboratory Studies

3. **Answer: B** This patient began experiencing confusion one week ago. This suggests that something changed at that time for the symptom to manifest itself. Such a development is consistent with delirium (option B), which typically has a specific etiology, is usually acute in onset, and is most often reversible.

   All of the other options (A, C, D, and E) describe a subtype of dementia. Dementia is more insidious in onset and in most cases, may be slowed in its progression but is not reversible. **Task:** A—History Taking and Performing Physical Examination

4. **Answer: E** Pneumoconiosis, option E, is a general term used to describe inflammatory lung disease in response to long-term exposure to mineral dust such as coal, silica, and many others. Silica (sand) is the main constituent of glass, which makes this the correct option.

   Brucellosis, option A, is a bacterial infection typically acquired by eating raw or unpasteurized dairy products or by working around infected domesticated ruminants and swine. Byssinosis (option B) is an occupational disease, also called brown lung disease, which is caused by long-term exposure to breathing dust from cotton, hemp, or flax processing. Hypersensitivity pneumonitis, option C, is an allergic lung disease caused by a reaction to any number of organic substances, such as moldy hay, organic dusts, animal or plant proteins, or fungal spores. Occupations where this type of pneumonitis occurs include mushroom worker's lung, cork worker's lung, and farmer's lung. Mesothelioma, option D, is a malignant cancer most often involving the pleura and, in approximately 80% of cases, is directly linked to exposure to asbestos. Since asbestos is not directly involved in the manufacturing of glass, option D is incorrect. **Task:** C—Formulating Most Likely Diagnosis

5. **Answer: D** An electrolyte study, option D, will provide information on the patient's sodium level. The sodium level is critical in the discussions of fluid balance, fatigue, and mentation. Also, given the patient's extensive smoking history and cough, a lung tumor affecting sodium balance is a very real possibility and could account for the hemoptysis.

   Apoceruloplasmin is a protein synthesized by the liver and, when bound to copper, is converted to ceruloplasmin. Ceruloplasmin, option A, is the primary copper-carrying protein in the body and is used as a measure of liver disease and copper-related disorders, such as Wilson disease. This does not explain the patient's symptoms of congestive heart failure nor the hemoptysis. Although complete blood cell count, option B, could help diagnose the fatigue and possible confusion, it does not provide an explanation for the weight gain or hemoptysis in this patient. A D-dimer assay, option C, is obtained when investigating an embolic event, such as a pulmonary embolism. While a pulmonary embolism would explain the hemoptysis, it does not account for or explain the patient's other symptoms. Thyroid-stimulating hormone level, option E, will identify hypothyroidism with the associated symptoms of fatigue and confusion. However, like the other incorrect options, thyroid function does not help explain this patient's cough and hemoptysis. **Task:** B—Using Diagnostic and Laboratory Studies

6. **Answer: A** Anasarca describes a condition of generalized edema. Bronchogenic carcinoma, option A, is correct because one form of bronchogenic carcinoma, namely small-cell carcinoma, is known for aberrant secretion of antidiuretic hormone (syndrome of inappropriate antidiuretic hormone secretion [SIADH]). SIADH presents with significant hyponatremia and edema consistent with this patient.

   Carcinoid syndrome, option B, is another form of paraneoplastic tumor that arises primarily not only in the gastrointestinal tract but also in the lungs. Vasoactive substances, such as serotonin, and other hormones like growth hormone and parathyroid hormone-related peptide are frequently secreted by carcinoid tumors. SIADH is not a typical finding with carcinoid tumors; therefore, this option is incorrect. The clinical, laboratory, and radiographic presentation of the patient is consistent with left and right congestive heart failure (CHF), option C. However, the findings that are not consistent with CHF include the absence of jugular venous distension and hepatojugular reflux. Emphysema, option D, typically does not result in anasarca. Rather, patients with emphysema are usually thin, barrel-chested, and do not have generalized edema as in this patient. Superior vena cava syndrome, option E, results from congestion due to a pulmonary or mediastinal neoplastic process obstructing venous return via the superior vena cava. The edema present in superior vena cava syndrome is confined to areas drained by the vessel including the head, neck, and upper torso. The dependent edema and laboratory results in this patient are not typical of this syndrome. **Task: C—** Formulating Most Likely Diagnosis

7. **Answer: E** Vasopressin, option E, also known as antidiuretic hormone (ADH), is correct. Osmoreceptors in the hypothalamus synthesize ADH in response to an increase in osmolality. ADH is then released at terminals in the posterior pituitary. The end result of ADH on fluid balance is to increase water reabsorption by the nephron. As ADH may be secreted by certain tumors, especially small-cell carcinoma of the lung, patients may become edematous with a concomitant dilutional hyponatremia as described in this patient.

   An increase in albumin, option A, has the opposite effect of anasarca. As the major constituent of the oncotic pressure of the blood, a decrease in albumin results in edema. Brain natriuretic peptide (option B), released from the ventricles in response to increased ventricular pressure, is more likely to result from anasarca rather than be a causative factor. Parathyroid hormone-related peptide (PTH-rp), option C, is a common aberrant secretion of certain tumors. PTH-rp is incorrect because overproduction of the hormone results in hypercalcemia and not anasarca.

Thyroxine, option D, is incorrect because an underproduction of thyroxine, not overproduction, likely results in an edematous state. **Task: E—**Applying Basic Scientific Concepts

8. **Answer: C** Pancoast syndrome, option C, results from extension of a lung cancer into the chest wall, particularly involving the low cervical and upper thoracic spinal nerves. This results in pain in the shoulder with radiation into the ipsilateral upper extremity. Pancoast syndrome and Horner syndrome often coexist with this type of cancerous invasion.

   The patient's signs and symptoms are originating in the lungs. Grey-Turner sign, option A, is ecchymosis of the flank resulting from retroperitoneal hemorrhage, particularly from acute necrotizing pancreatitis. Painless jaundice, option B, is typically observed with obstruction of the bile duct not related to a calculus. The classic disorder is cancer of the head of the pancreas. Sister Mary Joseph nodule, option D, presents as a firm, small mass occurring in the umbilicus and typically signals metastasis from a viscus of the gastrointestinal tract. Tic douloureux, option E, is an exquisitely painful paresthesia involving the trigeminal nerve. Since cranial nerve V does not extend into the chest, this option is incorrect. **Task: A—**History Taking and Performing Physical Examination

9. **Answer: D** Small-cell carcinoma of the lung, option D, has a well-documented association with aberrant secretion of antidiuretic hormone (ADH), resulting in syndrome of inapantidiuretic hormone secretion (SIADH). Hallmark features of SIADH include generalized edema and a dilutional hyponatremia. In fact, any person who smokes who has hyponatremia requires a thorough workup to rule out small-cell carcinoma of the lung.

   Human epidermal growth factor 2 (HER2), option A, is a growth-promoting protein normally present on all breast cells. Breast cancer cells typically express higher levels of HER2 and are thus termed HER2 positive. HER2 is not related to pulmonary cancer; therefore, this option is incorrect. Mesothelioma, option B, is a cancer originating in the pleura, pericardium, and/or peritoneum. It is uniquely associated with occupational exposure to asbestos; although it most commonly involves the pleura, mesothelioma is not associated with electrolyte balance. Reed-Sternberg cells, option C, are pathognomonic and diagnostic for Hodgkin lymphoma. While Hodgkin lymphoma commonly occurs in the chest cavity, the lymphoma itself does not cause a primary hyponatremia. Transitional cell carcinoma, option E, is incorrect because the cell type is only found in the urinary bladder. **Task: C—**Formulating Most Likely Diagnosis

10. **Answer: A** This patient has several signs of SIADH including volume overload, anasarca, dependent edema, pulmonary crackles, and what appears to be a dilutional hyponatremia. Such signs and symptoms are consistent with decreased serum osmolality, option A.

Since urine output is very concentrated, it has increased osmolality, which makes option B incorrect. As its name implies, SIADH results in decreased but concentrated urine output. These characteristics make options C, D, and E incorrect as well. **Task: B—Using Laboratory and Diagnostic Studies**

11. **Answer: C** The presence of cancer cells in a pleural effusion is a sign of an incurable malignancy. With the patient's disease state being incurable, palliative care, option C, is the most appropriate choice. Brachytherapy, option A, involves inserting radiotherapeutic pellets, and proton therapy, option D, is a directed form of radiation therapy. Either option could be directed at a specific tumor mass. However, these treatments are not appropriate for this patient, and both options are incorrect. Referral to a memory care center, option B, is appropriate for a patient with dementia. This patient has profound hyponatremia and is most likely experiencing delirium. Normalizing the serum sodium level will likely result in resolution of the confusion. The purpose of respite services, option E, is to provide caregivers with a temporary reprieve from their responsibilities. Such a reprieve might enable a caregiver the opportunity to go on vacation or simply have some time alone. While a respite service, along with hospice, may be in this patient's immediate future, neither he nor his wife appear to be at that point now. **Task: D2—Clinical Intervention**

12. **Answer: C** Patients with pneumonia caused by *Legionella*, option C, often present with hyponatremia; therefore, this option is correct.

Community-acquired pneumonia (CAP) with *H. influenzae*, option A, as the infecting organism presents with typical symptoms such as fever, cough, and congestion. Electrolyte disturbances are not consistent with this organism. *K. pneumoniae* infections, option B, are typically nosocomial in origin and often present in patients with alcohol use disorder. Also, electrolyte disturbance is not a hallmark of *Klebsiella* infections. Pneumonia caused by *S. aureus*, option D, typically follows influenza and is notorious for producing necrotizing lung damage. Also, electrolytes are not directly affected with this infection. CAP caused by *Streptococcus* is of course most frequently encountered. Interestingly, it has even become more common than *Klebsiella* in patients with alcohol use disorder. Since *S. pneumoniae* does not affect electrolytes extensively, option E is incorrect. **Task: E—Applying Basic Scientific Concepts**

13. **Answer: E** Posterior pituitary dysfunction, option E, includes SIADH, which is consistent with general hyponatremia.

Hyperaldosteronism (Conn syndrome), option A, can also result in weakness and fatigue, but its effect on electrolytes results in hypernatremia and hypokalemia. An increase in serum cortisol (Cushing syndrome), option B, can produce many of the symptoms displayed by this patient. However, hyponatremia and pneumonia are not related to Cushing syndrome. Similarly, many of this patient's symptoms are consistent with hypercalcemia associated with hyperparathyroidism, option C. However, pneumonia and hyponatremia are not associated with parathyroid disease, making this option incorrect. Multiple endocrine neoplasia type 1, option D, is a genetic disorder with an autosomal dominant inheritance pattern that results in sporadic tumors mostly of the parathyroid gland, pancreatic islet cells, adrenal cortex, and pituitary gland. The wide variety of symptoms depends on the hormone-specific tissue from which the tumors arise. Examples include prolactin, adrenocorticotropic hormone, growth hormone, gastrin, glucagon, vasoactive intestinal peptide, and parathyroid hormone. Despite the plethora of symptoms and hormone possibilities, hyponatremia and pneumonia are absent from the symptomatology, making option D incorrect. **Task: C—Formulating Most Likely Diagnosis**

14. **Answer: C** Regulation of sodium balance is a multiorgan task involving the osmoreceptors on neurons of the hypothalamus, antidiuretic hormone (ADH) release from the posterior pituitary, renal tubules, and the adrenal cortex. Given the patient's degree of hyponatremia, hypothalamic-induced release of ADH will be significantly decreased. Of the options presented, hypothalamus (option C) is the correct answer.

The adrenal medulla, option A, is incorrect because it is the adrenal cortex, not the catecholamine-secreting medulla, which serves a role in electrolyte balance. Alpha and beta cells of the pancreatic islets, option B, describes endocrine cells of the pancreas that secrete glucagon and insulin, respectively. Neither hormone has a significant role in regulating serum sodium. The role of the liver, option D, in human physiology and biochemistry is enormous. Interestingly, however, it leaves regulation of electrolyte levels to other visceral systems. The parathyroid glands, option E, are also incorrect. While parathyroid hormone functions in maintaining serum calcium and phosphorus balance, it does not participate in regulating sodium or potassium. **Task: E—Applying Basic Scientific Concepts**

15. **Answer: E** Vasopressin, option E, exerts its action on the renal tubules to increase reabsorption of water. The ensuing volume overload effectively results in a dilutional hyponatremia, making option E correct.

   Answer Key for this chapter begins on p. 313

Adrenocorticotropic hormone, aldosterone, angiotensin II, and cortisol (options A through D) all participate to some degree in serum sodium homeostasis. Each of these hormones activates directly or indirectly the renin–angiotensin–aldosterone system, resulting in a proportional reabsorption of sodium and water. Thus, none of the four hormones will produce a dilutional hyponatremia. **Task:** B—Using Diagnostic and Laboratory Studies

16. **Answer: E** Obtaining written certification that the patient is foregoing curative care, option E, is correct. In addition to being terminally ill with a life expectancy of less than six months, eligibility for hospice requires patients to accept palliative care for comfort instead of conventional care targeted toward a cure. Option A is incorrect because patients in hospice must opt to choose services provided by hospice care instead of all other Medicare-covered benefits and treatments that are designed more for chronic disease management, prolonging life, and improving the prognosis of a disease. Option B is incorrect because, for a Medicare beneficiary, hospice care is reimbursed under Part A. Note that Medicare Part A is provided to qualified individuals without cost and covers hospitalizations and related services. Part D is optional, must be purchased by the individual, and is intended to cover the cost of medications. Regarding option C, the initial hospice certification period is for six months. However, a patient may continue to receive hospice care as long as a physician recertifies that the patient is terminally ill. Option D is incorrect because

only an allopathic or osteopathic physician can certify that a patient is terminally ill and eligible for hospice care. While there have been many advancements in how physician assistants may participate in hospice care, certifying or recertifying a patient for hospice remains the privilege of physicians. **Task:** F—Entry-Level Professional Practice: Patient Care and Communication

17. **Answer: C** A living will (option C), also called an advanced directive, is a document originating directly from the patient for the specific purpose of guiding the type and extent of health care delivery during the end-of-life period. Therefore, this is correct.
Durable attorney for health care and health care proxy, options A and B, describe synonymous documents that identify a person to make end-of-life decisions when the patient is incapable of such. They are both incorrect choices because they describe not necessarily the patient's specific wishes, but the determinations of another individual appointed by the patient. A referral for palliative care, option D, does not necessarily equate to end-of-life care. While hospice care involves palliative care, the reverse is not always true in that individuals receiving palliative care can have a positive prognosis. A successor trustee, option E, is an individual designated to oversee a trust in the event the originator of the trust is no longer capable of making decisions for or managing the trust. As a successor trustee has no authority over health care issues, option E is incorrect. **Task:** F—Entry-level Professional Practice: Legal/Medical Ethics

BIBLIOGRAPHY

Arora, N., & Jefferson, J. (2021). Hyponatremia. In M. A. Papadakis, S. J. McPhee, & M. W. Rabow (Eds.), *Current medical diagnosis & treatment 2021*. McGraw Hill.

Durrani, T. S., & Harrison, R. J. (2014). Occupational infections. In J. LaDou & R. J. Harrison (Eds.), *Current diagnosis & treatment: Occupational & environmental medicine* (5th ed.). McGraw Hill.

Emanuel, E. J. (2018). Palliative and end-of-life care. In J. Jameson, A. S. Fauci, D. L. Kasper, S. L. Hauser, D. L. Longo, & J. Loscalzo (Eds.), *Harrison's principles of internal medicine* (20th ed.). McGraw Hill.

Horn, L., & Lovly, C. M. (2018). Neoplasms of the lung. In J. Jameson, A. S. Fauci, D. L. Kasper, S. L. Hauser, D. L. Longo, & J. Loscalzo (Eds.), *Harrison's principles of internal medicine* (20th ed.). McGraw Hill.

Jameson, J., & Longo, D. L. (2018). Paraneoplastic syndromes: Endocrinologic/hematologic. In J. Jameson, A. S. Fauci, D. L. Kasper, S. L. Hauser, D. L. Longo, & J. Loscalzo (Eds.), *Harrison's principles of internal medicine* (20th ed.). McGraw Hill.

Marder, K. (2019). Dementia & memory loss. In J. M. Brust (Ed.), *Current diagnosis & treatment neurology* (3rd ed.). McGraw Hill.

Mount, D. B. (2018). Sodium and water composition and physiology. In J. Jameson, A. S. Fauci, D. L. Kasper, S. L. Hauser, D. L. Longo, & J. Loscalzo (Eds.), *Harrison's principles of internal medicine* (20th ed.). McGraw Hill.

Robertson, G. L. (2018). Disorders of the neurohypophysis. In J. Jameson, A. S. Fauci, D. L. Kasper, S. L. Hauser, D. L. Longo, & J. Loscalzo (Eds.), *Harrison's principles of internal medicine* (20th ed.). McGraw Hill.

The mental status, psychiatric, and social evaluations. LeBlond R. F., & Brown D. D., & Suneja M, & Szot J. F.(Eds.), (2014). *DeGowin's Diagnostic Examination, 10e*. McGraw Hill.

Wang, S. (2021). Bronchogenic carcinoma. In M. A. Papadakis, S. J. McPhee, & M. W. Rabow (Eds.), *Current medical diagnosis & treatment 2021*. McGraw Hill.

Yu, V. L., Pedro-Botet, M., & Lin, Y. E. (2018). Legionella infections. In J. Jameson, A. S. Fauci, D. L. Kasper, S. L. Hauser, D. L. Longo, & J. Loscalzo (Eds.), *Harrison's principles of internal medicine* (20th ed.). McGraw Hill.

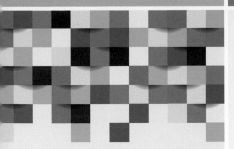

CASE STUDY 15

Renal System

Questions

Case Section I: Chief Complaint and History of Present Illness

A 67-year-old woman comes to the clinic because she has had nausea and dizziness for the past 12 hours. She says she also had severe diarrhea for the past three days that has since resolved and lower back pain for the past several months. The patient has no history of recent fever, chills, flank pain, or body aches. Medical history includes hypertension and type 2 diabetes mellitus. Medications include metformin 1000 mg twice daily, hydrochlorothiazide 25 mg daily, amlodipine 10 mg daily, lisinopril 20 mg daily, and ibuprofen 200 mg as needed for pain. She has no known drug allergies.

1. If malignancy of the kidney is suspected, which of the following is the most appropriate question to ask this patient?
   A. Do you engage in sexual intercourse?
   B. Have any other family members had diarrhea?
   C. Have you been drinking plenty of water?
   D. Have you noticed any blood in your urine?
   E. How often are you urinating?

2. Which of the following questions is most appropriate to ask in order to differentiate between polycystic kidney disease and other etiologies?
   A. Are you taking any over-the-counter or herbal supplements?
   B. Do you have a family history of kidney disorders?
   C. Do you have a history of hepatitis C?
   D. Do you smoke cigarettes, drink alcoholic beverages, or use illicit drugs?
   E. How often do you urinate?

3. If this patient also has malaise and altered mental status, which of the following is a possible diagnosis?
   A. Oliguria
   B. Proteinuria
   C. Pyrosis

D. Renal colic
E. Uremia

4. If this patient has azotemia, in addition to an elevated serum creatinine level, elevation of which of the following laboratory values is most likely?
   A. Hyaline casts
   B. Serum albumin
   C. Serum bicarbonate
   D. Serum blood urea nitrogen
   E. Urine protein

5. If this patient has an acute kidney injury, which of the following laboratory values is most likely to indicate the stage of injury?
   A. Red blood cell casts
   B. Serum blood urea nitrogen
   C. Serum creatinine
   D. Serum uric acid
   E. Urine protein

Case Section II: Objective Findings, Assessment, and Plan

Temperature is 37.1°C (98.8°F), pulse rate is 95/min, respirations are 16/min, and blood pressure is 156/92 mmHg. Oxygen saturation is 99% on room air. On physical examination, cardiac auscultation shows a regular rate and rhythm with no murmurs, rubs, or gallops. Auscultation of the lungs shows no wheezes, crackles, or rhonchi bilaterally. No pretibial edema is noted in the lower extremities. Laboratory findings include the following:

Serum	
Creatinine	2.5 mg/dL (N = 0.7–1.3 mg/dL)
Sodium	139 mEq/L (N = 135–145 mEq/L)
Chloride	103 mEq/L (N = 96–106 mEq/L)
Potassium	5.6 mEq/L (N = 3.5–5.0 mEq/L)
Bicarbonate	15 mEq/L (N = 23–29 mEq/L)

Glucose   110 mg/dL (N = 70–100 mg/dL)
Urea nitrogen 103 mg/dL (N = 6–24 mg/dL)
Urine
Osmolality   625 mOsm/kg (N = 500–850 mOsm/kg)
Hyaline casts Positive

6. Based on the findings in this patient thus far, which of the following is the most likely cause of the elevated renal waste products?
    A. Acute tubular necrosis
    B. Intrinsic renal disease
    C. Nephrotic syndrome
    D. Postrenal azotemia
    E. Prerenal azotemia

7. If this patient had waxing and waning flank pain, nausea and vomiting, as well as a serum creatinine of 2.9 mg/dL (N = 0.7-1.3 mg/dL), a serum urea nitrogen of 145 mg/dL (N = 6-24 mg/dL), and a urine osmolality of 233 mOsm/kg (N = 500-850 mOsm/kg), which of the following would be the most likely cause?
    A. Glomerulonephritis
    B. Intrinsic renal etiology
    C. Postrenal etiology
    D. Prerenal etiology
    E. Renal tubular acidosis

8. If this patient had an elevated serum creatinine level and microscopic urinalysis indicated red blood cells and red blood cell casts, which of the following would be the most likely diagnosis?
    A. Acute glomerulonephritis
    B. Acute interstitial nephritis
    C. Acute tubular necrosis
    D. Poor renal perfusion
    E. Renal artery stenosis

9. Which of the following drugs is most likely to alter the accuracy of fractional excretion of sodium in this patient?
    A. Amlodipine
    B. Hydrochlorothiazide
    C. Ibuprofen
    D. Lisinopril
    E. Metformin

10. If this patient had an elevated potassium level, which of the following would be the most likely cause?
    A. Diarrhea
    B. Hydrochlorothiazide
    C. Hypertension
    D. Lisinopril
    E. Metformin

11. If tapping on this patient's facial nerve during physical examination results in contraction of the facial muscle, which of the following electrolyte imbalances is most likely?
    A. Hyperkalemia
    B. Hypermagnesemia
    C. Hypernatremia
    D. Hypocalcemia
    E. Hypomagnesemia

12. Based on this patient's current potassium level of 5.6 mEq/L (N = 3.5-5.0 mEq/L), which of the following findings is most likely on electrocardiography?
    A. Peaked T waves and PR-interval elongation
    B. Prolonged QT interval
    C. Prolonged QT interval with ST-segment elongation
    D. Prominent U waves with broad T waves
    E. Shortened QT interval

13. Arterial blood gas analysis shows a pH of 7.30 (N = 7.35-7.45), pCO_2 of 30 mmHg (N = 35-45 mmHg), and HCO_3^- of 15 mEq/L (N = 23-29 mEq/L). This patient most likely has which of the following primary acid-base disorders?
    A. Metabolic acidosis
    B. Metabolic alkalosis
    C. Respiratory acidosis
    D. Respiratory alkalosis

Repeat urinalysis over the past six months has indicated continued proteinuria and hematuria as well as elevated urine creatinine. Results of complete blood cell count and complete metabolic panel are within normal limits except for elevated serum creatinine and blood urea nitrogen levels. Renal ultrasonography and a CT scan show no abnormalities.

14. Which of the following is the most appropriate next step?
    A. MRI of the kidneys
    B. Open biopsy of the kidneys
    C. Percutaneous needle biopsy of the kidneys
    D. PET scan of the kidneys

Six months later, the patient comes to the office because she has had weight gain, shortness of breath, and increased edema of her lower extremities. She has kept a log of her blood pressure which continues to be consistently above 150/90 mmHg despite the three-drug antihypertensive regimen.

15. If current laboratory studies show an elevated creatinine level and electron microscopy shows effacement of podocyte foot processes, which of the following is the most appropriate initial treatment?
    A. Corticosteroids
    B. Loop diuretic
    C. 0.9% Normal saline
    D. Plasma exchange therapy
    E. Salt restriction

16. Which of the following types of medications is most appropriate to help decrease hyperfiltration injury and slow the progression of chronic kidney disease in this patient?
    A. Angiotensin receptor blockers
    B. Beta-blockers
    C. Calcium channel blockers
    D. Loop diuretics
    E. Potassium-sparing diuretics

17. Laboratory studies show a decrease in glomerular filtration rate to 28 mL/min, which is most indicative of which of the following stages of chronic kidney disease?
    A. 1
    B. 2
    C. 3a
    D. 4
    E. 5

18. Given the patient's medical history of type 2 diabetes mellitus and the specific stage of her chronic kidney disease (CKD), which of the following is the most appropriate recommendation regarding management of diabetes mellitus secondary to CKD?
    A. Change to monthly hemoglobin A_{1c} checks
    B. Check the feet for sores or ulcers
    C. Continue yearly ophthalmic examinations
    D. Maintain aggressive control of hemoglobin A_{1c}
    E. Watch for hypoglycemic episodes

19. If the patient's glomerular filtration rate (GFR) continues to decrease to 25 mL/min, which of the following medications is most likely to increase the risk of lactic acidosis?
    A. Bicarbonate
    B. Carvedilol
    C. Furosemide
    D. Lisinopril
    E. Metformin

Six months later, the patient comes to the office for routine follow-up of chronic kidney disease. She says that she has increasing shortness of breath and nausea and vomiting even *after taking the prescribed oral thiazide diuretic. Current laboratory studies show a GFR of 8 mL/min. Chest x-ray study shows a left-sided mild pleural effusion.*

20. Which of the following is the most appropriate next step?
    A. Dialysis
    B. Inhalational ipratropium bromide/albuterol sulfate
    C. Intravenous furosemide
    D. Intravenous labetalol
    E. Thoracentesis

Case Section III: Comorbidity

Six months later, the patient comes to the office because she has had worsening pain in her long bones and proximal muscle weakness for the past two months. Laboratory findings include the following:

Hematocrit	28.6% (N = 35.5–44.9%)
Hemoglobin	7.4 g/dL (N = 13.2–16.6 g/dL)
Calcium	6.2 mg/dL (N = 8.6–10.3 mg/dL)
1,25 Dihydroxyvitamin D	5.6 pg/mL (N = 18–64 pg/mL)

Mean corpuscular volume and mean corpuscular hemoglobin level are within normal limits.

21. Based on these findings, this patient most likely has which of the following complications of CKD?
    A. Diabetic nephropathy
    B. Drug hypersensitivity
    C. Nephrolithiasis
    D. Renal vascular disease
    E. Secondary hyperparathyroidism

22. The patient's at-home blood pressure measurements have been 150/90 mmHg. According to current recommendations, it is most appropriate for this patient's blood pressure goal to be less than which of the following?
    A. 120/90 mmHg
    B. 130/80 mmHg
    C. 140/90 mmHg
    D. 145/80 mmHg
    E. 150/90 mmHg

23. Which of the following is the most appropriate treatment for the underlying cause of the anemia in this patient?
    A. Folate
    B. Intrinsic factor
    C. Iron infusion
    D. Recombinant erythropoietin
    E. Vitamin B_{12}

Answer Key for this chapter begins on p. 321

24. Which of the following findings on laboratory studies is the most likely cause of the bone pain and proximal muscle weakness in this patient?
    A. Decreased phosphorus level
    B. Decreased potassium level
    C. Decreased vitamin B_{12} level
    D. Elevated parathyroid hormone level
    E. Elevated potassium level

Case Section IV: Professional Practice

The patient, who now has end-stage renal disease and is on dialysis, comes to the emergency department because she is finding it more difficult to breathe. She says that she missed her last two dialysis appointments. Physical examination shows rhonchi throughout all lung fields and 2+ pitting pretibial edema. The patient is from Peru, South America and says that she wants to see her shaman and drink ayahuasca to help cure her disease.

25. Which of the following is the most appropriate response?
    A. Acknowledge her desire to seek alternatives, but recommend she keep up with the dialysis schedule
    B. Call the patient's shaman to discuss why ayahuasca treatment is wrong
    C. Explain that this is not a treatment that is recommended by the hospital
    D. Explain that this is not something that will help cure her disease

26. Which of the following is the best way to promote continuity of care with this patient?
    A. Ask the patient if she has transportation to office visits
    B. Check to make sure that the patient can pay for her office visits
    C. Discuss the patient's case with her family even though they are not approved for knowing this information
    D. Go over the patient's medication regimen with her to ensure proper use
    E. Tell the patient to make office visits for only when she is symptomatic

Answers

1. **Answer: D** It is most appropriate to ask this patient if she has noticed blood in her urine, option D, because gross hematuria without fever or renal colic is a possible indication of renal carcinoma. Renal cell carcinoma accounts for 10% of an upper tract source of hematuria. Most common presenting symptoms besides hematuria are an abdominal mass, abdominal pain, and/or weight loss. Asking this patient if she engages in sexual intercourse, has sick contacts, or if she has been drinking plenty of water (options A, B, and C) will not help identify symptoms of renal carcinoma. Asking how often the patient is urinating, option E, is important but is not specific nor sensitive for renal carcinoma. **Task:** A—History Taking and Performing Physical Examination

2. **Answer: B** Polycystic kidney disease (PCKD) is an autosomal dominant disorder; therefore, asking this patient if she has a family history of kidney disorders, option B, is the most appropriate question to ask. Finding out if the patient is taking over-the-counter or herbal supplements, option A, is important because different medications can cause renal disease; however, this does not impact the clinical reasoning for PCKD. Asking if she has a history of hepatitis C, option C, is important and can determine different types of kidney diseases, but it will not help determine if PCKD is a possible diagnosis. While knowing the patient's social history is important (option D), it will not help differentiate between PCKD and other etiologies as a possible diagnosis. Urinating frequently, option E, is not an indication of PCKD but is more common in medullary cystic kidney disease. **Task:** A—History Taking and Performing Physical Examination

3. **Answer: E** Malaise and altered mental status in addition to her current symptoms is most likely to indicate uremia, option E. This includes symptoms that are nonspecific but secondary to renal waste buildup. Oliguria, option A, is urinating/voiding less than 400 mL/d or less than 20 mL/hr. Proteinuria, option B, is a finding in urine with excessive protein. Pyrosis, option C, is the clinical term for heartburn. Renal colic, option D, is defined as waxing and waning pain secondary to renal stones. **Task:** C—Formulating Most Likely Diagnosis

4. **Answer: D** Azotemia is a diagnostic laboratory pattern that includes elevation of serum blood urea nitrogen and serum creatinine levels, option D. These waste products increase secondary to worsening kidney function.
Elevation of hyaline casts, serum albumin, serum bicarbonate, and urine protein (options A, B, C, and E) are not indicative of azotemia. **Task:** B—Using Diagnostic and Laboratory Studies

5. **Answer: C** The staging of acute kidney injury is based on either elevation of serum creatinine, option C, or decline in urinary output.
Staging of acute kidney injury is not based on red blood cell casts, serum blood urea nitrogen, serum uric acid, or urine protein (options A, B, D, and E). **Task:** B—Using Diagnostic and Laboratory Studies

6. **Answer: E** Patients who present with an acute kidney injury need to be classified under three different categories to help identify the cause and treat the disease. These three categories include prerenal, intrinsic, or postrenal. Prerenal azotemia, option E, is defined by a serum urea nitrogen (BUN)/creatinine ratio of greater than 20 with no indication of urinary obstruction.
Intrinsic renal disease, option B, includes a serum BUN/creatinine ratio of less than 20 unless a patient has acute glomerulonephritis. Acute tubular necrosis, option A, is a type of intrinsic renal disease. Nephrotic syndrome, option C, is a condition in which there is heavy proteinuria that leads to peripheral edema, which this patient does not have. Postrenal azotemia, option D, includes signs and symptoms of kidney or ureter obstruction. **Task:** C—Formulating Most Likely Diagnosis

7. **Answer: C** This patient's clinical symptoms of a serum BUN/creatinine ratio of greater than 20 with a urine osmolality of less than 300 mOsm/kg indicate possible obstruction. Obstruction of the urinary tract is an etiology of postrenal azotemia, option C.
Glomerulonephritis and renal tubular acidosis, options A and E, are forms of intrinsic renal disease and include corresponding diagnostic values. Intrinsic renal disease, option B, includes a serum BUN/creatinine ratio of less than 20 unless a patient has acute glomerulonephritis. Prerenal azotemia, option D, includes a BUN/creatinine ratio greater than 20 and a normal to high urine osmolality (N = 500-850 mOsm/kg). **Task:** C—Formulating Most Likely Diagnosis

Answer Key for this chapter begins on p. 321

8. **Answer: A** These laboratory findings are indicative of acute glomerulonephritis, option A.
Acute interstitial nephritis, option B, produces white blood cell casts. Acute tubular necrosis, option C, has granular or muddy brown casts/renal tubular casts. Poor renal perfusion and renal artery stenosis, options D and E, indicate dehydration and would produce benign or hyaline casts on microscopic urinalysis. **Task:** C—Formulating Most Likely Diagnosis

9. **Answer: B** The fractional excretion of sodium (FENa) is best used to differentiate between oliguric acute tubular necrosis and prerenal acute kidney injury. Normal physiological kidneys will have a FENa of less than 1%. A FENa can be calculated by using serum sodium and serum creatinine with random/spot urine sodium and urine creatinine. Diuretics can cause a FENa to be falsely elevated secondary to sodium excretion; therefore, hydrochlorothiazide (option B) is correct.
Amlodipine, option A, is metabolized in the liver and does not affect the kidney. Options C, D, and E are metabolized in the kidney; however, they do not affect the urine secretion of sodium in the kidney. **Task:** D3—Pharmaceutical Therapeutics

10. **Answer: D** Patients with hyperkalemia should have their medication list reviewed. Particular medications that can cause hyperkalemia include angiotensin-converting enzyme inhibitors such as lisinopril, option D. Other medications include angiotensin receptor antagonists, potassium-sparing diuretics, and medications containing trimethoprim.
Diarrhea, option A, can cause hypokalemia and not hyperkalemia. Hydrochlorothiazide, option B, decreases potassium. Hypertension, option C, is an important part of this patient's history but it does not cause hyperkalemia. Metformin, option E, has no effect on serum potassium. **Task:** D3—Pharmaceutical Therapeutics

11. **Answer: D** Facial muscle contraction upon tapping of the facial nerve is considered a positive Chvostek sign, which is an indication of hypocalcemia, option D. The Trousseau sign indicates hypocalcemia; however, it is indicated by carpal muscle movement after using a blood pressure cuff to occlude the brachial artery.
All the other options do not have an associated specific physical examination maneuver. Hyperkalemia, option A, includes muscle weakness or flaccid paralysis. Hypermagnesemia, option B, presents mildly with nausea and vomiting and facial flushing, and at severe levels, it presents with urinary retention, hyporeflexia, and muscle paralysis. Hypernatremia, option C, includes seizures, delirium, hyperthermia, and coma at severe levels (i.e., serum sodium level >158 mEq/L).

Hypomagnesemia, option E, can present as central nervous system hyperirritability, clonus, nystagmus, or a positive Babinski sign. **Task:** C—Formulating Most Likely Diagnosis

12. **Answer: A** This patient has hyperkalemia based on her potassium level; therefore, expected findings on electrocardiography include peaked T waves and/or PR-interval elongation, option A.
Prolonged QT interval (option B) indicates hypocalcemia; prolonged QT interval with ST-segment elongation (option C) indicates hypomagnesemia; prominent U waves with broad T waves (option D) indicates hypocalcemia; and a shortened QT interval (option E) indicates hypercalcemia. **Task:** B—Using Diagnostic and Laboratory Studies

13. **Answer: A** The renal system along with the respiratory system helps the body to maintain acid-base homeostasis with an arterial pH range of 7.35 to 7.45. To identify the acid-base disorder, it is appropriate to obtain arterial blood gases such as pH, pCO_2, and HCO_3^-. Once values are obtained, the pH can help to distinguish if the disease is an acidosis (pH < 7.4) or alkalosis (pH > 7.4) disorder. This patient has acidemia with a pH of 7.3.
The next step is to determine if the acidemia is of a metabolic or respiratory cause. This patient's HCO_3^- level is below normal as is her pCO_2. The decreased HCO_3^- represents the decrease in pH from a metabolic process. Therefore, this patient has metabolic acidosis, option A.
Metabolic alkalosis, option B, would show a pH greater than 7.4 and an elevated HCO_3^- level. The pCO_2 would also be elevated. Respiratory acidosis, option C, would have a pH less than 7.4, an elevated HCO_3^-, and a decreased pCO_2. Respiratory alkalosis, option D, would have a pH greater than 7.4, a decreased HCO_3^- level, and a decreased pCO_2. **Task:** E—Applying Basic Scientific Concepts

14. **Answer: C** Percutaneous needle biopsy, option C, is indicated when a patient has one of the following: unexplained acute kidney injury or chronic kidney disease; proteinuria and hematuria without a source; a previous lesion that was identified and treated to help guide therapy; systemic diseases like systemic lupus erythematosus or Goodpasture syndrome; or suspected kidney transplant rejection. This is a less invasive option for obtaining tissue than an open biopsy, option B, and so is the preferred option.
MRI and PET scanning of the kidneys, options A and D, are both types of imaging studies. Further imaging would not be indicated in this case based on the normal findings on ultrasonography and CT scan. **Task:** D2—Clinical Intervention